POCKET COMPANION
TO ACCOMPANY

—— NELSON ——
TEXTBOOK
of
PEDIATRICS

POCKET COMPANION
TO ACCOMPANY

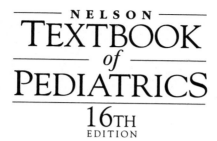

NELSON

TEXTBOOK
of
PEDIATRICS
16TH
EDITION

RICHARD E. BEHRMAN, MD
Clinical Professor of Pediatrics
Stanford University School of Medicine
University of California, San Francisco,
School of Medicine
Senior Vice President for Medical Affairs
The Lucile Packard Foundation for Children's Health
Palo Alto, California

ROBERT M. KLIEGMAN, MD
Professor and Chair
Department of Pediatrics
Medical College of Wisconsin
Pediatrician-in-Chief
Children's Hospital of Wisconsin
Milwaukee, Wisconsin

HAL B. JENSON, MD
Professor
Departments of Pediatrics and Microbiology
Chief, Pediatric Infectious Diseases
The University of Texas
Health Science Center at San Antonio
San Antonio, Texas

W.B. SAUNDERS COMPANY
A Harcourt Health Sciences Company
Philadelphia   London   New York   St. Louis   Sydney   Toronto

W.B. SAUNDERS COMPANY
A Harcourt Health Sciences Company

The Curtis Center
Independence Square West
Philadelphia, Pennsylvania 19106

Acquisitions Editor: Judith Fletcher
Developmental Editor: Heather J. Krehling
Project Manager: Tina Rebane
Production Manager: Norman Stellander
Illustration Specialist: John Needles
Book Designer: Marie Gardocky Clifton

POCKET COMPANION TO NELSON
TEXTBOOK OF PEDIATRICS

ISBN 0–7216–7770–3

Printed in the United States of America.

Last digit is the print number: 9   8   7   6   5   4   3   2   1

Preface

Medical students, residents, and others in training as health care professionals involved in caring for children may be overwhelmed by the quantity of medical knowledge potentially applicable to the prevention, diagnosis, and treatment of disorders that may affect children during their development from embryonic to adult life. The editors and contributors summarize this enormous amount of information and the relevant science on which it is based in *Nelson Textbook of Pediatrics,* which is completely revised and updated every 4 years.

Because of its necessary comprehensiveness, even as a distillate of the broad field of pediatrics, *Nelson Textbook of Pediatrics* cannot be kept in one's pocket wherever one is caring for children. Therefore, the editor has condensed the clinical portions of *Nelson Textbook of Pediatrics* into this pocket-sized companion handbook. This *Pocket Companion* consists of brief summaries of key features of growth and development and of the principal diseases and disorders the student or trainee is likely to encounter in caring for children.

This *Pocket Companion* should not and cannot be the replacement for a textbook of pediatrics. Each brief chapter is cross-referenced to the appropriate sections in *Nelson Textbook of Pediatrics,* 16th edition, except when the chapter numbers are the same. The *Pocket Companion* should be used only as a brief introduction to, or a reminder of, an aspect of clinical pediatrics when there is not immediate access to, or time to consult, the *Nelson Textbook.* Because the quantity of material presented is too brief to stand on its own, it is strongly recommended that the relevant subjects in the *Nelson Textbook* be consulted as soon as time permits. Both books should be used as a combined education activity.

Richard E. Behrman, MD

Acknowledgment

I am very appreciative of the assistance provided by my administrative assistant, Rolanda Fountain, in the preparation of *Pocket Companion to Accompany Nelson Textbook of Pediatrics,* 16th edition.

R.E.B.

NOTICE

Pediatrics is an ever-changing field. Standard safety precautions must be followed, but as new research and clinical experience broaden our knowledge, changes in treatment and drug therapy may become necessary or appropriate. Readers are advised to check the most current product information provided by the manufacturer of each drug to be administered to verify the recommended dose, the method and duration of administration, and contraindications. It is the responsibility of the treating physician, relying on experience and knowledge of the patient, to determine dosages and the best treatment for each individual patient. Neither the Publisher nor the editor assumes any liability for any injury and/or damage to persons or property arising from this publication.

THE PUBLISHER

Contents

PART 5

Children with Special Health Needs

PART 6

Nutrition

PART 7

Pathophysiology of Body Fluids and Fluid Therapy

PART 8

The Acutely Ill Child

PART 9
Genetics and Metabolic Diseases

PART 10
The Fetus and the Neonatal Infant
Noninfectious Disorders

Infections in Neonatal Infants

PART 11
Special Health Problems During Adolescence

PART 12
The Immunologic System and Disorders

PART 13
Allergic Disorders

PART 14
Rheumatic Diseases of Childhood

PART 15
Infectious Diseases

SECTION 13
Protozoan Diseases

SECTION 14
Helminthic Diseases

SECTION 15
Preventive Measures

PART 16
The Digestive System

SECTION 1
Clinical Manifestations of Gastrointestinal Disease

PART 24
The Endocrine System

PART 25
The Nervous System

PART 26
Neuromuscular Disorders

PART 27
Disorders of the Eye

PART 28
The Ear

PART 29
The Skin

PART 30
Bone and Joint Disorders

SECTION 1
Orthopedic Problems

SECTION 2
Sports Medicine

SECTION 3
Skeletal Dysplasia

PART 31
Unclassified Diseases

PART 32
Environmental Health Hazards

PART 1

The Field of Pediatrics

CHAPTER 1

Overview of Pediatrics
(Nelson Textbook, Chapters 1 and 4)

PEDIATRIC VITAL STATISTICS

The health problems of children and youth vary widely among the nations of the world depending on a number of factors, which are often interrelated. These factors include (1) the prevalence and ecology of infectious agents and their hosts; (2) climate and geography; (3) agricultural resources and practices; (4) educational, economic, social, and cultural considerations; (5) stage of industrialization and urbanization; and (6) in many instances the gene frequencies for some disorders.

Not only do problems differ in various parts of the world, but so do priorities, because they must reflect local concerns, resources, and needs. Assessment of the state of health of any community must begin with a description of the incidence of illness and must continue with studies that show the changes that occur with time and in response to programs of prevention, case finding, therapy, and adequate surveillance.

In the past half century the infant mortality rate in the United States has fallen from around 75/1000 live births in 1925 to approximately 7.2 in 1996. Both neonatal (<1 mo) and postneonatal (1–11 mo) mortality have had major reductions. However, most of the decline in infant mortality since 1970 is attributable to a decrease in the birth-weight-specific infant mortality rate related to pediatric care, not to the prevention of low-birthweight births. The majority of deaths of infants younger than 1 year of age occur within the first 28 days of life, most of these within the first 7 days; moreover, a large proportion of those within the first 7 days occur within the first day. However, an increasing number of severely ill infants born with very low birth weight survive the neonatal period and die later in infancy of neonatal disease, its sequelae, or its complications. Table 1–1 shows the persistent disproportionately high death rate within the 1st year, compared with the remainder of childhood.

Postneonatal infant mortality for the United States in 1996 was 2.5/1000 live births (5.0/1000 for black infants and 2.1/1000 for white infants). The leading cause of death in this age group was sudden infant death syndrome, followed in order by congenital anomalies, perinatal conditions, respiratory system diseases, acci-

TABLE 1–1 Death Rates* by Age, Sex, Race, and Hispanic Origin, 1996†

	White	Black	Hispanic	Asian/Pacific Islander	American Indian
Male					
<1 yr	683.4	1697.9	680.8	461.1	899.4
1–4 yr	37.3	72.8	37.8	27.2	74.1
5–14 yr	23.5	38.5	23.7	18.6	39.1
15–24 yr	115.1	234.7	140.3	72.4	176.2
Female					
<1 yr	557.1	1406.6	527.6	343.8	703.0
1–4	28.3	63.1	27.7	26.8	65.9
5–14	16.4	26.3	17.0	11.3	24.1
15–24 yr	42.8	66.5	38.8	31.1	64.0

*Per 100,000 U.S. Standard Population.
†Preliminary, National Center for Health Statistics.

dents, and infectious and parasitic diseases. Maternal risk characteristics, such as unmarried status, adolescence, high parity, and less than 12 yr of education, are correlated significantly with increased risk of postneonatal mortality and morbidity and low birth weight.

Table 1–2 shows the six leading causes of death in various age groups in 1996 and highlights the impact of violent deaths on mortality in older children, adolescents, and young adults.

Medical problems are exacerbated by social and demographic changes in the United States. By 1996, 26.4% of all children younger than 18 yr of age were living with one parent, about twice the number of such children in 1970. Of these one-parent families, 92% consisted of children living with their mother. There are substantial differences among children: 56.9% of black, 28.6% of Hispanic, 17.9% of white, and 36.5 of Native American children live with one parent. Furthermore, in 1995, 59% of women with children younger than 3 yr of age, 62% with children younger than 6, and 77% with children ages 6–17 yr, worked full time or part time outside the home.

Family income is central to the health and well-being of children. Children living in poor families are much more likely than children living in rich or middle class families to experience material deprivation and poor health, die during childhood, score lower on standardized tests, be retained in grade, drop out of school, have out-of-wedlock births, experience violent crime, end up as poor adults, and suffer other undesirable outcomes.

In 1991, children (birth–21 yr) made up 31.9% (80.3 million) of the population of the United States. The number of births has

TABLE 1–2 Causes of Death at Various Ages

Rank*	Causes	Sub-rank	Rate
	Under 1 Yr: All Causes		875†
1	Perinatal conditions		
	Intrauterine growth retardation/low birth weight	1	
	Respiratory distress syndrome	2	
	Newborn affected by maternal complications of pregnancy	3	
	Newborn affected by complications of placenta, cord, and membranes	4	
	Infections, perinatal	5	
	Intrauterine hypoxia/birth asphyxia	6	
2	Congenital anomalies		
3	Sudden infant death syndrome		
4	Accidents and adverse events		
5	Infections (respiratory)		
	1–4 Yr: All Causes		38†
1	Injuries		
2	Congenital anomalies		
3	Malignant neoplasms		
4	Homicide and legal intervention		
5	Diseases of the heart‡		
6	Respiratory infections		
	5–14 Yr: All Causes		22†
1	Injuries		
2	Malignant neoplasms		
3	Homicide and legal interventions		
4	Congenital anomalies		
5	Diseases of the heart‡		
6	Suicide		
	15–24 Yr: All Causes		90†
1	Injuries		
2	Homicide		
3	Suicide		
4	Malignant neoplasms		
5	Diseases of the heart‡		

*Adapted from Monthly Vital Statistics Report 46:2, 1997. Rates and rankings are for 1996 (Provisional). Source U.S. National Center for Health Statistics.
†Rate per 100,000 population.
‡Excludes congenital heart anomalies.

been increasing since 1976 and is expected to continue to increase at 1–2% annually. There were 3,899,589 live births in 1996. The racial, ethnic, and cultural diversity among children is increasing significantly. However, the proportion of children is decreasing relative to the adult population.

Child Health in the Developing World

More than 90% of the world's children are born each year in the developing world. Thirty-five thousand of them die each day, most of common and preventable problems. Health and illness for these children are a result of a complex dynamic of environmental, social, political, and economic factors. No single intervention will successfully interrupt the cycles of morbidity and mortality that plague them. Average infant and younger than age 5-yr mortality rates range from almost 200/1000 in least-developed countries to less than 9/1000 in developed countries. Each year, more than 10 million children die. Seven in 10 of these deaths are due to respiratory infections, diarrhea, measles and other vaccine-preventable illnesses, malaria, and/or malnutrition.

Pneumonia

Pneumonia causes the majority of deaths in children. Pathogens in developing countries are similar to those in economically advanced nations, but the frequency of primary and secondary bacterial infections is much greater. Respiratory viruses, in particular respiratory syncytial virus, cause the majority of acute respiratory tract infections. *Streptococcus pneumoniae, Haemophilus influenzae, Moraxella catarrhalis,* and *Staphylococcus aureus* account for the majority of bacterial infections. Cytomegalovirus, *Chlamydia, Mycoplasma pneumoniae,* and *Mycobacterium tuberculosis* also are common pathogens.

Vitamin A deficiency is clearly associated with increased incidence, morbidity, and mortality of respiratory tract disease. Supplementation with as little as a single 200,000 IU vitamin A capsule per year has been shown to decrease childhood mortality by 50%.

Diarrheal Diseases

The epidemiology of diarrheal disease in developing nations is similar to that in economically advanced countries. Rotavirus and other enteric viruses are the principal pathogens. Bacterial disease is usually caused by *Salmonella* and *Shigella.* Parasitic infections are endemic but generally result in nutritional deficiencies and not acute diarrheal disease. Cholera remains a problem throughout all regions of the developing world.

Oral rehydration solution saves the lives of millions of children and adults each year. When given in the right proportion, electrolytes and water are absorbed across the intestine despite ongoing diarrhea.

Immunization-Preventable Diseases

The six immunization-preventable diseases (measles, polio, diphtheria, pertussis, tetanus, and tuberculosis) kill, blind, cripple, and cause mental damage to some 10 million children each year.

Malnutrition

Malnutrition is a primary cause of morbidity and mortality and a complicating factor for other illnesses. In utero caloric deprivation results in some small-for-gestational-age births. Subsequent protein, calorie, and micronutrient malnutrition results in moderate to severe stunting in 50% of children, with concomitant deficiencies in cognitive development. Susceptibility to infectious diseases is increased.

Other Child Health Issues

Malaria, schistosomiasis, and dengue fever are examples of other infectious diseases common to children in developing countries. However, the medical, psychologic, and social impact of acquired immunodeficiency syndrome and violence is eclipsing all other causes of morbidity and mortality in many regions of the world. In areas of Central Africa as many as 40% of women are infected with human immunodeficiency virus (HIV). Without access to antiretroviral drugs that can greatly decrease rates of perinatal HIV transmission, approximately 25% of their offspring will be infected with HIV through vertical transmission.

War and natural disasters have always had a disproportionate effect on children. Conflicts persist in many regions of the world, exposing children to acts of violence and traumatic stress disorders. Violence directed at children, however, is not limited to war. Street children are routinely tortured and often killed; widespread childhood prostitution and forced labor persist, particularly in Southeast Asia and India; and patterns of abuse continue in all countries.

CHAPTER 2

Ethics in Pediatric Care
(Nelson Textbook, Chapters 2 and 3)

Ethical issues permeate all interactions between physicians and patients.

AUTONOMY. This is a central principle in medical ethics. Its purpose is to allow competent patients to make their own health care decisions based on their own values. In the United States and many other nations, competent patients almost have an absolute right to decide what shall be done to their own bodies. This principle is particularly relevant in adolescence, when a patient's competence begins to resemble that of an adult, but younger children are also sometimes competent to make their own health care decisions.

COMPETENCE. The principle of autonomy is intertwined inextricably with the concept of competence, because only competent patients are granted the right to make their own health care decisions. The most common definition of competence is based on patients' ability to understand the possible consequences of their decision and the available alternatives. Many adolescents meet this standard, creating potential conflicts when they are still under the supervision of their parents.

BENEFICENCE. This refers to the duties to avoid harm as well as to advance the welfare of others. A more complete principle would include some sense of not causing harm without a likelihood of compensating good, but individuals vary in respect to what they consider a "harm" or a "good" and how much harm they are willing to risk in exchange for a potential benefit.

PATERNALISM. This is defined as interfering with the liberty of another person for his or her benefit. It is generally considered to be a duty of parents, although this assumption has been questioned and is usually considered to be morally unjustified with regard to competent patients, with limited exceptions. There is general support for the opinion that paternalism is justified at least when there is a high probability of serious harm, when interference with the patient's liberty is likely to prevent the harm, and when there is a reasonable likelihood that the patient would want to be treated in this manner or will appreciate it later on.

TRUTH TELLING. The duty to tell the truth has special importance in the physician-patient relationship, in which trust is essential because of unequal power and because of the serious consequences of medical decisions.

CONFIDENTIALITY. Patients need to trust their physicians not to disclose private information to others because confidentiality facilitates full disclosure of information relevant for providing effective personal health care, may prevent disorders that threaten others in the community, and possibly reduces the total human and financial cost of illness and related disability through early treatment. There is an implied promise by the physician not to disclose information except with the consent of the patient, or of his or her representative, or when required by law. Exceptions to this principle are generally limited to circumstances carrying a high risk of serious physical harm to others that is most likely to be prevented only by unconsented disclosure.

CONFLICT OF INTEREST. Because a child patient is usually represented by someone else, the potential exists for a pediatrician to perceive the best interest of the child differently from the way in which it is perceived by the parent(s) or guardian(s). In addition, a physician's sense of responsibility for the rest of the family may result in conflicts between the interests of the family and the interest of the child patient.

ACCESS TO HEALTH CARE; RATIONING (DISTRIBUTIVE JUSTICE)

The most serious ethical problem in health care in the United States may be the inequality in access to care. No other major industrial country rations basic health care on the basis of ability to pay. Rationing of health care can be defined as limiting access to wanted and needed services of known benefit. The question is not whether to ration health care services but how to do so fairly.

CHAPTER 3

Preventive Pediatrics

(Nelson Textbook, Chapters 5 and 6)

Prevention in the health care of infants, children, and adolescents is at the core of pediatrics.

PERIODIC HEALTH SUPERVISION VISITS

The suggested sequence of health supervision visits is listed in Table 3–1. Beyond the traditional history and physical examination, screening, and immunizations, health supervision visits should include surveillance of developmental milestones, observations of parent-child interaction, counseling, anticipatory guidance, and an opportunity to meet the family's agenda with the use of open-ended or trigger questions. Table 3–2 provides a list of essential elements in health supervision visits.

TABLE 3–1 Suggested Schedule of Health Supervision Visits

Infancy 0–1 yr	Early Childhood 1–4 yr	Middle Childhood 5–10 yr	Adolescence 11–21 yr
Prenatal	15 mo	5 yr	11 yr
Neonatal	18 mo	6 yr	12 yr
First week	2 yr	8 yr	13 yr
1 mo	3 yr	10 yr	14 yr
2 mo	4 yr		15 yr
4 mo			16 yr
6 mo			17 yr
9 mo			18 yr
12 mo			19 yr
			20 yr
			21 yr

TABLE 3–2 Preventive Evaluation at Specific Ages*

Activity	1st Wk	1 Mo	2 Mo	4 Mo	6 Mo	9 Mo	12 Mo	15 Mo	18 Mo	2 Yr	3 Yr	4 Yr	5 Yr	6 Yr	8 Yr	10 Yr	11–14 Yr	15–17 Yr	18–21 Yr
Interview (for special attention)																			
Family history	✓	✓	✓	✓	✓	✓	✓	✓	✓	✓	✓	✓	✓	✓	✓	✓	✓	✓	✓
Pregnancy and delivery	✓	✓																	
Neonatal course	✓	✓																	
Developmental evaluation/ milestones	✓	✓	✓	✓	✓	✓	✓	✓	✓	✓	✓	✓	✓	✓	✓	✓	✓	✓	✓
Body systems (for special attention)																			
Hearing/vision	✓	✓	✓	✓	✓	✓	✓	✓	✓	✓	✓	✓	✓	✓	✓	✓	✓	✓	
CNS (including sleep)	✓	✓	✓	✓	✓	✓	✓	✓	✓	✓	✓	✓	✓	✓	✓	✓	✓	✓	
Gastrointestinal/feeding	✓	✓	✓	✓	✓	✓	✓	✓	✓	✓	✓	✓							
Urinary	✓	✓	✓			✓	✓	✓	✓	✓	✓	✓	✓	✓	✓	✓	✓	✓	✓
Dental care					✓		✓	✓	✓	✓	✓	✓	✓	✓	✓	✓	✓	✓	
Drugs, alcohol, tobacco															✓	✓	✓	✓	✓
Pica																			✓
Sexual behavior																	✓	✓	✓
Observations of parent-child interaction	✓	✓	✓	✓	✓	✓	✓	✓	✓	✓	✓	✓	✓	✓	✓	✓	✓	✓	✓
Physical Examination (complete) (for special attention)	✓	✓	✓	✓	✓	✓	✓	✓	✓	✓	✓	✓	✓	✓	✓	✓	✓	✓	✓
Height and weight	✓	✓	✓	✓	✓	✓	✓	✓	✓	✓	✓	✓	✓	✓	✓	✓	✓	✓	✓
Head circumference	✓	✓	✓	✓	✓	✓	✓	✓	✓	✓									
Blood pressure											✓	✓	✓	✓	✓	✓	✓	✓	✓
Skin	✓	✓	✓	✓	✓	✓	✓	✓	✓	✓	✓	✓	✓	✓	✓	✓	✓	✓	✓
Vision																			
Tear ducts	✓	✓	✓	✓	✓														
Fixed eyes	✓	✓	✓	✓															
Red reflex	✓	✓	✓	✓	✓	✓	✓												
Fundi	✓	✓	✓	✓	✓	✓											✓	✓	
Strabismus/eye movements	✓	✓	✓	✓	✓	✓				✓	✓								

8

Hearing	√	√	√	√	√	√			√	√	√	√	√	√	√	√	√	√	√	√
Speech				√	√	√	√	√	√	√		√	√							
Neurologic problems	√	√	√	√	√	√	√	√	√	√	√	√	√	√	√	√	√	√	√	√
Cardiac murmurs	√	√	√	√	√	√	√	√	√	√	√	√	√	√	√	√	√	√	√	√
Abdominal masses	√	√	√	√	√	√	√	√	√	√	√	√	√	√	√	√	√	√	√	√
External genitalia	√	√	√	√	√	√	√	√	√	√	√	√	√	√	√	√	√	√	√	√
Hip dysplasia/dislocation	√	√	√	√	√	√	√	√	√											
Gait						√	√	√	√	√	√	√								
Deformities (metatarsus adductus)	√	√	√	√	√	√														
Sexual development											√	√	√	√	√	√	√	√	√	√
Scoliosis											√	√	√	√	√	√	√	√	√	√
Evidence of neglect/abuse	√	√	√	√	√	√	√	√	√	√	√	√	√	√	√	√	√	√	√	√
Laboratory Testing and Screening																				
Hemoglobin/hematocrit		√ or	√ or																	
Urinalysis		√ or	√ or	√																
Urine culture (girls)		√ or	√ or	√																
Tuberculin		√ or	√ or	√																
Lipids							√ or			√ or		√ or		√ or		√ or		√ or		√ or
Metabolic	√	√																		
Lead		√ (Prior to 3 mo)		√ or	√ or	√ or	√ or													
Hearing screening									√	√	√	√	√	√						
Vision screening							√	√	√	√	√	√	√	√						
Sexually transmitted diseases				√																√
Immunizations (see Chapter 301 for details)	√	√	√	√	√	√	√	√	√	√	√	√	√	√	√	√	√	√	√	√
Anticipatory Guidance and Counseling (for special attention)																				
Parent-child interaction	√	√	√	√	√	√	√	√	√	√	√	√	√	√	√	√	√	√	√	√
Diet/nutrition	√	√	√	√	√	√	√	√	√	√	√	√	√	√	√	√	√	√	√	√
Sleep	√	√	√	√	√	√	√	√	√	√	√	√	√	√	√	√	√	√	√	√

Table continued on following page

9

TABLE 3–2 Preventive Evaluation at Specific Ages* *Continued*

Activity	1st Wk	1 Mo	2 Mo	4 Mo	6 Mo	9 Mo	12 Mo	15 Mo	18 Mo	2 Yr	3 Yr	4 Yr	5 Yr	6 Yr	8 Yr	10 Yr	11–14 Yr	15–17 Yr	18–21 Yr
Toilet training																			
Injury prevention	✓	✓	✓	✓	✓	✓	✓	✓	✓	✓	✓	✓	✓	✓	✓	✓	✓	✓	✓
Infant/child care (includes oral health)	✓	✓	✓	✓	✓	✓	✓	✓	✓	✓	✓								
School problems											✓	✓	✓	✓	✓	✓	✓	✓	✓
Puberty and sexuality															✓	✓	✓	✓	✓
Substance abuse														✓	✓	✓	✓	✓	✓
Family and social relationships	✓	✓	✓	✓	✓	✓	✓	✓	✓	✓	✓	✓	✓	✓	✓	✓	✓	✓	✓

*These suggestions or guidelines represent an analysis of recommendations by the American Academy of Pediatrics and Bright Futures. They are not intended to be all inclusive but rather to serve as reminders for some of the important preventive and health promotion activities that should be considered at various ages when physician-patient encounters may occur. The content and timing of visits will need to be altered according to special needs and the presence or absence of risk factors for the child and his or her family.

TOPICS OF FREQUENT CONCERN DURING HEALTH SUPERVISION

In the course of well child care visits, pediatricians provide specific advice in areas of behavior and parenting and educate families about common issues in normal growth and development. In the paragraphs that follow, some of the common topics of parenting and child care, chosen because of their prominence in health supervision visits, are discussed with an emphasis on prevention.

Diaper Dermatitis

As the most common skin disorder in infancy and one of the most visible problems in infant care, diaper rash is frequently discussed in well child care visits. Diaper dermatitis peaks at age 9–12 mo. Wearing diapers is the cause of most cases of diaper dermatitis. Diapers provide a warm, dark, moist environment where urine and feces are in contact with skin. Most diaper rashes are self-limited and respond to frequent diaper changes, a period of time without diapers, barrier creams to minimize the contact of urine and feces with skin, and appropriate cleansing of the diaper area with water and a mild, nonperfumed soap. Diarrheal disease is a major exacerbating factor.

Specific causes such as *Candida albicans* or underlying skin disorders such as atopic dermatitis, seborrheic dermatitis, or psoriasis may also have a role in the development of diaper dermatitis. Skin infections with bacteria such as *Staphylococcus aureus* occur as secondary infections when the protective barrier of the skin has been compromised. Parents should be alerted to seek additional advice if the diaper rash has been present for more than 5 days; if any exudates, vesicles, or pustules are present; if the rash spreads beyond the diaper area; or if there is cracking or bleeding.

Teething

Most infants have their first teeth erupt at age 6–8 mo and may have associated mild symptoms of gingival swelling and sensitivity, increased salivation, and irritability related to gum discomfort. No evidence shows that diarrhea, rhinorrhea, rashes, or fever is related to teething. Most infants tolerate teething without difficulty if offered a firm object to bite such as a teething ring. Rubbing the gums with a cool, wet washcloth can be comforting. If additional pain relief is needed, acetaminophen or ibuprofen may be administered.

Sleep Problems

In the first year, difficulties with transitions to sleep and with night awakening are commonly reported. Parents should be educated about separation anxiety, which develops in the latter half of the first year of life and is related to difficulty with night-time settling and night awakening. Older infants and children may experience nightmares or parasomnias such as night terrors, night walking, night talking, or bedwetting.

To help a child settle at night, parents should establish a bed-time routine starting with a quiet interaction like reading a bed-time story. Transitional objects, such as blankets and teddy bears, are integral parts of bedtime routines and facilitate falling asleep. It is important to allow infants to settle on their own, so that they are accomplishing a successful independent transition to sleep.

When parents experience difficulty with a child who wakes at night, the same approach of promoting night-time settling should be used. Parents should delay their response so that normal arousal states during sleep do not progress to complete awakening.

Nightmares are common and usually involve vivid, scary, or exciting events, which are easily recalled by the child on awakening. *Night terrors* are less common events, lasting 10–15 min, during which time the child is not easily aroused and may appear frightened and agitated. On awakening the next morning, a child who experienced a night terror will have amnesia for the event.

Bedwetting is one of the most common sleep problems facing school-aged children. By age 7, up to 7% of all children may experience occasional bedwetting episodes. Parents should be provided information about the prevalence of bedwetting to foster an understanding of enuresis as a developmental problem and thereby demystify the condition. If a child experiences "dry" nights (nights without bedwetting) on a weekly basis and is motivated to stop bedwetting, it may help to involve the child in keeping a record of wet and dry nights on a calendar.

Toilet Training

In the United States, the average age of successful toilet training is 27 mo, with a range of up to 3–4 yr. Early training (before age 2), because of its association with chronic stool retention and encopresis, should be discouraged. The key factor for parents to recognize in successful toilet training is the readiness of the child.

Temper Tantrums

A child's expression of anger in outbursts of rage is a significant challenge for parents. Identifying the type of tantrum may be helpful in offering advice about parental interventions (e.g., frustration or fatigue related, attention seeking or demanding, refusal, disruptive, potentially harmful, or ragelike). If a child is experiencing frustration related to excessive fatigue or hunger, he or she needs support, sleep, or food. Some positive remarks also may help the child with these feelings of frustration. For those tantrums in which a child is insistent and making unreasonable demands, it is best to ignore the demands and allow the child to regain composure over time. Refusal tantrums related to important issues such as bedtimes or going to school need to be met with firmness and consistency. Parents should be clear in their request for the child to comply and must allow opportunity for compliance. If this approach fails, it may be necessary to move the child physically to bed or into the car. When behavior is so disruptive and out of control or occurs in a public place such as the grocery store, physical removal followed by a time-out is most effective.

Discipline

The strategies suggested by the American Academy of Pediatrics include three essential elements: (1) a positive, supportive, loving relationship between parents and children; (2) use of positive reinforcement to increase desired behaviors; and (3) removing reinforcement of undesired behaviors and applying punishment to reduce or eliminate undesired behaviors.

PART 2

Growth and Development

CHAPTER 4

Overview and Assessment of Variability
(Nelson Textbook, Chapter 7)

Pediatricians need to understand growth and development in three ways. An understanding of the normative patterns of physical growth and the emergence of motor, cognitive, and emotional competence allows pediatricians to monitor children's progress and to identify delay or deviance. Understanding how biologic and environmental forces interact to shape development allows pediatricians to target factors that increase or decrease risk. Understanding how parents conceptualize development facilitates anticipatory guidance and remedial intervention. The beliefs of parents, like the theoretical models of Freud, Piaget, and Skinner, include implicit or explicit ideas about the nature of children, the characteristics of successful adults, and the processes that control the transformation from one to the other.

BIOPSYCHOSOCIAL MODELS OF DEVELOPMENT. Biopsychosocial models, now widely accepted, recognize the importance of both intrinsic and extrinsic forces. Height, for example, is a function of a child's genetic endowment (biologic), personal habits of eating (psychologic), and access to nutritious food (social).

Early experience has a direct effect on the physical properties of the brain, facilitating or impeding future learning. Early stressful experiences may also have long-standing effects on neurotransmitter and endocrine systems, possibly increasing the risk of mental illness later in life. Biologic, psychologic, and social influences on development are the focus, respectively, of the major theoretical perspectives described next.

BIOLOGIC INFLUENCES. Biologic influences on development include genetics, in utero exposure to teratogens, postpartum illnesses, exposure to hazardous substances, and maturation. Physical and neurologic maturation propels a child forward and sets lower limits for the emergence of most abilities. Maturational changes also create the potential for behavioral problems at predictable times. In addition to physical changes in size, body proportions, and strength, maturation is associated with hormonal influences.

A biologic influence of particular clinical importance is temperament. Temperament refers to a child's characteristic style of responding. Temperament is intrinsic to a child and relatively resistant to modification by parenting practices.

PSYCHOLOGIC INFLUENCES: ATTACHMENT AND CONTINGENCY. Attachment refers to a biologically determined tendency of a young child to seek proximity with the parent during times of stress. Children who are securely attached are able to use their parents to re-establish a sense of well-being after a stressful experience, such as physical examination or immunization.

At all stages of development and across multiple developmental lines, progress is fostered by adult caregivers who observe the child's verbal and nonverbal cues and respond accordingly. Contingent responses to nonverbal gestures create the groundwork for the shared attention and reciprocity critical for later language and social development. At all stages, learning is fostered when new challenges are made contingent on a child's current level of competence, being just slightly harder than what has already been mastered.

SOCIAL FACTORS: FAMILY SYSTEMS AND THE ECOLOGIC MODEL. Contemporary models of child development recognize the critical importance of influences outside of the mother-child dyad. Families function as systems, with more or less rigidly defined boundaries, subsystems, roles, and rules for interaction. The family system, in turn, functions within the larger systems of extended family, subculture, and society. The ecologic model depicts these relationships as concentric circles, with the parent-child dyad at the center and the larger society at the periphery.

UNIFYING CONCEPTS: THE TRANSACTIONAL MODEL, RISK AND RESILIENCE. Current thoughts have focused on understanding how biology and social interactions influence development. A child's status at any point in time is a function of both biologic and social influences. The influences are bidirectional: biologic factors such as temperament and health status both affect the child-rearing environment and are affected by it.

One implication of this model is that development assessment at any single point in time has limited ability to predict later outcome because at every stage the development trajectory is affected by both past and present conditions. As the number of risk factors increases, the percentage of children who developmentally thrive decreases but never reaches zero. Protective factors may make some children resilient, although not invulnerable. These factors, like risk factors, may be either biologic (temperamental persistence, athletic talent), or social.

DEVELOPMENTAL DOMAINS AND THEORIES OF EMOTION AND COGNITION. Another approach to child development tracks development within particular domains, such as gross motor, fine motor, social, emotional, language, and cognition. Within each of these categories are developmental lines or sequences of changes leading up

TABLE 4-1 Classic Stage Theories

Theory	Infancy (0–1 yr)	Toddlerhood (2–3 yr)	Preschool (3–6 yr)	School Age (6–12 yr)	Adolescence (12–20 yr)
Freud: psychosexual	Oral	Anal	Oedipal	Latency	Adolescence
Erikson: psychosocial	Basic trust	Autonomy vs. shame and doubt	Initiative vs. guilt	Industry vs. inferiority	Identity vs. identity diffusion
Piaget: cognitive	Sensorimotor (stages I–IV)	Sensorimotor (stages V, VI)	Preoperational	Concrete operations	Formal operations

to particular attainments. The concept of a developmental line implies that a child passes through successive stages. The psychoanalytical theories of Sigmund Freud and Erik Erikson and the cognitive theory of Jean Piaget share the idea of stages of qualitatively different epochs in the development of emotion and cognition (Table 4–1). In contrast, the behavioral theory of Skinner relies less on qualitative changes and more on gradual modification of behavior or accumulation of knowledge.

CHAPTER 5

Fetal Growth and Development

(Nelson Textbook, Chapter 8)

The most dramatic events in growth and development occur before birth. These changes are overwhelmingly somatic: the transformation of a single cell into an infant. Behavioral and psychologic developments in the fetus and the parents are also significant.

EMBRYONIC PERIOD. By 6 days postconceptual age, as implantation begins, the embryo consists of a spherical mass of cells with a central cavity (the blastocyst). By the 2nd wk, implantation is complete and uteroplacental circulation has begun. By the 3rd wk, along with primitive neural tube and blood vessels, paired heart tubes have begun to pump. During wk 4–8, the budding of arms and legs produces a human-like shape. By the end of wk 8, as the embryonic period closes, the rudiments of all major organ systems have developed.

FETAL PERIOD. From the 9th wk on (the fetal period), fetal somatic changes consist of increases in cell number and size and structural remodeling of several organ systems. By the 12th wk, the gender of the external genitalia becomes clearly distinguishable. By the 20th–24th wk, primitive alveoli have formed and surfactant production has begun; before that time, the absence of alveoli renders the lungs useless as organs of gas exchange. During the 3rd trimester, weight triples and length doubles as body stores of protein, fat, iron, and calcium increase.

PSYCHOLOGIC CHANGES IN THE PARENTS. Three changes of psychologic development may occur in a woman during pregnancy. Stage 1 begins when a woman first learns that she is pregnant. Ambivalent feelings are the norm, whether or not the pregnancy was planned. Stage 2 begins with awareness of fetal movements, or quickening, at approximately 20 wk or earlier with ultrasonic visualization. This palpable evidence that a fetus exists as a separate being often heightens a woman's feelings, both positive and negative. During stage 3, toward the end of pregnancy, a woman becomes aware of patterns of fetal activity and reactivity and begins to ascribe to her fetus an individual personality and an ability to survive independently.

CHAPTER 6

The Newborn
(Nelson Textbook, Chapter 9)

Infants survive physically and psychologically only in the context of their social relationships.

DETERMINANTS OF PARENTING

PRENATAL FACTORS. Pregnancy is a period of psychologic preparation for the profound demands of parenting. Most women experience ambivalence, particularly (but not exclusively) if their pregnancy was unplanned. The early experience of being mothered may establish unconsciously held expectations about nurturing relationships that permit mothers to "tune in" to their infants. Mothers whose early childhoods were marked by traumatic separations, abuse, or neglect may find it especially difficult to provide consistent, responsive care. Social support during pregnancy is also important. A supportive relationship with the child's father predicts satisfaction in mothering.

The Infant's Contribution

INTERACTIONAL ABILITIES. Almost immediately after birth, a neonate looks alert and readily suckles if given the opportunity. This first alert-wake period may be adversely modified by some maternal analgesics and anesthetics or fetal hypoxia. Nearsighted neonates have a fixed focal length of 8–12 in, approximately the distance from the breast to the mother's face, as well as an inborn visual preference for faces. Hearing is well developed, and infants preferentially turn toward a female voice. The initial period of social interaction, usually lasting about 40 min, is followed by a period of somnolence. After that, brief periods of alertness or excitation alternate with sleep.

MODULATION OF AROUSAL. Adaptation to extrauterine life requires rapid and profound physiologic changes, including aeration of the lungs, rerouting of the circulation, and activation of the intestinal tract. The necessary behavioral changes are no less profound. To obtain nourishment, to avoid hypothermia or hyperthermia, and to ensure safety, neonates must react appropriately to an expanded range of sensory stimuli. Infants must become aroused in response to stimulation but not so overaroused that behavior becomes random. Underaroused infants are not able to feed and interact; overaroused infants show signs of autonomic instability, including flushing or mottling, perioral pallor, hiccuping, vomiting, uncontrolled limb movements, and inconsolable crying.

BEHAVIORAL STATES. The organization of infant behavior into discrete behavioral states may reflect an infant's inborn ability to regulate arousal. Six states have been described: quiet sleep, active sleep, drowsy, alert, fussy, and crying. The behavioral state determines the infant's muscle tone, spontaneous movement, electroencephalographic pattern, and response to stimuli.

Mutual Regulation

Parents actively participate in an infant's state regulation, alternately stimulating or soothing to prolong the social interaction. In turn, the parents are regulated by the infant's signals, responding, for example, with a letdown of milk (or with a bottle) in response to cries of hunger. Such interactions constitute a system directed toward furthering the infant's physiologic homeostasis and physical growth. At the same time, they form the basis for the emerging psychologic relationship between parent and child.

Optimal Practices

A prenatal pediatric visit allows pediatricians to assess potential problems of bonding (e.g., a tense spousal relationship) and sources of social support and to try to allay unrealistic fears. Supportive hospital policies include use of birthing rooms; encouragement for the father or a trusted relative or friend to remain with the mother during labor or provision of a professional support person or doula; the practice of giving the newborn to the mother immediately after delivery or after brief stabilization and assessment; and placement of the newborn in the mother's room rather than in a central nursery. After discharge (often within 24 hr of delivery), home visits by nurses and lactation counselors may minimize early feeding problems and allow assessment of medical conditions that arise within the first week.

Assessing Parent-Infant Interactions

Observation during a feeding or when infants are alert and face to face with parents can be revealing. It is normal for infants and parents to appear absorbed in one another.

Teaching About Individual Competencies

The Newborn Behavior Scale (NBAS) provides a formal measure of an infant's neurodevelopmental competencies, including state control, autonomic reactivity, reflexes, habituation, and orientation (the ability to turn toward auditory and visual stimuli). This examination can also be used to demonstrate to parents an infant's capabilities and vulnerabilities.

CHAPTER 7

The First Year

(Nelson Textbook, Chapter 10)

During the first year of life, physical growth, maturation, acquisition of competence, and psychologic reorganization occur in rapid, discontinuous bursts. These changes qualitatively change a child's behavior and social relationships. Physical growth during this period is rapid; growth parameters for attained weight and length can be estimated as noted in Table 7–1. Table 7–2 presents an overview of milestones in the domains of gross motor, fine motor, and cognitive development.

AGE BIRTH–2 MO

The biologic and psychologic challenges facing neonates and their parents were described in Chapter 6. These consist of establishing effective feeding and a predictable sleep-wake cycle. The social interactions that occur when parents and infants accomplish these tasks lay the foundation for cognitive and emotional development.

PHYSICAL DEVELOPMENT. A newborn's weight may decrease 10% below birth weight in the first week as a result of excretion of excess extravascular fluid and possibly poor intake. Intake improves as colostrum is replaced by higher-fat milk, as infants learn to latch on and suck more efficiently, and as mothers become more comfortable with feeding techniques. Infants should regain or exceed birth weight by age 2 wk and should grow at approximately 30 g (1 oz)/day during the 1st mo (Table 7–3). Limb movements consist largely of uncontrolled writhing, with appar-

TABLE 7–1 Formulas for Approximate Average Height and Weight of Normal Infants and Children

Weight	Kilograms	(Pounds)
At birth	3.25	(7)
3–12 mo	$\dfrac{\text{age (mo)} + 9}{2}$	(age [mo] + 11)
1–6 yr	age (yr) $\times$ 2 + 8	(age [yr] $\times$ 5 + 17)
7–12 yr	$\dfrac{\text{age (yr)} \times 7 - 5}{2}$	(age [yr] $\times$ 7 + 5)
Height	**Centimeters**	**(Inches)**
At birth	50	(20)
At 1 yr	75	(30)
2–12 yr	age (yr) $\times$ 6 + 77	(age [yr] $\times$ 2½ + 30)

TABLE 7–2 Developmental Milestones in the First 2 Yr of Life

Milestone	Average Age of Attainment (mo)	Developmental Implications
Gross Motor		
Head steady in sitting	2.0	Allows more visual interaction
Pull to sit, no head lag	3.0	Muscle tone
Hands together in midline	3.0	Self-discovery
Asymmetric tonic neck reflex gone	4.0	Child can inspect hands in midline
Sits without support	6.0	Increasing exploration
Rolls back to stomach	6.5	Truncal flexion, risk of falls
Walks alone	12.0	Exploration, control of proximity to parents
Runs	16.0	Supervision more difficult
Fine Motor		
Grasps rattle	3.5	Object use
Reaches for objects	4.0	Visuomotor coordination
Palmar grasp gone	4.0	Voluntary release
Transfers object hand to hand	5.5	Comparison of objects
Thumb-finger grasp	8.0	Able to explore small objects
Turns pages of book	12.0	Increasing autonomy during book time
Scribbles	13.0	Visuomotor coordination
Builds tower of two cubes	15.0	Uses objects in combination
Builds tower of six cubes	22.0	Requires visual, gross, and fine motor coordination

Table continued on following page

21

TABLE 7–2 Developmental Milestones in the First 2 Yr of Life *Continued*

Milestone	Average Age of Attainment (mo)	Developmental Implications
Communication and Language		
Smiles in response to face, voice	1.5	Child more active social participant
Monosyllabic babble	6.0	Experimentation with sound, tactile sense
Inhibits to "no"	7.0	Response to tone (nonverbal)
Follows one-step command with gesture	7.0	Nonverbal communication
Follows one-step command without gesture (e.g., "Give it to me")	10.0	Verbal receptive language
Speaks first real word	12.0	Beginning of labeling
Speaks 4–6 words	15.0	Acquisition of object and personal names
Speaks 10–15 words	18.0	Acquisition of object and personal names
Speaks two-word sentences (e.g., "Mommy shoe")	19.0	Beginning grammaticization, corresponds with 50 + word vocabulary
Cognitive		
Stares momentarily at spot where object disappeared (e.g., yarn ball dropped)	2.0	Lack of object permanence (out of sight, out of mind)
Stares at own hand	4.0	Self-discovery, cause and effect
Bangs two cubes	8.0	Active comparison of objects
Uncovers toy (after seeing it hidden)	8.0	Object permanence
Egocentric pretend play (e.g., pretends to drink from cup)	12.0	Beginning symbolic thought
Uses stick to reach toy	17.0	Able to link actions to solve problems
Pretend play with doll (gives doll bottle)	17.0	Symbolic thought

TABLE 7-3 Growth and Caloric Requirements

Age	Approximate Daily Weight Gain (g)	Approximate Monthly Weight Gain	Growth in Length (cm/mo)	Growth in Head Circumference (cm/mo)	Recommended Daily Allowance (kcal/kg/day)
0–3 mo	30	2 lb	3.5	2.00	115
3–6 mo	20	1¼ lb	2.0	1.00	110
6–9 mo	15	1 lb	1.5	0.50	100
9–12 mo	12	13 oz	1.2	0.50	100
1–3 yr	8	8 oz	1.0	0.25	100
4–6 yr	6	6 oz	3 cm/yr	1 cm/yr	90–100

Adapted from National Research Council, Food and Nutrition Board: Recommended Daily Allowances. Washington, DC, National Academy of Sciences, 1989; Frank D, Silva M, Needlman R: Failure to thrive: Myth and method. Contemp Pediatr 10:114, 1993.

ently purposeless hand opening and closing. Smiling occurs involuntarily. In contrast, eye gaze, head turning, and sucking are under conscious control and thus can be used to demonstrate infant perception and cognition.

Initially, sleep and wakefulness are evenly distributed throughout the 24 hr. Neurologic maturation accounts for the consolidation of sleep periods into longer and longer blocks. By 2 mo of age, most infants are waking briefly two or three times to feed; some sleep 6 hr or more at a stretch. Crying normally peaks at about 6 wk of age, when healthy infants cry up to 3 hr/day, then decreases to 1 hr or less by 3 mo.

COGNITIVE DEVELOPMENT. Caretaking activities provide visual, tactile, olfactory, and auditory stimuli; all of these stimuli play an important part in the development of cognition. Infants habituate to the familiar, attending less and less to a stimulus that is repeated several times and then increasing their attention when the stimulus changes. Infants can differentiate among similar patterns, colors, and consonants. They can recognize facial expressions (smiles) as similar, even when they appear on different faces. They also can match abstract properties of stimuli, such as contour, intensity, or temporal pattern across sensory modalities. Infants appear to seek stimuli actively as though satisfying an innate need to make sense of the world.

EMOTIONAL DEVELOPMENT. Basic trust develops as infants learn that their urgent needs are met regularly. The consistent availability of a trusted adult creates a condition for a secure attachment. Infants who are consistently picked up and held in response to distress cry less at 1 yr and show less aggressive behavior at 2 yr. The emotional significance of any experience depends on an individual child's temperament as well as the parent's responses. Success or failure in establishing feeding and sleep cycles determines the parents' feelings of efficacy despite the unquestionable importance of infant temperament.

AGE 2–6 MO

At about 2 mo, the emergence of voluntary (social) smiles and increasing eye contact mark a change in the parent-child relationship, heightening the parents' sense of being loved back. During the next months, an infant's range of motor and social control and cognitive engagement increases dramatically. Mutual regulation takes the form of complex social interchanges.

PHYSICAL DEVELOPMENT. Between 3 and 4 mo, the rate of growth slows to approximately 20 g/day (see Table 7–3). Early reflexes that limited voluntary movement recede. A novel object may elicit purposeful although inefficient reaching. The quality of spontaneous movements also changes, from larger writhing to smaller, circular movements that have been described as "fidgety." Increasing control of truncal flexion makes intentional rolling possible. Head control improves, allowing infants to gaze across at things rather than merely up and to begin taking food from a spoon. At the same time, maturation of the visual system allows much greater depth of field. Total sleep requirements are 14–16 hr/24 hr, with 9–10 hr concentrated at night; about 70% of infants sleep for a 6- to 8-hr stretch by age 6 mo. The sleep cycle remains short, only 50–60 min, compared with the adult cycle of approximately 90 min.

COGNITIVE DEVELOPMENT. Four-month-old infants are described as "hatching" socially, becoming interested in a wider world. During feeding, infants no longer focus exclusively on the mother but become distracted. Infants at this age also explore their own bodies, staring intently at their hands, vocalizing, blowing bubbles, and touching their ears, cheeks, and genitalia. These explorations represent an early stage in the understanding of cause and effect as infants learn that voluntary muscle movements generate predictable tactile and visual sensations. They also have a role in the emergence of a sense of self.

EMOTIONAL DEVELOPMENT AND COMMUNICATION. The primary emotions of anger, interest, fear, disgust, and surprise appear in appropriate contexts as distinct facial expressions.

IMPLICATIONS FOR PARENTS AND PEDIATRICIANS. For most parents, this is a happy period. Most parents excitedly report that they can hold "conversations" with their infants, taking turns vocalizing and listening.

AGE 6–12 MO

Months 6–12 bring increased mobility and exploration of an inanimate world, advances in cognitive understanding and communicative competence, and new tensions around the themes of attachment and separation. Infants develop will and intentions, characteristics that most will welcome but will still find challenging to manage.

PHYSICAL DEVELOPMENT. Growth slows more (see Table 7–3). The ability to sit unsupported (about 7 mo) and to pivot while sitting (around 9–10 mo) provides increasing opportunities to manipulate several objects at a time and to experiment with novel combinations of objects. These explorations are aided by the emergence of a pincer grasp (around 9 mo). Many infants begin crawling and pulling to stand around 8 mo and walk before their first birthday either independently or in a walker. These ambulatory achievements expand infants' exploratory range and create new physical dangers as well as opportunities for learning. Tooth eruption occurs, usually starting with the mandibular central incisors. Tooth development also reflects, in part, skeletal maturation and bone age.

COGNITIVE DEVELOPMENT. At first, everything goes into the mouth; in time, novel objects are picked up, inspected, passed from hand to hand, banged, dropped, and then mouthed. The complexity of an infant's play, how many different schemata are bought to bear, is a useful index of cognitive development at this age. A major milestone is the achievement (at about 9 mo) of object constancy, in the understanding that objects continue to exist even when not seen.

EMOTIONAL DEVELOPMENT. The advent of object constancy corresponds with qualitative changes in social and communicative development. Separations also become more difficult. At the same time, a new demand for autonomy emerges. Infants no longer consent to be fed but turn away as the spoon approaches or insist on holding it themselves. Tantrums make their first appearance as the drives for autonomy and mastery come in conflict with parental controls and with infants' still-limited abilities.

COMMUNICATION. Infants at 7 mo are adept at nonverbal communication, expressing a range of emotions and responding to vocal tone and facial expressions. Around 9 mo, infants become aware that emotions can be shared between people. Between 8–10 mo, baby babbling takes on a new complexity, with many syllables ("ba-da-ma") and inflections that mimic the native language. The first true word, that is, a sound used consistently to refer to a specific object or person, appears in concert with an infant's discovery of object constancy. At this age, picture books provide an ideal context for verbal language acquisition.

IMPLICATIONS FOR PARENTS AND PEDIATRICIANS. With the developmental reorganization around 9 mo, previously resolved issues of feeding and sleeping re-emerge. Pediatricians can prepare parents at the 6-mo visit so that these problems can be understood as the result of developmental progress and not regression. Infants' wariness of strangers often make the 9-mo examination difficult, particularly if the infant is temperamentally prone to react negatively to unfamiliar situations.

CHAPTER 8

The Second Year

(Nelson Textbook, Chapter 11)

At approximately 18 mo of age, the emergence of symbolic thought causes a reorganization of behavior with implications in many developmental domains.

AGE 12–18 MO

PHYSICAL DEVELOPMENT. The growth rate slows further in the 2nd year of life (see Table 7–2), and appetite declines. "Baby fat" is burned up by the increased mobility; exaggerated lumbar lordosis makes the abdomen protrude. Brain growth continues, with myelinization throughout the 2nd yr. Most children begin to walk independently near their first birthday; some do not walk until 15 mo. At first, infants toddle with a wide-based gait, knees bent, and arms flexed at the elbow; the entire torso rotates with each stride; the toes may point in or out, and the feet strike the floor flat. After several months of practice, the center of gravity shifts back and the torso stays more stable, while knees extend and arms swing at the sides for balance. The toes are held in better alignment, and the child is able to stop, pivot, and stoop without toppling over.

COGNITIVE DEVELOPMENT. Object exploration accelerates because reaching, grasping, and releasing are nearly fully mature and walking increases access to interesting things. Toddlers combine objects in novel ways to create interesting effects, such as stacking blocks. Playthings are also more likely to be used for their intended purposes (combs for hair, cups for drinking). Imitation of parents and older children is an important mode of learning. Make-believe play centers on the child's own body (see Tables 8–1 and 7–2).

EMOTIONAL DEVELOPMENT. Infants developmentally approaching the milestone of their first steps may be irritable. Once they start walking, their predominant mood changes markedly. Toddlers are described as "intoxicated" with their new ability and with the power to control the distance between themselves and their parents. Toddlers often orbit around their parents. A child's ability to use the parent as a secure base for exploration depends on the attachment relationship. When the parents leave, most children stop playing, cry, and try to follow. On the parents' return, securely attached children instantly go to their parents to be picked up, or comforted, and then are able to return to play. Insecure response patterns may represent strategies infants develop to cope with punitive or unresponsive parenting styles and may predict later cognitive and emotional problems.

LINGUISTIC DEVELOPMENT. Receptive language precedes expressive language. By the time infants speak their first words, around 12 mo, they already respond appropriately to several simple statements such as "no," "bye-bye," and "give me." By 15 mo, the average child points to major body parts and uses four to six words spontaneously and correctly, including proper nouns. Toddlers also enjoy polysyllabic jargoning (see Tables 7–2 and 8–1) but do not seem upset that no one understands. Most communication of wants and ideas continues to be nonverbal.

IMPLICATIONS FOR PARENTS AND PEDIATRICIANS. A child's ability to wander out of sight increases the difficulty of providing supervision and the risks of injury. When walking is precluded by physical disability, parents and care providers should facilitate explora-

TABLE 8–1 Emerging Patterns of Behavior from 1 to 5 Yr of Age*

15 Mo

Motor:	Walks alone; crawls up stairs
Adaptive:	Makes tower of 3 cubes; makes a line with crayon; inserts pellet in bottle
Language:	Jargon; follows simple commands; may name a familiar object (ball)
Social:	Indicates some desires or needs by pointing; hugs parents

18 Mo

Motor:	Runs stiffly; sits on small chair; walks up stairs with one hand held; explores drawers and wastebaskets
Adaptive:	Makes a tower of 4 cubes; imitates scribbling; imitates vertical stroke; dumps pellet from bottle
Language:	10 words (average); names pictures; identifies one or more parts of body
Social:	Feeds self; seeks help when in trouble; may complain when wet or soiled; kisses parent with pucker

24 Mo

Motor:	Runs well, walks up and down stairs, one step at a time; opens doors; climbs on furniture; jumps
Adaptive:	Tower of 7 cubes (6 at 21 mo); circular scribbling; imitates horizontal stroke; folds paper once imitatively
Language:	Puts 3 words together (subject, verb, object)
Social:	Handles spoon well; often tells immediate experiences; helps to undress; listens to stories with pictures

30 Mo

Motor:	Goes up stairs alternating feet
Adaptive:	Tower of 9 cubes; makes vertical and horizontal strokes but generally will not join them to make a cross; imitates circular stroke, forming closed figure
Language:	Refers to self by pronoun "I"; knows full name
Social:	Helps put things away; pretends in play

36 Mo

Motor:	Rides tricycle; stands momentarily on one foot
Adaptive:	Tower of 10 cubes; imitates construction of "bridge" of 3 cubes; copies a circle; imitates a cross
Language:	Knows age and sex; counts 3 objects correctly; repeats 3 numbers or a sentence of 6 syllables
Social:	Plays simple games (in "parallel" with other children); helps in dressing (unbuttons clothing and puts on shoes); washes hands

48 Mo

Motor:	Hops on one foot; throws ball overhand; uses scissors to cut out pictures; climbs well
Adaptive:	Copies bridge from model; imitates construction of "gate" of 5 cubes; copies cross and square; draws a man with 2 to 4 parts besides head; names longer of 2 lines
Language:	Counts 4 pennies accurately; tells a story
Social:	Plays with several children with beginning of social interaction and role-playing; goes to toilet alone

60 Mo

Motor:	Skips
Adaptive:	Draws triangle from copy; names heavier of 2 weights
Language:	Names 4 colors; repeats sentence of 10 syllables; counts 10 pennies correctly
Social:	Dresses and undresses; asks questions about meaning of words; domestic role-playing

*Data are derived from those of Gesell (as revised by Knobloch), Shirley, Provence, Wolf, Bailey, and others. After 5 yr the Stanford-Binet, Wechsler-Bellevue, and other scales offer the most precise estimates of developmental level. To have their greatest value, they should be administered only by an experienced and qualified person.

tion and help the child attain greater control over separation and proximity.

AGE 18–24 MO

PHYSICAL DEVELOPMENT. Motor development is incremental at this age, with improvements in balance and agility and the emergence of running and stair climbing. Height and weight increase at a steady rate, although head growth slows slightly (see Table 7–3).

COGNITIVE DEVELOPMENT. Object permanence is firmly established; toddlers anticipate where an object may have been moved to even though the object was not visible while it was being moved. Cause and effect are better understood, and toddlers demonstrate flexibility in problem solving. Symbolic transformations in play are no longer tied to the toddler's own body, so that a doll can be "fed" from an empty plate.

EMOTIONAL DEVELOPMENT. In many children, the relative independence of the preceding period gives way to increased clinginess around 18 mo. Separations at bedtime are often difficult, with frequent false starts and tantrums. Many children use a special blanket or stuffed toy as a transitional object. Self-conscious awareness and internalized standards of evaluation first appear at this age. Toddlers looking in a mirror will, for the first time, reach for their own face rather than the mirror image if they notice a red dot on their nose or some other unusual appearance. They begin to recognize when toys are broken and may hand them to parents to fix.

LINGUISTIC DEVELOPMENT. Labeling of objects coincides with the advent of symbolic thought. Children may point at things with their index finger rather than their whole hand as though calling attention to objects not for the purpose of having them but for finding out their names. After the realization that words can stand for things, a child's vocabulary balloons from 10–15 words at 18 mo to 100 or more at 2 yr. After acquiring a vocabulary of about 50 words, toddlers begin to combine them to make simple sentences, the beginning of grammar. At this stage, toddlers understand two-step commands, such as "Give me the ball and then get your shoes." As toddlers learn to use symbols to express ideas and solve problems, the need for cognition based on direct sensation and motor manipulation wanes (see Table 8–1).

IMPLICATIONS FOR PARENTS AND PEDIATRICIANS. With children's increasing mobility, physical limits on their explorations become less effective; words become increasingly important for behavior control as well as cognition. Children with delayed language acquisition often have greater behavior problems. Language development is facilitated when parents and caregivers use clear, simple sentences, ask questions, and respond to children's incomplete sentences and gestural communication with the appropriate words.

CHAPTER 9

The Preschool Years

(Nelson Textbook, Chapter 12)

Between 2 and 5 yr of age, the core issues of attachment and separation are reshaped by the emergence of language and played out in the context of a widening social sphere. As a toddler, a child learned to walk away and come back. As a preschooler, he or she explores emotional separation, alternating between strident opposition and clinging dependence. Tension between a child's growing sense of autonomy and the awareness of internal and external limitations defines the central dynamic of this age.

PHYSICAL DEVELOPMENT

By the end of the 2nd yr, somatic and brain growth slows, with corresponding decreases in nutritional requirements and in appetite (see Table 7–3). Between the ages of 2 and 5 yr, the average child gains approximately 2 kg in weight and 7 cm in height per year. The toddler's prominent abdomen flattens, and the body becomes leaner. Physical energy peaks, and the need for sleep declines to 11–13 hr/24 hr, usually including one nap. Visual acuity reaches 20/30 by age 3 yr and 20/20 by age 4. All 20 primary teeth have erupted by 3 yr of age.

Most children walk with a mature gait and run steadily before the end of their 3rd yr. Beyond this basic level, there is wide variation in ability as the range of motor activities expands to include throwing, catching, and kicking balls; riding on bicycles; climbing on playground structures; dancing; and other complex-pattern behaviors. The effects of such individual differences on cognitive and emotional development depend in part on the demands of the social environment. Energetic, coordinated children may thrive emotionally with parents who encourage physical activity; lower energy, more cerebral children may thrive with parents who value quiet play. Handedness is usually established by the 3rd yr. Bowel and bladder control emerge during this period (average age 30 mo, with large individual and cultural variation). Day-time bladder control typically precedes bowel control, and girls precede boys in attaining this. Bedwetting is normal up to age 4 in girls, age 5 in boys. Many children master toileting with ease. For others, toilet training can involve a protracted power struggle. Refusal to defecate in the toilet or potty is relatively common and can lead to constipation and parental frustration. Defusing the situation by a temporary cessation of training (and return to diapers) often allows toilet mastery to proceed.

IMPLICATIONS FOR PARENTS AND PEDIATRICIANS. The normal decrease in appetite at this age often arouses worry about nutrition. For the most part, parents can be reassured that if growth is normal, the child's intake is adequate. Children normally modulate their food intake to match their somatic needs according to feelings of hunger or satiety. Daily intake fluctuates, at times widely, but intake during the period of a week is relatively stable. Motorically precocious, highly active children face increased risks of injury. Parents of such children benefit from early guidance about the need for childproofing the home, constant supervision, and bicycle helmet use (beginning with the tricycle).

LANGUAGE, COGNITION, AND PLAY

These three domains all involve symbolic function, a mode of dealing with the world that emerges during the preschool period.

LANGUAGE. Language development occurs most rapidly between 2 and 5 yr of age. Vocabulary increases from 50–100 words to more than 2000. Sentence structure advances from telegraphic phrases ("Baby cry") to sentences incorporating all of the major grammatical components. As a rule of thumb, between age 2 and 5, the number of words in a typical sentence equals the child's age (2 by age 2, 3 by age 3, and so on). By 2½, most children are using possessives ("My ball"), progressives (the "ing" construction, as in "I playing"), questions, and negatives. By 4 they can count to 4 and use the past tense; by 5 they can use the future tense. An important distinction is between speech, the production of intelligible sounds, and language, the underlying mental act. Language includes both expressive and receptive functions. Receptive language (understanding) varies less in its rate of acquisition than does expressive language and therefore has greater prognostic importance. Language acquisition depends critically on environmental input. Key determinants include the amount and variety of speech directed toward children and the frequency with which adults ask questions and encourage verbalization. Although experience determines the rate of language development, mental retardation may first become apparent with delayed speech at approximately 2 yr. Child abuse and neglect are correlated with delayed language, particularly the ability to convey emotional states. Language also allows children to express feelings, such as anger or frustration, without acting them out. Preschool language development lays the foundation for later success in school. Through repeated early exposure to written words, children learn about the uses of writing (telling stories or sending messages) and about its form (left to right, top to bottom).

Picture books have a special role not only in familiarizing young children with the printed word but also in the development of verbal language. Reading aloud with a young child is an interactive process in which a parent focuses the child's attention on a particular picture, requests a response (by asking "What's that"?), and then gives the child feedback ("Right, it's a dog.").

COGNITION. The preschool period corresponds to Piaget's preoperational (prelogical) stage, characterized by magical thinking, egocentrism, and thinking that is dominated by perception (see Table 4–1). Magical thinking includes a confusion of coincidence for causality, animism (attributing motivations to inanimate objects and events), and unrealistic beliefs about the power of wishes. Egocentrism refers to a child's inability to take another's point of view and does not connote selfishness.

PLAY. During the preschool period, play is marked by increasing complexity and imagination, from simple scripts replicating common experiences such as shopping and putting baby to bed (age 2 or 3 yr) to more extended scenarios involving singular events such as going to the zoo or going on a trip (age 3 or 4 yr) to creation of scenarios that have only been imagined, such as flying to the moon (age 4 or 5). A similar progression in socialization moves from minimal social interactions with peers during play (solo or parallel play, age 1 or 2 yr) to cooperative play such as building a tower of blocks together (age 3 or 4 yr) to organized group play with distinct role assignments, as in playing house. Play also becomes increasingly rule governed. Play allows children to experience mastery. Creativity, inherent in all play, is especially visible in drawing, painting, and other artistic activities. Themes and emotions that emerge in a child's drawings often reflect the emotional issues of greatest importance for the child. Moral thinking mirrors and is constrained by a child's cognition level. Emphatic responses to others' distress arise during the 2nd yr of life, but the ability to cognitively consider another child's point of view remains limited throughout the preschool period.

IMPLICATIONS FOR PARENTS AND PEDIATRICIANS. The significance of language as a target for assessment and intervention cannot be overestimated because of its central role as an indicator of cognitive and emotional development and as a key factor in behavioral regulation and later school success. Parents can support emotional development by using words that describe the child's feeling states ("You sound angry right now") and by using the child's words to express feelings rather than acting out the feelings. Parents should have a regular time each day for reading or looking at books with their children.

Preoperational thinking constrains how children understand experiences of illnesses and treatment. The imaginative intensity that fuels play and the magical, animist thinking characteristic of preoperational cognitive can also generate intense fears.

EMOTIONAL DEVELOPMENT

Emotional challenges facing preschool children include accepting limits while maintaining a sense of self direction, reining in aggressive and sexual impulses, and interacting with a widening circle of adults and peers. At age 2 yr, behavioral limits are predominantly external; by age 5 yr, these controls need to be internalized if a child is to function in a typical classroom. Success in achieving this goal relies on prior emotional development, particularly the ability to use internalized images of trusted adults to provide security in times of stress. Children need to believe themselves worthy of adult approval to be willing to work for it.

Children learn what behaviors are acceptable and how much power they wield vis-à-vis important adults by testing limits. Testing increases when it elicits an exceptional amount of attention, even though that attention is often negative, and when limits are inconsistent. Testing often arouses parental anger or inappropriate solicitude.

Control is a central issue. Inability to control some aspect of the external world, such as what to buy or when to leave, often results in a loss of internal control, that is, a temper tantrum. Fear, being overly tidy, or physical discomfort can also evoke tantrums. Tantrums normally appear toward the end of the 1st yr of life and peak in prevalence between ages 2 and 4 yr. Frequent tantrums after age 5 yr tend to persist throughout childhood.

Preschool children normally experience complicated feelings toward their parents: intense love and jealousy and resentment and fear that angry feelings might lead to abandonment. The resolution of this crisis, a process extending over years, involves a child's unspoken decision to emulate the parents rather than compete with them.

Curiosity about genitalia and adult sexual organs is normal, as is masturbation. Modesty appears gradually between ages 4 and 6 yr, with wide variations among cultures and families.

IMPLICATIONS FOR PARENTS AND PEDIATRICIANS. Most parents find it difficult to understand their preschool children at least some of the time. Rapid shifts between clinging dependence and defiant independence, between sophisticated-sounding language and infantile helplessness, and between angelic joy and uncontrollable rage can erode parents' self-confidence and patience. Guidance emphasizing appropriate expectations for behavioral and emotional development and acknowledging normal parental feelings of anger, guilt, and confusion can help lessen parents' worries both about their children and about themselves.

It may be difficult to decide whether a particular child's behavior is normally challenging or indicative of a true problem. Red flags include parents who do not volunteer any positive statements about their children, evidence of threatening or overtly punitive discipline, and the existence of problems (especially tantrums in day care or preschool, where most preschool-aged children manage to maintain self-control). The presence of chronic medical problems, development delays, or unusual family stresses signal the need for more detailed assessment.

Corporal punishment is accepted in many traditional cultures but may be inappropriate in the modern context in which most families now live (see Chapter 3). Children mimic the corporal punishment they receive, and it is not uncommon for preschool-aged children to strike their parents back. Parents may be helped to renounce spanking or at least reserve it for extreme circumstances if they learn more effective discipline techniques, including consistent limit setting, clear communication, and frequent approval. Time-out for approximately 1 min per year of age is a form of noncorporal punishment backed by extensive research.

CHAPTER 10

Early School Years
(Nelson Textbook, Chapter 13)

During middle childhood (6–12 yr), children face new challenges. The cognitive power to consider several factors simultaneously confers the ability to evaluate oneself and perceive others' evaluations. As a result, self-esteem becomes a central issue. School-aged children are judged according to their ability to produce socially valued outputs, such as good grades or home runs. Healthy development requires increasing separation from parents and the ability to find acceptance in the peer group and to negotiate challenges in the outside world.

PHYSICAL DEVELOPMENT. Growth during the period averages 3–3.5 kg (7 lb) and 6 cm (2.5 in) per year. Growth occurs discontinuously, in irregular spurts lasting on average 8 wk, three to six times per year. The head only grows 2–3 cm in circumference throughout the entire period, reflecting slowed brain growth; myelinization is complete by 7 yr of age. Body habitus tends to remain relatively stable throughout middle childhood.

Growth of the midface and lower face occurs gradually. Loss of deciduous (baby) teeth is a more dramatic sign of maturation, beginning about age 6 yr after eruption of the 1st molars. Replacement with adult teeth occurs at a rate of about 4 per year. Lymphoid tissues hypertrophy, often giving rise to impressive tonsils and adenoids, which occasionally require surgical treatment.

Muscular strength, coordination, and stamina increase progressively, as does the ability to perform complex movements, such as dancing or playing the piano.

The sexual organs remain physically immature, but interest in gender differences and sexual behavior remains active in many children and increases progressively until puberty. Masturbation is common, if not universal.

IMPLICATIONS FOR PARENTS AND PEDIATRICIANS. "Normality" encompasses a wide range of physical sizes, shapes, and abilities in school-aged children. Just as importantly, children's feelings about their physical attributes range from pride to shame to apparent nonchalance. The routine physical examination provides an opportunity to elicit concerns and allay fears.

Girls, in particular, often worry that they are overweight, and many engage in unhealthy dieting to achieve an abnormally thin cultural ideal. Shortness, particularly in boys, may be associated with decreased educational attainment and increased risks for behavior problems.

A child's physical appearance may also evoke strong feelings in parents, leading them to undermine the child's self-esteem inadvertently, or alternatively, to encourage vanity. Pediatricians can help parents distinguish between true health risks and individual variations that should be accepted.

COGNITIVE AND LANGUAGE DEVELOPMENT. In place of magical, egocentric, and perception-bound cognition, school-aged children increasingly apply rules based on observable phenomena, factor in multiple dimensions and points of view, and interpret their perceptions in view of realistic theories about physical laws. Mastery of the elementary curriculum requires that a large number of perceptual, cognitive, and language processes work efficiently. Attention and receptive language affect each other as well as every other aspect of learning.

The first 2 yr of elementary school are devoted to acquiring the fundamentals: reading, writing, and basic mathematics skills. By 3rd or 4th grade, the curriculum requires that children use those fundamentals to learn increasingly complex materials. The volume of work increases along with the complexity. Children can meet these demands only if they have mastered the basic skills to the point that their execution has become automatic.

Cognitive abilities interact with a wide array of attitudinal and emotional factors in determining classroom performance. A partial list of such factors includes eagerness to please adults, being cooperative, competitiveness, willingness to work for a delayed reward, belief in one's abilities, and ability to risk trying when success is not ensured.

Children's intellectual activity extends beyond the classroom. Beginning in the 3rd or 4th grade, children increasingly enjoy strategy games and word play (puns and insults) that exercise growing cognitive and linguistic mastery.

IMPLICATIONS FOR PARENTS AND PEDIATRICIANS. Children in the cognitive stage of concrete logical operations can understand simple explanations for illnesses and necessary treatments, although they may revert to prelogical thinking under stress (as may adults).

Academic and classroom behavior problems, like fever, are symptoms that require diagnosis. Among the broad range of possible causes are deficits in specific cognitive, perceptual, or linguistic functions (specific learning disabilities); global cognitive delay (mental retardation); primary attention deficit; and attention deficits secondary to emotional preoccupation, depression, anxiety, or any chronic illness. Remedial approaches depend on the underlying problem(s).

SOCIAL AND EMOTIONAL DEVELOPMENT. Social and emotional development proceeds in three contexts: the home, the school, and the neighborhood. Of these, the home remains the most influential. The beginning of school coincides with a child's further separation from the family and the increasing importance of teacher and peer relationships. Conformity is rewarded. Some children conform readily and enjoy easy social success; those who adopt individualistic styles or have visible differences may be stigmatized as "weird." In the neighborhood, real danger such as busy streets, bullies, and strangers tax school-aged children's common sense and resourcefulness.

IMPLICATIONS FOR PARENTS AND PEDIATRICIANS. Children need unconditional support as well as realistic demands as they venture into a world that is often frightening. Children who show unusual difficulty in separating from parents and in facing school and neighborhood challenges may be reacting to their parents' difficulty letting them go. Pediatricians need to be alert to children's functioning in all contexts (home, school, neighborhood) and consider how each of those environments either supports or overwhelms the child's ability to adapt and grow.

CHAPTER 11

Adolescence

(Nelson Textbook, Chapters 14 and 107–121)

Between the ages of 10 and 20 yr, children undergo rapid changes in body size, shape, physiology, and psychologic and social functioning. Hormones set the developmental agenda in conjunction with social structures designed to foster the transition from childhood to adulthood.

Adolescence proceeds across three distinct periods—early, middle, and late—each marked by a characteristic set of salient biologic, psychologic, and social issues (Table 11–1). However, individual variation is substantial, both in terms of the timing of somatic changes and the quality of the adolescent's experience. Gender and subculture profoundly affect the development course,

TABLE 11–1 Central Issues in Early, Middle, and Late Adolescence

Variable	Early Adolescence	Middle Adolescence	Late Adolescence
Age (yr)	10–13	14–16	17–20 and beyond
Sexual maturity rating	1–2	3–5	5
Somatic	Secondary sex characteristics; beginning of rapid growth; awkward	Height growth peaks; body shape and composition change; acne and odor; menarche; spermarche	Slower growth
Sexual	Sexual interest usually exceeds sexual activity	Sexual drive surges; experimentation; questions of sexual orientation	Consolidation of sexual identity
Cognitive and moral	Concrete operations; conventional morality	Emergence of abstract thought; questioning mores; self-centered	Idealism; absolutism
Self-concept	Preoccupation with changing body; self-consciousness	Concern with attractiveness, increasing introspection	Relatively stable body image
Family	Bids for increased independence; ambivalence	Continued struggle for acceptance of greater autonomy	Practical independence; family remains secure base
Peers	Same-sex groups; conformity; cliques	Dating; peer groups less important	Intimacy; possibly commitment
Relationship to society	Middle-school adjustment	Gauging skills and opportunities	Career decisions (e.g., drop out, college, work)

TABLE 11–2 Classification of Sex Maturity Stages in Girls

SMR Stage	Pubic Hair	Breasts
1	Preadolescent	Preadolescent
2	Sparse, lightly pigmented, straight, medial border of labia	Breast and papilla elevated as small mound; areolar diameter increased
3	Darker, beginning to curl, increased amount	Breast and areola enlarged, no contour separation
4	Coarse, curly, abundant but amount less than in adult	Areola and papilla form secondary mound
5	Adult feminine triangle, spread to medial surface of thighs	Mature, nipple projects, areola part of general breast contour

SMR = sexual maturity rating.
From Tanner JM: Growth at Adolescence, 2nd ed. Oxford, England, Blackwell Scientific Publications, 1962.

as do physical and social stressors such as cerebral palsy and parental alcoholism.

EARLY ADOLESCENCE

BIOLOGIC DEVELOPMENT. Adrenal production of androgen may occur as early as age 6, with development of underarm odor and faint genital hair (adrenarche). The rapid changes of puberty begin with increased sensitivity of the pituitary to gonadotropin-releasing hormone (GnRH); pulsatile release of GnRH, luteinizing hormone (LH), and follicle-stimulating hormone during sleep; and corresponding rises in gonadal androgens and estrogens. The resulting sequence of somatic and physiologic changes gives rise to the sexual maturity rating (SMR) or Tanner stages. Tables 11–2 and 11–3 describe the somatic changes used in the SMR scale.

TABLE 11–3 Classification of Sex Maturity Stages in Boys

SMR Stage	Pubic Hair	Penis	Testes
1	None	Preadolescent	Preadolescent
2	Scanty, long, slightly pigmented	Slight enlargement	Enlarged scrotum, pink, texture altered
3	Darker, starts to curl, small amount	Longer	Larger
4	Resembles adult type but less in quantity; coarse, curly	Larger; glans and breadth increase in size	Larger; scrotum dark
5	Adult distribution, spread to medial surface of thighs	Adult size	Adult size

SMR = sexual maturity rating.

TABLE 11–4 Variability in Timing of Sexual Maturation

SMR	Early (Mean − 2 SD Early)	Average (Median)	Late (Mean + 2 SD Late)
Timing of SMR Stages in Girls			
Pubic Hair			
SMR2	9.0	11.2	13.5
SMR3	9.6	11.9	14.1
SMR4	10.3	12.6	14.8
Breast Development			
SMR2	8.9	10.9	12.9
SMR3	9.8	11.9	13.9
SMR4	10.5	12.9	15.3
Timing of SMR Stages in Boys			
Pubic Hair			
SMR2	9.9	12.0	14.1
SMR3	11.2	13.1	14.9
SMR4	12.0	13.9	15.7
Penis Development			
SMR2	9.2	10.5	13.7
SMR3	10.1	12.4	14.6
SMR4	11.2	13.2	15.4

SMR = sexual maturity rating.

Data from Tanner JM, Davies PSW: Clinical longitudinal standards for height and height velocity for North American children. J Pediatr 107:317, 1985.

Table 11–4 lists median ages and normal ranges for key stages of breast, pubic hair, and penile development. The range of normal for progress through the stages of sexual maturity is wide.

In girls, the first visible sign of puberty is the appearance of breast buds, between 8 and 13 yr. Menses typically begin 2–2.5 yr later (normal range 9–16 yr), around the peak in height velocity. Less obvious changes include enlargement of the ovaries, uterus, labia, and clitoris; thickening of the endometrium and the vaginal mucosa; and increased vaginal glycogen, predisposing to yeast infections.

In boys, testicular enlargement begins as early as age 9½ yr. Peak growth occurs when testis volumes reach 9–10 cm^3. Under the influence of LH and testosterone, the seminiferous tubules, epididymis, seminal vesicles, and prostate enlarge. Some degree of breast hypertrophy occurs in 40–65% of pubertal boys as a result of a relative excess of estrogenic stimulation. Gynecomastia sufficient to cause embarrassment and social disability occurs in fewer than 10%. Obesity may exacerbate gynecomastia and should be addressed through diet and exercise.

For both sexes, growth acceleration begins in early adolescence, but peak growth velocities are not reached until SMR3 or SMR4. The growth spurt begins distally, with enlargement of hands and feet, followed by the arms and legs and finally by the trunk and chest. Adrenal androgens stimulate the sebaceous glands, promoting the development of acne. Dental changes include jaw growth, loss of the final deciduous teeth, and eruption of the permanent cuspids, premolars, and finally molars.

SEXUALITY. Interest in sex increases in early puberty. Ejaculation occurs for the first time, usually during masturbation and later spontaneously in sleep. Early adolescents sometimes masturbate socially; mutual sexual exploration is not necessarily a sign of homosexuality.

COGNITIVE AND MORAL DEVELOPMENT. In piagetian theory, adolescence marks the transition from the concrete operational thinking characteristic of school-aged children to formal logical operations. Formal operations include the ability to manipulate abstractions such as algebraic expressions, to reason from unknown principles, to weigh many points of view according to varying criteria, and to think about the process of thinking itself. Some early adolescents demonstrate formal thinking, others acquire the capability later, and others do not acquire it at all. It is unclear whether or not the hormonal changes of puberty directly affect cognitive development. The development of moral thinking roughly parallels general cognitive development.

SELF-CONCEPT. Self-consciousness increases exponentially in response to the somatic transformations of puberty. Self-awareness at this age tends to center on external characteristics in contrast to the introspection of later adolescence.

RELATIONSHIPS WITH FAMILY, PEERS, AND SOCIETY. In early adolescence, the trend toward separation from family with increasing involvement in peer activities accelerates. A symbolic expression of this shift is the renunciation of family norms of dress and grooming in favor of the peer group "uniform."

Early adolescents often socialize in same-sex peer groups. Scatologic jokes, teasing directed against the other gender, and rumor mongering about who likes whom attest to burgeoning sexual interest. An early adolescent's relationship to society centers on school.

IMPLICATIONS FOR PARENTS AND PEDIATRICIANS. Physical growth, body preoccupation, and sexual interest correlate with sexual maturity, whereas cognitive advancement, separation, and changes in social behavior may correlate more closely with chronologic age or grade in school.

Early adolescents often have questions about the somatic and sexual changes they are experiencing. During a physical examination, a pediatrician can anticipate concerns and volunteer information that the adolescent may have been too uncomfortable to request. Parents, too, may have concerns that they are hesitant to discuss.

MIDDLE ADOLESCENCE

BIOLOGIC DEVELOPMENT. In the average girl, the growth spurt peaks at 11.5 yr at a top velocity of 8.3 cm (3.8 in) per year and then slows to a stop at 16 yr. In the average boy, the growth spurt starts later, peaks at 13.5 yr at 9.5 cm (4.3 in) per year, and then slows to a stop at 18 yr. Weight gain parallels linear growth, with a delay of several months, so that adolescents seem first to stretch and then fill out. Pubertal weight gains account for approximately 40% of adult weight. Muscle mass also increases, followed several months later by an increase in strength; boys show greater gain in both.

Bone maturation correlates closely with SMR because epiphyseal closure is under androgenic control. Boys with SMR3 pubic hair and SMR4 genitalia normally have their peak growth spurt ahead of them; girls at the same SMR are usually past their peaks. Widening of the shoulders in boys and of the hips in girls is also hormonally determined. Other physiologic changes include a doubling in heart size and lung vital capacity from preadolescent norms. Blood pressure, blood volume, and hematocrit rise, particularly in boys. Androgenic stimulation of sebaceous and apocrine glands results in acne and body odor.

Sexual maturation in middle adolescence is dramatic, with the achievement of menarche in 30% of girls by SMR3 (mean age 11.9 yr) and in 90% by SMR4 (mean age 12.6–12.9 yr). Menarche usually follows approximately 1 yr after the growth spurt. Before menarche, the uterus achieves a mature configuration, vaginal lubrication increases, and a clear vaginal discharge appears, sometimes mistaken for a sign of infection. In boys, spermarche occurs and the penis lengthens and widens.

SEXUALITY. Dating becomes a normative activity during middle adolescence. The degree of sexual activity varies widely. Biologic maturation and social pressures combine to determine sexual activity. Homosexual experimentation is common and does not necessarily reflect a child's ultimate sexual orientation. Homosexual adolescents face increased risk of isolation and depression.

In addition to sexual orientation, middle adolescents begin to sort out other important aspects of sexual identity, including beliefs about love, honesty, and propriety. Dating relationships are often superficial at this age, emphasizing attractiveness and sexual experimentation rather than intimacy.

COGNITIVE AND MORAL DEVELOPMENT. With the transition to formal operational thought, middle adolescents question and analyze extensively. Questioning of moral conventions fosters the development of personal codes of ethics.

SELF-CONCEPT. The peer group exerts less influence over dress, activities, and behavior. Middle adolescents often experiment with different personae, changing styles of dress, groups of friends, and interests from month to month.

RELATIONSHIPS WITH FAMILIES, PEERS, AND SOCIETY. Puberty commonly results in strained relationships between adolescents and their parents. As a part of separation, adolescents may become distant from parents, redirecting emotional and sexual energies toward peer relationships. Middle adolescents often begin thinking seriously about what they want to do as adults, a question that formerly had been comfortably hypothetical.

IMPLICATIONS FOR PARENTS AND PEDIATRICIANS. Physical and sexual maturation, changes in sexual behavior and identity, emotional distance from parents, waning peer group influence, introspection, and growing cognizance of life after childhood all combine to make middle adolescence a time when the opportunity to talk confidentially with a nonjudgmental, informed adult can be particularly appreciated and helpful.

LATE ADOLESCENCE

BIOLOGIC DEVELOPMENT. The final stages of breast, penile, and pubic hair development occur by age 17–18 yr in 95% of males and females.

PSYCHOSOCIAL DEVELOPMENT. Sexual experimentation decreases as adolescents adopt more stable sexual identities. Cognition tends to be less self-centered, with increasing thoughts about concepts such as justice, patriotism, and history. Older adolescents are often idealistic but also may be absolutist and intolerant of opposing views. Intimate relationships are also an important component of identity for many older adolescents. Career decisions become pressing because an adolescent's self-concept is increasingly bound up in the emerging role in society (as student, worker, or parent).

IMPLICATIONS FOR PARENTS AND PEDIATRICIANS. Erikson identified the crucial task of adolescence as that of establishing a stable sense of identity, including separation from family of origin, initiation of intimacy, and realistic planning for economic independence. To achieve these milestones, developmental progress is required of both adolescents and their parents.

CHAPTER 12

Assessment of Growth and Development

(Nelson Textbook, Chapters 15 and 16)

Growth assessment is an essential component of pediatric health surveillance because almost any problem within the physiologic, interpersonal, and social domains can adversely affect growth. The most powerful tool in growth assessment is the growth chart.

GROWTH CHART DERIVATION AND INTERPRETATION. For infants, the measure of linear growth is length, taken by two examiners (one to position the child) with the child supine on a measuring board. For older children, the measure is stature, taken with a child standing on a stadiometer. The data are presented in four standard charts: (1) weight for age, (2) height for age, (3) head circumference for age, and (4) weight for height. Separate charts are provided for boys and girls.

Each chart is composed of seven percentile curves, representing the distribution of weight, length, stature, or head circumference values at each age. The percentile curve indicates the percentage of children at a given age on the *x*-axis whose measured value falls below the corresponding value on the *y*-axis. By definition, the 50th percentile is the median, the value above (and below) which 50% of the observed values fall. It is also termed the standard value in the sense that the standard height for a 7-mo-girl is 120 cm. The weight-for-height charts are constructed in an analogous fashion, with length or stature in the place of age.

It is important to appreciate both the strengths and limitations of these charts. The National Center for Health Statistics (NCHS) data, on which the charts are based, are representative of a population of well-nourished and healthy children in the United States. The NCHS curves are less appropriate for adolescents. Growth during adolescence is linked temporarily to the onset of puberty, which varies widely. The NCHS cross-sectional sample, based solely on chronologic age, lumps together subjects who are at different stages of maturation. Growth charts derived from longitudinal date are recommended for adolescents, when precision is necessary.

ANALYSIS OF GROWTH PATTERNS. Growth is a process rather than a static quality. An infant at the 5th percentile of weight for age may be growing normally, may be failing to grow, or may be recovering from growth failure, depending on the trajectory of the growth curve. Typically, infants and children stay within one or two growth channels. The canalization attests to the robust control that genes exert over body size.

A normal exception commonly occurs during the 1st 2 yr of life. For full-term infants, size at birth reflects the influence of the uterine environment; size at age 2 yr correlates with mean parental height, reflecting the influence of genes. Between birth and 18 mo, small infants often shift percentiles upward toward their parents' mean percentile. Large neonates with smaller parents often shift percentiles downward. For premature infants, overdiagnosis of growth failure can be avoided by subtracting the weeks of prematurity from the postnatal age when plotting growth parameters. Very-low-birth-weight (<1500 g) infants may continue to show catch-up growth through early school age. Special growth charts based on gestational rather than chronologic age have been developed for infants beginning at 26 wk gestational age.

Weight for height below the fifth percentile is the single best growth chart indicator of acute undernutrition. After several months of caloric deprivation, the height-for-age curve drops (stunting), whereas the weight-for-height curve may return toward normal. In infants, chronic, severe undernutrition also depresses head growth, an ominous predictor of later cognitive disability.

Nutritional insufficiency must be differentiated from congenital, constitutional, familial, and endocrine causes of decreased linear growth. In the latter cases, the length declines first or at the same time as the weight; weight for height is normal or elevated. In nutritional insufficiency, the weight declines before the length and the weight for height is low (unless there has been chronic stunting). Figure 12–1 depicts typical growth curves for four classes of decreased linear growth. In congenital pathologic short stature, an infant is born small and growth gradually tapers off throughout infancy. Causes include chromosomal abnormalities (Turner syndrome, trisomy 21), infection (TORCH [toxoplasmosis, other infections, rubella, cytomegalovirus infection, and herpes simplex] infections), teratogens (phenytoin [Dilantin], alcohol),

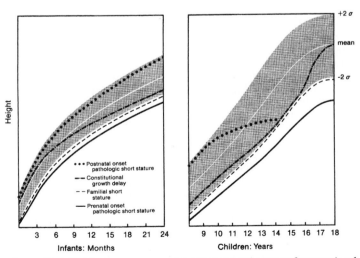

Figure 12–1 Height-for-age curves of the four general causes of proportional short stature: postnatal onset pathologic short stature, constitutional growth delay, familial short stature, and prenatal onset short stature. (From Mahoney CP: Evaluating the child with short stature. Pediatr Clin North Am 34:825, 1987.)

and extreme prematurity. In constitutional growth delay, weight and height decrease near the end of infancy, parallel the norm through middle childhood, and accelerate toward the end of adolescence. Adult size is normal. In familial short stature, both the infant and parents are small; growth runs parallel to and just below the normal curves.

OTHER INDICES OF GROWTH

BODY PROPORTIONS. Body proportions follow a sequence of regular changes with development. The head and trunk are relatively large at birth, with progressive lengthening of the limbs throughout development, particularly during puberty. Proportionality can be assessed by measuring the lower body segment, defined as the length from the symphysis pubis to the floor, and the upper body segment, defined as the height minus the lower body segment. The ratio for upper body segment divided by lower body segment (U/L ratio) equals approximately 1.7 at birth, 1.3 at 3 yr, and 1.0 after age 7 yr.

SKELETAL MATURATION. Reference standards for bone maturation facilitate estimation of bone age. Bone age correlates well with stage of pubertal development and can be helpful in predicting adult height in early- or late-maturing adolescents. In familial short stature, the bone age is normal (comparable to chronologic age). In constitutional delay, there is endocrinologic short stature and undernutrition.

DENTAL DEVELOPMENT. Dental development includes mineralization, eruption, and exfoliation. Initial mineralization begins as early as the second trimester (mean age for central incisors, 14 wk) and continues through age 3 yr for the primary (deciduous) teeth and age 25 yr for the permanent teeth. Eruption begins with the central incisors and progresses laterally. Exfoliation begins at about age 6 yr and continues through age 12 yr. Eruption of the permanent teeth may follow exfoliation immediately or may lag by 4–5 mo.

PHYSIOLOGIC AND STRUCTURAL GROWTH. Virtually every organ and physiologic process undergoes a predictable sequence of structural or functional changes, or both, during development. Reference values for developmental changes in a wide variety of systems (pituitary and rental function, electroencephalogram, electrocardiogram) have been published. Physiologic and structural changes of particular relevance to general pediatrics include the following:

1. Respiratory rate and pulse rate decrease sharply during the first 2 yr and then more gradually throughout childhood; blood pressure rises steadily beginning at approximately 6 yr of age.

2. Development of the paranasal sinuses continues throughout childhood. The ethmoidal, maxillary, and sphenoidal sinuses are present from birth; the frontal sinuses first appear radiologically

around age 6 yr. The ethmoidal sinuses reach their maximum size relatively early in childhood (age 7–14 yr); the others reach their maximum size after puberty.

3. Lymphoid tissues develop rapidly, reaching adult size by age 6 yr and continuing to hypertrophy throughout childhood and early adolescence before receding to adult size.

4. The metabolism of medications and a child's response to them change rapidly in the 1st mo of life and again under hormonal influences in puberty. No single pattern is characteristic of all medications, and individual variation is the rule.

5. Nutritional needs as well as a wide variety of biochemical and hematologic values undergo marked developmental changes.

DEVELOPMENT. Developmental assessment is the necessary prerequisite to intervention. The 1986 Amendments to the Education for All Handicapped Children Act (PL 99-457) require that every state create a system to identify and treat developmental disabilities in children age 3–5 yr. Most states have opted to extend these entitlements to children beginning at birth and to children deemed at risk for developmental problems as well as those with established delays.

Developmental assessment is a two-step process: (1) a screening procedure to pick out children in need of more in-depth assessment and (2) developmental diagnosis, the goal of which is to define the developmental problems and their significance in the context of a child's biologic, psychologic, and social strengths and vulnerabilities.

SCREENING AND SURVEILLANCE. The ideal screening test must be a highly sensitive (detect nearly all children with problems) and reasonably specific (not label many children as having problems when they do not in fact have them). It should also measure what it purports to measure (content validity), give similar results on repeat administration and on administration by different examiners (test-retest and inter-rater reliability), and be relatively quick and inexpensive.

The most widely used and researched test is the Denver-II. The test generates pass-fail ratings in four domains of development—personal-social, fine motor-adaptive, language, and gross motor—for children from birth to 6 yr. It can be administered in 20–30 min without extensive training or expensive equipment. Originally published in 1969 as the Denver Development Screening Test (DDST), the name was later changed to "The Denver" in recognition of its limited utility for screening, per se. The test may fail to identify children with subtle delays, and its ability to predict cognitive delays at a later age (predictive validity) is modest.

To increase the efficiency of screening, a series of brief parent questionnaires based on the DDST milestones has been recommended as a prescreen. The Denver Home Screening Questionnaire for parents provides information on the child-rearing environment, analogous to the well-validated Home Observation for Measurement of the Environment (HOME scale).

Screening for language delays is particularly important because of the strong links between language and cognitive development and later school performance. The Early Language Milestone (ELM) Scale provides pass-fail ratings in expressive, receptive, and visual language, using a format similar to that of the Denver.

Like the ELM, the Clinical Linguistic and Auditory Milestone Scale (CLAMS) is a sequence of language milestones that can be quickly administered, has been validated in infants and toddlers suspected of language delay and in those with known motor delays, and correlates well with standard diagnostic language tests.

The Ages and Stages Questionnaires (ASQ) are a series of 11 questionnaires designed to be completed at home by parents at several time points from 4 to 48 mo. Behavioral and psychiatric problems are common and often accompany developmental concerns. Screening for behavioral problems using the Pediatric Symptom Checklist is a simple, well-validated method.

LIMITATIONS OF SCREENING. Screening tests are subject to a number of abuses, including failure to follow the instructions for administration and scoring; overinterpretation of the results (essentially confusing screening with diagnosis); focusing on the screening test to the exclusion of other sources of information; screening too infrequently; using tests that are culturally biased; and failing to follow up with further assessments and treatment when indicated.

DEVELOPMENTAL SURVEILLANCE. Surveillance has been put forward as an antidote to the shortcomings of developmental screening. Developmental surveillance is a process that includes regular elicitation of the developmental history, attention to the parental concerns, careful developmental observations, and promotion of development. An approach combining ongoing surveillance with periodic use of screening tests may be the most effective and practical solution. Early identification of developmental and emotional problems will be maximized by keeping the following five principles in mind:

1. Parents, as a rule, are accurate observers of their children's behaviors; parental concerns about possible developmental delays are often appropriate and need to be taken seriously.

2. No child is too young for formal audiologic testing.

3. Risk factors are additive. Biologic impairments that may be relatively minor on their own (e.g., recurrent otitis) may have major impacts in the presence of environmental risk factors (e.g., maternal depression). Awareness of problems in one area should trigger increased vigilance in other areas.

4. Discomfort, fatigue, shyness, and oppositionality may adversely affect a child's performance on developmental testing.

5. Pediatricians and parents may worry about the adverse affects of labeling a child. Screening test results are not diagnosis. Follow-up assessment and intervention are critical.

DIAGNOSTIC ASSESSMENT

Once a child has been identified as having a potential problem, the next step is diagnostic assessment.

MEDICAL EVALUATION OF DEVELOPMENTAL DELAYS. The prevalence of more common developmental disabilities is listed in Table 12–1. The medical evaluation includes history, physical examination, and laboratory testing. Taking a thorough family history, including neurologic, psychiatric, and social difficulties (e.g., legal problems), is indispensable.

The prenatal history should include a search for potential teratogenic exposures, including radiation or medications, infectious illnesses, fever, addictive substances, and trauma. The perinatal history includes birth weight, gestational age, Apgar scores, and any medical complications. Postnatal medical factors that are sometimes overlooked include chronic respiratory or allergic illness, recurrent otitis, head trauma, and sleep problems (particularly signs of obstructive sleep apnea).

In the physical examination, points of particular importance include growth parameters and head circumference, facial and other dysmorphology, eye findings (e.g., cataracts in various inborn errors of metabolism), and signs of neurocutaneous disorders (café au lait spots in neurofibromatosis, hypopigmented macules in tuberous sclerosis).

No single set of laboratory tests is indicated in all cases. Most states screen for phenylketonuria, hypothyroidism, and other metabolic conditions in the neonatal period.

The medical evaluation for mental retardation and autism should include chromosomal and molecular biologic testing for

TABLE 12–1 Prevalence of Developmental Disabilities

Condition	Prevalence per 1000
Cerebral palsy	2–3
Visual impairment	0.3–0.6
Hearing impairment	0.8–2
Mental retardation	25
Learning disability	75
ADHD	150
Behavioral disorders	6–13%

ADHD = Attention deficit hyperactivity disorder.
Adapted from Levy SE, Hyman SL: Pediatric assessment of the child with developmental delay. Pediatr Clin North Am 40:465, 1993.

fragile X syndrome, the most commonly identified genetic cause of mental retardation.

DEVELOPMENTAL DIAGNOSIS FOR INFANTS AND PRESCHOOL-AGED CHILDREN. The most widely used newborn behavioral examination is the Brazelton Neonatal Behavioral Assessment Scale (NBAS). The NBAS allows quantitative estimation of an infant's neurologic intactness, adaptation to extrauterine life, primitive reflexes, state organization, self-regulatory ability, and interactive capacities from birth to 1 mo. The examination takes 30–45 min and requires extensive training for an examiner to reach proficiency. The NBAS is a poor predictor of later development, which is not surprising given the salience of environmental influences on development.

For older infants and preschool-aged children, the diagnostic process may include formal developmental testing, playroom observations, parent and family interviews, home observations, and team meetings. It often involves a multidisciplinary team of educators, psychologists, parents, social workers, therapists, and pediatricians.

For young children, intervention relies on parental participation. The federal Early Intervention Law (PL105-17) mandates family involvement at all stages of the process of assessment, construction of a service plan, and monitoring of a child's progress. For children who face predominantly social environmental risk factors (e.g., poverty), strong evidence shows that early intervention can raise IQ in the short term, as well as rates of school completion, job satisfaction, and social adjustment in the long term. For children at biologic risk because of prematurity, interventions combining direct therapy for a child with family support (home visiting, parent education) have resulted in significant gains in cognitive and emotional development. For children with established disabilities, the findings are more complex and controversial.

DIAGNOSTIC ASSESSMENT FOR SCHOOL-AGED CHILDREN. The medical evaluation includes the factors discussed in the prior chapters. Vision and hearing deficits, although seldom the sole causes of school problems, must be evaluated. The interview should assess functioning in the home, the school, and the neighborhood and with peers. Definitive diagnosis usually requires a team effort. Educational testing is indicated to define areas of academic strength and weakness. Psychologic evaluation is indicated to assess emotional problems, such as depression or anxiety, that may be either causes or consequences of the school problems. Assessment of family functioning is essential. Neuropsychologic testing may be indicated to assess specific functional deficits (short-term memory, verbal processing) that may cause a child to be inattentive. Pediatricians can facilitate these referrals and synthesize the information for parents and the school.

PART 3

Psychologic Disorders

CHAPTER 13

Psychiatric Considerations of Central Nervous System Injury
(Nelson Textbook, Chapter 18)

Psychiatric difficulties may follow infection; injury; intoxication; or genetic, metabolic, or idiopathic illness involving the central nervous system. Brain injury increases the risk of both intellectual impairment and psychiatric disorder, especially when the injury is severe. Social disinhibition appears to be a specific sequela of brain injury, but no typical psychiatric syndrome is associated. The development of novel psychiatric disorders presenting after brain injury is predicted by the severity of the injury, preinjury family functioning, and preinjury psychiatric history. Psychosis is not a typical result of brain injury or illness in childhood.

Brain-injured or epileptic children 5–15 yr old have five times the normal risk of psychiatric disorders. Mentally retarded children also are at increased risk of psychiatric disorders. Prematurity and neonatal complications place children at risk for such conditions as hyperactivity, impulsivity, difficulties in socialization, and poor control of emotions (especially anger) and for psychiatric disorders in general. Substance abuse during pregnancy may affect both prenatal and early childhood development.

The most significant factor in the child's adjustment to a chronic handicapping organic condition is the capacity of parents to adjust and cope. Most children with psychologic disturbances related to central nervous system injuries, as well as their families, benefit from understanding psychosocial support.

CHAPTER 14

Psychosomatic Illness
(Nelson Textbook, Chapter 19)

Psychologic conflict that significantly alters somatic function is the hallmark of psychosomatic disorder.

Conversion disorder, the loss or alteration of physical functioning without an demonstrable organic illness, is a type of somatoform disorder that usually presents in adolescence or adulthood. However, numerous childhood cases have occurred. Conversion reactions usually start suddenly, can often be traced to a precipitating environmental event, and end abruptly after a short duration. Voluntary musculature and organs of special sense are the most frequent target sites for the "hysterical" expressions of psychologic conflict. Physical examination often fails to reveal a close relationship with a person who exhibited similar symptoms or a recent episode of actual illness.

Hypochondriasis, preoccupation with the fear of having a serious illness, and *somatization disorder,* the use of multiple somatic complaints as a means of assuaging inner tension, are also somatoform disorders. Prevalence studies suggest that 11% of boys and 15% of girls are somatizers.

Psychophysiologic disorders have a more insidious onset than somatoform disorders. Chronic anxiety produces functional abnormalities within the autonomic nervous system that lead the structural changes within organ systems. Eczema, bronchial asthma, ulcerative colitis, and peptic ulcer are considered in some children to be psychophysiologic disorders or at least to have significant psychophysiologic components.

Reflex sympathetic dystrophy presents as chronic painful swelling in an extremity, decreased skin temperature, cyanosis, delayed capillary refilling, and limitation of function. It often follows injury to the involved limb.

CHAPTER 15

Vegetative Disorders

(Nelson Textbook, Chapter 20)

RUMINATION DISORDER

The hallmark of rumination disorder is a weight loss or failure to gain weight at the expected level because of repeated regurgitation of food without nausea or associated gastrointestinal illness. This rare disorder occurs more commonly in males and usually appears between 3 and 14 mo of age. Behavioral treatment is directed toward positively reinforcing correct eating behavior and negatively reinforcing rumination.

PICA

Pica involves repeated or chronic ingestion of non-nutrient substances, which may include plaster, charcoal, clay, wool, ashes, paint, and earth. The age at onset is usually 1–2 yr but may be earlier. Pica usually remits in childhood but can continue into adolescence and adulthood. Children with pica are at an increased risk for lead poisoning, iron-deficiency anemia, and parasitic infections.

ENURESIS (BEDWETTING)

Enuresis is defined as the voluntary or involuntary repeated discharge of urine into clothes or bedding after a developmental age when bladder control should be established. Most children have obtained bladder control during the day and night by age 5 yr. The diagnosis of enuresis is made when urine is voided for at least 3 consecutive months or clinically significant distress occurs in areas of the child's life as a result of the wetting.

CLINICAL MANIFESTATIONS. Bedwetting may be divided into the persistent (primary) type, in which the child has never been dry at night, and the regressive (secondary) type, in which a child who has been continent for at least 1 yr begins to wet the bed again. Primary enuresis represents approximately 90% of all cases. Secondary enuresis most frequently occurs between the age of 5 and 8 yr and is more common in late school-aged children.

TREATMENT. Some general suggestions are as follows:

1. It is important to enlist the cooperation of the child to deal with the problem. Rewarding the child for being dry at night is a useful step.

2. Older children should be expected to launder their own soiled bedclothes and pajamas.

3. The child should void before retiring.

4. Waking the child repeatedly to take him or her to the bathroom is useful in only a few children and may further engender or aggravate anger in the child or parents.

5. Punishment or humiliation of the child by parents or others should be strongly discouraged.

The use of conditioning devices (e.g., an alarm that rings when the child wets a special sheet) is usually not necessary and should be reserved for persistent and refractory cases in which the child's self-esteem has been seriously eroded. Imipramine (Tofranil) at a maximum dosage of 2.5 mg/kg/24 hr before bedtime has shown a success rate of approximately 50%, with a relapse rate of 30%, similar to that of the alarm system.

ENCOPRESIS

Encopresis refers to the passage of feces into inappropriate places after a chronologic age of 4 yr (or equivalent developmental level). Subtypes include encopresis with constipation and overflow incontinence and encopresis without constipation and overflow incontinence.

CLINICAL MANIFESTATIONS. Chronic soiling may persist from infancy onward (primary) or may appear as a regressive (secondary) phenomenon. It is often associated with chronic constipation, fecal impaction, and overflow incontinence (in about two thirds of cases) and may progress to psychogenic megacolon. School performance and attendance may be affected as the child becomes the target of scorn and derision from schoolmates because of the offensive odor.

TREATMENT. Management of encopresis should include educating and assisting the parents on how to re-establish normal toileting. For older children, relieving constipation and removing impactions can lead to significant improvement in about three fourths of cases. The use of mineral oil and a high-fiber diet helps prevent a recurrence of the constipation. Chronic use of enemas and laxatives should be avoided. Biofeedback, which is used to train the anal sphincter muscle, has been helpful. Rewards are offered for nonsoiling, and soiling is met with mild, nonjudgmental consequences. Failure to respond to supportive measures may require psychotherapeutic intervention with the child and family.

SLEEP DISORDERS

A sleep disorder may be characterized by too little or too much sleep than is normal for age; an abnormal type of sleep (e.g., narcolepsy, in which the regulation of sleep and wakefulness is abnormal); abnormal behavior during sleep (e.g., enuresis or sleepwalking); or a pathophysiologic event that occurs during sleep (e.g., obstructive sleep apnea syndrome).

Night-time awakenings are common in infancy. By 1–3 mo of age the longest daily sleep period should be between midnight and early morning. However, by 1 yr of age, 20–30% of infants are still waking at night.

Obstructive sleep apnea syndrome (OSAS) and *upper airway resistance syndrome* (UARS) are breathing-related sleep problems seen in infants, children, and adults. Adenotonsillar hypertrophy is a common cause of OSAS and UARS. Clinical manifestations include loud snoring (often continuous), difficulty breathing, marked paradoxical chest and abdominal motion, and retractions during sleep. Owing to sleep deprivation these patients have daytime sleepiness and performance deficits (e.g., behavioral and learning problems). Polysomnography recording evaluations are important in establishing the diagnosis. Obstructive apnea is defined by lack of (nasal/mouth) air flow despite continuous respiratory effort. Partial UARS is defined by a breathing pattern with diminished air flow, hyperventilation, and hypercarbia (increase in end-tidal and transcutaneous carbon dioxide); transcutaneous oxygen desaturation; and increase in transpleural esophagopharyngeal pressure. Central apnea is defined by no effort or air flow.

Mixed apnea usually starts with a central apnea followed by an obstructive event.

Adenotonsillectomy is effective treatment when adenotonsillar hypertrophy is the cause of OSAS and UARS. Other therapies for functional nonanatomic upper airway obstruction include nasal continuous positive airway pressure (CPAP) and bilevel positive airway pressure (BiPAP) during sleep. Craniofacial anomalies such as Pierre Robin syndrome sequence are characterized by abnormalities that can affect upper airway patency (micrognathia, glossoptosis, and cleft palate).

Gastroesophageal reflux (pH < 4 in the esophagus, 2 cm above the cardiac sphincter level) associated with sleep apnea may respond to prone sleep positioning and elevation of the head of a crib for infants, pharmacologic therapy, or surgery.

Narcolepsy is a disorder characterized by excessive daytime sleepiness, cataplexy, sleep paralysis, hypnagogic hallucinations, school academic and athletic failures, irritability, and emotional liability. Stimulants are used to decrease excessive daytime sleep.

CHAPTER 16

Habit Disorders

(Nelson Textbook, Chapter 21)

Habit disorders include tension-discharging phenomena, such as head banging, body rocking, thumb sucking, nail biting, hair pulling (trichotillomania), teeth grinding (bruxism), hitting or biting part of one's own body, body manipulations, repetitive vocalizations, breath holding, and air swallowing (aerophagia). Tics, which involve the involuntary movement of various muscle groups, are also included. Stuttering is discussed with the habit disorders, although it is not generally regarded as a tension-relieving activity.

All children at various developmental points show repetitive patterns of movement that can be described as habits. Whether they are considered disorders depends on the degree to which they interfere with the child's physical, emotional, or social functioning.

Teeth grinding, or bruxism, seems to result from tension that may originate in unexpressed anger or resentment. It may create problems in dental occlusion. Helping the child to find ways to express concerns may relieve the problem.

Thumb sucking is normal in early infancy. It makes the older child appear immature and may interfere with normal alignment of the teeth. The best strategy for dealing with thumb sucking is to provide the child with evidence of interest in his or her well-being and other forms of satisfaction. Parents should ignore the symptom, if possible, while giving attention to more positive aspects of the child's behavior.

Tics involve repetitive movements of muscle groups and represent discharges of tension originating in emotional and physical states that have no apparent useful function. They can be distinguished from dyskinetic movements and dystonias by their discontinuation during sleep and by virtue of the conscious control that can be achieved for short periods. Undue parental attention can reinforce tics, whereas ignoring them diminishes their occurrence.

Gilles de la Tourette syndrome appears before 7 yr of age in one half of cases. It is characterized by multiple tics, compulsive barking or grunting, or shouting obscene words. It can be fairly well managed with haloperidol (Haldol), a dopamine antagonist, or pimozide (Orap), a more powerful dopamine antagonist.

Primary stuttering usually begins as an atypical development during the learning of speech. It starts gradually, initially with the repetition of consonants, often followed by a repetition of words and phrases. As the child becomes aware of the dysfluency, anxiety and behavioral responses may occur. Most cases resolve spontaneously, although about 20% continue to suffer the disability in adulthood. Approaches to treatment include breath-control exercises and the use of a miniaturized metronome that "paces" the rhythm of speech.

CHAPTER 17

Anxiety Disorders
(Nelson Textbook, Chapter 22)

Anxiety, fearfulness, and worrying are regularly experienced as part of normal development. When they become disattached from specific situations or events or when they become disabling to the point that they negatively affect social interactions and development, they are pathologic and warrant intervention.

The antecedents of developmentally normal anxiety initially present at 7–8 mo of age. As infants begin to differentiate from their primary caregivers they often develop wariness and mood changes that did not exist when they were in the company of strangers. This *stranger reaction* is to be differentiated from *stranger anxiety,* which is a more intense discomfort that includes obvious psychologic and physiologic distress.

Children with *phobias* are anxious only under specific conditions. They try to avoid specific objects or situations that will automatically lead to anxiety. As with other forms of anxiety, phobias become pathologic when they interfere with social, professional, and interpersonal functioning. The parents of phobic children should remain calm in the presence of the child's anxiety or panic. Behavioral therapy is indicated, including systematic desensitization, the process of exposing the patient to the fear-inducing situation or object. Anxiety is managed through relaxation techniques.

School phobia, a syndrome in which a child will not attend school for various reasons, occurs in 1–2% of children. Management of the disorder involves treatment of the underlying psychiatric problems, family therapy, family management training, and liaison work with the child's school.

Separation anxiety disorder is characterized by unrealistic and persistent worries of possible harm befalling primary caregivers, reluctance to go to school or sleep without being near the parents, persistent avoidance of being alone, nightmares involving themes of separation, and numerous somatic symptoms and complaints of subjective distress. Psychiatric therapy is called for when the usual supportive approaches have failed to return the child to school or to reduce the symptoms. Parent training as well as family therapy is often necessary to delineate underlying motivations and to teach appropriate ways to help the child fulfill reasonable expectations regarding school attendance. A large percentage of children with separation anxiety disorder develop feelings of panic when they are coerced to separate from their parents. A judicious use of either antidepressant or antianxiety medicines is often necessary to facilitate treatment goals.

Childhood-onset social phobia is characterized by an excessive fear of contact with unfamiliar people that leads to social isolation. Buspirone, alprazolam, and phenelzine have been shown to be helpful in various types of studies.

Children who suffer from *generalized anxiety disorder* have unrealistic worries about future events, the appropriateness of past behavior, and concerns about competence. They frequently present with somatic complaints, are markedly self-conscious, need large amount of reassurance, and have trouble relaxing.

Many children present with repetitive thoughts that invade consciousness or repetitive rituals or movements that do not obviously contribute to a high level of adaptation in any given situation—an *obsessive-compulsive disorder* (OCD). These behaviors become part of a disorder when they cause distress, consume time, or interfere with accustomed occupational or social functioning. Treatment consists of behavioral therapy and pharmacotherapy. Overexposure of the patient to situations that lead to the symptoms and anxiety is a major therapeutic technique, used especially for rituals. Clomipramine (Anafranil), fluoxetine (Prozac), and fluvoxamine have all shown promise in ameliorating OCD symptoms.

POST-TRAUMATIC STRESS DISORDER (PTSD)

PTSD results from external traumatic events perceived by the child or adolescent as dangerous. Life-threatening situations that produce considerable stress predispose the child to the trauma.

CLINICAL MANIFESTATIONS. PTSD is characterized by recurrent and intrusive recollections and dreams of noxious events in addition to intermittently intense psychologic and physiologic distress in situations that symbolize the original trauma. Individuals with this disorder typically try to avoid stimuli associated with the original trauma. Symptoms and behaviors indicative of this disorder include re-experiencing the trauma through intrusive recollections and dreams and re-enactment through play and other behaviors; psychologic numbing by way of amnesia, isolation, avoidance, and reduced interest in activities; and increased states of arousal, as exemplified by sleep problems, agitated emotions, hypervigilance, extreme startle responses, and difficulty concentrating.

TREATMENT. Initial intervention should be directed toward determining the severity of the trauma, the child's vulnerability to the trauma, and the child's reaction to the trauma. Both early intervention and psychotherapy provide the child with an opportunity to talk about the trauma and express feelings of sadness, rage, and helplessness, among others. Family therapy and school consultations are often helpful. Pharmacotherapy designed to modify arousal behavior can be an important adjunctive treatment.

CHAPTER 18

Mood Disorders

(Nelson Textbook, Chapter 23)

Major depression is characterized by dysphoria and an obvious loss of interest and pleasure in usual activities, but it may also include a significant weight change secondary to decreased or increased food intake, insomnia or hypersomnia, psychomotor agitation or retardation, fatigue or loss of energy almost every day, feelings of worthlessness and excessive guilt, diminished ability to think and concentrate, and recurrent thoughts of death.

MAJOR DEPRESSION

EPIDEMIOLOGY. The prevalence of depression starting in childhood is 0.4–2.5%, and in adolescence it is 0.4–8.3%.

ETIOLOGY. Genetic factors play a role in 50% of mood disorders.

CLINICAL MANIFESTATIONS. Depressive symptoms vary according to age and development level. In the anaclitic depression of infancy, separation from a primary caregiver after 6–7 mo leads to protest (crying, searching, panic-like behavior, and hypermotility of both arms and legs). This is followed by the infant's close scrutiny of each approaching adult, looking for the caregiver. The child turns away from everyone else. The final phase involves apathy in which the infant becomes hypotonic and inactive, exhibiting an obviously sad facial expression. These babies cry silently and stare into space. When picked up, they search again for the familiar face; they cling to strangers and cry but are not consoled.

The clinical picture of depression in children somewhat parallels that of adults, except that children are more likely to present with separation anxiety, phobias, somatic complaints, and behavioral problems. The hallmark of psychotic depression in children is the occurrence of hallucinations; delusions, which require sophisticated cognitive development, are more common in adolescents and adults. Uncomplicated clinical depression in adolescents is similar phenomenologically to depression in adults.

The symptoms of a major depressive episode usually develop over a period of days or weeks. The duration of symptoms is variable. If untreated, symptoms often persist for 7–9 mo; 6–10% of cases are more protracted. Children and adolescents who are depressed are at risk of developing later episodes of depression.

DIAGNOSIS. The Children's Depression Inventory, Children's Depression Scale, Depression Self-Rating Scale, and the Center for Epidemiological Studies Depression Scale for Children have all been shown to be useful in diagnosing depression in children and adolescents. There are no biologic tests specific for depression.

TREATMENT. Fluoxetine (Prozac) is significantly more effective than placebo as an antidepressant medication for children and adolescents. A less favorable response has been found for tricyclic antidepressants. Cognitive behavior therapy (12–16 wk) is effective in about 70% of cases of adolescent depression.

DYSTHYMIC DISORDER

In this disorder, the dysphoria is generally more intermittent than in a major depression, with periods of normal mood lasting several days to several weeks. The dysphoria is less intense but more chronic, lasting up to several years.

ETIOLOGY. Dysthymia may be a partial phenotypic expression of an underlying genetic disorder or a different syndrome that has certain symptom clusters in common with major depression.

CLINICAL MANIFESTATIONS. With the exception of hallucinations and delusions, the symptoms of major depression may be present. Dysthymia frequently is the consequence of a pre-existing chronic condition such as anorexia nervosa, somatization disorder, or anxiety disorder. Patients often present the picture of helpless, passive, clinging, dependent, and lonely children. Others relate in a more hardened, aloof, negativistic manner. Such children frequently experience problems in school achievement and in their relationships with family and peers. They are at risk for the development of conduct disorders or substance abuse. Untreated dysthymic disorder lasts approximately 4 yr and is associated with increased risk for the subsequent development of major depression (70%), bipolar disorder (13%), and substance abuse disorder (15%).

TREATMENT. Antidepressant pharmacotherapy may be useful in the treatment of dysthymic patients. It is especially helpful for those who display vegetative symptoms of depression.

BIPOLAR DISORDER

Bipolar disorder is characterized by either alternating depression and mania (a typical adult presentation) or a rapid cycling of mood, which is more commonly seen in children and young adolescents. Twenty to 40% of adult bipolar patients report that their bipolar symptoms began in childhood.

Clinical manifestations include grandiose thoughts, high activity levels (often at bedtime), pressured speech, distractibility, increased pleasurable activities with high levels of danger, overspending, and extreme irritability and emotionality, among others.

Lithium carbonate has proved to be very effective in the treatment of bipolar illness and manic symptoms. The ideal therapeutic blood level for the initial treatment of acute symptoms is 1.0–1.2 mEq/L, and the recommended level for maintenance therapy is 0.5–0.8 Eq/L. During the acute manic phase, neuroleptic medication may also be required.

CHAPTER 19

Suicide and Attempted Suicide

(Nelson Textbook, Chapters 24 and 110)

Suicide is now the second leading cause of adolescent death. In addition, although few prepubertal children kill themselves, many in this age group consider suicide as a means of handling problems and conflicts.

EPIDEMIOLOGY. Nine to 18% of nonpsychiatrically disturbed preadolescents entertain suicidal ideas, whereas 1.5% actually make suicidal threats. Furthermore, it is estimated that there are 5 to 45 attempts for each completed act. The individual and family variables associated with suicidal ideation are different from those associated with suicide. Factors influencing suicidal thoughts include depression, preoccupation with death, and general psychopathologic factors. Ego functions such as impulsivity, poor reality testing, and ego mechanisms of defense such as projection, regression, and reaction formation are related to suicide attempts. In one third of suicides, a parent, a sibling, or other first-degree relative had previously shown overt suicidal behavior. Marital difficulties and child abuse are more likely in families of adolescent suicide victims. Drug use is a common family problem. Firearms serve as the major method of death in adolescent suicide. Males are more likely than females to use violent methods.

TREATMENT OF THREATS AND ATTEMPTS AT SUICIDE. Threats of suicide should be seen as acts of desperation, and all such threats or attempts should be taken seriously. The physician assessing suicidal behavior of a child or adolescent should carefully explore, in detail, the child's life during the 48–72 hr before either the threat or the suicide attempt. The precipitating events should be identified. The degree of premeditation or impulsivity should be assessed. It is important to understand whether the patient intended to stop or to be discovered and whether the behavior before or subsequent to the attempt promoted or impeded the patient's being discovered before or after the attempt. The physician should judge the margin of error allowed by the patient in terms of the method used or proposed; the closeness or remoteness of available help; whether the patient actually called for help after the attempt, if it was not immediately discovered; and whether the patient calculated correctly whether the family would return in time to discover the attempt. The most significant factor in assessing intent is the possibility and probability of rescue, as foreseen by the child or adolescent.

When the patient is able, the physician should investigate the child's frame of mind; the degree of hopelessness, helplessness, or overwhelming shame or guilt; and the presence or absence of anger (directed toward others or toward oneself). It is important to determine whether the child acted out a psychotic delusion or paranoid ideation or whether the act was the result of hallucinatory experiences that produce intolerable anxiety or panic.

When suicidal patients have been seen in the physician's office, the physician should enter into a nonsuicide contract with the patient. The parents should be notified, and a psychiatric consultation should be obtained. If possible, the patient and family should meet the therapist immediately after the examination by the physician. Suicide attempters who are seen in the emergency department should be admitted to the hospital for 1 day or more so that a more adequate evaluation can be made of the patient's frame of mind and of the circumstances of the family or environment.

CHAPTER 20

Disruptive Behavioral Disorders

(Nelson Textbook, Chapter 25)

Numerous behaviors considered appropriate at certain early developmental levels are obviously pathologic when they present at later ages.

Breath holding is not unusual during the first years of life. It is frequently used by infants and toddlers in an attempt to control their environment and their caregivers. Parents are best advised to ignore the behavior and leave the room in response. Without sufficient reinforcement, the behavior soon disappears.

Defiance, oppositionalism, and *temper tantrums* are often used by children 18 mo to 3 yr of age. In response to tantrums and oppositionalism, parents are advised to acknowledge verbally to the child that the reasons for frustration are understandable but that the particular response is not acceptable. The child should be given time and space to recover. If the child is unable to give up this behavior but instead presents with escalating oppositionalism, the parent should nonemotionally place the child on time-out or a room restriction until he or she is able to adjust more reasonably.

Lying is often used by 2–4 yr olds as a method of playing with the language. By observing the reactions of parents and caregivers, preschoolers learn cognitively and effectively about expectations for honesty in communication. In school-aged children, lying most often represents the child's attempt to avoid the pain of a relative loss of self-esteem. Many adolescents lie because they fear that their parents would disapprove of what they are doing. Chronic lying, however, often occurs in combination with several other antisocial behaviors and is a sign of an underlying psychopathologic condition. Regardless of the age or developmental level, when lying becomes a frequent way of managing conflict and anxiety, intervention is warranted. Initially, the parents should confront the child to give a clear message of what is acceptable. Sensitivity and support are necessary for a successful intervention, because children and adolescents are so developmentally vulnerable to shame and embarrassment.

Almost all children *steal* something at some point in their lives. It becomes a problem when it happens more than once or twice. It is important for parents to help the child undo the theft by returning the stolen articles or by rendering their equivalent either in money that the child can earn or in services.

Unlike the previous behaviors, *truancy* and *run-away* behavior are never developmentally appropriate. Most often, truancy represents disorganization within the home or developing personality problems, or both.

Genetic, social-cultural factors, temperament, some psychiatric conditions, and cognitive limitations can predispose individuals to antisocial acting out. *Aggression* is possibly the most serious of the disorders included in this group. Clinically, it is important to differentiate the causes and motives for childhood aggression. Many hyperactive, clumsy children are called aggressive because of the accidental results of their behavior. There is also a relationship between individual aggression and emotional disturbance, school failure, brain damage, overactivity, and character pathologic conditions. Psychopathologic conditions are also associated with conduct-disordered behavior; attention deficit hyperactivity disorder, depression, bipolar disorder, and borderline personality traits have been correlated with aggression.

The child aged 2–5 yr may show aggressive outbursts ranging from temper tantrums and screaming to hurting others or destroying toys and furniture. Verbal aggression increases between 2 and 4 yr, and after 3 yr of age, revenge and retaliation become more prominent as determinants of aggression. Aggressive behavior in boys is relatively consistent from the preschool period through adolescence; a boy with a high level of aggressive behavior from 3–6 yr of age has a high probability of carrying this behavior into adolescence.

Passive-aggressive behaviors are common in childhood and adolescence. Children with passive-aggressive behavior express hostility indirectly as procrastination, stubbornness, or resistance. Academic underachievement is common. Parents should be encouraged to handle passive-aggressive behavior by setting firm limits and expectations for the child. More refractory cases often require psychiatric intervention.

Conduct disorder is a distinct clinical entity manifested by several different antisocial behaviors: stealing, lying, fire setting, truancy, property destruction, cruelty to animals, rape, use of a weapon while fighting, armed robbery, physical cruelty to others, and repeated attempts to run away from home. A pattern of such behaviors that has existed for at least 6 mo warrants the diagnosis of a conduct disorder. At the very least, *fire setting* requires intervention by the parents but, most often, also intervention by mental health professionals. *Oppositional defiant disorder* is defined by less severe behavior than a conduct disorder: temper tantrums, continuous arguing, defiance of rules, continual blaming of others, angry and resentful affect, spiteful and vindictive behavior, and frequent use of obscene language. Many different approaches have been used in the treatment of children and adolescents with aggressive behavior, conduct disorder, and oppositional disorder. The most effective results have been obtained with parent management training, in which parents are trained directly to promote prosocial behaviors within the home and to place reasonable limits on unwanted, destructive behaviors. Pharmacotherapy is, by and large, not indicated for this problem. Some children present with such severe behavioral problems that residential treatment and psychiatric hospitalization are necessary for a successful outcome.

CHAPTER 21

Sexual Behavior and Its Variations

(Nelson Textbook, Chapter 26)

Gender identity refers to the individual's sense of self as a male or female. *Gender role,* on the other hand, refers to those behaviors within a culture commonly thought to be associated with maleness or femaleness. As the economics of family has changed—and both sexes have become potentially self-sufficient economically—gender roles, as they relate to job choices and performance, have changed dramatically or, in some cases, have simply disappeared.

Children identify themselves as boys or girls by about 18 mo of age (i.e., establish a gender identity). Between 18 and 30 mo of age, children establish *gender stability,* the concept that boys become men and girls become women. By 30 mo, gender constancy, the immutability of one's gender, is firmly established and resistant to change.

Transsexualism, the conviction by a person biologically of one gender that he or she is a member of the other gender, is the most obvious example of gender identity confusion. Transsexual adolescents feel discomfort and a sense of inappropriateness about their assigned sex. Gender roles of the opposite biologic sex are usually adopted. The prevalence of transsexualism is 1/30,000 for males and 1/100,000 for females. A preponderance of adult transsexuals had gender identity disorders as children and adolescents. Extreme femininity in boys is a predisposing factor. Treatment of transsexualism has taken two directions. Many transsexual adults have opted for hormonal and surgical therapies to produce primary and secondary sexual characteristics of the gender with which they identify. Follow-up studies consistently show continued distress after these treatments. Long-term dynamic and behavioral therapies also have been tried. Spontaneous remissions have been shown to occur.

Transvestism, cross-dressing, may occur transiently in preschool boys who dress up in their mother's clothing, or it may occur chronically in preschool-aged and school-aged boys who feel genuinely excited when dressed in women's clothing. Cross-dressing in girls is rarely an identified problem. Chronic cross-dressing might represent underlying transsexualism, although that is generally not the case.

GENDER IDENTITY DISORDER

Ten or more gender-atypical behaviors are exhibited in 22.8% of school-aged boys and 38.6% of girls. Persistent distress about being a particular gender while being preoccupied with cross-gender roles or repudiation of given anatomic genital structures is the hallmark of gender identity disorder. It encompasses transsexualism, transvestism, and effeminacy in boys. The etiology of gender identity disorder is unknown.

CLINICAL MANIFESTATIONS. Many children with gender identity disorder develop it before 4 yr of age. They are often ostracized by peers and have a difficult social adjustment, sometimes with subsequent depression. One half or more of the boys develop a homosexual orientation during adolescence and adulthood. Gender identity disorder is associated with numerous other childhood and adolescent disorders. It is probably not just an early manifestation of homosexuality.

TREATMENT. The relationship between gender identity disorder and separation anxiety disorder and other disturbances supports the importance of psychotherapy and possibly pharmacotherapy if behaviors satisfy criteria for separation anxiety disorder or other axis I disorders.

HOMOSEXUALITY

Homosexuality, the romantic and physical attraction to someone of the same gender, has occurred throughout the ages in about 5% of men and women.

ETIOLOGY. The cause is uncertain.

CLINICAL MANIFESTATIONS AND DIAGNOSIS. If a child is found to be engaging in homosexual behavior, parents should not immediately conclude that it means that the child is already homosexual. Sexual behavior during adolescence does not necessarily predict future sexual orientation. The first task of the physician after discovering that a child has engaged in homosexual activity is to help the younger child feel safe and less guilty. The physician can serve as a model for the parent through his or her own calm, sensitive, careful exploration of feeling and behavior with the child. If an older child is the initiator or seducer, he or she should be told clearly and firmly that such behavior will not be tolerated and that he or she will be expected to act with responsibility and control. The older child should talk with a physician or mental health professional; if concerns about emotional and social adjustment become evident, referral for a psychiatric evaluation is indicated. The physician may need to help the parents of exploited children refrain from ill-considered acts of revenge against the offenders.

TREATMENT. In spite of some anecdotal reports, very little can be done to change one's sexual orientation. Children need help in understanding how to cope with the reactions of others.

CHAPTER 22

Pervasive Developmental Disorders and Childhood Psychosis

(Nelson Textbook, Chapter 27)

AUTISTIC DISORDER

Autism develops before 30 mo of age. It is characterized by a qualitative impairment in verbal and nonverbal communication, in imaginative activity, and in reciprocal social interactions.

CLINICAL MANIFESTATIONS. Among the most noticeable symptoms and signs are nondeveloped or poorly developed verbal and non-verbal communication skills, abnormalities in speech patterns, impaired ability to sustain a conversation, abnormal social play, lack of empathy, and an inability to make friends. Stereotypical body movements, a marked need for sameness, very narrow interests, and a preoccupation with parts of the body are also frequent. The autistic child is withdrawn and often spends hours in solitary play. Ritualistic behavior prevails. Tantrum-like rages may accompany disruption of routine. Eye contact is minimal or absent. Visual scanning of hand and finger movements, mouthing of objects, and rubbing of surfaces may indicate a heightened awareness and sensitivity to some stimuli, whereas diminished responses to pain and lack of startle responses to sudden loud noises reflect lowered sensitivity to other stimuli. If speech is present, echolalia, pronomial reversal, nonsense rhyming, and other idiosyncratic language forms may be predominant.

Intelligence, measured by conventional psychologic testing, usually falls in the functionally retarded range; however, the deficits in language and socialization make it difficult to obtain an accurate estimate of the autistic child's intellectual potential. Deficits in verbal sequencing, abstraction, rote memory, and recip-rocal verbal exchange are typical in autistic children. Autistic children also show deficits in their understanding of what the other person might be feeling or thinking.

EPIDEMIOLOGY. The prevalence is 3–4/10,000 children. The disor-der is much more common in males than in females (3–4:1). Autism can be associated with other neurologic disorders, particu-larly tuberous sclerosis, seizure disorders, and, to a lesser extent, fragile X syndrome.

ETIOLOGY. The cause is unknown.

TREATMENT. Treatment is most successful when geared toward the individual's particular needs. Therapy with the very young often focuses on speech and language, special education, parent education, training and support, and pharmacotherapy for certain target symptoms. Older children and adolescents with relatively high intelligence but with poor social skills and psychiatric symptoms (e.g., depression, anxiety, and obsessive compulsive symptoms) may require psychotherapy, behavioral or cognitive therapy, and pharmacotherapy. Working with families of autistic children is vital to the child's overall care.

PROGNOSIS. The prognosis is guarded.

ASPERGER DISORDER

Children with this disorder have a qualitative impairment in the development of reciprocal social interaction, often demonstrating repetitive behaviors and restricted, obsessional, idiosyncratic interests. They do not, however, have the language impairments that characterize autism.

CHILDHOOD DISINTEGRATIVE DISORDER

This disorder, also known as Heller dementia, is a rare condition of unknown etiology. It is characterized by normal development up to 2–4 yr, followed by severe deterioration of mental and social functioning, with regression to a very impaired "autistic" state. Language, social skills, and imagination are profoundly affected; bowel and bladder control may be lost; and motor stereotypes are often present. The outcome appears to be worse than for autistic disorder.

RETT DISORDER

This is an X-linked dominant disorder affecting girls almost exclusively. Development proceeds normally until approximately 1 yr of age, at which time language and motor development regress and acquired microcephaly becomes apparent. These girls present with midline handwriting and unusual sighing. Autistic behaviors are typical. No specific etiology or treatment has been identified.

CHILDHOOD SCHIZOPHRENIA

In childhood schizophrenia, prominent symptoms include thought disorder, delusions, and hallucinations. The latter two symptoms, in addition to a later onset, higher intelligence scores, and fewer perinatal complications, differentiate schizophrenia from autism. As the symptoms imply, schizophrenic children often appear to be chaotic. They may have paranoid delusions, aggressive behavior, hebephrenic silliness, social withdrawal, and alternating moods not apparently related to environmental stimuli, among other possibilities. Because the typical age at onset in schizophrenia is late adolescence to early adulthood, a very small percentage of preschool and latency-aged children actually show symptoms that meet the criteria for a diagnosis of schizophrenia. The onset of the disorder is usually insidious. Auditory hallucinations are seen in 80% of schizophrenic children. Delusions and formal thought disorders usually do not present until mid adolescence. The prognosis is poor. Parent training is necessary to teach effective techniques to modify a schizophrenic child's behavior to a reasonable extent. Individual therapy designed to build a positive alliance is also very important. Neuroleptic therapy is often effective in managing hallucinations and psychotic delusions. School and community liaison work can establish and maintain a day-to-day schedule for the patient.

CHAPTER 23

Psychologic Treatment of Children and Adolescents

(Nelson Textbook, Chapter 28)

Using drugs to modify children's behavior is controversial. Only clinicians with appropriate training and experience should prescribe antipsychotics, mood stabilizers, and tricyclic antidepressants.

Neuroleptics are appropriately used for hallucinations, delusions, thought disorders, and severe agitation. They are primarily indicated for children and adolescents suffering with schizophrenic disorders, mood-congruent and mood-incongruent psychotic reactions secondary to major affective disorders, autism presenting with stereotypical and withdrawal symptoms and self-abuse, and Gilles de la Tourette syndrome. Serious questions have been raised about the efficacy of neuroleptics in childhood schizophrenia. This class of medicine is inappropriately used for anxiety, conduct disorder without extreme aggression, and attention deficit hyperactivity disorder. Both chlorpromazine and thioridazine are low-potency medicines and usually require a higher dose than the other neuroleptics for symptom remission. Both are rather sedating, producing numerous anticholinergic side effects but causing comparatively fewer extrapyramidal symptoms.

The most worrisome side effect of the neuroleptics is the development of tardive dyskinesia. This is characterized by choreoathetoid movements of the trunk, limbs, and facial musculature; these movements develop in 20–30% of children treated long term with neuroleptics. Dyskinesia can occur during the treatment with the drug or after it has been discontinued, in which case it is referred to as *withdrawal dyskinesia.* This latter type of dyskinesia, the symptoms of which can include nausea, vomiting, diaphoresis, ataxia, oral dyskinesia, and various dystonic movements, is reversible in most cases, whereas the dyskinesia developing during drug use may not be reversible. Treatment of tardive dyskinesia involves decreasing or discontinuing the medication if possible, despite the fact that it has been noted that increasing the neuroleptic causes a temporary diminution of dyskinesia symptoms. *Extrapyramidal symptoms,* a Parkinson-like syndrome (akathisia, bradykinesia, torticollis, drooling, and involuntary hand movements, among others), develop in at least one fourth of children treated with neuroleptics. The high-potency neuroleptics, which contain a few anticholinergic properties, are the most likely to produce extrapyramidal symptoms. This symptom can be treated by decreasing the neuroleptic or adding an anticholinergic agent (trihexyphenidyl HCl [Artane], benztropine mesylate [Cogentin]). *Neuroleptic malignant syndrome,* a rare side effect of neuroleptic use, can be fatal. Its development may be heralded by a high fever and a "lead pipe" stiffness of the extremities. The creatinine phosphokinase level is also markedly elevated. Immediate discontinuation of the medicine and supportive care are necessary during the early part of the syndrome.

Stimulant medications are used to treat the signs and symptoms of attention deficit hyperactivity disorder. These medications increase a child's ability to attend, improve classroom behavior, and increase social acceptance of affected children in various situations. Stimulants should be used concurrently with individual, family, and community therapy, but this often is not done. *Antidepressants* and *mood stabilizers* are useful in the treatment of affective disorders.

Antidepressants generally are effective for depression, whereas lithium, carbamazepine, and valproate have shown efficacy with mania. Before prescribing tricyclics in general and desipramine in particular, clinicians must procure a detailed medical history, including examination of a patient's cardiovascular system and ascertainment of any family history of cardiac disease (including unexplained syncope and sudden death).

Serotonin reuptake blockers, especially fluoxetine (Prozac), sertraline (Zoloft), and paroxetine (Paxil), have been shown to be effective in patients with mild depressive symptoms, anxiety, and compulsions. Clonidine has been partially successful in treating children with attention deficit hyperactivity disorder and in those who have a personal history of tics (including Gilles de la Tourette syndrome).

Carbamazepine, an antiepileptic medicine, is effective in the treatment of mania and episodic and dyscontrol syndrome. Clomipramine (Anafranil) is efficacious in the treatment of obsessive-compulsive disorder. Seizures have been reported secondary to its use, however.

If drugs are used, they should be used for as short a time as possible. Because psychotropic medications have significant biochemical effects on developing children, it is important for physicians to give an appropriate explanation to parents and children about the rationale for medication.

PSYCHOTHERAPY

There are many types of individual psychotherapy. Most involve the development of an alliance with patients that provides an opportunity to look at the problems precipitating therapy. There are also several types of *family therapy. Group therapy* is especially useful for children suffering from poorly developed social skills.

PSYCHIATRIC HOSPITALIZATION

Psychiatric hospitalization of a disturbed or emotionally ill child in a general, pediatric, or psychiatric hospital is at times helpful or necessary, and it may serve a number of functions.

CHAPTER 24

Neurodevelopmental Dysfunction in the School-Aged Child

(Nelson Textbook, Chapter 29)

PATTERNS OF DEVELOPMENT AND FUNCTION

Neurodevelopmental dysfunctions are central nervous system–mediated impairments that are commonly associated with academic underachievement, behavioral difficulties, and problems with social adjustment. It is estimated that 5–15% of schoolchildren harbor these so-called low severity/high prevalence handicaps.

ETIOLOGY. Diverse causes underlie these neurodevelopmental dysfunctions. Some reading and spelling disabilities have genetic causes. Many studies have uncovered etiologic associations between disorders of learning or attention and abnormal chromosome patterns, low-level lead intoxication, recurrent otitis media, meningitis, acquired immunodeficiency syndrome, intraventricular hemorrhage, serious head trauma, and low birth weight. Abnormalities of thyroid function have also been documented in a group of children with attentional dysfunction. Environmental and sociocultural deprivation have also been implicated as etiologic factors, or at least potentiators, of neurodevelopmental dysfunction. In individual cases, a definite cause usually cannot be ascertained.

CLINICAL MANIFESTATIONS. School-aged children with neurodevelopmental dysfunctions vary widely with regard to clinical symptoms. Their specific patterns of academic performance and behavior represent final common pathways, the convergence of many forces, including interacting cognitive strengths and deficits, environmental and cultural factors, temperament, educational experience, and intrinsic resiliency. Consequently, a memory dysfunction has different manifestations in a child with strong language skills, well-controlled attention, and a supportive home environment from those evident in an economically deprived youngster whose memory problems are accompanied by weakness of attention and difficulties with language.

TREATMENT. Treatment of children with neurodevelopmental dysfunctions often needs to be multidisciplinary.

ATTENTION DEFICIT HYPERACTIVITY DISORDER

Attention deficit hyperactivity disorder (ADHD) is characterized by poor ability to attend to a task, motoric overactivity, and impulsivity. Oppositional and aggressive behaviors are often seen in conjunction with ADHD. Tic disorder may coexist with ADHD. Many of these children are also afflicted by special learning disabilities. Appropriate management of ADHD requires careful delineation of all the problems in need of intervention.

ETIOLOGY. The cause of ADHD is unknown. Genetic factors as well as other factors affecting brain development during prenatal and early postnatal life are most likely responsible.

EPIDEMIOLOGY. The prevalence of ADHD depends on the precise definition adopted, the methods used to evaluate children, and more elusive factors that may ultimately be linked to culture. Estimates have ranged from as low as 1% to as high as 20%.

CLINICAL MANIFESTATIONS. ADHD-afflicted children display various behaviors indicative of problems with attention, hyperactivity, and impulsivity. According to the *Diagnostic and Statistical Manual of Mental Disorders*, 4th edition (DSM-IV), *inattentiveness* is manifested when a child (1) often makes careless mistakes, failing to give close attention; (2) often has difficulty sustaining attention; (3) often does not seem to listen; (4) often does not follow through on tasks; (5) often has difficulty getting organized; (6) often dislikes or avoids sustained mental effort; (7) often loses things; (8) often is easily distracted; and (9) often is forgetful. *Hyperactivity* is evidenced when a child (1) often fidgets; (2) often is out of his or her seat; (3) runs and climbs excessively; (4) often has difficulty playing quietly; (5) is always on the go as though driven by a motor; and (6) often talks excessively. *Impulsivity* is reflected in a child who (1) often blurts out answers, (2) often has difficulty awaiting his or her turn, and (3) often interrupts and intrudes on others. Diagnosis of ADHD requires the presence of at least six manifestations from the inattentiveness cluster, six from the hyperactivity/impulsivity cluster, or both.

TREATMENT. The approach most likely to be efficacious encompasses both psychosocial interventions and pharmacotherapy. Medications should be used as only part of a comprehensive treatment plan involving the child, parents, and school. Medication should not be used to compensate for an inadequate educational program or parenting deficits without directing therapeutic effort toward those aspects of the child's environment. Family psychotherapy may be required to help some families overcome interactional problems that hamper the implementation of structure and effective communication in a consistent manner.

Pharmacotherapy is especially effective in suppressing the core symptoms of ADHD. Stimulants, in particular, and various tricyclic antidepressants have been shown to be effective in reducing overactivity and impulsivity and increasing attention span. *Methylphenidate* is the most commonly used stimulant; it is efficacious in 75–80% of patients when administered in a dose ranging from 0.3–1.0 mg/kg. It generally has an effect for 2–4 hr, although the sustained-release form, available only in 20-mg tablets, lasts considerably longer. *Dextroamphetamine* is efficacious in 70–75% of patients. Its optimal dose range is 0.2–0.5 mg/kg. It has a longer half-life than methylphenidate, although the therapeutic effect of amphetamine preparations is reported to be no longer than 4 hr. Stimulant drugs can cause complications such as increased nervousness and jitteriness. Major short-term side effects include anorexia, upper abdominal pain, and difficulty sleeping. The abdominal discomfort usually remits spontaneously. Tics have been reported with stimulant use. *Tricyclic antidepressants* (e.g., imipramine, desipramine) are efficacious in 60–70% of children with ADHD. Unlike stimulants, tricyclic antidepressants have not been found to exacerbate tic disorder or Gilles de la Tourette syndrome.

SPECIFIC READING DISABILITY (DYSLEXIA)

Dyslexia is characterized by an unexpected difficulty in reading in children and adults who otherwise possess the intelligence, motivation, and opportunities to learn considered necessary for accurate and fluent reading.

ETIOLOGY. At a cognitive-linguistic level, dyslexia appears to reflect deficits within a specific component of the language system, the phonologic module, which is engaged in processing the sounds of speech. Dyslexia is both familial and heritable.

EPIDEMIOLOGY. Dyslexia may be the most common neurobehavioral disorder affecting children, with prevalence rates ranging from 5–10% in clinic-and school-identified samples to 17.5% in unselected population-based samples.

CLINICAL MANIFESTATIONS. Difficulties in decoding, word recognition, and reading comprehension may vary according to age and development level. However, the cardinal sign of dyslexia observed in school-aged children and adults is an inaccurate and labored approach to decoding, word recognition, and text reading. Listening comprehension is typically robust. Dyslexia may occur with ADHD.

DIAGNOSIS. Family history, teacher/classroom observation, and tests of language (particularly phonology), reading, spelling, and intellectual ability represent a core assessment for the diagnosis of dyslexia in children. No single test score is pathognomonic for dyslexia.

TREATMENT. No one treatment approach is equally efficacious to all children or adults with dyslexia. All studies point to the application of combined teaching methods that ensure mastery of phonologic skills, the accurate and fluent application of these skills when reading text, and direct instruction in reading comprehensive strategies. Early identification and early intensive intervention are critical to improving reading skills among dyslexic individuals.

PART 4

Social Issues

CHAPTER 25

Adoption
(Nelson Textbook, Chapter 30)

Adoption is a social, emotional, and legal process that creates a family for children when the birth family is unable or unwilling to parent. Approximately 1 million children in this country are adopted; 2–4% of all American families have adopted. In 1992, 127,441 children of all races and nationalities were adopted in the United States. Of these, 42% were stepparent or relative adoptions, 15.5% were children in foster care, and 5% were children from other countries adopted by U.S. families.

Pediatricians can help prospective adoptive parents evaluate the health and development history of the child and available background information from birth families to assess actual and potential problems or risks that children may have. Pediatricians can also promote positive adjustment of other children and the family by providing guidance and support at all stages in the adoption. In international adoptions, in particular, before traveling abroad, parents should try to learn as much as they can about the child's past experience and current condition. After the child is settled in the new home, pediatricians should encourage adoptive parents to seek comprehensive assessment of the child's health and developmental needs.

CHAPTER 26

Foster Care
(Nelson Textbook, Chapter 31)

Approximately 500,000 children in the United States were living in state-supported foster homes in 1995. Chronic underfunding of child welfare programs generally and worsening circumstances for the most disadvantaged segments of society have continued to plague this fragile system.

An increasing proportion of children entering foster care are young (nearly half are younger than 5 yr old at the time of placement) and from minority groups. Children who enter foster care have extraordinarily high rates of medical, developmental, and mental health problems. The majority suffer from behavioral and adjustment problems. Nearly three fourths of these children experience more than one foster home placement during their time in the foster care system. Changes of residences and caretakers may further disrupt the fragile care network, because the children usually change their health care provider with each move.

CHAPTER 27

Child Care
(Nelson Textbook, Chapter 32)

Profound social and demographic changes have resulted in an increasing number of children receiving a portion of their care from someone other than their parents. "Child care" is defined as care provided by an individual outside the nuclear family or in a setting separate from the child's home and is inclusive of such services as baby sitting, day care, preschool, early childhood programs, Head Start, and nursery school. Options for families generally include in-home care, family child care, and center child care. Child care is used for children of all ages.

The effect of child care on children's development depends on a number of interrelated factors, including the quality of the child care experience, as well as characteristics of the child and family. High-quality child care can favorably influence the cognitive and social development of children, especially those from disadvantaged populations. Conversely, poor-quality child care can adversely affect developmental outcomes. Good quality child care has been associated with a low adult-to-child ratio, small group size, and caregiver training in child development. Other important determinants include a caring and supportive staff that is stable and consistent; a developmentally appropriate curriculum that enables children to learn through a variety of fun activities; and a physical setting that affords cleanliness, sanitation, and adequate space for activities and rest as well as protection from environmental hazards.

CHAPTER 28

Separation and Death
(Nelson Textbook, Chapter 33)

Relatively brief separations of children from their parents, such as vacations, usually produce minor transient effects, but more enduring and frequent separations may cause significant sequelae. The potential impact of each event must be considered in light of the age and the stage of development of the child and the particular relationship with the absent person as well as the nature of the separation.

The initial reaction of young children to separation may involve crying, either of a tantrum-like, protesting type or of a quieter, sadder type. After a few hours or a day or so of separation, children may appear more subdued, withdrawn, and quiet or irritable, fussy, moody, and resistant to authority. Disturbance of appetite may occur, and there may be special difficulties at bedtime, such as reluctance about going to bed and problems in getting to sleep, with a resurgence of old fears and, in younger children, perhaps such regressive behavior as bedwetting. A child's response to reunion may surprise or alarm a parent who is not prepared. A parent who joyfully returns to the family may be met by wary or cautious children, who, after a brief interchange of affection, may move away from the parent and seem indifferent to his or her return. Such reactions are usually transient.

Experiences of loss such as divorce or placement in foster care can give rise to the same kinds of reactions listed earlier, but they are more intense and possibly more lasting. School-aged children may respond with evident depression, seem indifferent, or be markedly angry. Other children appear to deny or avoid the issue, behaviorally or verbally. Most children may cling to the hope or fantasy that the actual placement or separation is not real. Guilt may be generated by the child feeling that this loss, separation, or placement represents rejection and perhaps punishment for misbehavior. In response to separation and divorce of parents, older children and adolescents commonly show more intense anger. Almost all children cling to the magical belief that their parents will reunite after divorce.

Another version of separation experience occurs when a child's family moves. Children who move lose their old friends, the comfort of a familiar bedroom and house, and their ties to school and community. Frequent moves during the school years are likely to have adverse consequences on social and academic performance. Parents should prepare children well in advance of any move and allow them to express any unhappy feelings or misgivings. Parents should acknowledge their mixed feelings and agree that they will miss their old home while looking forward to a new one. Visits to the new home in advance are often useful preludes to the actual move.

As to the ultimate separation—death of a parent—most preadolescent children do not seem to go through a typical mourning process as psychoanalytically defined. The major mechanism in dealing with this catastrophe is denial, both overt and unconscious, and maintained by the magical wish and hope for a reunion and reappearance. Some children show hostile and angry feelings toward the surviving parent and tend to identify with and idealize the lost parent, sometimes with reunion fantasies accompanying denial. Children may feel guilty, reflecting their egocentric tendency. Alternatively, some children show considerable sorrow at the time of a parent's death or after a delay, when the defense of denial is longer effective.

Children younger than 5 yr view death as reversible, possibly with belief in the dead coming back to life and in ghosts. In the next stage, up to 8–9 yr, death is personified, for example, the Grim Reaper who punishes and avenges. Only after this age do children realistically understand death as a universal and final biologic process.

Physicians can help children and surviving caretakers through a period of separation or adjustment to death of a parent or sibling, first by helping them recognize that the adults themselves are going through a period of grief and mourning. When a parent dies, the child needs the support and reassurance of having the remaining parent or other important caretakers available. Close physical contact and emotional exchange, with verbal explanations and reassurance for those children who can understand, are important aspects of support. Children should not be expected or forced to discuss all their feelings or to put into words their reactions to a parent's death. Continuance of usual activities should not be interpreted by adults or older children as callousness or indifference but rather as a child's way of dealing, at his or her stage of development, with what is as much a catastrophe for him or her as it is for an adult. In most cases, it seems helpful for children to participate appropriately in the rituals that generally surround the death and burial of a parent.

CHAPTER 29

Impact of Violence on Children
(Nelson Textbook, Chapter 34)

The source of first exposure to violence for children is often *domestic violence*. Occasional wife battering is estimated to exist in 16% of all families, and 3.4% (or 1.8 million women) are beaten regularly by their husbands. Family violence is most likely to be perpetrated by those between ages 18 and 30 yr—"the child-rearing years." One study estimated that 3 million children witness domestic violence every year. In a series of 62 domestic incidents, children were victims in 15% of domestic violence incidents. Witnessing violence is only now being recognized as detrimental to children.

Another source of witnessed violence is *community violence*. Children living in high crime and violent areas observe death more frequently and at younger ages than children growing up in more secure surroundings.

The most ubiquitous source of exposure to violence for children in the United States is television. Many studies confirm that media violence desensitizes children to the meaning and impact of violent behavior.

The violence children experience and witness has a profound impact on health and development. Beyond injuries, violence affects children psychologically and behaviorally; it may influence how they view the world and their place in it. Fear may thwart their exploration of the environment, which is essential to learning in childhood. Children who grow up in violent homes are more likely to be aggressive with their peers. Infants chronically exposed to violence may have difficulties sleeping and exploring their environment. Toddlers may become more "clingy," finding it hard to separate from caregivers. Young and middle-school children may have difficulty concentrating at school and may be easily distracted or hyperactive. Growth may be slowed in infants, toddlers, and young children. Adolescents may become more easily aroused and "develop a short fuse," quickly resorting to violence to solve conflicts. Finally, some children exposed to severe and/or chronic violence may suffer from post-traumatic stress disorder, exhibiting constricted emotions, difficulty concentrating, autonomic disturbances, and re-enactment of the trauma through play or action.

Many parents and children who have been exposed to violence can be effectively counseled by the pediatrician. Matters to be covered include gathering the facts and details of the event; gaining access to support services; providing information about the symptoms and behaviors common in children exposed to violence; and helping parents talk to their children about the event.

CHAPTER 30

Abuse and Neglect of Children
(Nelson Textbook, Chapter 35)

Child maltreatment encompasses a spectrum of abusive actions, or acts of commission, and lack of action, or acts of omission, that result in morbidity or death. Physical abuse may be narrowly defined as intentional injuries to a child by a caregiver that result in bruises, burns, fractures, lacerations, punctures, or organ damage. A broader definition would include short- and long-term emotional consequences, which can be more debilitating than the physical effects. Physical neglect, and other acts of omission, may result in failure to thrive, develop, and learn. Nutritional neglect is the most common cause of underweight in infancy and may account for more than half the cases of failure to thrive. Physicians are most likely to identify medical neglect that results from the failure of a parent to provide appropriate medical care, whereas failure to provide shelter, schooling, adequate clothing, and protection from environmental hazards tends to be observed by neighbors, relatives, teachers, and social workers. Medical neglect of a child with an acute or chronic disease may result in worsening of the condition and death.

Psychologic maltreatment includes intentional verbal or behavioral acts of omission that result in adverse emotional consequences. A caregiver may intentionally fail to provide nurturing verbal and behavioral actions that are necessary for healthy development. Sexual abuse, or involving a child in any act intended for the sexual gratification of an adult, accounts for the major proportion of the continued increase in abuse reports that are made to agencies.

EPIDEMIOLOGY. The number of reports to children's protective services (CPS) and law enforcement agencies in the county in which the alleged abuse or neglect occurred have steadily increased since mandated reporting began in the 1960s. This increase in reports is attributed primarily to improved case finding and reporting. In 1995, 36% (1 million) reports were "substantiated" by CPS. It is estimated that 2000 children die each year of abuse. More than 90% of abusing parents have neither psychotic nor criminal personalities. Rather, they tend to be lonely, unhappy, angry, young, single parents who do not plan their pregnancies, have little or no knowledge of child development, and have unrealistic expectations for child behavior. The occasion precipitating the abuse may be associated with a family crisis, such as a loss of a job or home, marital strife, death of a sibling, physical exhaustion, or development of an acute or chronic physical or mental illness in the parent or child.

CLINICAL MANIFESTATIONS. Physical abuse is suspected when an injury is unexplained, unexplainable, or implausible. If an injury is incompatible with the history given or with the child's development, suspected abuse should be reported. Before reporting suspected medical neglect, the physician should determine whether the parents have an understanding of the disease process and the intellectual, emotional, and physical resources needed to provide for their children. A report of neglect should bring needed services.

Bruises are the most common manifestation of child abuse and may be found on any body surface. Accidental bruises, from impact trauma, are most likely to be found on leading surfaces overlying superficial bone edges, such as the shins, forearms, and brows. Bruises to the buttocks, genitals, back, and back of the hands are less likely to be due to an accident. The shape of the injury may suggest the object used. Bilateral, symmetric, or geometric injuries should raise suspicion of child abuse. Bruises of different colors on the same body surface generally are not compatible with a single event.

Hair that is pulled causes alopecia in which the hairs are broken at various lengths. Infants who are left to lie on their backs may have a flattened occiput with an overlying area of missing hair.

Approximately 10% of cases of physical abuse involve *burns*. The shape or pattern of a burn may be diagnostic when it reflects the pattern of an object or method of injury. Cigarette burns produce circular, punched-out lesions of uniform size. An immersion burn occurs when a child is placed in hot water by accident or as punishment. Extremity immersions result in glove or stocking burn patterns. When a child's body is placed in hot water, the level of burn demarcation is uniform and distinct.

The most common cause of death from physical abuse is *head trauma*. Twenty-nine percent of child abuse reports from a children's hospital recorded injuries to the head, face, or cranial contents. More than 95% of serious intracranial injuries during the 1st yr of life are the result of abuse. Injured infants may present with coma, convulsions, apnea, and increased intracranial pressure.

Intra-abdominal injuries from impacts are the second most common cause of death in battered children. Affected children may present with recurrent vomiting, abdominal distention, absent bowel sounds, localized tenderness, or shock.

LABORATORY DATA. Screening tests should be performed in all cases of bruising to rule out a bleeding diathesis. When physical abuse is suggested in a child younger than 2 yr, a *radiographic bone survey* consisting of multiple views of the skull, thorax, long bones, hands, feet, pelvis, and spine is necessary. These films should be repeated in 7–10 days to reveal healing of fractures not seen on the initial films. For verbal children older than 4–5 yr, radiographs may only need to be obtained if there is bone tenderness or a limited range of motion on physical examination. If films of a tender site are initially negative, they should be repeated in 7–10 days to detect any calcification, subperiosteal bleeding, or nondisplaced epiphyseal separations that were initially undetected. Bone trauma is found in 10–20% of physically abused children.

DIAGNOSIS. Suspicion of physical abuse or neglect is usually based on a history that is not in keeping with physical findings of the child's developmental stage. An analysis of the circumstance of the injury is critical.

After separation from caretakers, a child older than age 3 yr may be able to tell a sensitive and skillful interviewer that a particular adult hurt him or her. However, verbal children may not give a history of intentional injury if they are concerned about retribution from the perpetrator or separation from their home, school, siblings, friends, or a nonoffending parent.

TREATMENT. Appropriate medical, surgical, and psychiatric treatment should be promptly initiated. The law requires that a child *suspected* of being abused or neglected be reported immediately to CPS. Children with suspected abuse should not be discharged from the clinic or office without first consulting the county CPS agency.

Hospital admission is indicated for children (1) whose medical or surgical condition requires inpatient management; (2) in whom the diagnosis is unclear; and (3) when no alternative safe place for custody is immediately available. If the safety of the child is in doubt, the physician, agency, and court should err on the side of protecting the child. If the parents refuse hospitalization or treatment, an emergency court order must be obtained.

Professionals should expect anger from abusing or neglectful parents; however, expressing anger toward them damages rapport, increases defensiveness, and makes their cooperation less likely. Hospitals caring for children should have a team of professionals who are trained and skilled in child abuse recognition, reporting, and services. Child welfare agencies are responsible for developing and monitoring a case plan for the child and family. The pediatrician should continue to coordinate the health care of the abused child.

PREVENTION. The pediatrician's role in primary abuse prevention includes identifying parents at high risk for being unable to accept, love, or properly discipline and care for their offspring. Parental risks include a history of family violence or child abuse, drug addiction, depression, lack of support, socioeconomic problems, serious psychiatric illness, mental retardation, young parental age, closely spaced pregnancies, single-parent status of the mother, negative parental comments about the newborn, lack of evidence of maternal attachment, infrequent visits to a new infant whose discharge is delayed because of prematurity or illness, inappropriate anger toward or spanking of an infant younger than 18 mo or a handicapped child, and neglect of infant hygiene. Child risks include mental or physical handicap, chronic illness, prematurity, being a twin, and learning or behavior problems. Abuse and serious neglect may be prevented when at-risk families receive intensive training and support during pregnancy and after delivery.

PROGNOSIS. Early studies of abused children returned to their parents without any intervention indicated that about 5% were killed and that 25% were seriously reinjured. With comprehensive, intensive family treatment, 80–90% of families involved in child maltreatment may be rehabilitated to provide adequate care for their children.

SEXUAL ABUSE

Sexual abuse includes any activity with a child, before the age of legal consent, that is for the sexual gratification of an adult or significantly older child. Sexual abuse includes oral-genital, genital-rectal, hand-genital, hand-rectal, or hand-breast contact; exposure of sexual anatomy; forced viewing of sexual anatomy; and showing pornography to a child or using a child in the production of pornography. Sexual mistreatment by family members (incest) and nonrelatives known to the child is the most common type of sexual abuse. The least common offender is a stranger.

EPIDEMIOLOGY. Most of the increase in child abuse reports is due to increased reporting of sexual abuse. In 1995, 13% of confirmed reports were of sexual abuse. Surveys of adult women indicate that from 12–38% were sexually abused by 18 yr of age. Reported offenders are 97% male. Females are more often perpetrators in child care settings, including baby sitting.

CLINICAL MANIFESTATIONS. A child may disclose sexual abuse to the mother and be brought to the physician at that time. If the mother does not believe the child, the child may delay further comment indefinitely or later tell a friend, relative, friend's mother, teacher, or school counselor. Children, given the opportunity, may disclose their abuse to a physician in a private interview or during physical examination. The possibility of sexual abuse should be considered as the result of associated physical symptoms, including (1) vaginal, penile, or rectal pain, discharge, or bleeding; (2) chronic dysuria, enuresis, constipation, or encopresis; and (3) rarely, premature puberty in a female. Behaviors more likely to be associated with sexual abuse include sexualized activity with peers, animals, or objects; seductive behavior; and age-inappropriate sexual knowledge and curiosity.

Investigating the possibility of sexual abuse requires supportive, sensitive, and detailed *history taking.* Because of variance in the type of abuse, the ages of the victim and perpetrator, and the time since abuse, less than 15% of cases yield physical or laboratory findings. Ideally, the videotaped forensic interview, which uses open-ended, nonleading questions, should be conducted by one or two experienced interviewers in the presence of law enforcement and social service workers who observe behind a one-way mirror.

A thorough *physical examination* should be conducted, with special attention to the neck and mouth. If present, bite marks should be measured, and wax impressions and wiping for saliva should be done to aid in identification of the perpetrator. The abdominal examination should assess the possibility of pregnancy.

The mouth should be examined for redness, abrasions, or purpura that may be due to recent trauma. The rectum should be examined for signs of trauma and laxity. The external genitalia should be examined for signs of trauma and discharge with the aid of a colposcope or strong light and magnifier. Drawings of trauma should be supplemented with photographs or video recordings using the colposcope or photographs from a hand-held 35-mm camera and macro lens.

LABORATORY DATA. Laboratory investigation depends on the history and the time from the injury. The body of a victim seen within 72 hr of sexual abuse should be examined under a Wood lamp for ejaculatory evidence. In addition, specimens of possible offender blood and hair and the victim's nail clippings and clothing should be collected. If there is a history of contact with the perpetrator's genitalia, gonorrhea and *Chlamydia* cultures should be obtained from the mouth, anus, and genitalia. In the vagina, motile sperm can be found for 6 hr; nonmotile sperm exist for longer than 72 hours.

DIAGNOSIS. It is most common for the diagnosis of sexual abuse to depend on the history offered by the victim. False accusations are rare except in unusual cases involving adolescents, emotionally disturbed patients, or patients in custody disputes. The physical or laboratory examination may corroborate a child's history, but normal physical and laboratory examination findings are compatible with sexual abuse. Laboratory findings of pregnancy, sperm, semen, and nonpregnancy- or delivery-related syphilis, gonorrhea, *Chlamydia*, herpesvirus type 2 (genital), and human immunodeficiency virus may be considered diagnostic of sexual abuse and reported.

TREATMENT. Sexual abuse is a criminal offense and is investigated by the police. All victims of sexual abuse require psychologic support. The consequences and appropriate therapy of sexual abuse vary, depending on the type of abuse, the age and other physical and emotional factors of the victim, the frequency of abuse, and the identity of the abuser. Medication to prevent pregnancy may be given to postmenarchal girls in mid cycle who have experienced vaginal intercourse within the previous 72 hr. Treatment with antibiotics is initiated to prevent sexually transmitted diseases if the perpetrator is known to be infected, if the victim has signs of infection, or if the likelihood of follow-up is poor.

PREVENTION. The primary prevention of sexual abuse is related, in part, to normal developmental education and sexual behavior. Teaching children the proper names of all body parts, including the names, function, and significance of "private parts" (nipples, genitalia, and rectum) should begin in the home and pediatrician's office and continue in school. Children should be taught to say "no" to inappropriate touches to these areas by anyone and to report to a trusted adult any actions that make them uncomfortable. Caregivers, including baby sitters and their companions, should be carefully screened by parents and agencies.

PROGNOSIS. With early and adequate intervention, victims may lead normal adult lives. However, even with intervention, certain adolescent victims may run away from home and fall prey to adolescent prostitution, violence, drug addiction, and unprepared parenthood. Others who remain at home may manifest a variety of emotional problems.

MUNCHAUSEN SYNDROME BY PROXY

In Munchausen syndrome by proxy, a parent, invariably the mother, simulates or causes disease in a child. The parent may (1) fabricate a medical history; (2) cause symptoms by repeatedly exposing the child to a toxin, medication, infectious agent, or physical trauma; or (3) alter laboratory samples or temperature measurements. The syndrome is inflicted on children who are either unable to or unwilling to identify the true offense and offender.

CLINICAL MANIFESTATIONS. The child's symptoms, their pattern, or the response to treatment may not be compatible with a recognized disease. They may involve any organ system and suggest a panoply of disease processes. Although generally reported in preverbal children, cases have been recognized in children up to 16 yr of age. There may be an associated actual disease. Symptoms are always associated with the proximity of the mother to the child. The mother may have a background in health care. She may have a history of Munchausen syndrome and seem relatively unconcerned about the child's illness.

Apnea and seizures, two common manifestations, the observation of which may be falsified, may also be created by partial suffocation. Symptoms created by toxins, medications, water, and salts require familiarity with those substances available to families and the wide array of consequences from misuse of these substances. The clinical pattern is variable, depending on the agent.

DIAGNOSIS. Investigations should be based on a high index of suspicion of this diagnosis so that unpleasant, dangerous, or unnecessary tests are not undertaken on the child. Specimens should be analyzed for potentially harmful agents and for "foreign" blood. Hospitalized children should be under constant surveillance.

TREATMENT. After all laboratory information is collected and the diagnosis is established, the offending parent should be confronted by a nonaccusatory physician and staff who offer help. All cases should be reported promptly and with careful documentation to the CPS.

PART 5

Children with Special Health Needs

CHAPTER 31

Failure to Thrive

(Nelson Textbook, Chapter 36)

Failure to thrive (FTT) is diagnosed in an infant or child whose physical growth is significantly less than that of his or her peers. It often is associated with poor developmental and socioemotional functioning. FTT usually refers to growth below the 3rd or 5th percentile or a change in growth that has crossed two major growth percentiles. Organic FTT is marked by an underlying medical condition; nonorganic or psychosocial FTT occurs in a child who is usually younger than age 5 yr and has no known medical condition that causes poor growth.

EPIDEMIOLOGY AND ETIOLOGY. From 5–10% of low-birth-weight children and children living in poverty may have FTT. Family discord, neonatal problems other than low birth weight, and maternal depression are also associated with FTT. The causes of FTT are numerous (Table 31–1). Psychosocial FTT is most often due to poverty or poor child-parent interaction. It occasionally occurs with severe stress such as child abuse. Organic and nonorganic etiologic factors may also occur together.

CLINICAL MANIFESTATIONS. The clinical presentation of FTT ranges from failure to meet expected age norms for height and weight to alopecia, loss of subcutaneous fat, reduced muscle mass, dermatitis, recurrent infections, marasmus, and kwashiorkor. In developed countries, the most common presentation is poor growth detected in an ambulatory setting; in developing countries, recurrent infections, marasmus, and kwashiorkor are more common presentations.

The degree of FTT is usually measured by calculating each growth parameter (weight, height, and weight/height ratio) as a percentage of the median value for age based on appropriate growth charts. Appropriate growth charts are often not available for children with specific medical problems; serial measurements are especially important for these children. For premature infants, correction must be made for the extent of prematurity. For weight, mild, moderate, and severe FTT is equivalent to 75–90%, 60–74%, and less than 60% of standard, respectively. For height, the corresponding values are 90–95%, 85–89%, and less than

TABLE 31–1 Major Organic Causes of Failure to Thrive

System	Cause
Gastrointestinal	Gastroesophageal reflux, celiac disease, pyloric stenosis, cleft palate/cleft lip, lactose intolerance, Hirschsprung disease, milk protein intolerance, hepatitis, cirrhosis, pancreatic insufficiency, biliary disease, inflammatory bowel disease, malabsorption
Renal	Urinary tract infection, renal tubular acidosis, diabetes insipidus, chronic renal insufficiency
Cardiopulmonary	Cardiac diseases leading to congestive heart failure, asthma, bronchopulmonary dysplasia, cystic fibrosis, anatomic abnormalities of the upper airway, obstructive sleep apnea
Endocrine	Hypothyroidism, diabetes mellitus, adrenal insufficiency or excess, parathyroid disorders, pituitary disorders, growth hormone deficiency
Neurologic	Mental retardation, cerebral hemorrhages, degenerative disorders
Infectious	Parasitic or bacterial infections of the gastrointestinal tract, tuberculosis, human immunodeficiency virus disease
Metabolic	Inborn errors of metabolism
Congenital	Chromosomal abnormalities, congenital syndromes (fetal alcohol syndrome), perinatal infections
Miscellaneous	Lead poisoning, malignancy, collagen vascular disease, recurrently infected adenoids and tonsils

85%. The laboratory evaluation for children with FTT is often not helpful and, therefore, should be done judiciously.

DIAGNOSIS. The history, physical examination, and observation of the parent-child interaction usually suggest the diagnosis. The latter observation, especially with feeding, is often critical to the diagnosis of psychosocial FTT. The causes of insufficient growth include (1) failure of a parent to offer adequate calories, (2) failure of the child to take sufficient calories, and (3) failure of the child to retain sufficient calories. With young infants, it is particularly important to obtain a detailed dietary history, including what the diet consists of, how often the infant is fed, and how the parents respond when the child cries or sleeps for prolonged periods.

TREATMENT. Regardless of cause, an appropriate feeding atmosphere at home is important. Children with severe malnutrition must be re-fed carefully. For children with organic FTT, the underlying medical condition should be treated. For older infants and young children with psychosocial FTT, mealtimes should be 20–30 min, solid foods should be offered before liquids, environmental distractions should be minimized, and children should eat with other people and not be force fed. The intake of water, juice, and low-calorie beverages should be limited. High-calorie foods, such as peanut butter, whole milk, cheese, and dried fruits, should be emphasized. High-calorie supplementation, such as Polycose, or high-calorie liquids, such as Carnation Instant Breakfast with whole milk, or formulas containing more than 20 calories per ounce are sometimes necessary. Weight gain in response to adequate caloric feedings usually establishes the diagnosis of psychosocial FTT. Indications for hospitalization include severe malnutrition, need for further diagnostic and laboratory evaluation, lack of catch-up growth, and evaluation of parent-child feeding interaction. The goals of hospitalization are to obtain sustained catch-up growth and educate parents about appropriate foods and feeding styles.

PROGNOSIS. FTT in the 1st yr of life, regardless of cause, is particularly ominous. Approximately one third of children with psychosocial FTT are developmentally delayed and have social and emotional problems. The prognosis for children with organic FTT is more variable, depending on the specific diagnosis and severity of FTT.

CHAPTER 32

Developmental Disabilities and Chronic Illness: An Overview
(Nelson Textbook, Chapter 37)

Children with special health care needs constitute a heterogeneous population that includes youngsters with a wide variety of developmental disabilities and chronic illness. Fifteen to 18% of children and adolescents have some form of chronic condition, including physical conditions, developmental disabilities, disorders of learning, and primary mental health conditions. Adding speech defects, visual and hearing impairments, repeated ear infections, skin allergies, and other common conditions raises the prevalence to over 30%. Six to 7% of all children and adolescents have some limitation of activity due to a chronic health condition. Within these groups, approximately 40% of children have disorders of development and learning; 35%, chronic physical conditions; and 25%, chronic mental health conditions. Early detection of persistent conditions, amelioration of the functional consequences of specific disabilities, and prevention of secondary psychosocial handicaps are central to the provision of care for children with special health needs.

CHRONIC ILLNESS IN CHILDHOOD

EPIDEMIOLOGY, SEVERITY, AND OUTCOME. The epidemiology of chronic illness in childhood differs in important ways from that of long-term illness in adults. Children face a wide variety of

TABLE 32–1 Estimated Prevalence of Representative Childhood Chronic Conditions, Ages Birth–20, United States

Chronic Conditions	Rates/1000
Asthma (moderate and severe)	15.00
Congenital heart disease	10.00
Seizure disorder	3.00
Arthritis	3.00
Diabetes mellitus	1.40
Cleft lip/palate	1.40
Sickle cell anemia	1.20
Down syndrome	1.00
Cystic fibrosis	0.20
Hemophilia	0.15
Acute lymphocytic leukemia	0.11
Muscular dystrophy	0.06

Adapted from Gortmaker SL, Sappenfield W: Chronic childhood disorders: Prevalence and impact. Pediatr Clin North Am 31:3, 1984; and Newacheck PW, Taylor WR: Childhood chronic illness: Prevalence, severity, and impact. Am J Public Health 82:364, 1992.

mainly quite rare diseases. Only two groups of chronic physical conditions in childhood are common: allergic disorders (mainly asthma, eczema, and hay fever) and neurologic disorders (mainly seizure disorders and neuromuscular conditions such as cerebral palsy). Table 32–1 indicates prevalence rates for representative childhood conditions.

The aggregate number of children with all types of chronic health conditions is high, despite the rarity of individual conditions, mainly because the number of different conditions that affect children is very large. The percentage of children with severe, long-term illnesses has more than doubled in the past 2 decades. This change reflects major advances in the technology of medical and surgical care and marked improvements in survival more than increased incidence of chronic conditions.

ISSUES COMMON TO DIVERSE CHRONIC CONDITIONS. Families of children with a variety of long-term illnesses face several issues in common, reflecting chronicity itself rather than aspects of the specific disease. Many chronic childhood illnesses are high-cost health conditions. The daily burden of care rests with the families, and that burden can be extensive. Children with long-term health conditions frequently have multiple providers and multiple treatments. The comparative rarity of most childhood chronic conditions makes families feel isolated. Many of these conditions are unpredictable in their implications, longevity, complications, and developmental impact on the child. Chronic illness has a pervasive influence on a child's daily life. Finally, a chronic illness creates additional stress and demands on families and on children that apparently healthy children do not face.

DEVELOPMENTAL ASPECTS OF LONG-TERM ILLNESS. Two issues are central to an understanding of the developmental implications of long-term childhood illness: the development of children's understanding of illness mechanisms and the impact of illness at different stages of child development.

MENTAL RETARDATION

Mental retardation is characterized by limitations in performance that result from significant impairments in measured intelligence and adaptive behavior. It also confers a social status that can be more handicapping than the specific disability itself. The pediatric identification evaluation and care of children with cognitive difficulties and their families require a considerable level of both technical sophistication and interpersonal sensitivity. Categories of mild, moderate, severe, and profound retardation have been replaced by a classification system that specifies four levels of support systems needed for daily functioning (i.e., intermittent, limited, extensive, and pervasive).

ETIOLOGY AND PATHOGENESIS. The neurobiologic roots of mental retardation may be found among such diverse factors as structural malformations of the brain, metabolic abnormalities, and central nervous system deficits related to infection, malnutrition, or hypoxic/ischemic injury. The environmental precursors of retardation may be identified in histories of impaired caregiving related to parental psychopathology, extreme family disorganization, or economic hardship.

EPIDEMIOLOGY. Approximately 3% of the general population has an IQ less than 2 standard deviations below the mean. It has been estimated that 80–90% of persons with mental retardation function within the mild range, whereas only 5% of the population with mental retardation is severely to profoundly impaired.

CLINICAL MANIFESTATIONS. Children with physical findings suggestive of recognizable syndromes that are associated with mental retardation should be identified at birth or during early infancy. These disorders, however, represent a small percentage of the population of youngsters with intellectual impairment. The overwhelming majority are identified because of their failure to meet age-appropriate expectations.

Delayed achievement of developmental milestones is the cardinal symptom of mental retardation. The natural history of mental retardation is highly variable and influenced by the availability of appropriate educational and therapeutic experiences as well by neuromaturation and the presence of associated disabilities. Although many youngsters may experience transient "plateau periods" during which measurable progress appears to be minimal, most individuals with mental retardation acquire new skills and continue to learn throughout their lifetimes. In general, children within the relatively mild range of retardation who receive appropriate education can achieve 4th to 6th grade reading levels and may be able to function relatively independently as adults. Individuals with more significant intellectual limitations require greater degrees of supervision, depending on their range of adaptive abilities. A thorough pediatric history is essential to identify relevant contributing factors as well as to document the evolving pattern of the child's developmental skills over time. The product of the history should be a comprehensive inventory of risk factors that increase the likelihood of developmental impairment as well as protective factors that may contribute to more adaptive functioning. A systematic physical examination may reveal findings that help explain the etiology of the child's disability or that identify particular treatment needs.

DIAGNOSIS. The primary care pediatrician is strategically situated to identify young children with possible mental retardation through routine developmental surveillance in the context of general pediatric care. Parental reports of a child's typical skills and behaviors in conjunction with in-office screening procedures are important complementary sources of information. For young children involved in a program outside the home the impressions of the caregiver or teacher are most valuable.

Ultimately, the diagnosis of mental retardation requires confirmation of significantly subaverage general intellectual functioning (i.e., an IQ standard score of 70–75 or below) in association with deficits in two or more of the following 10 adaptive skill areas: communication, self-care, home living, social skills, community use, self-direction, health and safety, functional academics, leisure, and work. A range of laboratory studies must be considered in the medical evaluation of a youngster with retardation. A comprehensive history, physical examination, and laboratory evaluation often lead to identification of specific factors that contribute to the phenomenon of mental retardation. More commonly, however, the results of the medical evaluation are nonspecific and inconclusive.

TREATMENT. Management of a child with mental retardation is multidimensional and highly individualized. One of the critical and most demanding roles played by the physician involves the initial synthesis and presentation of diagnostic findings to the family. Specialized education and therapeutic services are central elements in the multidisciplinary care of children with mental retardation. During the adolescent years, issues related to sexuality, vocational training, and community living become more prominent.

PREVENTION. Although most pathogenetic mechanisms remain unknown, an increasing number of disorders can be detected through prenatal diagnostic studies such as ultrasonography, amniocentesis, or chorionic villus biopsy. The provision of complete information and sensitive medical management are therefore essential to ensure informed family decisions about all available prenatal intervention options.

CHAPTER 33

Pediatric Palliative Care: The Care of Children with Life-Limiting Illness
(Nelson Textbook, Chapter 38)

The care of the dying child represents a personal and professional challenge to the physician that is never easy, but it also represents a unique and privileged opportunity to guide, comfort, and lay the groundwork for true healing to occur.

SCOPE OF THE PROBLEM: A DIVERSITY OF NEEDS. There are smaller numbers of dying children compared with adults. This means that even professionals specializing in the care of children may only rarely encounter the death of a child.

COMMUNICATION ISSUES AND ANTICIPATORY GUIDANCE. A child's perception of death depends on his or her concepts of universality (the recognition that all things inevitably die), irreversibility (the ability to understand that dead people cannot come back to life), nonfunctionality (the understanding that being dead means that all biologic functions cease with death), and causality (the ability to understand the objective causes of death). Children up to 6 yr of age have difficulty with the concepts of irreversibility and nonfunctionality. Children 6–8 yr old begin to understand that not only do others die but they, too, will die, and they begin to acknowledge the concepts of irreversibility and nonfunctionality. The last concept to become clear is causality.

It is also important to recognize that a child's expressed questions may have different levels of meaning. Many children find nonverbal expression much easier; art, play therapy, and storytelling may bring out more than direct conversation does.

Siblings are at special risk both during the course of the illness and after death. Because of the stress on parents to meet the needs of their ill child, siblings may feel that their needs are not being acknowledged.

Parents may blame themselves for their child's illness and may spend considerable energy and resources looking for "miracle cures." The physician should be sensitive to these concerns and realize that parents need an effective listener who is engaged and attentive. Anticipatory guidance involves exploring a variety of options and formulating a care plan. Parents need to know about the availability of home care, respite services, educational books and videotapes, and support groups. It is important to discuss how parents envision their child's death and to address myths surrounding pain control and the benefit of involving siblings.

In communications with the child and family the physician should avoid giving estimates of survival length, even when explicitly asked for. Decision-making should remain focused on the goals of therapy, rather than on specific limitations of care.

SYMPTOM MANAGEMENT. *Pain control* is of paramount importance in reducing the suffering of the child, family, and caregivers. It is important to form and initiate a pain treatment plan even without a confirmed diagnosis. *Respiratory symptoms* such as dyspnea are common, and many children with chronic life-threatening diseases have symptomatic airway secretions. Excessive secretions and salivation due to poor swallowing may be treated with oral glycopyrrolate. Dyspnea can be relieved with the use of opioids, and oxygen may be helpful in certain cases to relieve hypoxemia-related headaches.

Neurologic symptoms include seizures that are often part of the antecedent illness but that may increase in frequency and severity toward the end of life. Anticonvulsants should be administered, and parents can be taught to use rectal diazepam at home.

Feeding and hydration issues raise ethical questions that include the use of nasogastric and gastrostomy feeding for the child who can no longer feed by mouth. These complex issues require evaluating the risks and benefits of artificial feedings, taking into consideration the child's functional level and prognosis.

Nausea demands prompt treatment after a search for common causes (drug effects, constipation, primary disease, metabolic disturbance). Drugs such as metoclopramide, phenothiazines, ondansetron, and corticosteroids may be used depending on the etiology and desired secondary effects.

Constipation is common, and the first step is to assess stool frequency and quantity. Children on regular opioids should routinely be placed on stool softeners (docusate) and may also need the addition of laxative agents (senna derivatives, lactulose).

Skin care issues include the prevention of problems such as bedsores by the early use of inexpensive egg-crate type foam mattresses and careful attention to turning the child. Pruritus may be secondary to systemic disorders or drug therapy. Treatment includes avoiding excessive use of soap, using moisturizers, trimming fingernails, and wearing loose-fitting clothing, in addition to administering topical or systemic corticosteroids. Oral antihistamines and other specific therapies may also be indicated.

THE TERMINAL PHASE. As death approaches, the major task of the physician is to help prepare the child and family for expected problems and issues. If the child is cared for at home, arrangements must be made to manage new symptoms as they occur (terminal airway secretions, seizures, irritability, myoclonus, vomiting). Legal issues such as who will perform the declaration of death may be addressed, and the necessary documents can be partially filled out and left in a sealed envelope in the child's home. In the hospital, the care plan should be clear to all involved professionals and should include an understanding of the specific needs and requests of the child and family.

For the family, the moment of death is an event that is recalled in detail for years to come. After death, they should be given the option of remaining with their child for as long as they need to.

CHAPTER 34

Children at Special Risk
(Nelson Textbook, Chapter 39)

CHILDREN IN POVERTY

Poverty and economic loss diminish the capacity of parents to be supportive, consistent, and involved with their children. Children who are poor have higher than average rates of death and illness from almost all causes. Although physicians cannot cure poverty, they have a obligation to ask parents about their economic resources, adverse changes in their financial situation, and the family's attempts to cope. Encouraging concrete methods of coping, suggesting ways to reduce stressful social circumstances while increasing social networks that are supportive, and referring patients and their families to appropriate welfare, job training, and family agencies can significantly improve the health and functioning of children at risk when their families live in poverty.

NATIVE AMERICANS, INCLUDING ALASKAN ESKIMOS AND ALEUTS

The unemployment and poverty levels of Native Americans are, respectively, three-fold and four-fold that of the white population, and far fewer Native Americans graduate from high school or go on to college. Deaths during the 1st yr of life due to sudden infant death syndrome, pneumonia, and influenza are higher than the average in the United States. Accidental death among Native Americans occurs at twice the rate for other U.S. populations. During adolescence and young adulthood, suicide and homicide are the second and third causes of death in this population and occur at about twice the rates of the rest of the population. As many as three fourths of these children have recurrent otitis media and high rates of hearing loss. This results in learning problems for many children. Psychosocial problems are more prevalent in these populations than in the general population and include depression, alcoholism, drug abuse, out-of-wedlock teenage pregnancy, school failure and dropout, and child abuse and neglect.

CHILDREN OF MIGRANT FARM WORKERS

Many children travel with their parents in the migrant seasons. The circumstances of migrants often include poor housing and frequent moves. Children often go without schooling because of the moves, and medical care is usually limited. The medical problems of children of migrant farm workers are similar to those of children of homeless families: increased frequency of infections (including human immunodeficiency virus and acquired immunodeficiency syndrome), trauma, poor nutrition, poor dental care, low immunization rates, exposure to toxic chemicals, anemia, and developmental delays.

CHILDREN OF IMMIGRANTS

Families of different origins obviously bring different health problems and different cultural backgrounds, which influence health practices and use of medical care and need to be understood to provide appropriate services. Children from Southeast Asia and South America have growth patterns that are generally below the norms established for children of Western European origin, and high rates of hepatitis, parasitic diseases, and nutritional deficiencies are prevalent, as well as high degrees of psychosocial stress. The high prevalence of hepatitis among women from Southeast Asia makes use of hepatitis B vaccine necessary for newborns in this group.

HOMELESS CHILDREN

Families with children are the fastest growing segment of the homeless population (36–38%), with an estimated 100,000 children living in shelters on a given night and about 500,000 homeless each year. In addition, an unknown number of thrown-away and runaway children and adolescents are homeless, living in shelters, on the streets, and elsewhere. Homeless children have an increased frequency of illness, including intestinal infections, anemia, neurologic disorders, seizures, behavior disorders, mental illness, and dental problems, as well as increased frequency of trauma and substance abuse. Homeless children are admitted to hospitals at a much higher rate than the national average. They have higher school failure rates, and the likelihood of their being victims of abuse and neglect is much higher. Because families tend to break apart under the strain of poverty and homelessness, many homeless children end up in foster care.

RUNAWAY AND THROWN-AWAY CHILDREN

The number of runaway and thrown-away children and youths in 1988 (the most recent national survey) was 577,800, and at least 192,700 of these children had no secure and safe place to stay. Teenagers make up most of both groups. The usual definition of a runaway is a youth younger than 18 yr who is gone for at least one night from his or her home without parental permission. Most runaways leave home only once, stay overnight with friends, and have no contact with the police or other agencies. This group is no different from their "healthy" peers in psychologic status. A smaller but unknown number become multiple or permanent "runners" and are significantly different from the one-time runners.

The same constellation of causes common to many of the other special-risk groups is characteristic of permanent runaways. The causes include environmental problems (family dysfunction, abuse, poverty), as well as personal problems of the young person (poor impulse control, psychopathology, substance abuse, or school failure). Thrown-aways experienced more violence and conflicts within their families.

The minority of runaway youths who become homeless street people have a high frequency of problem behaviors. Three fourths engage in some type of criminal activity and half engage in prostitution as a means of support. A majority of permanent runaways have serious mental problems; more than one third are the product of families who engage in repeated physical and sexual abuse. These children also have a high frequency of medical problems, including traditional infections, hepatitis, sexually transmitted diseases, and drug abuse.

INHERENT STRENGTHS IN VULNERABLE CHILDREN AND INTERVENTIONS

By age 20–30 yr, many children who were at special risk will have made moderate successes of their lives. Certain biologic characteristics are associated with success over the long term, such as being born with an accepting temperament. Avoidance of additional social risks is even more important. Children generally do better if they can gain social support, either from family members or from a nonjudgmental adult outside the family, especially an older mentor or peer.

PART 6

Nutrition

CHAPTER 35

Nutritional Requirements

(Nelson Textbook, Chapter 40)

Individual nutrition requirements vary with genetic and metabolic differences. For infants and children, the basic goals are achievement of satisfactory growth and avoidance of deficiency states. Good nutrition helps to prevent acute and chronic illness, to develop physical and mental potential, and to provide reserves for stress.

Because some essential substances remain unidentifiable, a varied diet may be the only prudent way of providing them after early infancy. Only human milk appears to supply all essentials for a prolonged time. Although some food essentials should be included in the early diet, others are stored by the body and may be supplied periodically. Although any diet producing good nutrition varies considerably, mild excess of nutrients or calories may be as undesirable as mild deficiencies.

WATER

Water is essential for existence; lack of it results in death in a matter of days. The water content of infants is relatively higher (75–80% of body weight) than that of adults (55–60%). Although dietary fluids provide the principal source of water, some water is obtained from the oxidation of foods.

Human needs for water are related to caloric consumption, to insensible loss, and to the specific gravity of the urine. The infant must consume much larger amounts of water per unit of body weight compared with adults (Table 35–1). The daily consumption of fluid by the healthy infant is equivalent to 10–15% of body weight compared with 2–4% in the adult.

ENERGY

The unit of heat in metabolism is the large calorie, or kilocalorie (1 Cal = 1 kcal); it is used to refer to the energy content of food. Energy needs of children at different ages and under various conditions vary greatly. The approximate average expenditures of energy by the child 6–12 yr of age are basal metabolism 50%; growth 12%; physical activity 25%; fecal loss about 8%, mainly as unabsorbed fat; and thermic effect of food 5%. For each centi-

TABLE 35–1 Range of Average Water Requirements of Children at Different Ages Under Ordinary Conditions

Age	Average Body Weight (kg)	Total Water in 24 hr (mL)	Water per Kilogram of Body Weight in 24 hr (mL)
3 days	3.0	250–300	80–100
10 days	3.2	400–500	125–150
3 mo	5.4	750–850	140–160
6 mo	7.3	950–1100	130–155
9 mo	8.6	1100–1250	125–145
1 yr	9.5	1150–1300	120–135
2 yr	11.8	1350–1500	115–125
4 yr	16.2	1600–1800	100–110
6 yr	20.0	1800–2000	90–100
10 yr	28.7	2000–2500	70–85
14 yr	45.0	2200–2700	50–60
18 yr	54.0	2200–2700	40–50

grade degree of fever, basal metabolism increases approximately 10%. The basal requirement in infants is about 55 kcal/kg/24 hr; it decreases to 25–30 kcal/kg/24 hr at maturity. The average requirement for physical activity is 15–25 kcal/kg/24 hr, with peak utilizations as high as 50–80 kcal/kg/24 hr for short periods. The daily caloric requirement is 80–120 kcal/kg for the 1st yr of life, with subsequent decreases of about 10 kcal/kg for each succeeding 3-yr period. Periods of rapid growth and development near puberty require increased caloric consumption. Each gram of ingested protein or carbohydrate provides 4 kcal. One gram of short-chain fatty acids provides 5.3 kcal; 1 g of medium-chain fatty acid gives 8.3 kcal; and 1 g of long-chain fatty acids provides 9 kcal.

PROTEINS

Protein constitutes about 20% of adult body weight. Its amino acids are essential nutrients in forming cell protoplasm. Twenty-four amino acids have been identified; nine were found to be essential for infants (threonine, valine, leucine, isoleucine, lysine, tryptophan, phenylalanine, methionine, and histidine). Arginine, cystine, and taurine are essential for low-birth-weight infants. Nonessential amino acids can be synthesized and need not be supplied in the diet.

Proteins are broken down in the digestive process. The amino acids are carried to the liver by the portal circulation, and from there they are distributed to other tissues. Amino acids are reconstituted to functional human proteins (e.g., albumin, hemoglobin, hormones). Abundant protein is available for children in the United States, but the supply in many developing countries is limited, and specific disorders of inadequate quality or quantity of protein intake may be encountered.

CARBOHYDRATES

Carbohydrates, while supplying the necessary bulk of the diet, supply most of the body's energy needs. In their absence, the body uses proteins and fats for energy. Stored chiefly as glycogen in the liver and muscles, carbohydrates probably constitute no more than 1% of the body weight. Because the size of the infant's liver is 10% that of the adult and the muscle mass is 2%, the infant's glycogen reserve is a fraction (approximately 3.5%) of that of the adult.

Carbohydrates are oxidized as glucose (dextrose) but are consumed in various forms. Through a series of enzymatic and chemical reactions in the digestive tract, complex carbohydrates are split into simpler structures. Some glucose may be oxidized directly, such as in the brain and heart. Most of the absorbed sugar is converted to glycogen in the liver, although glycogenesis also occurs in other tissues. Up to 15% of the weight of the liver and 3% of the muscle may be glycogen; small amounts are also found in practically all other organs. Glycogenolysis in the liver yields glucose as the chief product, whereas glycogen breakdown in the muscle yields lactic acid.

FATS

Fats or their metabolic products form an integral part of cellular membranes and are efficient stores of energy. They impart palatability to food and serve as vehicles for fat-soluble vitamins A, D, E, and K. Approximately 98% of natural fats are triglycerides, three fatty acids combined with glycerol. The remaining 2% include free fatty acids, monoglycerides, diglycerides, cholesterol, and phospholipids (including lecithin, cephalin, sphingomyelin, and cerebrosides).

Ingested triglycerides are partially hydrolyzed by lingual lipase and emulsified in the stomach. In the duodenum, pancreatic lipase hydrolyzes the triglycerides to monoglycerides and fatty acids and, with bile salts, forms micelles, which increase fatty solubility. Long-chain fatty acids and monoglycerides (those with more than 10 carbon atoms) in micelles are presumably absorbed into the mucosal cell by diffusion. Transport across the cell involves re-esterification of these fatty acids and monoglycerides to triglycerides, which are then "coated" with lipoprotein to form the chylomicron, in which the fat is transported in the lymph system to the venous circulation through the thoracic duct. Short- and medium-chain triglycerides are readily hydrolyzed by pancreatic lipase to free fatty acids, which are transported through the cell. These free fatty acids directly enter the intestinal veins and pass to the liver through the portal system. The alternative pathway for short- and medium-chain triglycerides is used in nutritional formulations for children with severe absorptive problems.

ESSENTIAL FATTY ACIDS. Humans do not synthesize linoleic or linolenic acid. Both must be supplied in the diet and are, therefore, "essential." Essential fatty acids are necessary for growth, skin and hair integrity, regulation of cholesterol metabolism, lipotropic activity, decreased platelet adhesiveness, and reproduction.

MINERALS

The ash content of the fetus is about 3% of the body weight at birth. It increases continuously throughout childhood. Adult ash content is 4.35% of body weight; 83% is in the skeleton, and 10% in the muscle. For each gram of protein retained, 0.3 g of mineral matter is deposited. The principal cations are calcium, magnesium, potassium, and sodium; the comparable anions are phosphorus, sulfur, and chloride. Iron, iodine, and cobalt appear in important organic complexes. The trace elements fluorine, copper, zinc, chromium, manganese, selenium, and molybdenum have known metabolic roles; silicon, boron, nickel, aluminum, arsenic, bromine, and strontium are also present in the diet and in the body.

VITAMINS

The word "vitamin" refers to organic compounds required in minute amounts to catalyze cellular metabolism essential for growth or maintenance of the organism.

EVALUATION OF DIET

See Table 35–2. The recall interview for determining children's food habits is usually satisfactory, but for a more accurate ac-

TABLE 35–2 Recommended Food Intake for Good Nutrition According to Food Groups

Food Group	Serving Size	Servings/day	1 yr	2–3 yr	4+ yr
Bread, cereal, rice, pasta	1 slice 1 oz (cereal)	6–11	1–2	2–4	3–11
Vegetables	½ cup	3–5	1/2	1	3–5
Fruit	1 apple, banana	2–4	1/2	1	2–4
Milk, cheese	1 cup 1½ oz cheese	2–3	1/2	1	1–3
Meat, poultry, etc	2–3 oz	2–3	1/2–1	1/2–1	1–3

After age 2 yr, fats, oils, and sweets should be consumed sparingly.
C = 1 cup or 8 oz or 240 mL.
Tbsp = tablespoon (1 Tbsp = 15 mL = ½ oz).

counting the parent should observe and record the actual food intake and convert to "servings" appropriate to the child's age. A food intake record can indicate possible nutritional imbalances.

CHAPTER 36

The Feeding of Infants and Children
(Nelson Textbook, Chapter 41)

Successful infant feeding requires cooperation between the mother and her infant, beginning with the initial feeding experience and continuing throughout the child's period of dependency. Promptly establishing comfortable, satisfying feeding practices contributes greatly to the infant's and mother's well-being.

As soon after birth as an infant can safely tolerate enteral nutrition, as judged by normal activity, alertness, suck, and cry, feedings should be initiated to maintain normal metabolism and growth during the transition from fetal to extrauterine life; to promote maternal-infant bonding; and to decrease the risk of hypoglycemia, hyperkalemia, hyperbilirubinemia, and azotemia. Mistakes are made by feeding the infant too much or too little. Inadequate fluid intake, particularly in hot environments, may result in "dehydration fever." Most infants may start breast-feeding shortly after birth, and others do so within 4–6 hr. When any question about the tolerance of feeding arises because of physical or neurologic status, feeding should be withheld until the newborn is carefully evaluated, and parenteral fluids or other means of enteral feeding may be substituted. Subsequent formula or breast feedings are given every 3–4 hr/day and night by the mother. Artificially fed infants should receive sterile water for the first feeding because regurgitation and aspiration of this liquid are less likely to cause significant irritation of the respiratory tract. Ideally, the feeding schedule should be based on this reasonable "self-regulation." Variation in the times between feedings and in the amount taken per feeding is to be expected in the first few weeks during the establishment of the self-regulation plan. By the end of the first month, more than 90% of infants will have established a suitable and reasonable regular schedule. Most healthy bottle-fed infants will want 6–9 feedings/24 hr by the end of the first week of life. Some will take enough at one feeding to satisfy themselves for approximately 4 hr; others who are smaller or whose gastric emptying time is more rapid will want formula about every 2–3 hr; breast-fed infants often prefer shorter intervals. Most term infants will rapidly increase their intake from 30 mL to 80–90 mL every 3–4 hr at 4–5 days of life. Feedings should be considered as having progressed satisfactorily if the infant is no longer losing weight by 5–7 days and is gaining weight by 12–14 days.

BREAST-FEEDING

Breast-feeding continues to have practical and psychologic advantages that should be considered when the mother selects the method for feeding. Human milk is the most appropriate of all available milks for the human infant because it is uniquely adapted to his or her needs.

PREPARATION OF THE PROSPECTIVE MOTHER. Most women are physically capable of breast-feeding, provided they receive sufficient encouragement and are protected from discouraging experiences and comments while the secretion of breast milk is becoming established. Physical factors conducive to a good breast-feeding experience include establishing and maintaining a state of good health, proper balance of rest and exercise, freedom from worry, early and sufficient treatment of any intercurrent disease, and adequate nutrition.

ESTABLISHING AND MAINTAINING THE MILK SUPPLY. The most satisfactory stimulus to the secretion of human milk is regular and complete emptying of the breasts; milk production is reduced when the secreted milk is not drained. Once lactation is well established, mothers are capable of producing more milk than their infants need. There are many reasons for incomplete nursing, but the principal ones are lack of support, weakness of the infant, and failure to initiate the natural hunger cycle.

Breast-feeding should begin soon after delivery as the condition of the mother and of the baby permits, preferably within the first hours. Appropriate care for tender or sore nipples should be instituted before severe pain from abrasions and cracking develops.

PSYCHOLOGIC FACTORS. No factor is more important than a happy, relaxed state of mind. Worry and unhappiness are the most effective means for decreasing or abolishing breast secretions.

HYGIENE. Once a day, the breasts should be washed. If soap is drying to the nipple and areolar area, its use should be discontinued. The nipple area should be kept dry.

DIET. The nursing mother needs a varied diet, sufficient to maintain her weight and high in fluids, vitamins, and minerals. She should avoid weight-reducing diets. Whenever possible, nursing mothers should not take drugs, because many preparations are harmful to the neonate and many have not been evaluated.

TECHNIQUE OF BREAST-FEEDING. At feeding time, the infant should be hungry, dry, neither too cold or too warm, and held in a comfortable, semisitting position for his or her enjoyment and for ease of eructation without vomiting. The mother, too, must be comfortable and completely at ease. The infant is supported comfortably with the face held close to the mother's breast by one arm and hand while the other hand supports the breast so that the nipple is easily accessible to the infant's mouth and yet does not obstruct the infant's breathing. The infant's lips should engage considerable areola as well as nipple.

The infant's rooting reflex brings the entire areola area into the mouth; the contact of the nipple against the palate and posterior tongue elicits sucking or "milking," and the buccal fat pads help keep the nipple in place. This *sucking reflex* is a process of squeezing the sinuses of the areola rather than simply suction on the nipple. The infant's sucking results in afferent impulses to the mother's hypothalamus and then to both anterior and posterior pituitary. Prolactin from the anterior pituitary stimulates milk secretion in the cuboidal cells in the acini or alveoli of the breast. Finally, milk in the infant's mouth triggers the *swallowing reflex.* In contrast, bottle-feeding requires the infant to compress the nipple to avoid choking.

Some infants will empty a breast within 5 min; others nurse more leisurely for 20 min. Most of the milk is obtained early in the feeding: 50% in the first 2 min and 80–90% in the first 4 min. The infant should be permitted to suck until satisfied unless the mother has sore nipples. At the end of the nursing period, the infant should be held erect over the mother's shoulder or on her lap with or without gently rubbing or patting the back to assist in expelling swallowed air; often this "burping" procedure is necessary one or more times during the feeding as well as 5–10 min after the infant has been put into the crib.

ONE OR BOTH BREASTS PER FEEDING. The infant should empty at least one breast per feeding; otherwise, it will not be stimulated to refill. Both breasts should be used at each feeding in the early weeks to encourage maximal production of milk. After the milk supply has been established, the breasts may be alternated at successive feedings, and the infant will usually be satisfied with the amount obtained from one.

DETERMINING ADEQUACY OF MILK SUPPLY. If the infant is satisfied after each nursing period, sleeps 2–4 hr, and gains weight adequately, the milk supply is sufficient. The "let-down" or *milk rejection reflex* in the mother is an important sign of successful nursing. When this reflex functions well, milk flows from the opposite breast as the infant begins to nurse.

SUPPLEMENTARY FEEDINGS. It is acceptable to feed the infant a commercial formula during the day and to continue nursing in the evening and throughout the night. The breast milk production will gradually decrease so that the mother is not plagued by engorged, leaking breasts.

WEANING. Most infants gradually reduce the volume and frequency of their demand for breast-feedings at 6–12 mo of age, and they become accustomed to increasing amounts of solid foods and liquids by bottle and cup. As they demand less breast milk, the mother's supply gradually diminishes, causing the mother no discomfort from engorgement. Over several days, one of the breast-feedings is replaced and then subsequently another, and so on, until the infant is weaned completely.

FORMULA FEEDING

Whole cow's milk or its modified form is the basis for most formulas, although other milks and milk substitutes are available for infants who cannot tolerate it. Sterilization and refrigeration of the formula greatly reduce morbidity and mortality from gastrointestinal infections. Conventional formulas of whole and evaporated cow's milk provide 3–4 g of protein/kg/24 hr ("high protein" intake largely exceeding the basic need), whereas breast milk and many commercially prepared feedings simulating the composition of breast milk supply 1.5–2.5 g/kg/24 hr ("low protein" intake supplying a smaller degree of excess). Commercial formulas are modified from a cow's milk base, and their protein and ash levels are reduced nearer to those of human milk.

TECHNIQUE OF ARTIFICIAL FEEDING. The setting should be similar to that for breast-feeding. The bottle should be held so that milk, not air, channels through the nipple. The bottle of milk is customarily warmed to body temperature. The nipple holes should be of a size that milk will drop slowly. Especially during the first 6–7 mo of life, the eructation of air swallowed during feeding is important for avoiding regurgitation and abdominal discomfort.

MILK USED IN FORMULAS

Pasteurized Milk. Pasteurization destroys many pathogenic bacteria and modifies casein so that smaller, less tough curds are produced in the stomach. Pasteurized milk should be boiled when used for infant feeding. If it is allowed to stand in the refrigerator for as long as 48 hr, its bacterial count may increase significantly.

Homogenized Milk. The principal advantage of homogenized milk is the smaller, less tough curd produced in the stomach.

Evaporated Milk. The unopened can will keep for months without refrigeration. The casein curd produced in the stomach is softer and smaller than that of boiled whole milk; homogenization of the fat also contributes to smaller curd formation. The whey protein or lactoglobulin appears to be less allergenic than that of fresh milk.

Prepared Milks. The composition of the majority simulates breast milk in various ways. All are fortified with vitamin D and other vitamins, and some have added iron.

Milk Substitutes and Hypoallergenic Milks. A number of milks and milk substitutes are available for infants allergic to cow's milk. These include evaporated goat's milk, a preparation in which nutrient nitrogen is supplied as an amino acid mixture (casein or whey hydrolysate), and nonmilk foods in which the protein is derived from soybeans. Those not containing lactose are useful for infants with galactosemia. Powdered casein in medium-chain triglycerides (MCT oil) is available for special purposes.

MILK FORMULAS. The formulas combine milk, sugar, and water and some modification for a more desirable, smaller curd formation. They should contain about 20 kcal/oz.

Caloric Requirements. The average caloric requirements of full-term infants are 45–55 kcal/lb or 80–120 kcal/kg during the first few months of life and about 45 kcal/lb or 100 kcal/kg by 1 yr of age; individual variations are significant, and for many infants intakes of this order exceed caloric need.

Fluid Requirements. Fluid requirements are high during infancy. During the first 6 mo of life, they range from 2–3 oz/lb/24 hr or 130–190 mL/kg/24 hr and may increase during the hot weather. Most of the fluid required is in the formula, but some is supplied in juice and other foods and by water between feedings.

Number of Feedings Daily. The number of feedings required per day decreases throughout the first year; by 1 yr of age, most infants are satisfied with 3 meals/day. The interval between feedings differs considerably among infants but, in general, ranges from 3–5 hr during the first year of life, averaging 4 hr for full-term infants.

Quantity of Formula. The quantity taken at a feeding varies with different infants of the same age and with the same infant at different feedings. Each infant must be primarily responsible for determining the quantity of intake (Table 36–1).

OTHER FOODS

VITAMINS. Most marketed and whole artificial milks are fortified with 10 g of vitamin D per reconstituted quart; commercially prepared milks vary in the content of other vitamins. Orange and other citrus fruit juices are natural sources of vitamin C, but because many young infants do not seem to tolerate them in amounts large enough to supply an adequate vitamin intake, it is preferable to give 35 mg of ascorbic acid.

TABLE 36–1 Average Quantity of Feedings

Age	Average Quantity Taken in Individual Feedings
1st and 2nd wk	2–3 oz (60–90 mL)
3 wk–2 mo	4–5 oz (120–150 mL)
2–3 mo	5–6 oz (150–180 mL)
3–4 mo	6–7 oz (180–210 mL)
5–12 mo	7–8 oz (210–240 mL)

IRON. The most effective way to prevent iron deficiency is to provide iron supplementation in the form of an iron-fortified milk formula or medicinal iron (2 mg/kg up to a total of 15 mg/24 hr) beginning at 6 wk of age.

"SOLID" FOODS. The inclusion of solid foods in the diet before 4–6 mo of age does not contribute significantly to the health of the normal infant nor does it increase the likelihood of the infant's sleeping through the night, providing hunger is avoided. Any new food should be initially offered once a day in small amounts (1–2 teaspoonfuls).

Cereal. The various precooked cereals on the market provide in a conventional form a variety of grains excellent for infants. Most contain iron and factors of the vitamin B complex.

Fruits. Strained or pureed cooked fruits furnish minerals and some water-soluble vitamins and usually have a mild laxative effect.

Vegetables. Vegetables are moderately good sources of iron and other minerals and of the B-complex vitamins. They should be freshly cooked and strained or commercially prepared. Vegetables are usually added to the infant's diet by about 7 mo of age.

Meats, Eggs, and Starch Foods. Eggs and starchy foods are usually introduced during the second 6 mo of life. Potatoes, rice, spaghetti, bread, and similar starchy foods have a principally caloric value. They are not included in the infant's diet until the more essential foods mentioned earlier are being taken regularly. Meat is an excellent source of protein as well as of iron and vitamins. Ground fresh beef or liver or the strained canned meats may be used initially by about 6 mo of age.

FIRST-YEAR FEEDING PROBLEMS

UNDERFEEDING. Underfeeding is suggested by restlessness and by crying and failure to gain weight adequately, despite complete emptying of the breast or bottle. The extent and duration of underfeeding determine the clinical manifestations. Constipation, failure to sleep, irritability, and excessive crying are to be expected. There may be poor gain in weight or an actual loss. Treatment consists of increasing the fluid and caloric intake, correcting deficiencies in vitamin and mineral intake, and instructing the mother in the art of infant feeding.

OVERFEEDING. Regurgitation and vomiting are frequent symptoms or overfeeding. Diets too high in fat delay gastric emptying, cause distention and abdominal discomfort, and may cause excessive gain in weight. Diets too high in carbohydrates are likely to cause undue fermentation in the intestine, resulting in distention and flatulence and in too rapid a gain in weight. Such diets may be deficient in essential protein, vitamins, and minerals. Formulas too high in caloric content in the first 1–2 wk of life are likely to result in loose or diarrheal stools.

REGURGITATION AND VOMITING. The return of small amounts of swallowed food during or shortly after eating is called regurgitation or spitting up. More complete emptying of the stomach, especially that occurring some time after feeding, is called vomiting. Within limits, regurgitation is a natural occurrence, especially during the first 6 mo or so of life. It can be reduced to a negligible amount, however, by adequate eructation of swallowed air during and after eating, by gentle handling, by avoiding emotional conflicts, and by placing the infant on the right side for a nap immediately after eating. Vomiting, one of the most common symptoms in infancy, may be associated with a variety of disturbances, both trivial and serious.

LOOSE OR DIARRHEAL STOOLS. The stool of the breast-fed infant is naturally softer than that of the infant fed cow's milk. From the 4th to the 6th day of life, the stools go through a transitional stage in which they are rather loose and greenish yellow and contain mucus; within a few days, the typical "milk stool" appears. Subsequently, the use of laxatives or the ingestion of certain foods by the mother may be temporarily responsible for an infant's loose stools. Excessive intake of breast milk may also increase the frequency and the water content of the stool. Actual diarrhea in a breast-fed infant is unusual and should be considered infectious until proved otherwise.

Although the stools of artificially fed infants tend to be firmer than those of breast-fed infants, loose stools may result from artificial feeding. In the first 2 wk or so of life, overfeeding is likely to cause loose, frequent stools. Later, formulas too concentrated or too high in sugar content, especially in lactose, may also produce loose, frequent stools.

CONSTIPATION. Constipation is practically unknown in breast-fed infants receiving an adequate amount of milk and is rare in artificially fed infants receiving an adequate diet. The nature of the stool, not its frequency, is the basis for diagnosing constipation. Although most infants have one or more stools daily, an infant will occasionally have a stool of normal consistency only at intervals of 36–48 hr.

Whenever constipation or obstipation is present from birth or shortly thereafter, a rectal examination should be performed. Tight or spastic anal sphincters may occasionally be responsible for obstipation, and correction usually follows finger dilatation. Anal fissures or cracks may also cause constipation. Aganglionic megacolon may be manifested by constipation in early infancy.

Constipation in the artificially fed infant may be caused by an insufficient amount of food or fluid. In other cases, it may result from diets too high in fat or protein or deficient in bulk. Simply increasing the amount of fluid or sugar in the formula may be corrective in the first few months of life. After this age, better results are obtained by adding or increasing the amounts of cereal, vegetables, and fruits.

COLIC. The term *colic* describes a frequent symptom-complex of paroxysmal abdominal pain, presumably of intestinal origin, and of severe crying. It occurs usually in infants younger than 3 mo.

The clinical manifestations are characteristic: the attack usually begins suddenly; the cry is loud and more or less continuous; so-called paroxysms may persist for several hours; the face may be flushed, or there may be circumoral pallor; the abdomen is distended and tense; the legs are drawn up on the abdomen, although they may be momentarily extended; the feet are often cold; the hands are clenched. The attack may terminate only when the infant is completely exhausted, but often there is apparent temporary relief with the passage of feces or flatus. Colic rarely persists after 3 mo of age. A supportive, sympathetic physician is important in successfully resolving the problem.

FEEDING DURING THE SECOND YEAR OF LIFE

Most infants naturally adapt themselves to a schedule of three meals a day by about the end of the 1st yr of life.

REDUCED CALORIC INTAKE. Toward the end of the 1st yr and during the 2nd yr, because of the constantly decelerating rate of growth, there is a gradual reduction in the infant's caloric intake per unit of body weight. In addition, it is not unusual to have temporary periods of lack of interest in certain foods or even in food in general.

SELF-SELECTION OF DIET. Children's strong likes or dislikes of particular foods should be respected whenever possible and practicable.

SELF-FEEDING BY INFANTS. Before 1 yr of age, the infant should be permitted to participate in the act of feeding. By approximately 6 mo, the infant can hold a bottle; within another 2–3 mo, a cup. By the end of the 2nd yr, infants should be largely responsible for feeding themselves.

EATING HABITS. Eating habits formed in the 1st or 2nd yr of life distinctly affect those of the subsequent years.

SNACKS BETWEEN MEALS. During the 2nd yr and even for several years thereafter, orange juice or other fruit juice or fruit, together with a cracker, may be given in either or both of the between-meal periods.

VEGETARIAN DIET. All-vegetable diets supply all necessary nutrients when vegetables are selected from different classes. Those who consume eggs are ovovegetarians. Those who consume milk are lactovegetarians. Those who consume neither are vegans. Vegans may develop vitamin B_{12} deficiency and, because of high fiber intake, may develop trace mineral deficiency.

LATER CHILDHOOD AND ADOLESCENCE

As the child reaches age 2 yr, diet is similar to that of the family. All the known nutrients are supplied by a varied diet and should include selections from each of the food groups: cereals, fruits, vegetables, proteins, and dairy.

CHAPTER 37

Malnutrition

(Nelson Textbook, Chapter 42)

Worldwide, malnutrition is one of the leading causes of morbidity and mortality in childhood. Malnutrition may be due to improper or inadequate food intake or may result from inadequate absorption of food. It may be acute or chronic, reversible or irreversible.

MARASMUS (INFANTILE ATROPHY, INANITION, ATHREPSIA)

ETIOLOGY. The clinical picture of marasmus originates from an inadequate caloric intake due to insufficient diet, to improper feeding habits such as those of disturbed parent-child relations, or to metabolic abnormalities or congenital malformations.

CLINICAL MANIFESTATIONS. Initially there is failure to gain weight, followed by loss of weight until emaciation results, with loss of turgor in skin that becomes wrinkled and loose as subcutaneous fat disappears. The abdomen may be distended or flat, and the intestinal pattern may be readily visible. Atrophy of muscle occurs, with resultant hypotonia. The temperature is usually subnormal; the pulse may be slow; and the basal metabolic rate tends to be reduced. At first, the infant may be fretful but later becomes listless, and the appetite diminishes. The infant is usually constipated, but the so-called starvation type of diarrhea may appear, with frequent small stools containing mucus.

PROTEIN MALNUTRITION (PROTEIN-CALORIE MALNUTRITION, KWASHIORKOR)

The principal symptoms of protein malnutrition are due to insufficient intake of protein of good biologic value. There may also be impaired absorption of protein, such as in chronic diarrheal states; abnormal losses of protein in proteinuria (nephrosis), infection, hemorrhage, or burns; and failure of protein synthesis, such as in chronic liver disease.

Kwashiorkor is a clinical syndrome that results from a severe deficiency of protein and an inadequate caloric intake. Secondary vitamin and mineral deficiency may contribute to the signs and symptoms.

CLINICAL MANIFESTATIONS. Early clinical evidence of protein malnutrition is vague but does include lethargy, apathy, or irritability. When well advanced, it results in inadequate growth, lack of stamina, loss of muscular tissue, increased susceptibility to infections, and edema. Secondary immunodeficiency is one of the most serious and constant manifestations.

The child may develop anorexia, flabbiness of subcutaneous tissue, and loss of muscle tone. The liver may enlarge early or late; fatty infiltration is common, and hepatic export proteins are reduced. Edema usually develops early; failure to gain weight may be masked by edema, which is often present in internal organs before it can be recognized in the face and limbs. Renal plasma flow, glomerular filtration rate, and renal tubular function are decreased. The heart may be small in the early stages of the disease but is usually enlarged later.

Dermatitis is common. Darkening of the skin appears in irritated areas but not in areas exposed to sunlight, a contrast to the situation in pellagra. Dyspigmentation may occur in these areas after desquamation, or it may be generalized. The hair is often sparse and thin and loses its elasticity.

Infections, both acute and chronic (tuberculosis and human immunodeficiency virus infection), and parasitic infestations are common, as are anorexia, vomiting, and continued diarrhea. Mental changes, especially irritability and apathy, are common. Stupor, coma, and death may follow with a substantial case-fatality rate (~30–40%) even when the disease is diagnosed and appropriately treated.

LABORATORY DATA. Decrease in the concentration of serum albumin is the most characteristic change. Potassium and magnesium deficiencies are frequent. Severe hypophosphatemia (<0.32 mmol/L) is associated with increased mortality. Anemia may be normocytic, microcytic, or macrocytic. Signs of vitamin (particularly vitamin A) and mineral deficiencies are usually evident. Bone growth is usually delayed.

PREVENTION. This requires a diet containing an adequate quantity of protein of good biologic quality.

TREATMENT. Immediate management of any acute problems such as severe diarrhea, renal failure, and shock and, ultimately, the replacement of missing nutrients are essential. Initial management consists of administration of low-volume, dilute milk feedings with nutrient supplementation such as Nutriset. The routine administration of antibiotics such as co-trimoxazole has also been advocated. Moderate or severe dehydration, manifest or suspected infection, eye signs of severe vitamin A deficiency, severe anemia, hypoglycemia, continuing or recurrent diarrhea, skin and other mucous membrane lesions, anorexia, and hypothermia all must be treated. Intravenous fluids are necessary for the treatment of severe dehydration. When dehydration is corrected, oral and nasogastric feeding starts with small, frequent feedings of dilute milk (66 kcal and 1.0 g protein/100 mL at ~120 mL/kg/24 hr) with nutrient supplementation; strength and volume are gradually increased and frequency decreased over the next 5–7 days. By day 6–8, the child should receive 150 mL/kg/24 hr in about 6 feedings of high-energy milk (114 kcal and 4.1 g protein/100 mL). Vitamins and minerals, especially vitamin A, potassium, and magnesium, are necessary from the outset of treatment. Iron and folic acid usually correct the anemia. Bacterial infections should be treated concomitantly with the dietary therapy, whereas treatment of parasitic infestations, if they are not severe, may be postponed until recovery begins. If growth and development have been extensively impaired, mental and physical retardation may be permanent.

MALNUTRITION IN CHILDREN BEYOND INFANCY

ETIOLOGY. Malnutrition in children may be a continuation of an undernourished state begun in infancy, or it may arise from factors that become operative during childhood. In general, the causes are the same as those for malnutrition in infants.

CLINICAL MANIFESTATIONS. Malnutrition does not invariably result in underweight. Fatigue, lassitude, restlessness, and irritability are frequent manifestations. Restlessness and overactivity are frequently misinterpreted by parents as evidence of lack of fatigue. Anorexia, easily induced digestive disturbances, and constipation are common complaints, and even in older children the starvation type of mucoid diarrheal stool may be observed. Malnourished children often have a limited attention span and do poorly in school. They have increased susceptibility to infections. Muscular development is inadequate, and the flabby muscles result in a posture of fatigue, with rounded shoulders, flat chest, and protuberant abdomen. Hypochromic anemia is common.

TREATMENT. Individualized treatment is aimed at correcting underlying psychologic and physical disturbances. An adequate diet should be outlined; vitamin concentrates may be added and continued for a time after the dietary intake has become adequate.

PROTEIN EXCESS

Excessive protein intake, especially in the absence of sufficient water, may lead to signs of dehydration-protein fever. Premature infants fed a high-protein diet may have an increased morbidity. Marasmic infants fed high-protein diets during the recovery phase may develop hyperammonemia; protein intoxication has also been noted in children with other liver disease.

CHAPTER 38

Obesity

(Nelson Textbook, Chapter 43)

Obesity in childhood is not a disease but rather a symptom-complex having a weak association with adult obesity with its correlates of increased mortality, cardiovascular disease, hypertension, hyperlipidemias, liver disease, cholelithiasis, and adult-onset diabetes.

ETIOLOGY. Factors related to the occurrence of overweight and obesity are multifactorial with the exception of certain single-gene disorders associated with human obesity (Prader-Willi, Bardet-Biedl, Ahlstrom, and Cohen syndromes). Some of the unknown factors include excessive intake of high-energy foods, inadequate exercise in relation to age and activity and more sedentary lifestyle, low metabolic rate relative to body composition and mass, increased respiratory quotient in the resting state, and increased insulin sensitivity.

EPIDEMIOLOGY. Longitudinal studies in industrialized societies during the past century have shown growth in height and weight compared with previous generations. Individual studies have described a prevalence of children who are overweight of 7–43% in Canada, 7.3% in the United Kingdom, and approximately 25% for children and adolescents in the United States. The incidence of childhood obesity relates strongly to family variables, including parental obesity, small family size, and family patterns of inactivity.

CLINICAL MANIFESTATIONS. Obesity may become evident at any age, but it appears most frequently in the 1st yr of life, at 5–6 yr of age, and during adolescence. Children whose obesity is due to excessively high caloric intake are usually not only heavier than others in their own cohort but also taller, and bone age is advanced. The adiposity in the mammary regions in boys is often suggestive of breast development and, therefore, may be an embarrassing feature. The abdomen tends to be pendulous, and white or purple striae are often present. The external genitalia of boys appear disproportionately small but actually are most often of average size; the penis is often embedded in the pubic fat. The development of the external genitalia is normal in most girls, and menarche is usually not delayed and may be advanced. Genu valgum is common.

DIAGNOSIS. The body mass index (BMI) is recommended for definition of obesity and overweight populations.

DIFFERENTIAL DIAGNOSIS. Children with obesity defined by an elevated BMI should receive careful medical evaluation for disorders that may have a primary medical association with obesity. Most of these disorders are rare (Table 38–1).

TABLE 38–1 Differential Diagnosis of Childhood Obesity

Endocrine Causes

Cushing syndrome
Hypothyroidism
Hyperinsulinemia
Growth hormone deficiency
Hypothalamic dysfunction
Prader-Willi syndrome
Stein-Leventhal syndrome (polycystic ovary)
Pseudohypoparathyroidism type I

Genetic Syndromes

Turner syndrome
Laurence-Moon-Biedl syndrome
Alstrom-Hallgren syndrome

Other Syndromes

Cohen syndrome
Carpenter syndrome

Adapted from Dietz WH, Robinson TN: Assessment and treatment of childhood obesity. Pediatr Rev 14:337, 1993.

COMPLICATIONS AND MORBID OBESITY

Children with obesity or overweight experience significant social and psychologic stresses and difficulties. Glucose intolerance and non–insulin-dependent diabetes mellitus occur in obese children and adolescents. Obese children and adolescents characteristically have elevated serum levels of low-density lipoprotein cholesterol and triglycerides and lowered high-density lipoprotein cholesterol. Sleep apnea is increasingly identified in obese children and adolescents and may mandate aggressive forms of therapy. Orthopedic complications of obesity include Blount disease (overgrowth of the proximal medial tibial metaphysis) and slipped capital femoral epiphysis in adolescents.

Obese infants and children are at moderately increased risk of becoming obese adults. The increased risk is associated with greater severity of childhood obesity, decreased time interval to adult age, and greater number of obese family members. There is an association between childhood obesity and cardiovascular risk factors.

The *pickwickian syndrome* is a rare complication of extreme exogenous obesity in which patients have severe cardiorespiratory distress with alveolar hypoventilation and a decrease in pulmonary, tidal, and expiratory reserve volumes. The manifestations include polycythemia, hypoxemia, cyanosis, cardiac enlargement, congestive cardiac failure, and somnolence.

PREVENTION AND TREATMENT. Because obesity may be self-perpetuating for psychologic or physiologic reasons, obese children, children of obese parents, or those with obese siblings should be encouraged to adhere to a systematic program of energetic exercise and a balanced diet appropriate to their energy expenditure level. After childhood obesity is established, it is extremely difficult to implement an effective plan for weight reduction and maintenance without active participation and motivation of both the child and the family. Successful treatment of childhood obesity requires attention to at least the following components: (1) modification of diet and caloric content, (2) definition and use of appropriate exercise programs, (3) behavior modification for the child, and (4) involvement of the family in therapy.

PROGNOSIS. Results with dietary or exercise modification have been successful only for the short term; follow-up studies of adequate duration show a higher rate of relapse at 4–10 yr, with successful maintenance of reduced (but not normal) weight in only 50% of patients.

CHAPTER 39

Vitamin Deficiencies and Excesses
(Nelson Textbook, Chapter 44)

VITAMIN A DEFICIENCY

The term *vitamin A* is a generic label for all β-ionone derivatives other than provitamin A carotenoids. Retinol signifies vitamin A alcohol; retinal ester, vitamin A ester; retinal, vitamin A aldehyde; and retinoic acid (vitamin A acid). *Provitamin A carotenoids* is the generic term for all carotenoids that have the biologic activity of β-carotene.

Ingested carotenoids are nontoxic and may result in yellow discoloration of the skin but not of the sclera. The disorder, *carotenemia,* is especially likely to occur in children with liver disease, diabetes mellitus, or hypothyroidism and in those who have congenital absence of enzymes that convert provitamin A carotenoids.

ETIOLOGY. The risk of vitamin A deficiency is small in healthy children with balanced diets. Deficient diets commonly cause disease by age 2–3 yr. Vitamin A deficiency also results from inadequate intestinal absorption. Low intake of dietary fat results in low vitamin A absorption.

CLINICAL MANIFESTATIONS. Ocular lesions develop insidiously. The posterior segment of the eye is initially affected, with impairment of dark adaptation resulting in night blindness. Later, drying of the conjunctiva (xerosis conjunctivae) and of the cornea (xerosis corneae) is followed by wrinkling and cloudiness of the cornea (keratomalacia). Dry silver-gray plaques may appear on the bulbar conjunctiva (Bitot spots), with follicular hyperkeratosis and photophobia.

Vitamin A deficiency may result in retardation of mental and physical growth and in apathy. Anemia with or without hepatosplenomegaly is usually present. The skin is dry and scaly, and follicular hyperkeratosis may at times be found on the shoulders, buttocks, and extensor surface of the extremities. Increased intracranial pressure with wide separation of cranial bones at the sutures may occur.

DIAGNOSIS. Dark adaptation tests may be helpful. Xerosis conjunctivae can be detected by biomicroscopic examination of the conjunctiva.

PREVENTION. Infants should receive at least 500 μg of vitamin A daily; older children and adults should receive 600–1500 μg of vitamin A or carotene.

For therapeutic reasons, low-fat diets should be supplemented with vitamin A. In disorders with poor absorption of fat or increased excretion of vitamin A, water-miscible preparations should be administered in amounts several times the usual daily requirement.

TREATMENT. In case of latent vitamin A deficiency, a daily supplement of 1500 μg/kg/24 hr is given orally for 5 days and then continued with intramuscular injection of 7500 μg of vitamin A in oil daily until recovery occurs.

HYPERVITAMINOSIS A. Acute hypervitaminosis A may occur in infants after ingesting 100,000 μg or more. The symptoms are nausea, vomiting, drowsiness, and bulging of the fontanel. Diplopia, papilledema, cranial nerve palsies, and other symptoms suggestive of brain tumor (pseudotumor cerebri) may also occur.

Chronic hypervitaminosis A appears after ingestion of excessive doses for several weeks or months. An affected child has anorexia, pruritus, and a lack of weight gain. Also noted are increased irritability, limitation of motion, and tender swelling of the bones. Alopecia, seborrheic cutaneous lesions, fissuring of the corners of the mouth, increased intracranial pressure, and hepatomegaly may develop. Craniotabes and desquamation of the palms and soles are common. Radiographs reveal hyperostosis affecting several long bones; it is most notable at the middle of the shafts.

Severe congenital malformations may occur in infants of mothers consuming large amounts of oral retinoids used in treating acne.

VITAMIN B COMPLEX DEFICIENCY

Diets deficient in any one factor of the B complex are frequently poor sources of other B vitamins. Because manifestation of several B deficiencies can usually be found in the same patient, it is generally practical to treat the patient with the entire B complex.

THIAMINE DEFICIENCY (BERIBERI)

Breast milk or cow's milk, vegetables, cereals, fruits, and eggs are sources of thiamine. Infants whose source of food is the milk of thiamine-deficient mothers may develop beriberi. Thiamine is easily destroyed by heat in neutral or alkaline media and is readily extracted from foodstuffs by cooking water. Because the covering of grains of cereals contains most of the vitamin, polishing reduces its availability. Thiamine absorption decreases with gastrointestinal or liver disease.

CLINICAL MANIFESTATIONS. Early manifestations of deficiency include fatigue, apathy, irritability, depression, drowsiness, poor mental concentration, anorexia, nausea, and abdominal discomfort. Signs of progression include peripheral neuritis with tingling, burning, and paresthesias of the toe and feet; decreased tendon reflexes; loss of vibration sense; tenderness and cramping of leg muscles; congestive heart failure; and psychic disturbances. Patients may have ptosis of the eyelids and atrophy of the optic nerve. Hoarseness or aphonia due to paralysis of the laryngeal nerve is a characteristic sign. Muscle atrophy and tenderness of nerve trunks are followed by ataxia, loss of coordination, and loss of deep sensation.

In dry beriberi, the child may appear plump but is pale, flabby, listless, and dyspneic; the heart rate is rapid, and the liver is enlarged. In wet beriberi, the child is undernourished, pale, and edematous and has dyspnea, vomiting, and tachycardia. The skin appears waxy. The urine may contain albumin and casts.

The cardiac signs at first are slight cyanosis and dyspnea. Tachycardia, enlargement of the liver, loss of consciousness, and convulsions may develop rapidly. The heart is enlarged, especially on the right. The electrocardiogram shows an increased QT interval, inversion of T waves, and low voltage, changes that rapidly revert to normal with treatment. Cardiac failure may lead to death in either chronic or acute beriberi.

WERNICKE'S ENCEPHALOPATHY. This is characterized by irritability, somnolence, and ocular signs and less commonly by mental confusion and ataxias; it occurs infrequently in malnourished infants and children.

DIAGNOSIS. Demonstrations of lowered red blood cell transketolase and high blood or urinary glyoxylate values have been proposed as diagnostic tests. Clinical response to administration of thiamine remains the best test for thiamine deficiency.

PREVENTION. A maternal diet containing sufficient amounts of thiamine prevents this deficiency in breast-fed infants. Thiamine requirements increase with a high-carbohydrate content of the diet.

TREATMENT. If beriberi occurs in a breast-fed infant, both the mother and child should be treated with thiamine. The daily dose for adults is 50 mg and for children 10 mg or more. Oral administration is effective unless gastrointestinal disturbances prevent absorption. Thiamine should be given intramuscularly or intravenously to children with cardiac failure. Because patients with beriberi often have other B complex deficiencies, all other vitamins of the B complex should be administered, in addition to large doses of thiamine chloride.

RIBOFLAVIN DEFICIENCY (ARIBOFLAVINOSIS)

Riboflavin deficiency without deficiencies of other members of the B complex is rare. Riboflavin deficiency is usually caused by inadequate intake.

CLINICAL MANIFESTATIONS. Evidence of riboflavin deficiency include cheilosis (perlèche), glossitis, keratitis, conjunctivitis, photophobia, lacrimation, marked corneal vascularization, and seborrheic dermatitis.

DIAGNOSIS. Urinary excretion of riboflavin below 30 μg/24 hr is abnormally low.

PREVENTION. Riboflavin deficiency is usually prevented by a diet that contains adequate amounts of milk, eggs, leafy vegetables, and lean meats.

TREATMENT. Treatment is the oral administration of 3–10 mg of riboflavin daily. If no response occurs within a few days, intramuscular injections of 2 mg of riboflavin in saline solution may be made three times daily.

NIACIN DEFICIENCY (PELLAGRA)

ETIOLOGY. Pellagra (*pellis,* "skin"; *agra,* "rough"), a deficiency disease caused mainly by a lack of niacin (nicotinic acid), affects all tissues of the body. Although dietary tryptophan can partially substitute for niacin, other sources of niacin are necessary. Pellagra occurs chiefly in countries where corn (maize), a poor source of tryptophan, is a basic foodstuff. Milk and eggs, which contain little niacin, are good pellagra-preventive foods because of their high content of tryptophan

CLINICAL MANIFESTATIONS. The early symptoms of pellagra are vague. Anorexia, lassitude, weakness, burning sensations, numbness, and dizziness may be prodromal symptoms. After a long period of niacin deficiency, the characteristic symptoms appear. The classic triad, which is usually not well developed in infants and children, consists of dermatitis, diarrhea, and dementia. Manifestations in children with parasites or chronic disorders may be especially severe.

The most characteristic manifestations are the cutaneous ones, which may develop suddenly or insidiously and may be elicited by irritants, particularly by intense sunlight. They first appear as symmetric erythema of the exposed surfaces that may resemble sunburn and in mild cases may escape recognition. The cutaneous lesions are sometimes preceded by stomatitis, glossitis, vomiting, or diarrhea.

DIAGNOSIS. Diagnosis is usually made from the physical signs of glossitis, gastrointestinal symptoms, and a symmetric dermatitis. Rapid clinical response to niacin is an important confirming test.

PREVENTION. A well-balanced diet containing meat, vegetables, eggs, and milk is usually effective.

TREATMENT. Children respond rapidly to antipellagral therapy. A liberal and well-balanced diet should be supplemented with 50–300 mg/24 hr of niacin; 100 mg may be given intravenously in severe cases or in cases of poor intestinal absorption. The diet should always be supplemented with other vitamins, especially with other members of vitamin B complex. Sun exposure should be avoided during the active phase.

PYRIDOXINE (VITAMIN B_6) DEFICIENCY

Vitamin B_6 includes pyridoxal, pyridoxine, and pyridoxamine.

ETIOLOGY. Pyridoxine is adequate in human and cow's milk and cereals, but prolonged heat processing of the latter two destroys it. Diseases with malabsorption, such as celiac syndrome, may contribute to vitamin B_6 deficiency.

There are several types of *vitamin B_6 dependence syndromes*, presumably a result of errors in enzyme structure or function, in which patients respond to very large amounts of pyridoxine. These syndromes include vitamin B_6-dependent convulsions, a vitamin B_6–responsive anemia, xanthurenic aciduria, cystathioninuria, and homocystinuria.

CLINICAL MANIFESTATIONS. Four clinical disturbances caused by vitamin B_6 deficiency have been described in humans: convulsions in infants, peripheral neuritis, dermatitis, and anemia. Infants fed a formula deficient in vitamin B_6 for 1–6 mo exhibit irritability and generalized seizures. Gastrointestinal distress and an aggravated startle response are common. Peripheral neuropathy may occur during treatment of tuberculosis with isoniazid. The neuropathy responds to administration of pyridoxine or to a decrease in the dose of the drug. Skin lesions include cheilosis, glossitis, and seborrhea around the eyes, nose, and mouth. Microcytic anemia, oxaluria, oxalic acid bladder stones, hyperglycinemia, lymphopenia, decreased antibody formation, and infections also occur. *Convulsion due to vitamin B_6 dependence* may occur several hours to as long as 6 mo after birth. Seizures are typically myoclonic, with hypsarrhythmic patterns on the electroencephalogram. In vitamin B_6–dependent anemia, the red blood cells are microcytic and hypochromic.

LABORATORY DATA. After administration of 100 mg/kg of tryptophan, large amounts of xanthurenic acid are found in the urine of patients with pyridoxine deficiency; in normal persons, none is detected. The result of this test may be normal in patients with pyridoxine dependence.

DIAGNOSIS. Infants with seizures should be suspected of having vitamin B_6 deficiency or dependence. If more common causes of infantile seizures, such as hypocalcemia, hypoglycemia, and infection, can be eliminated, 100 mg of pyridoxine should be injected. If the seizure stops, vitamin B_6 deficiency should be suspected, and a tryptophan loading test is indicated.

PREVENTION. Balanced diets usually contain enough pyridoxine so that deficiency is rare. Daily intake of 0.3–0.5 mg of pyridoxine in an infant, 0.5–1.5 mg in a child, and 1.5–2.0 mg in an adult prevents deficiency states.

TREATMENT. For convulsions possibly due to pyridoxine deficiency, 100 mg of the vitamin should be given intramuscularly. One dose should suffice if the diet is adequate. For pyridoxine-dependent children, 2–10 mg intramuscularly or 10–100 mg orally may be necessary daily.

TOXICITY. Excessive intake may cause neuropathy.

BIOTIN DEFICIENCY

Biotin deficiency is rare. It is found in those consuming the biotin antagonist avidin, found in raw egg white.

CLINICAL MANIFESTATION. Brawny dermatitis, orofacial lesions, alopecia, somnolence, hallucinations, hypotonia, and hyperesthesia with accumulation of organic acids are common. Other neurologic signs and defective immunity may occur.

DIAGNOSIS. Biotin deficiency is suggested by organic aciduria.

PREVENTION AND TREATMENT. Parenteral solutions should contain biotin. Deficient patients respond to oral administration of 10 mg.

FOLATE DEFICIENCY

Deficiency of folic acid is best recognized for its hematologic effects. Folate deficiency in a pregnant woman results in serious dysmorphologic effects in her fetus and newborn. Consumption of 400 μg/24 hr of folic acid in the periconceptual period decreases the incidence of neurotubular and other anatomic defects. Food may be fortified with folate as a preventive measure to decrease the incidence of neural tube defect.

VITAMIN C (ASCORBIC ACID) DEFICIENCY (SCURVY)

Ascorbic acid is essential for the formation of normal collagen; the defects in collagen structure arising from deficiency of the vitamin produce many of the metabolic and clinical manifestations of scurvy.

ETIOLOGY. An infant is born with adequate stores of vitamin C if the mother's intake has been adequate. Under these circumstances, breast milk is an adequate source of vitamin C. Deficiency of vitamin C in the mother's diet may result in scurvy in her breast-fed infant. Infants fed with evaporated milk formula must receive vitamin C supplements. The need for vitamin C is increased by febrile illnesses and by iron deficiency, cold exposure, protein depletion, or smoking.

CLINICAL MANIFESTATIONS. Scurvy may occur at any age but is rare in newborns. The majority of cases occur in infants age 6–24 mo. Clinical manifestations require time to develop; after a variable period of vitamin C depletion, vague symptoms of irritability, tachypnea, digestive disturbances, and loss of appetite appear. There is evidence of general tenderness, especially noticeable in the legs when the infant is picked up or when the diaper is changed. The pain results in pseudoparalysis, and the legs assume the typical frog-leg position, in which the hips and knees are semiflexed with the feet rotated outward. Edematous swelling along the shafts of the legs may be present. In some cases, a subperiosteal hemorrhage can be palpated at the end of the femur. The facial expression is apprehensive. Changes in the gums, most noticeable when the teeth are erupted, are characterized by bluish purple, spongy swellings of the mucous membrane, usually over the upper incisors. A "rosary" at the costochondral junctions and a depression of the sternum may be noted. Petechial hemorrhages may occur in the skin and mucous membranes. Hematuria, melena, and orbital or subdural hemorrhages may be found. Low-grade fever is usually present. Wound healing is delayed, and apparently healed wounds may break down. Swollen joints and follicular hyperkeratosis may develop, as well as the sicca syndrome of Sjögren.

RADIOGRAPHIC MANIFESTATIONS. The diagnosis of scurvy is usually based on radiographic changes in the long bones, especially at their distal ends and greatest in the area of the knee.

DIAGNOSIS. Diagnosis is based mainly on the characteristic clinical picture, the radiographic appearance of the long bones, and the history of poor intake of vitamin C.

DIFFERENTIAL DIAGNOSIS. The tenderness of the limbs and the pain elicited by movement have often led to a false diagnosis of arthritis or acrodynia.

PROGNOSIS. With proper treatment, recovery occurs rapidly in infants, but the swelling of the subperiosteal hemorrhage may require months to disappear.

PREVENTION. Scurvy is prevented by a diet adequate in vitamin C; citrus fruits and juices are excellent sources.

TREATMENT. Daily administration of 3–4 oz of orange juice or tomato juice quickly produces healing, but ascorbic acid is preferable. The daily therapeutic dose is 100–200 mg or more, orally or parenterally.

RICKETS OF VITAMIN D DEFICIENCY

Rickets is the term signifying a failure in mineralization of growing bone or osteoid tissue. Subsequently, if healing is not initiated, clinical manifestations appear. Failure of mature bone to mineralize is called *osteomalacia*.

ETIOLOGY. During the first third of this century, the predominant cause of rickets was nutritional deficiency of vitamin D due to inadequate direct exposure to ultraviolet rays in sunlight or to inadequate intake of vitamin D, or both.

In industrialized countries, conditions besides inadequate nutritional prophylaxis with vitamin D collectively produce most of the observed rachitic lesions. These conditions include clinical entities that interfere with the metabolic conversion and activation of vitamin D, such as hepatic and renal lesions, or that disrupt calcium and phosphorus homeostasis in other ways.

The diet of infants may contain only small amounts of vitamin D. Most marketed cow's milk is fortified with vitamin D 10 μg/qt of milk, and most commercially prepared milks for infant formulas are also fortified. Rickets and epiphyseal dysplasia are particularly likely to develop during rapid growth, such as in low-birth-weight infants and in adolescents. Darkly pigmented children are singularly susceptible to rickets.

Children with disorders such as celiac disease, steatorrhea, or cystic fibrosis may acquire rickets because of deficient absorption of vitamin D or calcium or both. Anticonvulsant therapy, as with the phenytoins or phenobarbital, may interfere in the metabolism of vitamin D.

CLINICAL MANIFESTATIONS. Osseous changes of rickets can be recognized after several months of vitamin D deficiency. In breast-fed infants whose mothers have osteomalacia, rickets may develop within 2 mo. Florid rickets appears toward the end of the 1st and during the 2nd yr of life. Later in childhood, manifest vitamin D–deficient rickets is rare. One of the early signs of rickets, craniotabes, is due to thinning of the outer table of the skull and detected by pressing firmly over the occiput or posterior parietal bones. A Ping-Pong ball sensation is felt. Palpable enlargement of the costochondral junctions (the rachitic rosary) and thickening of the wrists and ankles are other early evidences of osseous changes. Increased sweating, particularly around the head, may be present.

The softness of the skull may result in flattening and, at times, permanent asymmetry of the head. The anterior fontanel is larger than normal; its closure may be delayed until after the 2nd yr of life. The central parts of the parietal and frontal bones are often thickened, forming prominences or bosses, which give the head a boxlike appearance. Eruption of the temporary teeth may be delayed, and there may be defects of the enamel and extensive caries. The permanent teeth that are calcifying may also be affected.

Enlargement of the costochondral junctions may become prominent; the beading of the ribs is not only palpable but also visible. The sternum with its adjacent cartilage appears to be projected forward, producing the so-called pigeon breast deformity. Affected children frequently have a concomitant deformity of the pelvis, which is also retarded in growth. As the rachitic process continues, the epiphyseal enlargement at the wrists and ankles becomes more noticeable. Bending of the softened shafts of the femur, tibia, and fibula results in bowlegs or knock-knees. Greenstick fractures occur in the large bones; there are often no clinical symptoms. Deformities of the spine, pelvis, and legs result in reduced stature (rachitic dwarfism). Relaxation of ligaments helps to produce deformities and partly accounts for knock-knees, overextension of the knee joints, weak ankles, kyphosis, and scoliosis.

DIAGNOSIS. The diagnosis of rickets is based on a history of inadequate intake of vitamin D and on clinical observation; it is confirmed chemically and by radiographic examination. The serum calcium level may be normal or low, the serum phosphorus level is below 4 mg/dL, and the serum alkaline phosphatase level is elevated.

COMPLICATIONS. Respiratory infections such as bronchitis and bronchopneumonia are common in rachitic infants, and pulmonary atelectasis is frequently associated with severe deformities of the chest.

PROGNOSIS. If sufficient amounts of vitamin D are administered, healing begins within a few days and progresses slowly until the normal bony structure is restored.

PREVENTION. Rickets can be prevented by exposure to ultraviolet light or administration of vitamin D. The daily requirement of vitamin D is 10 μg or 400 IU.

TREATMENT. Natural and artificial light are effective therapeutically, but oral administration of vitamin D is preferred. Daily administration of 50–150 μg of vitamin D_3 or 0.5–2 μg of 1,25-dihydroxycholecalciferol produces healing demonstrable on radiographs within 2–4 wk, except in cases of vitamin D refractory rickets. Administering 15,000 μg of vitamin D in a single dose without further therapy for several months may be advantageous. If no healing occurs, the rickets is probably resistant to vitamin D. After healing is complete, the dose of vitamin D should be lowered to 10 μg/24 hr.

TETANY OF VITAMIN D DEFICIENCY (INFANTILE TETANY)

CHEMICAL PATHOLOGY. When the serum ionized calcium concentration falls below 3–4 mg/dL, muscular irritability occurs, apparently owing to the loss of the inhibitory control that calcium exerts on the neuromuscular junctions.

CLINICAL MANIFESTATIONS. The symptoms and signs of tetany are manifested, and rickets usually occurs concurrently. Vitamin D–deficient tetany may exist in either a latent or a clinical manifest stage.

LATENT TETANY. Symptoms are not evident, but they can be elicited by means of the Chvostek, Trousseau, and Erb procedures. The serum calcium level is less than 7–7.5 mg/dL (3–4 mg/dL ionized).

MANIFEST TETANY. Spontaneous clinical manifestations include carpopedal spasm, laryngospasm, and convulsions. The serum calcium level is well under 7 mg/dL.

DIAGNOSIS. This is based on the combined presence of rickets, low serum calcium level, and symptoms of tetany. The serum phosphorus level is usually low; the serum alkaline phosphatase level is increased.

TREATMENT. Active treatment raises the serum calcium above the tetany level. This level may be attained by administration of calcium chloride in 1–2% solution in milk. For the first 1–2 days, 4–6 g/24 hr may be given in 1-g doses, the initial dose being 2–3 g; smaller doses of 1–3 g/24 hr should then be continued for 1–2 wk. Calcium lactate may be added to milk in doses of 10–12 g/24 hr for 10 days. When oral medication is impractical, calcium gluconate (5–10 mL of a 10% solution) can be administered intravenously.

Oxygen inhalation is indicated during convulsive seizures. When intravenously administered calcium gluconate does not quickly control the attacks, sodium phenobarbital may be given intramuscularly. Prolonged attacks of laryngospasm are usually controlled by sedation and by administering calcium salts. After the acute manifestations have been controlled, vitamin D in daily doses of 50–100 μg should be started with the oral administration of calcium.

HYPERVITAMINOSIS D

Symptoms develop after 1–3 mo of large intakes of vitamin D; they include hypotonia, anorexia, irritability, constipation, polydipsia, polyuria, and pallor. Hypercalcemia and hypercalciuria are notable. Aortic valvular stenosis, vomiting, hypertension, retinopathy, and clouding of the cornea and conjunctiva occur. The urine may show proteinuria. With continued excessive intake, renal damage and metastatic calcification occur. Radiographs of the long bones reveal metastatic calcification and generalized osteopetrosis.

PREVENTION. Prevention requires careful evaluation of vitamin D dosage.

TREATMENT. This includes discontinuing vitamin D intake and decreasing the intake of calcium. For severely affected infants, aluminum hydroxide by mouth, cortisone, or sodium versenate may be used.

VITAMIN E DEFICIENCY

Deficiency may occur in malabsorption states such as cystic fibrosis and acanthocytosis. Diets in high unsaturated fatty acids increase the vitamin E requirements in premature infants. Excessive iron administration exaggerates signs of vitamin E deficiency.

CLINICAL MANIFESTATIONS. Some patients deficient in vitamin E have creatinuria, ceroid deposition in smooth muscle, focal necrosis of striated muscle, and muscle weakness. Some improvement may occur after administration of vitamin E. Patients with malabsorption and vitamin E deficiency due to biliary atresia develop a degenerative, potentially reversible, neurologic syndrome consisting of cerebellar ataxia, peripheral neuropathy, and posterior column abnormalities.

PREVENTION. Minimal daily requirements of vitamin E are not known; 7 mg/g of unsaturated fat in the diet appears adequate. Children with deficient fat absorption should take more. Large oral or parenteral doses of vitamin E may prevent permanent neurologic abnormalities in children with biliary atresia or abetalipoproteinemia.

VITAMIN K DEFICIENCY

Vitamin K is a naphthoquinone that participates in oxidative phosphorylation. Its absence or its failure to be absorbed from the intestinal tract results in hypoprothrombinemia and decreased hepatic synthesis of proconvertin.

SOURCE OF VITAMIN K. Natural-occurring vitamin K is fat soluble; it is found in high concentrations of hog's liver, soybeans, and alfalfa and in smaller amounts in some vegetables, such as spinach, tomatoes, and kale. Suppression of intestinal bacteria by various antibiotics may be responsible for vitamin K deficiency, which results in diminution of prothrombin.

CLINICAL MANIFESTATIONS. Deficiency of vitamin K or hypoprothrombinemia should be considered in all patients with a hemorrhagic disturbance. The incidence of the hemorrhagic disease of the newborn has been sharply decreased by prophylactic administration of vitamin K. In childhood, the deficiency is usually due to factors affecting absorption or utilization of fat or to factors limiting its synthesis in the intestine, such as prolonged use of antibiotics. Diarrhea in infants, particularly breast-fed ones, may cause vitamin K deficiency. Disease of the liver may lead to hypoprothrombinemia, which usually does not respond to administration of vitamin K. Hypoprothrombinemia may also result from administering certain drugs.

TREATMENT. Oral administration of vitamin K may correct mild prothrombin deficiency. One to 2 mg/24 hr for an infant usually suffices. If prothrombin deficiency is severe and hemorrhagic manifestations have appeared, 5 mg/24 hr of vitamin K should be given parenterally.

PART 7

Pathophysiology of Body Fluids and Fluid Therapy

CHAPTER 40

Water

(Nelson Textbook, Chapter 45)

Diabetes insipidus is a specific disease state caused by an inability to effectively conserve urinary water. The clinical result of excessive urinary water loss is increased concentration of extracellular fluid solute (mainly sodium), or hypernatremia. Central diabetes insipidus occurs if antidiuretic hormone (ADH) is not released into the circulation. This abnormality is produced by an interruption of the supraoptic-osmoreceptor-hypophyseal axis, preventing the release of ADH into the circulation despite appropriate physiologic stimuli, such as increases in plasma osmolality. In nephrogenic diabetes insipidus, ADH is normally released in response to plasma osmolality changes, but the renal collecting ducts fail to respond to the ADH, often because of a defect in the epithelial cell membrane receptor for ADH.

Factors altering ADH release disrupt the normal mechanisms that regulate it. ADH release may be stimulated or inhibited by emotional factors. Stressful stimuli such as pain or the mass discharge of peripheral receptors resulting from trauma, burns, or surgery increase ADH output and are important considerations in devising appropriate fluid therapy. Nicotine, prostaglandins, and cholinergic and α-adrenergic drugs are potent stimulators of ADH output. Meperidine (Demerol), morphine, and barbiturates are probably antidiuretic in this way. Alcohol is a potent inhibitor of ADH release, with a consistent dose-response relationship. Phenytoin and possibly glucocorticoids also inhibit ADH release.

Factors altering the renal response to ADH produce increased urinary excretion of water despite appropriate ADH levels. Anesthesia reduces urinary flow, probably by altering renal hemodynamics. The presence of nonabsorbable, osmotically active solutes in the renal tubular lumen (e.g., glucose in diabetes mellitus) reduces the amount of water that can diffuse into the hypertonic medulla and limits the ability of ADH to conserve water. Intrinsic renal conditions, such as urinary tract obstruction (particularly if it occurs in utero), tubular damage from nephrotoxins or tubular necrosis, and advanced renal disease, can reduce renal responsiveness to ADH.

Chapter 41

Sodium

(Nelson Textbook, Chapter 46)

Changes in serum sodium concentration in the absence of serum solids excess, such as hyperlipidemia or hyperglycemia, usually result from changes in body water or sodium, or a combination of the two. The serum sodium concentration does not necessarily reflect the status of total body sodium contents. A particular abnormality of serum sodium concentration must be understood in the context of sodium and water regulation.

HYPERNATREMIA. Hypernatremia (serum sodium > 150 mEq/L) is caused by conditions that produce an excessive gain of sodium or result in an excessive loss of body water that is greater than the loss of sodium. Hypernatremia due to an excessive gain of sodium, primary sodium excess (Table 41–1), is usually associated with iatrogenic causes. The more commonly encountered causes of hypernatremia are those related to a primary water deficit (see Table 41–1), in which the loss of total body water exceeds any loss of sodium.

TABLE 41–1 Pediatric Causes of Hypernatremia

Primary Sodium Excess

Improperly mixed formula or rehydration solution
Accidental substitution of NaCl for glucose in infant formulas
Excessive sodium bicarbonate during resuscitation
Hypernatremic enemas
Ingestion of seawater
Hypertonic saline intravenous administration
NaCl used to induce vomiting
Intentional salt poisoning (i.e., Munchausen by proxy)
High breast milk sodium

Primary Water Deficit

Diabetes insipidus
　Central
　Nephrogenic
Diabetes mellitus or other solute diuresis
Gastroenteritis (i.e., water loss greater than solute loss)
Inadequate breast-feeding
Intentional withholding of water intake
Increased insensible water loss (i.e., premature infant)
Adipsia
Inadequate access to free water

TABLE 41–2 Pediatric Causes of Hyponatremia

Sodium Deficit with Sodium Depletion

Renal Losses

Prematurity
Acute tubular necrosis, recovery phase
Diuretics
Renal salt-wasting
Mineralocorticoid deficiency
Expanded extracellular fluid
Osmotic diuresis
Renal tubular acidosis

Extrarenal Losses

Vomiting and diarrhea
Third-spacing
Burns
Nasogastric drainage
Cystic fibrosis
Excess sweating

Nutritional Deficits

WIC syndrome (i.e., inadequate oral sodium intake)
Inadequate sodium in parenteral fluids
Cerebrospinal fluid drainage
Burns
Paracentesis

Water Excess with Water Gain

Syndrome of inappropriate antidiuretic hormone secretion
Glucocorticoid deficiency
Hypothyroidism
Drugs
Excess parenteral fluid administration
Psychogenic polydipsia
Tap water enemas

Excess of Sodium and Water

Nephrotic syndrome
Cirrhosis
Cardiac failure
Acute and chronic renal failure

HYPONATREMIA. Hyponatremia (serum sodium < 130 mEq/L) is caused by conditions that create primary sodium deficits resulting in the depletion of sodium; produce a gain in total body water; or combine sodium and water abnormalities (Table 41–2).

CHAPTER 42

Potassium

(Nelson Textbook, Chapter 47)

CONSEQUENCES OF HYPERKALEMIA. The major consequences of hyperkalemia result from its neuromuscular effects. Hyperkalemia reduces transmembrane potential toward threshold levels, producing delayed depolarization, faster repolarization, and a slower conduction velocity. Paresthesias are followed by weakness and eventually by flaccid paralysis if treatment is not instituted. The heart is particularly vulnerable to hyperkalemia. The electrocardiogram typically shows peaking of the T waves. Lengthening of the PR interval and widening of the QRS complex develop later and are particularly ominous, because they often herald the development of ventricular fibrillation. Because the sequence of cardiotoxic events often progresses rapidly, hyperkalemia should be treated as a medical emergency.

CAUSES OF HYPERKALEMIA. Acute increases in potassium intake, usually through parenteral administration, may result in hyperkalemia, although it is typically transient. Because the kidney has a large capacity to excrete excess potassium and to prevent hyperkalemia, this electrolyte abnormality is most often seen when renal excretory mechanisms are impaired. It may occur in acute or chronic renal failure, in adrenal insufficiency, in hyporeninemic hypoaldosteronism, and with the use of potassium-sparing diuretics.

Sources of potassium include the potassium salts of penicillin (1.7 mEq/1 million units) and salt substitutes by patients on a salt-restricted diet. Acute tissue breakdown, such as from trauma, major surgery, burns, and cell lysis from chemotherapeutic agents, can release sufficient potassium into the extracellular fluid to cause hyperkalemia. An elevated serum potassium level may occur with transcellular redistribution of potassium, which occurs typically in metabolic acidosis and shortly before death or in severely ill patients. Certain drugs may increase the serum potassium level by similar mechanisms. Succinylcholine inhibits membrane repolarization, which requires cellular uptake of potassium. Severe digitalis overdose may cause severe hyperkalemia, presumably by inhibiting sodium-potassium exchange by cell membranes. Because intracellular levels of potassium are 30 times as high as those in the extracellular fluid, lysis of red blood cells during the collection or handling of a blood sample or release of potassium from platelets during clotting may result in pseudohyperkalemia.

CONSEQUENCES OF HYPOKALEMIA. Hypokalemia produces functional alterations in skeletal muscle, smooth muscle, and the heart. The most observable cardiac manifestations of hypokalemia are electrocardiographic changes, including a prolonged QT interval and flattened T waves. Hypokalemia also can produce serious neurologic symptoms, including autonomic insufficiency, manifested by orthostatic hypotension, tetany, and decreased neuromuscular excitability. The last results in weakness and decreased bowel motility. Weakness is an early manifestation, typically noticed first in limb muscles before trunk and respiratory muscles. Areflexia, paralysis, and death from respiratory muscle failure can develop.

Paralytic ileus and *gastric dilatation* reflect smooth muscle dysfunction. Hypokalemia affects protein metabolism and diminishes growth hormone release, contributing to the failure to thrive of children with chronic hypokalemia, most notable in Bartter syndrome. *Rhabdomyolysis* is a dramatic complication of hypokalemia.

In the kidney, potassium deficiency may result in vacuolar changes in the tubular epithelium. If sustained for a long time, it leads to *nephrosclerosis* and *interstitial fibrosis*. The kidney has a reduced ability to concentrate or dilute the urine, with polyuria and polydipsia developing. An increase in bicarbonate reabsorption and hydrogen ion secretion results in *systemic alkalosis*. External losses of potassium also result in a shift of potassium from the intracellular to the extracellular fluid. Intracellular potassium is replaced in part by hydrogen ions and by dibasic amino adds. If these changes become severe, intracellular acidosis in the renal tubular cells may result in excessive exchange of intracellular hydrogen for sodium in the distal tubular fluid, leading to aciduria, with the increased urinary excretion of ammonia, and to systemic alkalosis.

CAUSES OF HYPOKALEMIA. Abnormally low amounts of total body potassium occur in various disease states (e.g., muscular dystrophy) that are characterized by a decrease in muscle mass. These disorders are not necessarily accompanied by hypokalemia. A low serum potassium level may result from a prolonged decreased intake, from increased renal excretion, or from increased extrarenal losses. Renal losses may be increased by the use of diuretics, including osmotic diuretics and carbonic anhydrase inhibitors; by tubular defects, such as renal tubular acidosis; by acid-base disturbances; in endocrinopathies such as Cushing syndrome, primary aldosteronism, and thyrotoxicosis; and in diabetic ketoacidosis, Bartter syndrome, and magnesium deficiency.

Extrarenal losses may osccur from the bowel (e.g., diarrhea, chronic catharsis, frequent enemas, protracted vomiting, biliary drainage, enterocutaneous fistulas) or from the skin if there is profuse sweating. Movement of potassium into cells during correction of a metabolic acidosis, for example, may also result in hypokalemia, as may familial hypokalemic periodic paralysis, a rare disorder in which episodes of paralysis are usually accompanied by an abrupt and marked hypokalemia caused by movement of potassium into an extravascular body compartment. A urine concentration of 15 mEq/L or less indicates renal conservation of potassium and suggests that the loss occurred from a nonrenal source.

CHAPTER 43

Chloride

(Nelson Textbook, Chapter 48)

Hypochloremia and hyperchloremia are usually associated with comparable degrees of hyponatremia and hypernatremia, respectively, and are seen most often in patients with dehydration secondary to diarrhea.

HYPOCHLOREMIA. Hypochloremia is typically seen in metabolic alkalosis. Chloride depletion as a cause of metabolic alkalosis occurs when chloride is lost from the body in excess of sodium losses. Examples include a loss from the bowel with vomiting or gastric drainage or in chloride diarrhea, and sweat loss in cystic fibrosis.

Administering chloride is necessary to correct most cases of metabolic alkalosis whether or not the disorder is associated with potassium deficiency. In cases of potassium deficiency, both potassium and chloride must be given before the potassium deficits can be corrected. Treating patients with metabolic alkalosis with potassium or sodium chloride, as appropriate, results in the prompt excretion of bicarbonate into the urine and correction of the alkalosis. Hypochloremia also results from a protracted, inadequate intake of chloride. Infants fed a chloride-deficient milk formula for several months have developed chronic depletion of body chloride, severe hypochloremia (serum sodium levels usually remained normal), severe hypokalemic metabolic alkalosis, loss of appetite, failure to thrive, muscle weakness, and lethargy. Although adding chloride to the diet quickly reverses the electrolyte abnormalities, long-term sequelae may develop, including disturbed behavioral patterns.

HYPERCHLOREMIA. Hyperchloremia may result when chloride is conserved by the kidney in excess of sodium and potassium or when alkaline urine is formed during the renal correction of alkalosis. An increased fractional reabsorption of chloride in the renal proximal tubule in distal renal tubular acidosis also results in hyperchloremia. Hyperchloremia may occur when large amounts of parenteral fluids containing chloride, such as normal saline and lactated Ringer's solution, are administered during acute fluid resuscitation.

ANION GAP. The concentration of the most abundant serum cation (i.e., sodium) is greater than the sum of the two most abundant serum anions (i.e., chloride and bicarbonate). The difference is referred to as the anion gap:

$$\text{Anion gap} = [\text{Na}] - ([\text{HCO}_3] + [\text{Cl}]).$$

It is normally about 12 mEq/L (range, 8–16 mEq/L). The anion gap results from the effect of the combined concentrations of the unmeasured anions, such as phosphate, sulfate, proteins, and organic acids, which exceed those of the unmeasured cations, primarily potassium, calcium, and magnesium. An abnormal condition in which a *normal anion* gap exists is the metabolic acidosis due to renal tubular acidosis or stool losses of bicarbonate.

An *increased anion gap* in renal failure is a result of increased concentrations of phosphate and sulfate; in diabetic ketoacidosis, to 3-hydroxybutyrate and acetoacetate; in lactic acidosis, to lactate; in hyperglycemic nonketotic coma, to unidentified organic acids; and in disorders of amino acid metabolism, to various organic acids. Increased anion gap also follows the administration of large amounts of penicillin. After ethylene glycol ingestion, it is caused by glycolate production; after methanol ingestion, by formate production; and after salicylate poisoning, by the salicylate anion and various organic anions secondary to the uncoupling of oxidative phosphorylation. A *decreased anion gap* occurs less frequently. It may be found in nephrotic syndrome, in which it is caused by a decreased serum concentration of albumin.

CHAPTER 44

Calcium

(Nelson Textbook, Chapter 49)

Symptomatic *hypocalcemia* may be caused by a low concentration of ionized calcium resulting from vitamin D deficiency, which is caused by nutritional deficiency, malabsorption, or abnormal metabolism of vitamin D. Hypocalcemia may also be a result of hypoparathyroidism, pseudohypoparathyroidism, hyperphosphatemia, magnesium deficiency, and acute pancreatitis. Because acidosis increases and alkalosis decreases the proportion of calcium that is ionized, symptomatic hypocalcemia may occur during rapid correction or overcorrection of acidosis or with alkalosis. The neonate is particularly susceptible to hypocalcemia associated with hypoparathyroidism, abnormal vitamin D metabolism, a low calcium intake, or a high phosphate intake.

The causes of *hypercalcermia* include primary or tertiary hyperparathyroidism, hyperthyroidism, vitamin D intoxication, immobilization, malignancies (especially those that metastasize to bone), use of thiazide diuretics, excessive calcium in total paren-teral nutrition fluid, milk-alkali syndrome, and sarcoidosis. An idiopathic form may occur in infancy associated with typical elfin facies and supravalvular aortic stenosis; this Williams syndrome may be caused by hypersensitivity to vitamin D. If their dietary intake of phosphorus is inadequate, low-birth-weight infants may develop hypercalcemia as a result of resorption of phosphorus and calcium from bone.

CHAPTER 45

Magnesium
(Nelson Textbook, Chapter 50)

HYPOMAGNESEMIA. Hypomagnesemia occurs in various clinical states, including malabsorption syndromes, hypoparathyroidism, diuretic therapy, hypercalcemia, renal tubular acidosis, primary aldosteronism, alcoholism, and prolonged intravenous fluid ther-apy with magnesium-free fluids. Nephrotoxic agents may produce hypomagnesemia through increased urinary losses. Infants with early or late neonatal tetany also often have hypomagnesemia. When associated with early neonatal tetany, hypomagnesemia tends to be mild and transient and may not require treatment with magnesium. In late neonatal tetany, hypocalcemia may fail to respond to treatment until magnesium levels have been re-turned to normal. The symptoms of hypomagnesemia are primar-ily those of increased neuromuscular irritability and include tet-any, severe seizures, and tremors. Personality changes, nausea, anorexia, abnormal cardiac rhythms, and electrocardiographic changes may also be seen.

HYPERMAGNESEMIA. Hypermagnesemia, which is an increase in total body magnesium, rarely occurs in the absence of decreased renal function. The usual sources of a magnesium load include magnesium-containing laxatives, enemas, intravenous fluids, and magnesium-containing antacids used as phosphate binders in pa-tients with chronic renal failure. Severe hypermagnesemia may occur in neonates born of mothers who were treated with intra-muscular injections of magnesium sulfate for the hypertension of pre-eclampsia. There is also an increased incidence of hypermag-nesemia in patients with Addison disease.

The symptoms of hypermagnesemia occur when magnesium levels exceed 5 mg/dL. Hyporeflexia antedates respiratory depres-sion, drowsiness, and coma. Manifestations are rapidly reversed by intravenous administration of calcium. Coma and death usu-ally occur when the serum magnesium level increases above 15 mg/dL.

CHAPTER 46

Phosphorus

(Nelson Textbook, Chapter 51)

HYPERPHOSPHATEMIA. Hyperphosphatemia is characteristic of hypoparathyroidism but rarely occurs in the absence of renal insufficiency. Hyperphosphatemia may also result from the excessive administration of phosphate by oral or intravenous routes or of phosphate-containing enemas. Using cytotoxic drugs to treat malignancies, especially lymphomas or leukemias, results in cytolysis, with hyperphosphatemia caused by the release of phosphate into the circulation. The major clinical consequences of hyperphosphatemia are symptoms of the resulting hypocalcemia.

HYPOPHOSPHATEMIA. Hypophosphatemia may result from the phosphate deficiency associated with starvation, protein-calorie malnutrition, and malabsorption syndromes. It may result from intracellular shifts of phosphate, such as those that occur with respiratory or metabolic alkalosis, during the treatment of diabetic ketoacidosis (typically during the first 24 hr), and after the administration of corticosteroids. Increased urinary losses of phosphate may be sufficiently severe to reduce the plasma concentration; this reduction is observed in primary and tertiary hyperparathyroidism, in renal tubular defects, after extracellular fluid volume expansion, or after the administration of diuretics. A combination of pathophysiologic mechanisms often is responsible for the hypophosphatemia.

The very-low-birth-weight infant requires a high phosphorus intake at the time of rapid postnatal growth. Inadequate intake results in phosphorus depletion and hypophosphatemia. Insufficient phosphorus intake occurs particularly in patients receiving total parenteral nutrition when the physician fails to recognize the need to achieve relatively higher levels of serum phosphorus in premature infants. Bone demineralization, hypercalcemia, and calciuria may occur.

In most instances, hypophosphatemia is mild or moderate and asymptomatic. Occasionally, plasma phosphate concentrations may fall to very low levels (<0.3 mM/L [>1.0 mg/dL]). Such low levels have been observed with the prolonged use of intravenous alimentation without phosphate supplements and may produce a very severe, well-defined syndrome. Red cell concentrations of 2,3-diphosphoglycerate and adenosine triphosphate are decreased. The resultant decreased release of oxygen by the red blood cells produces tissue anoxia. Increased hemolysis may occur, as may leukocyte and platelet dysfunction. Some patients display the symptoms of a metabolic encephalopathy, including irritability, paresthesias, confusion, seizures, and coma; some may develop abnormalities revealed by the electroencephalogram. Hypercalcemia (thought to result from the increased release of calcium from bone), rhabdomyolysis, cardiopathy, and possibly hepatocellular dysfunction also have been reported. Renal tubular defects may occur, and the kidney's ability to excrete hydrogen ions is impaired. Promptly recognizing and treating this syndrome, preferably by oral administration of phosphate salts, is beneficial, but permanent defects may result.

CHAPTER 47

Hydrogen Ion
(Nelson Textbook, Chapter 52)

TERMINOLOGY. An acid is a proton (i.e., hydrogen ion) donor. Hydrochloric, sulfuric, phosphoric, and carbonic acids are conventional acids, each dissociating to liberate protons. A strong acid is one that is highly dissociated and therefore produces a high concentration of hydrogen ions; a weak acid is one that is poorly dissociated. A base is a hydrogen ion acceptor. Bases bind free hydrogen ions, reducing their concentration. Examples include hydroxyl ions, ammonia, and the anions of weak acids. A buffer is defined as a substance that reduces the change in free hydrogen ion concentration of a solution on the addition of an acid or base. The presence of a buffer in a solution increases the amount of acid or alkali that must be added to cause a change in pH. The addition of a strong acid to any of these buffer systems produces a neutral salt and a weak acid.

DISTURBANCES OF ACID-BASE BALANCE

Definitions. Abnormalities in blood pH occur when the hydrogen ion concentration increases above normal, called acidemia, or decreases below normal, called alkalemia. The suffix "-emia" refers to changes in blood pH. The abnormal clinical processes that cause acid or alkali to accumulate are called acidosis and alkalosis, respectively.

Metabolic Acidosis. This results from an alteration in the balance between production and excretion of acid. Systemic acidosis may result from increased blood hydrogen ion concentration due to accumulation caused by increased intake from an exogenous source or increased endogenous production or by inadequate excretion of hydrogen ions or excessive loss of bicarbonate in the urine or stools. Rapid expansion of the extracellular fluid (ECF) space by a bicarbonate-free solution may also produce metabolic acidosis by diluting the bicarbonate in the ECF. The hydrogen ion load is buffered initially by bicarbonate in the ECF and by intracellular buffers such as hemoglobin and phosphate.

The resulting systemic acidosis and increased Pco_2 stimulate the respiratory center (and possibly peripheral chemoreceptors in the carotid artery and aorta) to increase the respiratory rate, which increases the rate of excretion of CO_2. Plasma P_{CO_2} and H_2CO_3 levels fall, partially or almost totally correcting the acidosis but at the expense of lowering both plasma bicarbonate and P_{CO_2}. The blood pH is decreased but rarely drops as low as might be predicted from the low level of plasma bicarbonate.

The acidosis also stimulates the kidneys to increase ammonia production and hydrogen ion excretion into the urine. In the distal nephron, the secretion of hydrogen ion is accompanied by the return of a bicarbonate to the circulation, increasing the generation of bicarbonate and returning the plasma bicarbonate level to normal if the primary disease process has been alleviated. The respiratory rate subsequently decreases, with the P_{CO_2} returning to normal.

The clinical manifestations of metabolic acidosis are often nonspecific. The most important physical sign is hyperventilation, the extreme of which is the deep, rapid respirations (i.e., Kussmaul breathing) needed for respiratory compensation. However, severe acidosis itself may cause a decrease in peripheral vascular resistance and cardiac ventricular function, resulting in hypotension, pulmonary edema, and tissue hypoxia. The laboratory findings are decreased serum pH and decreased levels of HCO_3, and P_{CO_2}. In general, metabolic acidosis associated with an elevated anion gap results from overproduction of endogenous acids, such as ketoacids in diabetic ketoacidosis or lactic acidosis; underexcretion of fixed acids with advanced renal failure; or the ingestion of excess exogenous acids, such as salicylates. A normal anion gap (i.e., hyperchloremic) results from the net loss of bicarbonate from the kidneys (e.g., renal tubular acidosis, nephrotoxin related) or the gastrointestinal tract, mainly from diarrhea.

RENAL CAUSES. The renal causes of metabolic acidosis are numerous. Diseases involving the proximal tubules may limit the ability of this segment of the nephron to secrete hydrogen ions and cause incomplete bicarbonate reabsorption. In distal renal tubular acidosis, the distal tubule cannot maintain a normal hydrogen ion gradient to promote hydrogen ion secretion into the distal tubular lumen. With chronic renal insufficiency, acidification mechanisms work normally or at supranormal rates. However, the reduced tubular mass limits the ability of the kidneys to generate sufficient ammonia and to excrete adequate amounts of hydrogen ions.

OTHER CAUSES. Metabolic acidosis may also develop in diabetic ketoacidosis from incomplete metabolism of body lipids and catabolism of body protein, accompanied by the production of large amounts of acetoacetic, 3-hydroxybutyric, phosphoric, and sulfuric acids. In salicylism, metabolic acidosis results from hydrogen ions derived from salicylic acid and from the uncoupling of oxidative phosphorylation by salicylate. In severe diarrhea, the increased losses of bicarbonate in diarrheal fluid and possibly the formation of organic acids from the incomplete breakdown of carbohydrate in the stools result in metabolic acidosis.

Metabolic Alkalosis. Three basic mechanisms may produce alkalosis: excessive loss of hydrogen ion, as in prolonged gastric aspiration or persistent vomiting associated with pyloric stenosis; increased addition of bicarbonate to the ECF, which may result from excessive administration by the parenteral route or by oral intake, as in the milk-alkali syndrome, or from increased renal reabsorption of bicarbonate caused by profound potassium depletion, primary hyperaldosteronism, Cushing syndrome, Bartter syndrome, or excessive intake of licorice; and contraction of the ECF volume, which increases bicarbonate concentration in this fluid space and increases bicarbonate reabsorption in the proximal tubule.

Respiration may be depressed with some increase in plasma P_{CO_2}, but this response is limited by increasing hypoxia so that respiratory compensation is always incomplete and never restores the pH to normal. The renal threshold for bicarbonate is exceeded, and bicarbonate appears in the urine, which may have a pH as high as 8.5–9.0.

The diagnosis of metabolic alkalosis should be considered in any patient with an appropriate history; there are no pathognomonic clinical manifestations of this electrolyte disturbance. Patients may have cramps or feel weak and may have the signs of tetany if ionized calcium has been reduced by the alkalosis.

Characteristically, the pH, plasma bicarbonate level, and P_{CO_2} of arterial blood are elevated. Hypochloremia and hypokalemia are usually present. Classically, the urine pH is alkaline, but in the case of severe depletion of potassium, the urinary potassium level is low and paradoxical aciduria exists.

Respiratory Acidosis. Inadequate pulmonary excretion of CO_2, in the case of normal production of this gas, produces acidosis. It may occur acutely in neuromuscular disorders, such as brain stem injury, Guillain-Barré syndrome, or sedative overdose; in airway obstruction, such as that caused by a foreign body, severe bronchospasm, or laryngeal edema; in vascular diseases, such as massive pulmonary embolism; and in other conditions, such as pneumothorax, pulmonary edema, or severe pneumonia. Chronic respiratory acidosis may accompany the pickwickian syndrome, poliomyelitis, chronic obstructive airway disease, kyphoscoliosis, or chronic administration of sedatives.

In any of the disease states causing respiratory acidosis, the level of P_{CO_2} increases until it is elevated sufficiently to cause pulmonary excretion of CO_2 equal to its production. Although a new steady state is reached, the increase in P_{CO_2} (i.e., hypercapnia) causes a systemic acidosis by increasing serum concentrations of H_2CO_3 and, therefore, of hydrogen ions.

The rise in P_{CO_2} must be buffered initially by the nonbicarbonate buffers—the proteins in the ECF and phosphate, hemoglobin, other proteins, and lactate in the cells. The acidosis and increased P_{CO_2} stimulate the kidneys to increase hydrogen ion excretion as ammonium and titratable acid and to generate and reabsorb more bicarbonate; the plasma bicarbonate levels may be increased somewhat above normal.

The causes of acute respiratory acidosis are often associated with hypoxemia, which usually dominates the clinical manifestations, along with the signs of respiratory distress. Hypercapnia results in vasodilatation and increased cerebral blood flow and may be responsible for the headaches and raised intracranial pressure sometimes found in these patients.

Respiratory Alkalosis. Excessive pulmonary losses of CO_2 in the presence of normal production result in a fall in P_{CO_2} and produce respiratory alkalosis. This process may be observed with hyperventilation of psychogenic origin, with overventilation from mechanically assisted ventilation, and in the early stages of salicylate overdose as a result of stimulation of the respiratory center by salicylate or of increased sensitivity of the respiratory center to P_{CO_2}. Plasma P_{CO_2} falls, and pH rises.

The clinical manifestations are usually those of the underlying disease process. However, acute hypercapnia may result in neuromuscular irritability and paresthesias in the extremities and periorally because of a decrease in the concentration of ionized calcium. Arterial pH is elevated, and the P_{CO_2} and plasma bicarbonate levels are decreased.

Mixed Disorders. Under certain circumstances, mixed disturbances may occur; in these, more than a single primary cause is responsible for the abnormal acid-base balance.

CHAPTER 48

Fluid Therapy

(Nelson Textbook, Chapter 53)

Parenteral or oral fluid therapy is employed to maintain or restore the normal volume and composition of body fluids. It should be administered in a safe and efficient manner that maximizes the corrective capability of normal physiologic mechanisms within the body.

DETERMINATION OF REQUIREMENTS. Fluid therapy consists of three categories: maintenance, deficit replacement, and supplemental replacement of ongoing losses.

MAINTENANCE THERAPY. Maintenance fluid and electrolyte requirements are directly related to metabolic rate. Changes in

TABLE 48–1 Simplified Method for Calculating Maintenance Fluid Requirements from Body Weight (based on 100 mL for each 100 kcal expended)

Body Weight (kg)	mL/day*
Up to 10	100 mL/kg
11–20	1000 mL + 50 mL/kg for each kg above 10 kg
Above 20	1500 mL + 20 mL/kg for each kg above 20 kg

*Maintenance fluid and electrolytes: 100 mL water (35 mL insensible water loss, 65 mL urinary water loss) and 2–4 mEq of Na and K for every 100 calories expended.

metabolic rate affect endogenous water production through the oxidation of carbohydrate, fats, and protein; urinary solute excretion, which influences urinary fluid losses; and heat production, 25% of which must be dissipated through the mechanism of insensible water loss. The simplified scheme by Holliday and Segar (Table 48–1) that relates caloric expenditure to body weight for a resting, hospitalized patient is easy to use, physiologic, and applicable over the range of pediatric and adult weights.

Because fecal water losses are usually negligible, fluid requirements of 100 mL/100 calories primarily address insensible and renal water losses. Approximately one third of this water requirement is for insensible water loss, and two thirds are for renal water loss. Insensible water loss occurs through pulmonary and cutaneous routes, with the latter accounting for two thirds and the former for one third of insensible water loss. Conditions that may increase or decrease insensible water loss requirements are associated with changes in caloric expenditure, heat production, and the need for changes in insensible water loss to modulate dissipation of body heat. Insensible water loss increases with increased activity (<30%), with fever (i.e., 12% increase for each 1°C rise in body temperature), and with reduced vapor tension in the environment. Conversely, insensible water loss decreases with decreased activity, as in comatose states, and with hypothermia, by 12% for every 1°C fall in body temperature. Pulmonary insensible water loss increases with hyperventilation, as in asthma or diabetic ketoacidosis, and decreases with exposure to highly humidified atmospheres or humidified ventilator systems. Cutaneous losses may be especially high in the low-birth-weight and very-low-birth-weight infant with a large surface area and decreased skin thickness.

Urinary water requirements may be increased when renal concentrating ability is diminished by an increased solute load or by diminished secretion of or response to antidiuretic hormone. The solute load may be increased in diabetes mellitus, after the infusion of mannitol or radiocontrast agents, in electrolyte wasting, or by high-protein diets. Urinary water losses are diminished in conditions associated with oligoanuria, such as the syndrome of inappropriate antidiuretic hormone secretion, acute or chronic renal failure, or genitourinary tract obstruction. If urinary water loss is abnormal, maintenance fluid therapy should be adjusted accordingly by replacing insensible water loss plus urinary output on a milliliter for milliliter basis with free water.

Maintenance requirements for sodium and potassium may also be modified for certain patients. Sodium requirements may be higher in patients with increased cutaneous losses from cystic fibrosis; in patients with increased urinary losses from salt-losing nephritis, obstructive uropathy, chronic pyelonephritis, or diuretic therapy; and in patients with increased gastrointestinal losses from fistulas, diversions, nasogastric drainage, or inflammatory bowel disease. Sodium requirements are diminished in edematous states owing to hepatic, cardiac, or renal disease; edema indicates excess body sodium.

Maintenance potassium requirements may also be higher in patients with ongoing abnormal gastrointestinal or genitourinary losses. Potassium-losing states generally parallel sodium-losing states and may occur with chronic renal disease associated with renal medullary injury, with gastric or intestinal drainage, and with chronic laxative or diuretic abuse. Increased renal potassium loss accompanies the alkalosis associated with gastric drainage and loss of hydrochloric acid. In conditions of diminished potassium-excreting ability, such as chronic renal failure and adrenal insufficiency, potassium intake may have to be modified. In cases of acute anuric renal failure, adrenal insufficiency, or severe acidosis with hyperkalemia, no potassium should be administered. Further maintenance requirements are created by internal shifts of body fluid. In certain clinical situations, third spacing, the shift of extracellular fluid from the plasma compartment elsewhere, such as interstitial or transcellular spaces, may necessitate changes in the provision of fluid and electrolytes.

Maintenance fluid and electrolytes may be given orally or parenterally. A 5% dextrose solution usually provides enough calories to have some sparing effect on catabolism of protein, but for patients with diminished glycogen and fat storage or those in highly catabolic states, this amount of dextrose may be calorically insufficient. In these patients and in those on parenteral therapy for more than a few days, additional nutrition is provided by parenteral alimentation with 5% or higher dextrose solutions, with or without the addition of amino acids, or by the use of total parenteral nutrition.

DEFICIT THERAPY. Deficits in fluid and electrolytes (Table 48–2) represent the cumulative net impact of oral or parenteral dietary intake, pathologic body losses resulting from disease processes, or physiologic body losses including corrective attempts to modify

TABLE 48–2 Estimated Deficits of Water and Electrolytes in Infants with Moderately Severe Dehydration

Condition	H₂O (mL)*	Na (mEq)	K (mEq)†	Cl (mEq)
Fasting and thirsting	100–120	5–7	1–2	4–6
Diarrhea				
Isonatremic	100–120	8–10	8–10	8–10
Hypernatremic	100–120	2–4	0–4	−2 to −6‡
Hyponatremic	100–120	10–12	8–10	10–12
Pyloric stenosis	100–120	8–10	10–12	10–12
Diabetic acidosis	100–120	8–10	5–7	6–8

*All estimated deficits are per kilogram of body weight.
†Converted for breakdown of tissue cells: −1 g of N = 3 mEq of K.
‡Negative balance of chloride indicates an excess at the beginning of therapy.

the volume and composition of losses through normal excretory routes.

Severity of Deficit. The severity of fluid deficit is represented as a percentage of body weight lost (Table 48–3). In older children and adults, total body water is a smaller percentage of body weight; mild, moderate, and severe dehydration represent 5%, 7%, and 10%, respectively, of body weight lost.

The type of dehydration (Table 48–4) is a reflection of the relative net losses of water and electrolytes and is based on serum sodium concentration or plasma osmolality. Hypertonic dehydration may occur with serum sodium levels less than 150 mEq/L in the presence of other abnormal osmol levels, such as glucose in diabetic ketoacidosis or mannitol.

Changes in the osmolality in one compartment lead to compensatory shifts in water, which is freely diffusible across cell membranes, from one compartment to the other, to restore equality of osmolality between body water compartments. In *isotonic* or *isonatremic* dehydration, no osmotic gradient across cell walls exists and intracellular fluid volume remains unchanged. In *hypotonic* or *hyponatremic* dehydration, the extracellular fluid is hypotonic relative to the intracellular fluid, and water shifts from the extracellular to the intracellular compartments. Volume depletion through external losses in this form of dehydration is exacerbated by an internal shift of extracellular fluid to the intracellular compartment. The resultant marked decrease in extracellular volume may be manifested clinically as profound dehydration leading to circulatory collapse. In patients with *hypertonic* or *hypernatremic* dehydration, the converse occurs; water shifts from the intracellular space to the extracellular space to restore equality of osmolality between compartments.

A careful history can provide information for estimating the magnitude and type of deficit. Careful attention must be paid

TABLE 48–3 Clinical Assessment of Severity of Dehydration

Signs and Symptoms	Mild Dehydration	Moderate Dehydration	Severe Dehydration
Body weight loss (%)	3–5%	6–9%	10% or more
General appearance and condition; infants and young children	Alert, restless	Thirsty, restless or lethargic, irritable to touch	Lethargic or comatose; limp, cold, sweaty, cyanotic; poor peripheral perfusion
Older children and adults	Thirsty, alert, restless	Thirsty, alert, postural hypotension	Usually conscious; apprehensive; cold, sweaty, cyanotic; wrinkled skin of fingers and toes; muscle cramps
Radial pulse	Normal rate and strength	Rapid and weak	Rapid, feeble, sometimes impalpable
Respiration	Normal	Deep, may be rapid	Deep and rapid
Anterior fontanel	Normal	Sunken	Very sunken
Systolic blood pressure	Normal	Normal or low; orthostatic hypotension	Low, may be unrecordable
Skin elasticity	Pinch retracts immediately	Pinch retracts slowly	Pinch retracts very slowly
Eyes	Normal	Sunken	Grossly sunken
Tears	Present	Absent to reduced	Absent
Mucous membranes	Moist	Dry	Very dry
Urine flow	Normal	Reduced amount and dark	Anuria/severe oliguria
Capillary refill	Normal	± 2 sec	>3 sec
Estimated fluid deficit (mL/kg)	30–50	60–90	100 or more

TABLE 48–4 Dehydration and Serum Sodium Concentration

Type of Dehydration	Electrolyte Status
Hypotonic or hyponatremic	Serum Na <130 mEq/L
Isotonic or isonatremic	Serum Na 130–150 mEq/L
Hypertonic or hypernatremic	Serum Na >150 mEq/L

to the types and quantities of fluid intake and output, to any documented changes in body weight or in the frequency and appearance of urine, and to the general appearance and behavior of the child.

CLINICAL MANIFESTATIONS. Table 48–3 summarizes the physical findings in children with mild, moderate, and severe dehydration. Laboratory tests can be useful in evaluating the nature and extent of dehydration and in guiding therapy, but they cannot substitute for careful bedside observation of the patient. Identifying hemoconcentration, indicated by elevated hemoglobin, hematocrit, and plasma proteins, may help in estimating the severity of dehydration and in monitoring the response to rehydration. Serum sodium concentration defines the type of dehydration and reflects the relative losses of water and electrolytes, not of total body sodium stores. Serum potassium values are usually normal or elevated in diarrheal dehydration. Hyperkalemia may be related to acidosis or diminished renal function. Hypokalemia may occur with significant stool losses; with gastric losses associated with alkalosis, as in pyloric stenosis; or with acute intracellular shifts in potassium with the administration of glucose or alkali. Serum bicarbonate concentrations are helpful in detecting metabolic acidosis or alkalosis. Blood urea nitrogen and serum creatinine levels may be elevated in severe dehydration because of a decreased glomerular filtration rate.

CHAPTER 49

Principles of Therapy
(Nelson Textbook, Chapter 54)

In patients with profound dehydration, intravenous fluid should be administered on an emergent basis, even before a complete evaluation of the patient is undertaken. In less urgent situations, before administration of fluids the patient should be evaluated clinically and the type and quantity of fluids calculated.

Oral rehydration therapy is usually successful in patients with mild to moderate dehydration. Such therapy requires both the close and consistent attention of a caregiver and patient compliance.

TRADITIONAL FLUID THERAPY. Parenteral therapy is indicated for patients with severe dehydration and those who refuse oral intake or have persistent vomiting. Although the intravenous route is preferable for parenteral therapy, in unusual situations ample fluids may be given intraperitoneally or intraosseously.

Initial Therapy. The goal of initial therapy is to expand extracellular fluid volume, especially plasma volume, rapidly to prevent or treat shock (Table 49–1). Isotonic saline (i.e., 0.9%; sodium and chloride, both 154 mEq/L) containing glucose (5 g/dL) is useful, especially in a dehydrated patient with metabolic alkalosis. In patients with severe metabolic acidosis, the acidosis may be worsened with the additional chloride load and by dilution of serum bicarbonate levels. In this situation, an isotonic solution in which some chloride is replaced by bicarbonate (e.g., containing 140 mEq/L of sodium, 115 mEq/L of chloride, 25 mEq/L of bicarbonate) may be used.

In the initial phase, 20–40 mL/kg of isotonic solution should be given by rapid bolus and *repeated* a second or, occasionally, a third time, until the patient is hemodynamically stable. At this time, laboratory values are usually available and the physician can proceed with a logical and well-planned approach. This initial therapy applies to all forms of dehydration: hypernatremic, hyponatremic, or isotonic. The physician must never initially rehydrate a patient with hypotonic solution. Potassium is usually withheld from intravenous fluids unless the patient is hypokalemic or renal function is well established. In desperate situations in which electrolyte solutions are unavailable, pure plasma expansion is needed, and a severe coexisting anemia complicates the patient's clinical condition, blood may be used in the amount of 10 mL/kg.

Subsequent Therapy. The subsequent phase of therapy is devoted to continued replacement of existing deficit, provision of maintenance fluid and electrolytes, and replacement of ongoing losses. It is possible to calculate over 8-hr intervals (see Table 49–1) the water and sodium requirements for deficit, maintenance, and ongoing losses and arrive at a volume and composition of replacement fluid to be used.

Total-body potassium deficits are not fully restored to normal until the patient is on oral feedings or, in cases of protracted parenteral therapy, on total parenteral nutrition. Large amounts of parenterally provided potassium can lead to hyperkalemia, which may have serious cardiac sequelae. Potassium is usually not provided unless the patient has voided and demonstrated acceptable renal function.

CORRECTION OF DEFICITS

Isonatremic Dehydration. Table 49–1 indicates approaches to treatment and estimations of the range of sodium deficit in a child

TABLE 49-1 Treatment of 10% Isotonic Dehydration in a 10-kg Infant during the First 24 Hours

Hours	First 8 Hours		Second 8 Hours		Third 8 Hours	
	Water (mL)	Sodium (mEq/L)	Water (mL)	Sodium (mEq/L)	Water (mL)	Sodium (mEq/L)
Deficit	500	70	250	35	250	35
Isotonic boluses	−250	−35				
Maintenance	333	10	333	10	333	10
Ongoing losses	150	7	150	7	150	7
Total loss	733	52	733	52	733	52
Electrolyte* solution	1,000	70	1,000	70	1,000	70

*Approximate electrolyte solution for each 8-hr period is one-half isotonic (after isotonic boluses are given).

with moderate to severe dehydration. Full repletion of deficit is calculated over 24 hr, with one half provided in the first 6–8 hr of therapy. Initial rehydration with fluid boluses is subtracted from the totals for the first 8-hr period. Some experts propose replacement of deficit in 8–12 hr if patients are not hypernatremic. Maintenance requirements exist on an hourly basis and must be met regardless of the deficit and ongoing losses. Ongoing losses represent estimates of continued pathologic losses. The patient must be observed carefully, because losses may be less than or more than expected; not recognizing the latter may lead to serious delays in restoration of the extracellular fluid volume.

Hyponatremic Dehydration. Relatively greater losses of sodium than of water produce hyponatremic dehydration. The extra sodium loss can be calculated from the formula:

$$\text{Sodium deficit [mEq]} = (\text{Desired } S_{Na} - \text{Actual } S_{Na}) \times \text{Total body water [in L] } (0.6 \times \text{weight in kg})$$

in which Actual S_{Na} represents the measured serum sodium concentration and Desired S_{Na} is the targeted serum sodium.

Treatment of hyponatremic dehydration is similar to that for isonatremic dehydration except that the extra losses of sodium should be taken into account when calculating electrolyte administration. Hyponatremia, with emergent symptoms, such as seizures, is usually treated by intravenous administration of a 3% solution of sodium chloride at a rate of 1 mL/min to a maximum of 12 mL/kg of body weight.

Hypernatremic Dehydration. Fluid therapy for hypernatremic dehydration can be difficult, because severe hyperosmolality may result in cerebral damage with widespread cerebral hemorrhages, thromboses, and subdural effusions. This cerebral injury may result in permanent neurologic deficit. Even in the absence of obvious pathologic lesions, patients with severe hypernatremia are vulnerable to seizures. Frequently, seizures occur during treatment as the serum sodium is returning to normal. The incidence of such complications may be reduced by correcting dehydration and hypernatremia slowly over a period of days. Therapy is adjusted to return the serum sodium levels toward normal by not more than 10 mEq/L/24 hr. A suitable regimen is a 5% dextrose solution containing 25 mEq/L of sodium as a combination of the bicarbonate and chloride. Others have suggested 40 mEq/L of sodium and 40 mEq/L of potassium. Hypocalcemia occasionally occurs during treatment of hypernatremic dehydration and may require intravenous administration of calcium.

SUPPLEMENTAL FLUIDS. These are mainly needed to replace ongoing losses from diarrhea or from procedures such as nasogastric drainage.

NUTRITIONAL DEFICIENCIES. Although parenteral fluid therapy results in a caloric intake inadequate to meet the patient's needs, this is rarely a cause for concern because of the short duration of therapy.

CHAPTER 50

Fluid and Electrolyte Treatment of Specific Disorders

(Nelson Textbook, Chapter 55)

ACUTE DIARRHEA AND ORAL REHYDRATION

The administration of intravenous fluids for treating profound dehydration from severe diarrhea is discussed in Chapter 49. Mild to moderate dehydration from diarrhea of any cause can be treated very effectively in a wide range of age groups using a simple, oral glucose-electrolyte solution. Oral rehydration is used in many countries and has significantly reduced the morbidity and mortality from acute diarrhea and lessened diarrhea-associated malnutrition. Intravenous therapy may still be required for patients with severe dehydration in shock; those with uncontrollable vomiting; those unable to drink because of extreme fatigue, stupor, or coma; or those with gastric or intestinal distention.

As a guideline for oral rehydration, 50 mL/kg of the oral rehydration solution (ORS) should be given within 4 hr to patients with mild dehydration and 100 mL/kg over 4 hr to those with moderate dehydration. The amounts and rates should be increased if the patient continues to have diarrhea or if rehydration does not appear complete; fluids should be decreased if the patient appears fully hydrated earlier than expected or develops periorbital edema.

When rehydration is complete, maintenance therapy should be started. Patients with mild diarrhea usually can then be treated at home using 100 mL of ORS/kg/24 hr until the diarrhea stops. Breast-feeding or supplemental water intake should be maintained. Patients with more severe diarrhea require continued supervision. The volume of ORS ingested should equal the volume of stool losses. If stool volume cannot be measured, an intake of 10–15 mL of ORS/kg/hr is appropriate. Regimens for treating acute diarrhea, including that recommended by the American Academy of Pediatrics, now encourage continued oral intake of nutrients.

In patients treated with intravenous therapy, oral feeding of one of the carbohydrate and electrolyte mixtures may be initiated shortly after rehydration if gastric distention and vomiting are absent. As soon as oral feeding is tolerated the caloric intake may be increased gradually by substituting mixtures that also contain fat and protein until the usual dietary intake is attained, usually within 7–8 days. Drugs such as opiates, which inhibit peristaltic activity of the bowel; absorbents such as kaolin or pectin; or bismuth subsalicylate, which alters secretion, have little or no effect on the course of infantile diarrhea and are not recommended.

Diarrhea in Chronically Malnourished Children

Severe malnutrition complicated by diarrheal dehydration is common in tropical and subtropical countries and occurs occasionally in the temperate zones. Therapy should be adapted to meet the specific disturbances in body composition characteristic of the dehydrated and malnourished infant, in whom there appears to be an overexpansion of the extracellular space, accompanied by extracellular and presumably intracellular hypo-osmolality. Serum sodium, potassium, and magnesium levels tend to be low, and tetany occasionally may result from a magnesium or calcium deficiency. Serum protein levels are frequently below 3.6 g/dL. The electrocardiogram frequently shows tachycardia, low amplitude, and flat or inverted T waves. Cardiac reserve seems lowered, and heart failure is a common complication. Despite clinical signs of dehydration and reduced body water, urinary osmolality may be low in the chronically malnourished child.

Survival of the malnourished infant with diarrhea is limited by caloric deficit to a greater extent than by water and electrolyte deficit. Reparative calories can be given by slow drip through an indwelling nasogastric tube in conjunction with oral or, when necessary, intravenous rehydration.

Pyloric Stenosis

The therapy differs little from that for other causes of dehydration, except that potassium replacement should begin early, as soon as the child has urinated. In addition, relatively more sodium and potassium should be given as the chloride salt than is usual in treating dehydration; this is partly because of the larger deficit of chloride in pyloric stenosis and partly because this results in some correction of the alkalosis as the volume is expanded. Except in the mildly ill infant without signs of dehydration, it is preferable to delay surgery for at least 24–48 hr to achieve optimal readjustment of body functions.

Fasting and Thirsting

Parenteral fluid therapy is usually required in initially treating the fasting infant or child who has taken little or no water and food for 1 or more days. Therapy is begun with an isotonic solution to produce rapid and safe expansion of extracellular volume and to improve renal function.

Electrolyte Disturbances Associated with Central Nervous System Disorders

Diseases of the central nervous system are frequently associated with disturbances in sodium concentration. A decrease in serum sodium is almost entirely the result of retention of water.

The diagnosis of the syndrome of inappropriate antidiuretic hormone secretion (SIADH) is considered in the absence of hypovolemia, edema, endocrine dysfunction (including primary and secondary adrenal insufficiency and hypothyroidism), renal failure, and drugs impairing water excretion. Along with central nervous system causes, and neonatal hypoxia or hydrocephalus, this syndrome is also found in patients with pulmonary disorders, including pneumonia, tuberculosis, and asthma, as well as in those on positive-pressure ventilation and with certain carcinomas. Patients with this syndrome generally have a concentrated urine despite the presence of hyponatremia and a urinary sodium concentration greater than 20 mEq/L.

Treatment of acute symptomatic hyponatremia should be prompt. One may use hypertonic saline in combination with furosemide to enhance free water excretion. Chronic and/or asymptomatic hyponatremia is best managed conservatively by water restriction to allow a gradual increase of serum sodium over 24–48 hr.

Hypernatremia is a consequence of central diabetes insipidus and may be treated by increased oral or parenteral free water, by vasopressin boluses, or by continuous vasopressin infusion at 1.5 to 2.5 mU/kg/hr.

PERIOPERATIVE FLUIDS

Preoperatively, preparing a patient having no pre-existing deficit or in whom the deficit has been repaired consists mainly of supplying adequate carbohydrate for sustenance and protein sparing and the usual maintenance requirements of water and electrolytes. Deficits of water and electrolytes from vomiting or from stasis caused by intestinal obstruction should be replaced before the surgery.

During surgery, blood, plasma, saline, or other volume expanders may be given if blood loss, tissue trauma, third spacing, or excessive evaporative loss occurs. *The most common error in administering parenteral fluid during and after surgery is excessive administration, particularly of dextrose in water rather than use of isotonic solutions.*

Postoperatively, fluid intake should be limited for 24 hr. Thereafter, the usual maintenance therapy is gradually resumed. The water intake should not exceed 85 mL/100 kcal metabolized, because of antidiuresis resulting from trauma, circulatory readjustment, general anesthesia, or narcotic pain relief, unless renal ability to concentrate the urine is limited, as in patients with sickle cell disease, chronic pyelonephritis, or obstructive uropathy. If the intake of water is not limited, whether given parenterally or orally, water intoxication may occur associated with severe hyponatremia and even fatal cerebral edema.

ISOLATED DISTURBANCES IN BLOOD pH AND CONCENTRATIONS OF ELECTROLYTES

ACIDOSIS. Respiratory acidosis, in which the pH may be markedly lowered, primarily owing to retention of carbon dioxide, may be seen with severe respiratory insufficiency as in severe bronchiolitis and asthma, with neonatal respiratory distress syndrome, and in patients receiving assisted ventilation for any reason, who may be inadequately ventilated or have airway blockage. Mild metabolic acidosis may coexist because hypoxia leads to the accumulation of lactic and other organic acids in the extracellular fluid. The appropriate treatment is to improve ventilation by assisting respiration rather than by administering sodium bicarbonate, which may produce hyperosmolality and cardiac failure.

Metabolic acidosis, which can result from renal tubular acidosis, renal insufficiency, or accumulation of organic acids, may require the administration of alkali, especially if symptoms are evident. The usual initial dose is 1–2 mEq/kg. However, a more precise estimate of the dosage required is given by the general formula:

$$(C_d - C_a) \times k \times \text{body weight [in kg]} = \text{mEq required}$$

in which C_d and C_a represent, respectively, the serum bicarbonate concentration desired and the one measured, expressed in units of mEq/L; k represents that fraction of the total body weight in which the administered material is apparently (not actually) distributed. The k for bicarbonate or potential bicarbonate approximates 0.5–0.6. Treating acidosis with sodium bicarbonate should always be considered a temporizing measure. Every attempt should be made to treat the underlying causes.

ALKALOSIS. Typically, *metabolic alkalosis* is caused by the administration of excess amounts of alkali, intravenously or orally as in milk-alkali syndrome; by the loss of hydrogen ion through emesis from pyloric stenosis or nasogastric drainage; or by acute volume contraction with disproportionate losses of chloride. Severe hypokalemia can result in alkalosis or may perpetuate it.

When the plasma bicarbonate level is elevated, respiratory compensation may result in hypoventilation and an increase in P_{CO_2}. Severe alkalotic tetany may also occur. In such instances, administering ammonium chloride may effect symptomatic improvement; the dose may be calculated from the general formula presented under metabolic acidosis, with a probable k of 0.2–0.3. Metabolic alkalosis associated with volume contraction responds to measures designed to expand volume and replace the chloride and potassium deficits.

Respiratory alkalosis occurs in salicylate intoxication; in various central nervous system diseases, such as severe hypoxic insult, trauma, infection, or tumors; with hysterical hyperventilation or fever; with overventilation on a respirator; and in congestive heart failure, hepatic insufficiency, and gram-negative septicemia. Treatment should be directed at removing the underlying cause, although measures designed to return the P_{CO_2} to normal may be indicated.

HYPONATREMIA. The serum sodium level is usually reduced as a result of true sodium depletion or water intoxication, or a combination of the two. *Apparent* hyponatremia, an artifact, may be seen in diabetic ketoacidosis and nephrotic syndrome, when the water content of plasma is reduced by the presence of increased quantities of lipids. Patients with a serum sodium level below 120 mEq/L are often symptomatic (e.g., convulsions, shock, lethargy). In infants younger than 6 mo of age, hyponatremia is a common cause of convulsions.

The treatment of *asymptomatic hyponatremia* depends on its cause. With water overload, fluid restriction is the appropriate measure. Adding extra salt to the diet or increasing the sodium concentration of parenterally administered fluid often corrects a sodium deficit. Urinary sodium concentration is often greater than 20 mmol/L in renal salt-losing conditions and less than 10 mmol/L in other situations. Correction requires administration of isotonic saline. In patients in whom hyponatremia is caused by an excess of total body water (e.g., SIADH, hypothyroidism, pain, use of certain drugs such as morphine, desmopressin, selective serotonin reuptake inhibitors, and street drugs such as ecstasy), urinary sodium concentration usually exceeds 20 mmol/L, and therapy consists of water restriction.

In patients who have excesses of sodium and water, edematous states such as nephrotic syndrome, cirrhosis, or cardiac failure, the urinary sodium level is usually less than 10 mmol/L; however, in edematous patients with acute and chronic renal failure, the urinary sodium level may be in excess of 20 mmol/L. Treatment of hyponatremia associated with edema due to excess water and salt retention is usually water and salt restriction.

Treatment of *symptomatic hyponatremia* consists of administering a hypertonic saline solution, calculated according to the formula in the preceding section on acidosis, with k representing serum sodium rather than bicarbonate. The value for k should be 0.6–0.7 for the child and adolescent and 0.7–0.8 for the newborn or premature infant. The initial rapid therapeutic increase in the serum sodium level should be to a value of only about 125 mEq/L; only the symptomatic individual should be treated; and no more than 10 mEq/L should be used in any 24-hr period.

HYPERNATREMIA. The excessive intake of sodium is accompanied by increases in total body sodium and in the volume of extracellular water. Severe acidosis results from a shift of organic acids and free hydrogen ions to extracellular fluid. With the shift of water from brain cells, distention of cerebral vessels occurs, leading to subdural, subarachnoid, and intracerebral hemorrhage. Hypernatremia is associated with a high mortality rate, especially if the serum sodium concentration exceeds 158 mEq/L. Treatment is directed toward the removal of excess sodium from the body. Intravenous fluids should consist of glucose in water, potassium acetate, and calcium as needed. In patients with salt poisoning, *peritoneal dialysis* with glucose solutions can remove large quantities of sodium and correct hyperosmolality without the danger of pulmonary edema and heart failure.

HYPOKALEMIA. Severe hypokalemia may result in weakness of skeletal muscles, decreased peristalsis, ileus, an inability of the kidney to concentrate urine, and excessive thirst. Patients may present with frank paralysis and significant respiratory difficulty.

Treatment consists of administration of adequate amounts of potassium (usually up to 3 mEq/kg/24 hr); in Bartter syndrome or other causes of hypokalemia associated with massive urinary losses, 10 mEq/kg or more may have to be given orally.

HYPERKALEMIA. Marked elevation of the serum potassium level results in ventricular fibrillation and death. Levels above 6.5 g/mEq/L should be treated promptly, although such levels are often reasonably well tolerated by premature newborns. The presence or absence of electrocardiographic changes may be helpful in deciding when to initiate therapy.

Rapid intravenous administration of sodium bicarbonate (1–3 mEq/kg) or glucose and insulin (0.5–1 g of glucose/kg with 1 U crystalline insulin/3 g of glucose) results in the movement of potassium into cells and lowers the serum potassium level. Intravenous calcium gluconate (up to 0.5 mL of a 10% solution/kg given slowly over several minutes) counters the cardiotoxicity of potassium, but the electrocardiogram should be monitored while the calcium gluconate is being administered. These are temporizing measures until a negative potassium balance can be established by the use of ion exchange resins, such as Kayexalate (1 g/kg/dose given by oral or rectal routes every 6–12 hr) or by hemodialysis or peritoneal dialysis.

HYPOMAGNESEMIA. The only definitive symptom-complex associated with hypomagnesemia (i.e., serum magnesium level < 1.3 mEq/L) is that of latent or manifest tetany. Convulsions, muscular twitching, disorientation, athetoid movements, carpopedal spasm, and hyperreactivity to mechanical and auditory stimulation have been observed. The intramuscular injection of 0.1 mL of a 24% solution of $MgSO_4 \cdot 7H_2O$ (0.2 mEq/kg) repeated every 6 hr for three or four doses produces symptomatic and biochemical improvement.

HYPERMAGNESEMIA. Levels of serum magnesium higher than 10 mEq/L are accompanied by drowsiness and occasionally produce coma. Intravenously administering calcium gluconate rapidly reverses the depressant effects of hypermagnesemia and the associated cardiac abnormalities.

TETANY

Tetany, the state of hyperexcitability of the central and peripheral nervous systems, results from abnormal concentrations of ions in the fluid bathing nerve cells. These abnormalities may include decreases of H^+ (alkalosis), Ca^{2+}, or Mg^{2+}.

At physiologic concentrations of H^+ and K^+, tetany may develop at Ca^{2+} concentrations of less than 3.0 mg/dL. Tetany usually is manifested at Ca^{2+} concentrations less than 2.5 mg/dL. At normal concentrations of serum albumin, these levels correspond to total serum calcium concentrations of approximately 7 mg/dL and 5 mg/dL, respectively. The normal range of magnesium in serum is 1.6–2.6 mg/dL, of which about 75% is Mg^{2+}. Total serum magnesium reduced to less than 1.0 mg/dL may be associated with hyperexcitability of the nervous system.

MANIFEST TETANY. The classic signs of peripheral hyperexcitability of motor nerves are spasms of the muscles of the wrists and ankles (i.e., carpopedal spasm) and of the vocal cords (i.e., laryngospasm). In carpopedal spasm the wrists are flexed, the fingers extended, the thumbs adducted over the palms, and the feet extended and adducted. *Laryngospasm* causes inspiratory obstruction accompanied by a high-pitched inspiratory crow. The sensory manifestations are paresthesias, particularly numbness and tingling of the hands and feet. Motor excitability of the central nervous system may be manifested by brief but recurrent convulsions, which are usually generalized but may be localized to one side of the body.

LATENT TETANY. This is the condition in which ischemia or mechanical or electrical stimulation of motor nerves is required to produce the motor response characteristic of tetany.

ALKALOTIC TETANY. Alkalotic tetany can be induced through spontaneous overventilation, producing respiratory alkalosis; such hyperventilation is most often of psychogenic origin. The treatment of alkalotic tetany resulting from spontaneous hyperventilation is to have the patient rebreathe into a bag or a balloon to increase the P_{CO_2}. In patients with low Ca^{2+} concentrations, tetany may be precipitated by overventilation or by a metabolic alkalosis after the administration of sodium bicarbonate. Correcting acidosis can cause tetany and convulsions.

HYPOCALCEMIC TETANY

Disorders of Parathyroid Function. The most common disorder of parathyroid function is transient physiologic hypoparathyroidism of the newborn infant, sometimes referred to as neonatal hypocalcemia. Clinically, these infants can be separated into two groups: one group with hypocalcemia during the first 72 hr of life, usually before achieving a significant oral intake of milk; and a second group in whom hypocalcemia results from a high phosphate load that develops only after ingestion of cow's milk for several days. The onset of symptoms in the second group occurs most commonly during the first 5–10 days of life; clinical manifestations have occasionally appeared as late as 6 wk of age.

Early Hypocalcemia. The infants at greatest risk are low-birthweight infants, especially those with intrauterine growth retardation; infants born of diabetic mothers; and infants who have been subjected to prolonged, difficult deliveries.

Asymptomatic hypocalcemia of premature infants usually resolves spontaneously. However, when possible, oral calcium gluconate should be given, because it usually obviates the subsequent need for intravenous therapy and its attendant complications. *Treatment* of clinical manifestations requires the intravenous injection of a 10% solution of calcium gluconate in a dose of about 2 mL/kg (18 mg Ca/kg), which must be given slowly while monitoring the cardiac rate for bradycardia. Tissue necrosis and calcification may occur if this solution extravasates or is given intramuscularly. The intravenous dose of calcium gluconate can be repeated at 6- to 8-hr intervals until calcium homeostasis becomes stable, or the calcium gluconate (50–75 mg elemental Ca/kg/24 hr) can be added to a constant intravenous infusion.

Late Hypocalcemia. After a feeding of high-phosphate milk, tetany can occur in full-term and prematurely born infants and in infants whose clinical histories have been benign. The intake of a highphosphate food, such as cow's milk, in a relatively large volume leads to an elevated serum phosphate level. The elevated serum phosphate level depresses the serum calcium level through deposition of calcium phosphate in bone and possibly in other tissues.

CLINICAL MANIFESTATIONS. The most important presentation of hypocalcemia in infants is convulsions, usually generalized, short, and without loss of consciousness. Irritability, muscular twitching, jitteriness, and tremors are common clinical manifestations in the newborn. A serum calcium concentration below 7 mg/dL establishes the diagnosis; a level below 7.5 mg/dL is suggestive. The serum phosphate level is increased, sometimes to 10–12 mg/dL.

TREATMENT. Initial treatment of the convulsing infant is intravenous injection of a 10% solution of calcium gluconate (2 mL/kg), with the precautions given previously. The response may be dramatic. After this, specific treatment of late hypocalcemia aims at reducing the serum phosphate level.

Phosphate absorption from food can be suppressed by adding calcium lactate powder to milk. As treatment decreases the serum phosphorus level, the serum calcium level returns to normal. In most infants, restoration of normal calcium homeostasis and presumably normal parathyroid responsiveness occurs in 1–2 wk. Occasionally, a more prolonged calcium supplementation period is needed, in which case the treatment must be individualized by serial measurements of calcium and phosphate concentrations.

HYPOMAGNESEMIC TETANY. Hypomagnesemia has reportedly caused tetany associated with low or normal serum calcium concentrations. This hypomagnesemia usually responds to treatment directed at reducing the serum phosphate concentration.

Hypomagnesemic tetany and convulsions beyond the newborn period may result from prolonged parenteral nutrition with magnesium-free solutions or congenital disorders of magnesium transport, causing a failure of absorption of dietary magnesium or failure of tubular reabsorption of magnesium with excessive urinary loss. Treatment requires magnesium administered intramuscularly, intravenously (2–10 mL/kg of 1 % magnesium sulfate solution) by slow infusion, or orally in the form of magnesium salts.

PART 8

The Acutely Ill Child

CHAPTER 51

Evaluation of the Sick Child in the Office and Clinic

(Nelson Textbook, Chapter 56)

Most sick child visits are made because of acute intercurrent infections, and often the child is febrile. Both the risk for and the cause of serious illness in children with acute febrile illness vary depending on the child's age. The infant in the first 3 mo of life is more susceptible to sepsis and meningitis caused by group B streptococci and gram-negative organisms. Urinary tract infections are more frequent in male infants. As the infant matures beyond 3 mo, the bacterial pathogens that usually cause sepsis and meningitis are *Streptococcus pneumoniae, Haemophilus influenzae* type b (if the child has not been immunized or has been only partially immunized), and *Neisseria meningitidis.* After infancy, urinary tract infections are seen more often in girls. In children older than 36 mo, pharyngitis caused by group A streptococci is a common bacterial infection. *Mycoplasma pneumoniae* assumes increasing importance as a cause for pulmonary infiltrates in children older than 5 yr of age.

Observation is a key factor in the evaluation of children with acute problems for the possibility of a serious illness. The child should be observed for specific evidence of a serious illness, such as grunting, which might indicate pneumonia or sepsis, or a bulging fontanel, which might indicate bacterial meningitis. Most observational data that the pediatrician gathers during an acute illness should focus, however, on assessing the child's response to stimuli.

Six observation items and their scales (the Acute Illness Observation Scales) that have reliably and validly identified serious illness in febrile children are shown in Figure 51–1. A normal finding is scored as 1, moderate impairment as 3, and severe impairment as 5. The best possible score is 6 items $\times$ 1 = 6; the worst score is 6 items $\times$ 5 = 30. The chance of serious illness is 1–2% if the total score is less than 10; if the score is more than 10, the risk of serious illness increases by at least 10-fold. It is not clear whether these scales can be used in the first 2–3 mo of life, because infants may not have developed the skills required to score some of these items.

In addition to the general level of interaction, color, and hydra-

Acute Illness Observational Scales *(Please check boxes that describe your child's appearance and behavior)*

OBSERVATION ITEM	NORMAL	MODERATE IMPAIRMENT	SEVERE IMPAIRMENT
1. Quality of Cry	Strong with normal tone ☐ *or* Content and not crying ☐	Whimpering ☐ *or* Sobbing ☐	Weak ☐ *or* Moaning ☐ *or* High Pitched ☐
2. Reaction to Parent Stimulation (Effect on crying when held, patted on back, jiggled on lap, or carried)	Cries briefly, then stops ☐ *or* Content and not crying ☐	Cries off and on ☐	Continual cry ☐ *or* Hardly responds ☐
3. State Variation (Going from awake to asleep or asleep to awake)	If awake, then stays awake ☐ *or* If asleep, and stimulated, then wakes up quickly ☐	Eyes close briefly, then awakens ☐ *or* Awakens with prolonged stimulation ☐	Will not rouse ☐ *or* Falls to sleep ☐
4. Color	Pink ☐	Pale hands, feet *and* Acrocyanosis (blue hands and feet) ☐	Pale ☐ *or* Blue ☐ *or* Ashen (grey) ☐ *or* Mottled ☐
5. Hydration (Moisture in skin, eyes, mouth)	Skin normal *and* Eyes, mouth moist ☐	Skin, eyes normal *and* Mouth slightly dry ☐	Skin doughy or tented *and* Eyes may be sunken *and* Dry eyes and mouth ☐
6. Response to Social Overtures (Being held, kissed, hugged, touched, talked to, comforted)	Smiles ☐ *or* Alerts (2 months or less) ☐	Brief smiles ☐ *or* Alerts briefly (2 months or less) ☐	No smile, face anxious ☐ *or* Dull, expressionless ☐ *or* No alerting (2 months or less) ☐

Figure 51–1 Acute illness observational scales for clinical evaluation of the well and sick child. (From McCarthy PL, Sharpe MR, Spiesel SZ, et al: Observation scales to identify serious illness in febrile children. Pediatrics 70:802, 1982. Reproduced by permission of Pediatrics.)

tion, the child's respiratory status is evaluated. This evaluation includes determining respiratory rate and noting any evidence of inspiratory stridor, expiratory wheezing, grunting, or coughing. Evidence of increased work of breathing (retractions, nasal flaring, and use of abdominal musculature) is also sought.

The skin examination may also yield evidence of more serious infections, such as bacterial cellulitis or petechiae associated with bacteremia. When the child is seated and is least perturbed, an assessment of fontanel tension can be completed; it can be determined if the fontanel is depressed, flat, or bulging. It is also important at this time to assess the child's willingness to move and ease of movement. Usually the child with meningitis will hold the neck stiffly and often cry when any attempt is made to move the neck, even during cuddling by the parent. The child with cellulitis, osteomyelitis, or septic arthritis in an extremity will resist movement of that limb. The child with peritoneal inflammation will sit quietly and become irritable during movement. The sensitivity of the carefully performed clinical assessment, observation, history, and physical examination for the presence of serious illness is approximately 90%.

Chapter 52

Injury Control
(Nelson Textbook, Chapter 56)

Injuries are the most common cause of death during childhood beyond the first few months of life and represent one of the most important causes of preventable pediatric morbidity and mortality.

INJURY CONTROL. Reduction in morbidity and mortality from injuries can be accomplished not only through primary prevention (averting the event or injury in the first place) but also through secondary and tertiary prevention. The latter approaches include appropriate emergency medical services for injured children; regionalized trauma care for the multiply injured, severely burned, or head-injured child; and specialized pediatric rehabilitation services that attempt to return children to their prior level of functioning.

SCOPE OF THE PROBLEM
Mortality. Injuries cause almost 40% of the deaths among children aged 1–4 yr and three times more deaths than the next leading cause, congenital anomalies.

Motor vehicle injuries lead the list of causes of death due to injury at all ages during childhood and adolescence, even in children younger than 1 yr of age.

Drowning ranks second overall as a cause of unintentional

trauma deaths, with peaks in the preschool and later teenage years.

Fire and burn deaths account for nearly 10% of all trauma deaths and more than 20% in those younger than 5 yr of age.

Asphyxiation and choking account for approximately 40% of all unintentional deaths in children younger than 1 yr of age.

Homicide is the leading cause of injury death for infants younger than 1 yr, the fourth leading cause of injury death for ages 1–14 yr, and the second leading cause of injury death in adolescents (15–19 yr).

Suicide is rare in children younger than age 10 yr; only 1% of all suicides occur in children younger than 15 yr of age. The suicide rate increases markedly after the age of 10 yr, with the result that suicide is now the third leading cause of death for 15- to 19-yr-olds, accounting for more than 100,000 potential years of life lost.

Morbidity. Twenty to 25% of children and adolescents receive medical care for an injury each year in hospital emergency departments, and at least an equal number are treated in physician offices. Falls are the leading causes of both emergency department visits and hospitalizations. Bicycle-related trauma is the most common type of sports and recreational injury, accounting for more than 300,000 emergency department visits annually.

PRINCIPLES OF INJURY CONTROL. Efforts to control injuries include education or persuasion, changes in product design, and modification of the social or physical environment.

CHAPTER 53

Emergency Medical Services for Children

(Nelson Textbook, Chapter 58)

ANTICIPATORY GUIDANCE. Early recognition and treatment of many illnesses can prevent the need for emergency care. Equally important is education for parents and caregivers on the importance of first aid training, the recognition of signs and symptoms of serious illness or significant injury, and indications for seeking immediate care.

OFFICE PREPAREDNESS. Emergency preparedness in the office requires training and continuing education for staff members, policies and procedures for emergency intervention, ready availability of appropriate resuscitation equipment, knowledge of local resources for emergency medical services (EMS) response and transport, and a working relationship with area emergency departments to ensure that children are cared for in facilities with expertise in pediatric emergency care.

POLICIES AND PROCEDURES. Written policies and procedures for the management of status asthmaticus, upper airway obstruction, seizures, ingestions, shock, sepsis/meningitis, trauma, head injury, anaphylaxis, and cardiopulmonary arrest should be generated and made available to all potentially involved staff members.

RESUSCITATION EQUIPMENT. Every physician's office should have essential resuscitation equipment and medications packaged in a pediatric resuscitation cart or kit

TRANSPORT. Every office should be prepared to initiate resuscitation on a child with a life-threatening medical problem. A decision must be made on how to transport a child to a facility capable of providing definitive care once the child's condition has been stabilized.

PEDIATRIC PREHOSPITAL CARE

ACCESS TO THE EMS SYSTEM. Most metropolitan and many rural communities in the United States have a "911" telephone system that provides direct access to a dispatcher who coordinates police, fire, and EMS response. In activating the 911 system, it is important for physicians to make it clear to the dispatcher the nature of the medical emergency and the condition of the child.

PROVIDER CAPABILITY. There are many levels of training for prehospital EMS providers, ranging from individuals capable of providing only first aid to those trained and licensed to provide advanced life support (ALS) in the field. The Pediatric Trauma Score (PTS) can be used to assess the severity of injury (Table 53–1).

TABLE 53–1 Pediatric Trauma Score

Clinical Category	Score		
	+2	**+1**	**−1**
Size	≥20 kg	10–20 kg	<10 kg
Airway	Normal	Maintainable	Unmaintainable
Systolic blood pressure	≤90 mm Hg	50–90 mm Hg	<50 mm Hg
Central nervous system	Awake	Obtunded/loss of consciousness	Coma/decerebrate
Open wound	None	Minor	Major/penetrating
Skeletal	None	Closed fracture	Open/multiple fractures

From Ford EG: Trauma triage. *In:* Ford EG, Andrassy RJ (eds): Pediatric Trauma Initial Assessment and Management. Philadelphia, WB Saunders, 1994, p 112.

THE PEDIATRIC PATIENT IN THE HOSPITAL EMERGENCY DEPARTMENT: PRIORITIES IN PEDIATRIC RESUSCITATION

Cardiopulmonary arrest in children is rarely the result of a primary cardiac event. Rather, full arrest in children is usually a result of prolonged myocardial ischemia related to untreated hypoxemia or untreated shock. By the time the heart has sustained a sufficient hypoxic insult to result in asystole, the central nervous system has sustained a severe asphyxial insult as well. This accounts for the poor outcome for children who are brought into the emergency department with ongoing cardiopulmonary resuscitation (CPR).

Whether a child presents with a primary cardiovascular, respiratory, neurologic, infectious, or metabolic disorder, the goal is early recognition of respiratory and circulatory insufficiency. Early intervention is geared toward preventing the progression of hypoxemia and hypoperfusion to full cardiopulmonary arrest, with its attendant poor prognosis. During the primary survey (Table 53–2), life-threatening conditions are identified and resuscitation is begun simultaneously. Interventions should be undertaken in a graded progression, from least to most invasive, with careful reassessment after each intervention. A head-to-toe physical assessment, or secondary survey, and definitive care should be undertaken only after the primary survey is complete and appropriate resuscitation is underway.

A: AIRWAY/SPINAL IMMOBILIZATION. In assessing the airway, look for evidence of appropriate chest rise and for signs of increased work of breathing, such as retractions and accessory muscle use. Listen over the trachea for abnormal sounds, such as snoring, gurgling, or stridor, and over the peripheral lung fields for the adequacy of inspiratory effort. Feel for movement of air on expiration and ascertain that the trachea is midline.

If the airway is patent, without evidence of obstruction, the child is allowed to maintain a position of comfort and supplemental oxygen is administered as needed, preferably by mask or nasal prongs. If the child has evidence of partial or complete airway obstruction, the head is repositioned, placing it in the "sniff" position by using the chin lift or, in trauma patients, jaw thrust, and taking care not to hyperextend the neck. Blood, secretions, or gastric contents should be removed from the mouth with a rigid suction device. If a patent airway cannot be established or maintained with these maneuvers, consideration must be given to placing an oral or nasal airway. These devices are rarely tolerated by a conscious child; placement may lead to gagging, vomiting, and the possibility of aspiration. In managing a child's airway, it is important to remember that adult airway equipment cannot be adapted for use in a pediatric patient.

The cervical spine must be immobilized in any child who has

TABLE 53–2 Pediatric Primary Survey and Resuscitation Measures

A = Airway/Cervical Spine Control

1. Assess airway patency
   If patent and patient conscious—maintain position of comfort
   If compromised—position, suction,? oral airway
   If unmaintainable—oral endotracheal intubation
2. Maintain cervical spine in neutral position with manual immobilization if head/facial trauma or high-risk injury mechanism

B = Breathing

Assess respiratory rate, color, work of breathing, mental status
   If respiratory effort adequate—administer high-flow supplemental oxygen
   If respiratory effort inadequate—bag-valve-mask ventilation with 100% oxygen, naso/orogastric tube; consider intubation

C = Circulation/Hemorrhage Control

Assess heart rate, pulse quality, color, skin signs, mental status
   If perfusion adequate—apply cardiac monitor, establish IV access, direct pressure to bleeding sites
   If signs of shock—establish vascular access (IV/IO), isotonic fluid bolus, baseline laboratory studies, cardiac monitor, urinary catheter
   If ongoing hemorrhage suspected and continued signs of shock—perform blood transfusion and surgical consultation

D = Disability (Neurologic Status)

Assess pupillary function, mental status (AVPU)
   If decreased level of consciousness—reassess and optimize oxygenation, ventilation, circulation
   If increased ICP suspected, elevate head of bed, consider mild hyperventilation, neurosurgical consultation

E = Exposure

Remove clothing for complete evaluation. Prevent heat loss with blankets, heat lamps, radiant warmer.

AVPU = alertness, response to voice, response to pain, unresponsive; ICP = intracranial pressure; IO = intraosseous; IV = intravenous.

sustained a high-velocity injury or has evidence of multiple trauma or of significant injury above the level of the clavicles. A child must then be immobilized on a backboard, using towel or blanket rolls to eliminate dead space and 2-in. adhesive tape across the forehead to secure the child's head to the board. Care must be taken to ensure neutral alignment of the head and neck on the backboard.

B: BREATHING. Once the patency of a patient's airway is established, the evaluation proceeds to assess the adequacy of the child's minute ventilation, a function of respiratory rate and tidal volume. In a conscious child with spontaneous respiratory effort, one should look before touching. Observation alone permits evaluation of respiratory rate, skin color, mental status, and work of breathing. Listen over the trachea and over the peripheral lung fields for the adequacy of air entry, symmetry, and abnormal breath sounds such as crackles or wheezing. Placement of a pulse oximetry probe, when available, permits continuous assessment of oxygenation.

If the airway is patent and minute ventilation appears adequate, high-flow supplemental oxygen should be administered pending objective evaluation of arterial oxygen levels. All seriously ill and injured patients should receive supplemental oxygen. If the airway is patent but spontaneous respiratory effort appears to be inadequate, *positive-pressure ventilation* by means of a bag-valve-mask device with an oxygen reservoir should be initiated. If a child fails to respond to positive-pressure ventilation with improved color, heart rate, and level of consciousness, equipment and technique should be checked to ensure that the child is being effectively ventilated. If bag-valve-mask ventilation is unsuccessful or prolonged, positive-pressure ventilation is required, then endotracheal intubation must be undertaken.

Pneumothorax must be considered in trauma victims presenting with respiratory failure, especially one who does not improve with supplemental oxygen and positive-pressure ventilation. Classically, tension pneumothorax produces decreased breath sounds and hyperresonance in the affected hemithorax, mediastinal shift, cyanosis, and distended neck veins, as well as compromised cardiac output caused by decreased venous return to the heart. If the diagnosis is suspected, one can insert a needle or over-the-needle catheter into the second intercostal space at the midclavicular line, aspirate with a syringe to confirm the presence of free air, and immediately decompress the chest. Definitive treatment involves placing a chest tube in the fifth intercostal space, anterior to the midaxillary line.

C: CIRCULATION. The evaluation of circulation involves assessment of cardiac output and, in cases of trauma, identification and control of exsanguinating hemorrhage. Hypovolemia is the most common cause of shock in children, followed by septic and cardiogenic shock. The early signs and symptoms of shock may be subtle, and tachycardia may be the only objective finding. Cool extremities, mottled or pale skin color, delayed capillary refill time, and effortless tachypnea are relatively early signs of shock, which may be followed by the development of weak or absent peripheral pulses, altered mental status, and hypotension if the shock state is not recognized and treated.

Initial priorities in the treatment of shock are directed at restoring adequate perfusion of the vital organs. In trauma victims, shock is almost always due to blood loss. Initial resuscitation efforts should include control of hemorrhage, elevation of the lower extremities, prevention of heat loss, and volume resuscitation. Volume resuscitation is also the cornerstone of therapy in children with hypovolemic shock of medical etiology.

Achieving vascular access in a child in shock may be difficult.

The preferred site is the antecubital fossa, using a short, over the-needle intravenous catheter. If initial attempts to establish one or, preferably, two large-bore peripheral intravenous lines are not successful within 2–5 min, alternate methods of vascular access must be undertaken to prevent a dangerous delay in initiating resuscitation. Depending on the experience and expertise of the provider, this might take the form of a surgical venous cutdown, central venous line, or intraosseous line.

Initial volume resuscitation of patients in shock should be with isotonic crystalloid fluids. Unless a patient has cardiogenic shock, an initial bolus of 20 mL/kg administered as rapidly as possible should be given. Further fluid boluses are administered if reassessment of a patient's response to therapy so warrants, with frequent vital sign checks and attention to signs of end-organ perfusion (skin color and warmth, mental status, and urine output).

D: DISABILITY. Rapid assessment of both cortical and brain stem function is an important part of the initial assessment of a seriously ill or injured child. Head injury is the most common cause of death due to trauma, accounting for 75% of fatal injuries. The Glasgow Coma Scale or one of the several children's coma scales adapted from that tool may be used to document serial neurologic assessments. A more abbreviated initial examination consists of an evaluation of papillary responses and categorization of mental status based on the acronym AVPU—is the patient *A*lert? Responsive to *V*oice? Responsive to *P*ain? or *U*nresponsive? Frequent reassessment of neurologic status is of utmost importance. If signs of elevated intracranial pressure are identified, immediate stabilizing measures should be undertaken.

E: EXPOSURE. Undressing and exposing the patient are necessary to perform a thorough examination and to identify all injuries. Attention must be paid to preventing heat loss during the emergency evaluation and treatment phase.

CHAPTER 54

Pediatric Critical Care

(Nelson Textbook, Chapters 54, 60, 61, and 72)

Pediatric critical care represents a convergence of knowledge, technologies, and approaches to multisystem organ failure from the operating room, neonatal intensive care areas, and adult intensive care units. Children having acute neurologic deterioration, respiratory distress, cardiovascular compromise, or life-threatening traumatic injuries constitute the most common admissions to a pediatric intensive care unit (PICU). Patients are admitted to a PICU because they require a very high level of monitoring of vital signs and other body functions not available in other parts of the hospital.

As PICUs have developed in selected sites, specialized transport programs (interfacility transport) to bring patients from community facilities to the PICU have evolved. The members of the transport team must have the cognitive and technical skills required for the needs of pediatric patients and should be supervised by an attending physician (medical control physician) who has expertise in either pediatric emergency medicine or pediatric critical care.

DISPATCH CENTER/TRANSFER CENTER. The regional pediatric center or PICU should provide phone consultation and deploy a team of specialized health care providers to assist in stabilization of patients to transport them in a safe mobile environment to the PICU. The selection of the vehicle is made by the medical control physician in coordination with the referring hospital and those who will participate in transport of the child. Once the transport team arrives at the referring facility, the team leader should reassess the patient's condition, review all the pertinent laboratory data and medications, and discuss the situation with the parents and referring physicians.

THE PEDIATRIC PATIENT IN AN UNFAMILIAR ENVIRONMENT. It is difficult to imagine a situation producing more terror, sadness, fright, and anger in families than a child's serious illness that requires admission to a PICU. Although patients in a PICU may not be fully alert or able to interact normally with those around them, the goal of PICU care should be to allow the maximum amount of time for parents to be with their child and to participate actively in their child's care.

IDENTIFYING PERSONNEL AND THEIR ROLES. Large medical centers, especially teaching hospitals, are environments in which many physicians, students, nurses, respiratory therapists, social workers, chaplains, and others are involved in the care of a patient in a PICU. A single physician (usually the senior attending physician) should assume primary responsibility for communication with the family. This physician should have sufficient experience to place individual pieces of information about a patient in context and to avoid hasty and incompletely supported conclusions. He or she should communicate at least daily with the family.

INFORMED CONSENT. The goal of informed consent is to provide patients or parents or other adults who are responsible for representing the interests of a child with a full understanding of their choices and the benefits and risks of each potential course of action. The concept should guide virtually all interactions between the physician, the patient, and the patient's family.

PROVIDING HEALTH INFORMATION CONSISTENTLY AND ACCURATELY. The goal should be to speak to the family with simple honesty and compassion about the child's condition and prognosis, unless certain circumstances would make such a frank discussion problematic (e.g., psychiatric or other serious illness in a parent).

Chapter 55

Monitoring the Critically Ill Infant and Child; Scoring Systems

(Nelson Textbook, Chapters 62 and 63)

The ability to provide advanced technologic therapies to critically ill patients makes physiologic monitoring essential.

HEMODYNAMIC MONITORING. This is indicated for any patient who is admitted to the intensive care unit and who may be in shock, has respiratory failure or impending respiratory failure, or has sustained an acute neurologic insult. Included in hemodynamic monitoring are heart rate, blood pressure, central venous pressure, pulmonary capillary wedge pressure, and, less commonly (e.g., in postoperative cardiovascular patients), left atrial pressure. Complications from arterial catheterization are infrequent but may be serious. Bleeding and infection are relatively rare. The most serious complication is probably arterial thrombosis. Complications of central venous catheters include dysrhythmias, pneumothorax, hydrothorax, hemothorax, air embolism, shearing of the catheter, losing the guide wire, bleeding, or apnea. Infection is associated with longer duration of catheter placement and percutaneous (vs. tunneled) catheters.

PULMONARY MONITORING. Patients receiving respiratory support require monitoring of blood gases. Arterial blood gas sampling requires techniques similar to inserting an arterial line. Noninvasive blood gas devices are frequently used to monitor critically ill infants and children in pediatric intensive care units (PICUs). Capnography measures the P_{CO_2} in exhaled gas and end-tidal carbon dioxide, using a spectrometric instrument. Pulse oximetry is the standard method for noninvasive bedside monitoring of oxygen saturation.

NEUROPHYSIOLOGIC MONITORING. Frequent clinical observations should include evaluation of the cranial nerves, especially the pupillary reflexes, and use of a modified Glasgow Coma Scale (GCS) for infants and children. Most patients with a GCS score less than 12 should be observed in a PICU. Neurophysiologic monitoring involves careful clinical observation accompanied by highly technical noninvasive devices (e.g., electroencephalography, evoked potentials, near-infrared spectroscopy) or invasive catheters (to monitor intracranial pressure [ICP]). Invasive neuro-

TABLE 55–1 Physiologic Factors Considered in PRISM Scoring

Vital Signs	*Hematology*
Systolic blood pressure Heart rate Stupor/coma (GCS <8) Pupillary reflexes	White blood cell count (<3000 cells/mm³) Platelet count (<50,000 or 50,000–200,000/mm³) PT (>22 seconds) or PTT (>57 seconds)
Acid-Base Status	*Other Factors*
pH <7.28 or >7.48 Total CO_2 > 34 mmol/L Pao_2 (<50 mm Hg) $Paco_2$ (>50 mm Hg)	Nonoperative disease Chromosomal anomaly Cancer Previous PICU admission
Chemistry	Pre-ICU resuscitation (CPR) Postoperative
Glucose (>200 mg/dL or >11 nmol/L) Potassium (>6.9 mmol/L) Creatinine increase Blood urea nitrogen increase	Acute diabetes (e.g., ketoacidosis) Transfer from inpatient unit

CPR = cardiopulmonary resuscitation; GCS = Glasgow Coma Scale; ICU = intensive care unit; PICU = pediatric intensive care unit; PT = prothrombin time; PTT = partial thromboplastin time.

logic monitoring includes ICP monitoring and jugular bulb catheterization. The indications for ICP monitoring include any acute neurologic deterioration in which elevated ICP may produce further injury to the patient.

PEDIATRIC RISK OF MORTALITY (PRISM). This scoring system assesses the severity of illness in a population of pediatric patients (Table 55–1). The PRISM has demonstrated a consistent relationship between the number of malfunctioning organ systems (the score) at 12 and 24 hr and the mortality risk in a given PICU. However, it is of limited predictive value for a single patient.

CHAPTER 56

Stabilization of the Critically Ill Child

(Nelson Textbook, Chapters 64, 66, 67, and 68)

LIFE-THREATENING EMERGENCIES AND PRE-ARREST STATES IN CHILDREN

The most common life-threatening illnesses in children are those involving respiratory, cardiac, or neurologic failure. Acute failure of the liver, kidneys, or adrenals also may place pediatric patients in peril and requires early recognition. Pinpointing the cause of all of these various organ failures may take considerable

TABLE 56–1 Vital Signs at Various Ages

Age	Heart Rate (beats/min)	Blood Pressure (mm Hg)	Respiratory Rate (breaths/min)
Premature	120–170*	55–75/35–45†	40–70‡
0–3 mo	100–150*	65–85/45–55	35–55
3–6 mo	90–120	70–90/50–65	30–45
6–12 mo	80–120	80–100/55–65	25–40
1–3 yr	70–110	90–105/55–70	20–30
3–6 yr	65–110	95–110/60–75	20–25
6–12 yr	60–95	100–120/60–75	14–22
12* yr	55–85	110–135/65–85	12–18

*In sleep, infant heart rates may drop significantly lower, but if perfusion is maintained, no intervention is required.

†A blood pressure cuff should cover approximately two thirds of the arm; too small a cuff yields spuriously high pressure readings, and too large a cuff yields spuriously low pressure readings.

‡Many premature infants require mechanical ventilatory support, making their spontaneous respiratory rate less relevant.

time, but treatment to stabilize a child physiologically should begin immediately.

DETECTING AND ASSESSING PHYSIOLOGIC INSTABILITY. A simple and consistent approach is necessary for rapid and efficient evaluation of a pediatric patient who may be in serious distress. Observation begins with determination of the alertness of the patient, including response to stimuli, spontaneous vocalization or movement, and muscle tone. This is followed by assessment of the *vital signs* (Table 56–1) and other basic indicators of the physiologic state.

HEART RATE. When a child's heart rate lies outside the physiologic parameters, cardiac output may be affected. A rapid heart rate (e.g., supraventricular tachycardia) may be associated with a serious reduction in stroke volume as reflected in poor perfusion, increased fussiness, and poor appetite. Cardiac failure may develop with pulmonary edema. Bradycardia also may represent a serious pre-arrest condition.

ORGAN PERFUSION. Skin perfusion is assessed by the temperature of the extremities and capillary refill time. Normal capillary refill time is 2 sec or less.

RESPIRATORY EFFORT. Muscle *retractions* in the chest and neck and flaring of the nostrils at inspiration are signs of an abnormally high level of effort required to move air into the lungs. Grunting is a moaning noise at expiration, associated with generation of positive pressure to maintain alveolar patency. A child who is inadequately oxygenated demonstrates *cyanosis* (a blue or dusky color of the skin and mucous membranes).

CARDIAC DYSRHYTHMIAS. Disturbances in cardiac rate and rhythm are not rare in children, but the majority are fleeting and not pathologic. Life-threatening cardiac emergencies in children are far more likely to involve bradycardia or asystole than they are to involve ventricular fibrillation, which is more common in adults. However *asystole* and *bradycardia* present two distinct resuscitative paradigms that require swift recognition and intervention; offices, clinics, and inpatient areas need to be prepared to manage these complicated situations (Figs. 56–1 and 56–2). Electrolyte imbalances also may produce life-threatening dysrhythmias.

ASSESSING METABOLIC STATUS. Two of the most important acute destabilizing metabolic disorders are acidosis and hypoglycemia.

ASSESSING CENTRAL NERVOUS SYSTEM (CNS) FUNCTION. The integrity of the CNS may be assessed through interviewing patients, when feasible, and through various physical examination techniques. See Table 56–2 for an example of encephalopathy.

GLASGOW COMA SCALE (GCS). Although this scale has not been validated as a prognostic scoring system for infants and young children, the GCS is commonly used in assessment of pediatric patients with an altered level of consciousness, especially those who have sustained a traumatic head injury (Table 56–3). The GCS provides very rapid assessment of cortical function. Patients with a GCS score of 8 or less may require aggressive management including intracranial pressure monitoring as well as mechanical ventilation.

RESUSCITATION

The goal in pediatric resuscitation is to maintain adequate oxygenation and perfusion of blood throughout the body while steps are taken to stabilize a child's condition and establish long-term homeostasis. An orderly sequence of events similar to those used in adult resuscitation should be instituted, beginning with the ABC principles: airway, breathing, and circulation (see Chapter 53). About 90% of pediatric patients undergoing resuscitation recover to a substantial degree. However, if a patient is asystolic on arrival at the hospital or in the advanced stages of a disease process before he or she receives medical care, then the chances for success decline dramatically.

RESPIRATORY SUPPORT. If no obstruction by a foreign body is found and if a child has no spontaneous respirations, steps should be immediately taken to breathe for the child. This should be done by *mouth-to-mouth* or *mouth-to-nose* breathing, a mask over the patient's nose and mouth and *mouth-to-mask* breathing, or bag-mask respirations. If air does not move easily, then head-tilt, chin-lift, and placement of an oral airway or nasal trumpet may be elected. If these measures do not facilitate adequate air entry, then endotracheal intubation is indicated. *Foreign-body aspiration* always should be suspected if respiratory distress has had a sud-

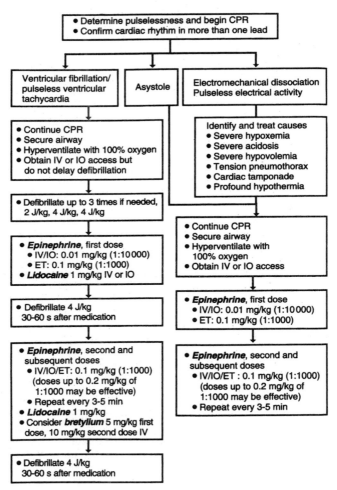

Figure 56–1 Asystole and pulseless arrest decision tree. CPR = cardiopulmonary resuscitation; ET = endotracheal; IO = intraosseous; IV = intravenous. (From Emergency Cardiac Care Committee and Subcommittees, American Heart Association. Pediatric advanced life support, part VI. JAMA 268:2262, 1992. Copyright 1992, American Medical Association.)

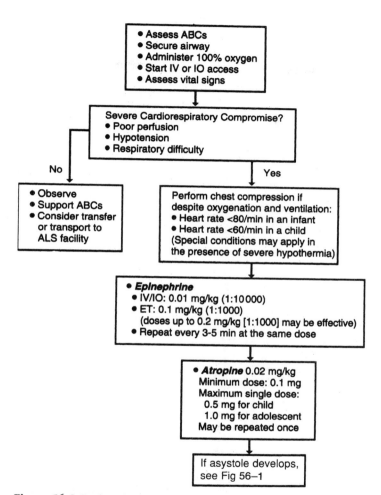

Figure 56–2 Bradycardia decision tree. ABCs = airway, breathing, and circulation; ALS = advanced life support; ET = endotracheal; IO = intraosseous; IV = intravenous. (From Emergency Cardiac Care Committee and Subcommittees, American Heart Association. Pediatric advanced life support, part VI. JAMA 268:2262, 1992. Copyright 1992, American Medical Association.)

TABLE 56-2 Clinical Staging of Encephalopathy

	Clinical Stage			
1	**2**	**3**	**4**	**5**
Lethargic	Combative	Comatose	Comatose	Comatose
Follows commands	Inconsistent following of commands	Occasional response to commands	Responds only to pain	No response to pain
Pupils reactive	Pupils sluggish	Eyes may deviate	Weak pupillary response	No pupillary response
Breathing normal	May hyperventilate	Irregular breathing	Very irregular breathing	Requires mechanical ventilation
Normal muscle tone	Reflexes inconsistent	Decorticate posturing	Decerebrate posturing	Absent tendon reflexes—flaccid

TABLE 56–3 Glasgow Coma Scale

Eye Opening (total points 4)	
Spontaneous	4
To voice	3
To pain	2
None	1

Verbal Response (total points 5)

Older Children		*Infants and Young Children*	
Oriented	5	Appropriate words; smiles, fixes, and follows	5
Confused	4	Consolable crying	4
Inappropriate	3	Persistently irritable	3
Incomprehensible	2	Restless, agitated	2
None	1	None	1

Motor Response (total points 6)

Obeys	6
Localizes pain	5
Withdraws	4
Flexion	3
Extension	2
None	1

Adapted and modified from Teasdale G, Jennett B: Assessment of coma and impaired consciousness: A practical scale. Lancet 2:81, 1974.

den onset or if the chest does not rise when ventilation is first attempted in an unconscious, apneic infant or child.

CARDIOVASCULAR SUPPORT. As resuscitation proceeds and ventilation is started, support of the *heart rate* also should be provided to sustain adequate blood flow to deliver oxygen to the tissues. The rate and depth of chest compressions vary with age and size (Table 56–4). Chest compressions in small infants and newborns

TABLE 56–4 Parameters for Optimal Cardiorespiratory Resuscitation

Age	Chest Compression Rate	Respiration Rate (breaths/min)	Endotracheal Tube Size
Newborn	100/min; 1 inch deep	20–24	3.5–4.0 mm inner diameter
Child	80/min; 1.5 inches deep	16–20	4.5–6 mm inner diameter
Teen	60/min; 2 inches deep	12–18	6–7.5 mm inner diameter

From Rogers MC: Textbook of Pediatric Intensive Care, 2nd ed. Baltimore, Williams & Wilkins, 1992.

may be performed by placing two fingers over the midsternum and compressing or by holding the child in the supine posture on one's lap, with fingers wrapped around the chest wall to the vertebral column and thumbs positioned over the midportion of the sternum, to perform the compressions. With children, the ratio of chest compressions to breaths should be approximately 5:1.

INTUBATION AND MECHANICAL VENTILATION. Although it is possible to intubate infants without sedation, analgesia, or paralysis, analgesia is recommended to reduce metabolic stress.

CRICOTHYROTOMY. When the airway is obstructed and tracheal intubation has not succeeded, *needle cricothyrotomy* is indicated.

VENOUS ACCESS. Veins suitable for cannulation are numerous, but there is considerable anatomic variation. A large vein on the *lateral side of the foot,* running in the horizontal plane, usually about 1–2 cm dorsal to the lower margin of the foot is preferable.

ARTERIAL ACCESS. Arterial catheters require special care for insertion and subsequent management because the blood flow to tissue can be compromised and considerable hemorrhage can occur if a catheter is dislodged. In most hospitals, the child should be in the pediatric intensive care unit. The adequacy of perfusion distal to the catheter must be monitored (warmth, capillary filling, edema, and so on). Catheters usually need to be heparinized ($\frac{1}{2}$–1 unit/mL) to minimize clotting.

THORACENTESIS AND CHEST TUBE PLACEMENT. *Thoracentesis* is the placement of a needle or catheter (chest tube) into the pleural space to evacuate fluid, blood, or air. Most insertions are performed between the 4th and 9th ribs along the midclavicular line in the anterior chest wall (in adolescents and adults) or in the plane of the midaxillary line.

PERICARDIOCENTESIS. When fluid, blood, or gas accumulates in the pericardial sac, a danger is that the heart will be compressed and will not be able to fill and empty with normal volumes of blood, leading to diminution in cardiac output. Pericardiocentesis is needle aspiration of the sac performed with or without ultrasound verification of needle placement or attachment of a recording electrode.

SHOCK

Shock is an acute syndrome characterized by inadequate circulatory perfusion of tissue to meet the metabolic demands of vital organs. If inadequate tissue perfusion continues, various metabolic and systemic responses occur as the patient becomes more physiologically unstable. The specific pattern of response and related pathophysiology, clinical manifestations, and treatments varies with the etiology of shock.

CLINICAL MANIFESTATIONS. A classification of shock is presented in (Table 56–5). There is significant overlap in these categories,

TABLE 56–5 Clinical Classification of Shock

	Type of Shock				
	Septic	*Cardiogenic*	*Distributive*	*Hypovolemic*	*Miscellaneous*
Characteristics	Infectious organisms release toxins that affect fluid distribution, cardiac output and so on	Primary pump failure produces inadequate tissue perfusion; resultant metabolic acidosis further impairs cardiac function	Neurologic disturbances may cause uneven distribution of fluids, leading to acidosis Overdose of drugs can alter fluid distribution	Reduced fluid volume reduces cardiac output; metabolic acidosis can result from low intravascular volume and poor tissue perfusion; serious electrolyte abnormalities may occur	Various disturbances that lead to fluid loss, pump failure, or maldistribution of fluid
Sample Causes	Bacterial Viral Fungal (all are more likely in immuno-compromised)	Ischemic insult Cardiomyopathy Congenital heart disease Tamponade	Neurogenic (disturbance of vasomotor tone) Anaphylaxis Toxic Allergic reactions	Enteritis Hemorrhage Extensive burns Diabetes insipidus Nephrotic syndrome	Major vascular obstruction Hypothermia

173

especially between septic and distributive shock. The clinical presentations of shock depend, in part, on the cause; however, if shock is unrecognized and untreated, a very similar untoward progression of clinical signs and pathophysiologic changes occurs (Table 56–6). The clinical features of shock may also relate to the stage of the process (e.g., early vs. late).

Hypovolemic shock usually presents as changes in mental status, tachypnea, tachycardia, hypotension, cool extremities, and oliguria. However, hypovolemic shock may initially present as normal or only mild to moderate changes in heart rate and blood pressure and slightly cool distal extremities. Septic shock may initially present as *compensated* or "warm shock," with warm extremities (due to peripheral vasodilatation secondary to low systemic vascular resistance), bounding pulses and tachycardia (due to high stroke volume and cardiac output), tachypnea, adequate urination, and mild metabolic acidosis. In contrast, cardiogenic shock presents as cool extremities, delayed (>2 sec) capillary filling, hypotension, tachypnea, increasing obtundation, and decreased urination (all due to peripheral vasoconstriction and decreased cardiac output). *Uncompensated* or "cool shock" (high vascular resistance, decreased cardiac output, oliguria) occurs in the late stage of shock due to almost all causes.

TREATMENT

Initial Management. In most cases of early shock, a fluid bolus of 20 mL/kg of normal saline or lactated Ringer's solution should be given rapidly. If it is not possible to insert an intravenous catheter into a peripheral vein within 90 sec or within three attempts, an intraosseous needle should be inserted to administer fluids. After this infusion, the patient is reassessed to determine if more fluid is required or other forms of therapy should be initiated (i.e., antibiotics, vasoactive agents, or other types of fluids). Children in severe hypovolemic shock may require and tolerate a fluid bolus of 60–80 mL/kg within the first 1–2 hr of presentation. However, the risk of fluid overload must be continually reassessed.

Cardiovascular Management. Septic, cardiogenic, distributive, and, rarely, hypovolemic shock may require various drugs to stimulate both heart rate (*chronotropic*) and cardiac contractility (*inotropic*). These agents should be infused through a central venous catheter in an intensive care unit. These drugs increase oxygen consumption and the risk of dysrhythmias. Dopamine is probably the most frequently used agent and is preferred for cardiogenic shock.

RESPIRATORY DISTRESS AND FAILURE

Respiratory distress/failure is the primary diagnosis in close to 50% of the children admitted to pediatric intensive care units. The causes of these respiratory problems may be classified by age,

TABLE 56–6 Signs of Decreased Perfusion

Organ System	↓ Perfusion	↓ ↓ Perfusion	↓ ↓ ↓ Perfusion
CNS	—	Restless, apathetic	Agitated/confused, stuporous
Respiration	—	↑ Ventilation	↑ ↑ Ventilation
Metabolism	—	Compensated metabolic acidemia	Uncompensated metabolic acidemia
Gut	—	↓ Motility	Ileus
Kidney	↓ Urine volume	Oliguria	Oliguria/anuria
	↑ Urinary specific gravity		
Skin	Delayed capillary refill	Cool extremities	Mottled, cyanotic, cold extremities
CVS	↑ Heart rate	↑ ↑ Heart rate, ↓ Peripheral pulses	↑ ↑ Heart rate, ↓ blood pressure, central pulses only

CNS = central nervous system; CVS = cardiovascular system; ↑ = increased; ↓ = decreased.
Adapted with permission from Lister G, Apkon M, Fabry JT: Shock. *In*: Emmanouilides GC, Riemenschneider TA, Allen HD, Gutgesell HP (eds): Moss & Adam's Heart Disease in Infants, Children and Adolescents: Including the Fetus and Young Adult, 5th ed. Baltimore, Williams & Wilkins, 1994, pp 1725–1746.

TABLE 56–7 Anatomic Classification of Respiratory Failure

Lung	Respiratory Pump
Central Airway Obstruction	***Chest Wall Deformity***
Tracheomalacia	Kyphoscoliosis
Subglottic stenosis	Diaphragmatic hernia
Epiglottitis	Flail chest
Croup	Eventration of diaphragm
Vocal cord paralysis	Prune-belly syndrome
Foreign body aspiration	***Brain Stem***
Vascular ring	
Adenotonsillar hypertrophy	Sleep apnea
Near-strangulation	Poisoning
Peripheral Airway Obstruction	Trauma
	Central nervous system infection
Bronchiolitis	***Spinal Cord***
Asthma	
Aspiration	Trauma
Cystic fibrosis	Poliomyelitis
Bronchomalacia	Werdnig-Hoffmann disease
Diffuse Alveolar Damage (Adult [Acute] Respiratory Distress Syndrome)	***Neuromuscular***
	Postoperative nerve injury
	Birth trauma
Sepsis	Infantile botulism
Pneumonia	Guillain-Barré syndrome
Pulmonary edema	
Near-drowning	
Pulmonary embolism	
Lung contusion	
Shock	

Adapted from Helfaer M, Nichols D, Rogers M: Developmental physiology of the respiratory system. *In*: Rogers MC (ed): Textbook of Pediatric Intensive Care, 2nd ed. Baltimore, Williams & Wilkins, 1992, pp 104–133.

anatomic lesions, or abnormalities as involving (1) lung and chest wall mechanics, (2) neuromuscular systems, and (3) CNS control or drive. Increased respiratory rate and effort (tachypnea and dyspnea) suggest mechanical problems of the lung or chest wall. Neuromuscular disease may result in progressively weaker respiratory efforts and eventually fatigue. CNS pathology may present as various respiratory patterns, including bradypnea, apnea, and Cheyne-Stokes respirations. The heterogeneous group of pediatric diseases that can cause respiratory distress and failure requiring mechanical ventilation is presented in Table 56–7.

CLINICAL MANIFESTATIONS. Children with impending respiratory failure due to lung disease have respiratory distress characterized by rapid breathing, or *tachypnea*; exaggerated use of accessory muscles *(retractions, nasal flaring)*; and *grunting* due to closing of the glottis at the end of expiration to generate positive end-expiratory pressure. Impending respiratory failure caused by respiratory pump dysfunction may be more difficult to recognize because these children may not have any signs of respiratory distress. Other causes of respiratory pump failure, such as a narcotic ingestion or a brain tumor, cause decreased ventilatory drive and hypoventilation. An abnormally low respiratory rate or the shallowness of the breathing may identify these children.

DIAGNOSIS. Severe respiratory distress in children is usually diagnosed by history and physical examination, and very severe distress may need treatment initiated before performing diagnostic procedures or tests.

LABORATORY FINDINGS. Hypoxemic respiratory failure is defined as a Pao_2 less than 60 mm Hg with Fio_2 greater than 0.6 (in the absence of cyanotic heart disease), and hypercarbic respiratory failure is defined as an acute $Paco_2$ greater than 50 mm Hg.

TREATMENT. Respiratory arrest or repeated apnea requires immediate respiratory support. Severe shock also may require mechanical ventilation, even if arterial blood gases are within acceptable range, because patients need increased oxygen delivery to vital organs.

MECHANICAL VENTILATION

UNDERLYING CONCEPTS AND TERMINOLOGY. Since the 1960s, positive-pressure ventilators have been predominately used in adult, pediatric, and neonatal intensive care units, and this discussion focuses on these ventilators (Table 56–8).

Pressures. Peak inspiratory pressure (PIP) occurs during inspiration. Positive end-expiratory pressure (PEEP) helps maintain the end-expiratory resting lung volume. Thus, the maximum pressure gradient is the difference between PIP and PEEP. The mean airway ure is a measure of the average pressure to which the lungs are exposed during the respiratory cycle. Adjusting the ventilator to increase mean airway pressure is the therapy for hypoxemia that is not responding to an increasing Fio_2.

Components of the Ventilator Breath. Each complete ventilator breath has an allotted time for inspiration (I time) before the ventilator must cycle into exhalation time (E time). The sum of the I time

TABLE 56–8 Commonly Used Abbreviations for Ventilator Terminology

Fio_2	Fraction of inspired oxygen (% oxygen)
IT	Inspiratory time (I time seconds)
I:E	Inspiratory to expiratory ratio (I:E)
FRC	Functional residual capacity (mL)
PIP	Peak inspiratory pressure (cm H_2O)
PEEP	Positive end-expiratory pressure (cm H_2O)
SIMV	Synchronized intermittent mandatory ventilation
V_T	Tidal volume (mL)

and E time equals the allotted time per breath. The ventilator delivers a set number of breaths per minute, the ventilator frequency. The frequency determines the length of each breath. The change in lung volume during the inspiratory period is defined as the tidal volume (V_T). It is the volume above the functional residual capacity (FRC), that is, the volume above the end-expiratory lung volume.

Pressure-Controlled versus Volume-Controlled Ventilation. Pressure-controlled ventilators allow a clinician to set the PIP and PEEP. The increase in airway pressure occurs swiftly at the initiation of inspiration to achieve the set PIP. This PIP is then maintained throughout the I time. In pressure-controlled ventilation, the lung volume rises until it reaches its capacity at that PIP or until the ventilator cycles into exhalation. Thus, V_T is not set but rather is determined by both the pressure gradient of the ventilator and the pulmonary mechanics of the patient. In volume-controlled ventilation, the V_T is preset as a product of setting flow and I time. The airway pressure rises throughout inspiration and reaches its peak when the entire V_T has been delivered.

Ventilator-Patient Interactions. When children are not attempting to breathe spontaneously, the ventilator completely controls the respiratory pattern. For children who can attempt to breathe, the degree to which a ventilator is able to synchronize with the patient's own respiratory efforts may have significant clinical repercussions.

Synchronized Intermittent Mandatory Ventilation (SIMV). SIMV is a ventilator mode that was developed to allow better response by the ventilator to the patient. During SIMV, the ventilator allows the child to trigger a breath by spontaneously attempting to inspire.

Monitoring and Alarms. What is not controllable is monitored. In pressure-controlled ventilation, the V_T is monitored. In volume-controlled ventilation, the airway pressure is monitored; safety precautions include pop-off limits to the peak airway pressure. An oxygen analyzer allows monitoring of F_{IO_2}.

APPROACH TO MECHANICAL VENTILATION. The pressure gradient that inflates the lungs must overcome the pulmonary mechanics of the patient's respiratory system.

Diseases of Decreased Compliance. Compliance is decreased in various diseases that affect the lung parenchyma, such as adult respiratory distress syndrome, atelectasis, pneumonia, pulmonary edema, pulmonary hemorrhage, and respiratory distress syndrome. Decreased compliance requires a higher pressure gradient to achieve a given V_T. This means that with volume-controlled ventilation, the PIP will be higher than it would for a patient with normal lungs.

Diseases of Increased Resistance. Resistance is increased in various diseases that decrease the caliber of the airway lumen by edema, spasm, or obstructing material. Because airways decrease in caliber during exhalation, increased resistance affects expiratory flow more than inspiratory flow. Diseases in which airway resistance is increased include asthma, bronchiolitis, bronchopulmonary dysplasia, and cystic fibrosis. Increased resistance requires that a higher pressure must occur for the flow of gas to reach the terminal air sacs. Therefore, if volume-controlled ventilation is used, an increase in PIP is required to deliver a given V_T. If pressure-controlled ventilation is used, tidal volume is lower than in a normal lung at the same pressure.

Initial Settings. When initiating mechanical ventilation, there are three approaches: providing support for lungs that function normally, for diseases of decreased compliance, or for diseases of increased resistance (Table 56–9).

RENAL STABILIZATION

STRATEGIES TO IMPROVE RENAL FUNCTION. Although oliguria is common in the pediatric intensive care unit and may be associated with poor outcomes, often only fluids or low doses of diuretics are needed for correction. In patients with oliguric renal failure, adequate intravascular fluid volumes estimated by the heart rate (within 20% of normal for age) and central venous pressure (at least 4–9 cm H_2O) should be maintained. In addition to treating the underlying cause, loop diuretics may be helpful.

VASOACTIVE MEDICATIONS AND RENAL PRESERVATION. Dopamine at doses of 1–3 µg/kg/min often improves urine output and natriuresis.

RENAL REPLACEMENT THERAPIES. Continuous venovenous hemofiltration is the modality of choice for renal replacement therapy in critically ill children.

NUTRITIONAL STABILIZATION

Critically ill children need nutritional support to ameliorate negative nitrogen balance resulting from catabolism (Table 56–10). Carbohydrate (glucose infusion of 3–5 mg/kg/min) also is given to inhibit the breakdown of endogenous protein. Generally, 70% of calories should be derived from carbohydrates and 30% from lipids. Vitamins, particularly water-soluble vitamins B complex and C, are best administered enterally.

ENTERAL FEEDING. Early enteral feeding in critically ill children, particularly those with sepsis, may avert ulcerative complications, preserve the indigenous intestinal flora, avoid overgrowth by pathogens, and prevent atrophy of the mucosa. If the gastrointestinal tract cannot be used, parenteral nutrition is necessary.

NEUROLOGIC STABILIZATION

Acute neurologic deterioration in children may be a life-threatening event with numerous causes and diverse clinical presenta-

TABLE 56-9 Guidelines for Initiating Mechanical Ventilation

	Normal Lungs	Decreased Compliance	Increased Resistance
Tidal volume(V_T)	8–12 mL/kg (set if volume-controlled and derived if pressure-controlled ventilation)	10–12 mL/kg (may need to use less if the inflating pressures are too high; i.e., risk for volutrauma)	10–12 mL/kg (may need to use less volume if the inflating pressures required are too high; i.e., barotrauma)
Rate (breaths/min)	Physiologic norm for age or lower (depending on the V_T used; e.g., infant rate = 30, toddler rate = 20, adolescent rate = 16)	May require higher rates to maintain adequate minute ventilation	Often requires lower rates to allow adequate emptying time
Peak inspiratory pressure (cm H_2O)	Initial PIP = 20–25 H_2O; monitor for adequate chest expansion and V_T	May require higher PIP to obtain acceptable V_T	May require higher PIP to obtain acceptable V_T
Positive end-expiratory pressure	2–4 cm H_2O to prevent atelectasis	Frequently requires higher PEEP to achieve oxygenation and improved compliance (e.g., 6–10 cm H_2O) Anticipate decreased venous return and cardiac output	May need to maintain low PEEP to avoid exacerbation of gas trapping and overinflation
Oxygen concentration (FIO_2)	May not need supplemental oxygen; however, one usually begins with FIO_2 of 1.0 and may then quickly wean to an FIO_2 ≤0.5	Begin with an FIO_2 of 1.0 Attempt to wean to ≤ 0.6 by adjusting mean airway pressure/PEEP	Begin with an FIO_2 of 1, wean to maintain adequate oxygenation and avoid oxygen toxicity
Inspiratory time (I time)	Normal for age I:E = 1:2, 1:3	Generous I time to allow recruitment of collapsed lung segments (e.g., 1:1.2)	Ensure adequate I time and E time, especially E time, to avoid gas trapping (e.g., I:E of 1:3 or 1:4)

TABLE 56–10 Caloric and Protein Requirements in the Critically Ill Child

Critical illness	25–30 kcal/kg/24 hr
Mechanical ventilation	20–25 kcal/kg/24 hr
Receiving growth hormone	15–20 kcal/kg/24 hr as carbohydrate
Burn or trauma	40–45 kcal/kg/24 hr
Protein	1.5–2.5 g/kg/24 hr
Protein (burn >20%)	2.0–3.0 g/kg/24 hr

tions. Children with an evolving neurologic illness must be quickly stabilized to avoid further injury to the brain. The most common causes of global neurologic dysfunction in children are head trauma, hypoxic ischemia, CNS infection, and encephalopathies due to endogenous metabolites or exogenous toxins.

CLINICAL MANIFESTATIONS

Head Trauma. This diagnosis usually is fairly obvious. A head CT scan is indicated to identify subdural and epidural hematoma, effusions, punctate intracerebral hemorrhages, skull fractures, atrophy, or hydrocephalus.

Hypoxia-Ischemia. Encephalopathy due to poor or absent cerebral circulatory perfusion often heralds a poor outcome, especially if the child has experienced a period of asystole and required cardiopulmonary resuscitation, as may occur after near-drowning episodes, near-miss sudden infant death syndrome, and other life-threatening events.

CNS Infection. CNS infections include meningitis, meningoencephalitis, and brain abscess.

Encephalopathies from Endogenous Metabolites or Exogenous Toxins. Profound encephalopathy with obtundation, stupor, or coma may result from metabolic defects (e.g., those that result in hyperammonemia), fulminant hepatic failure (in which NH_3 acts as a marker of other neurodepressant toxins), hypoglycemia, diabetic ketoacidosis, or ingestion of certain drugs or substances.

Herniation. Coma may precede herniation of intracranial contents as brain stem herniation proceeds from higher to lower brain centers. Coma is followed by decorticate rigidity, small pupils, and Cheyne-Stokes breathing. As the midbrain and pons become involved, posturing is decerebrate, pupils are midposition and nonreactive, and the breathing pattern is hyperpneic. As the medulla is compromised, the blood pressure and heart rate fluctuate greatly, the patient becomes flaccid, and breathing is irregular and then absent.

TREATMENT OF GLOBAL NEUROLOGIC DYSFUNCTION

Normalize the Circulation and Respiration. The basics of neurologic stabilization include the ABCs and maintenance of adequate oxygenation and perfusion during the various diagnostic tests that must be performed.

Reduction of Intracranial Hypertension: Positioning and Hyperventilation. The head should be positioned in the midline and elevated about 30 degrees to allow optimal venous drainage. Movement should be minimized with sedation (e.g., intermittent or continuous benzodiazepines and narcotics). Hyperventilation is helpful: cerebral vessels constrict in response to a falling PCO_2. The PCO_2 should be maintained between 25 and 30 mm Hg.

Diuretics and Corticosteroids. Mannitol (0.5 g/kg) promotes a shift of fluid from the intracellular to the intravascular CNS space, from which it can be removed by renal excretion. Furosemide is a safer but less effective alternative. The combination is often prescribed.

Seizures: Benzodiazepines versus Antiepileptics. Both benzodiazepines and antiepileptics reduce cerebral metabolism, but the antiepileptics are more effective at suppressing subsequent seizure activity. Both phenobarbital and phenytoin are effective. If necessary in refractory status epilepticus, phenobarbital can be infused at a very high dose (e.g., to a serum level of 50–200 mg/dL) with very little effect on the cardiovascular system.

CHAPTER 57

Acute (Adult) Respiratory Distress Syndrome

(Nelson Textbook, Chapter 65)

Acute or "adult" respiratory distress syndrome (ARDS) is diagnosed in 2.5–3% of children in the pediatric intensive care unit. The syndrome consists of (1) hypoxemia ($PaO_2/FIO_2 < 200$), (2) diffuse pulmonary infiltrates on chest radiograph, (3) normal pulmonary artery occlusion pressure, and (4) normal cardiac function.

CLINICAL MANIFESTATIONS. The acute pulmonary deterioration of ARDS may not be appreciated initially. During this latent period, patients may exhibit mild respiratory distress, evidenced by tachypnea, and an increased oxygen requirement. Auscultation of the lungs may reveal clear breath sounds or scattered rales. Within a few hours, patients begin to develop more severe hypoxia accompanied by carbon dioxide retention. The onset of ARDS may be quite variable in sepsis, very sudden with pulmonary aspiration, or insidious in acute neurologic injury or shock.

LABORATORY FINDINGS. These patients usually are initially monitored with a pulse oximeter; and when an FIO_2 greater than 0.5

is required to maintain the arterial oxygen saturation above 92%, the diagnosis of ARDS is considered. During the next few hours, the chest radiographs begin to demonstrate interstitial and alveolar pulmonary edema. Positive-pressure ventilation may alter the radiographic features of pulmonary edema, but the abnormalities in pulmonary function and blood gases coupled with a worsening respiratory status support the diagnosis.

TREATMENT. The underlying disease (e.g., sepsis, aspiration, shock) should be treated. A minority of patients respond to oxygen therapy and meticulous fluid management. However, most patients progress to severe respiratory failure and require endotracheal intubation and mechanical ventilation in a pediatric intensive care unit. The duration of respiratory support may be prolonged, accompanied by numerous complications and a very high mortality rate.

CHAPTER **58**

Drowning and Near-Drowning
(Nelson Textbook, Chapter 69)

After submersion in a liquid medium, suffocation and asphyxia may occur, with or without pulmonary aspiration. Irreversible multisystemic injury occurs very rapidly, often leading to death. Death within 24 hr of submersion is termed *drowning*, which may be immediate or may follow resuscitation. Survival of more than 24 hr is termed *near-drowning*, regardless of whether the victim later dies or recovers.

EPIDEMIOLOGY. Children are particularly at risk for drowning. In the United States, drowning is the fourth leading cause of death for children younger than 19 yr old and the single leading cause of injury death for children younger than 5 yr of age. Two age groups are at particular risk: toddlers, who commonly drown in residential swimming pools during brief periods of inadequate supervision, and older adolescent males (15–19 yr old), who often drown in natural bodies of water. Residential swimming pools account for half of all drowning in the United States but are the site of almost 90% of submersion events in children younger than 5 yr old.

CLINICAL MANIFESTATIONS AND TREATMENT. A submersion victim's clinical course and outcome are primarily determined by the circumstances of the incident, the duration of submersion, the speed of the rescue, and the effectiveness of resuscitative efforts.

Initial Evaluation and Resuscitation. Once a submersion has occurred, extrication and immediate institution of cardiopulmonary resuscitation (CPR) at the scene potentially have the greatest chance of improving outcome. The initial out-of-hospital resuscitation of submersion victims must focus on rapidly restoring oxygenation, ventilation, and adequate circulation. The airway should be clear of vomitus or foreign material, which may result in obstruction or aspiration. Abdominal thrusts should not be routinely used for lung fluid removal, because their effectiveness is not established. They may increase the risk of regurgitation, aspiration, and loss of airway control; they may delay or interrupt CPR; and they have the potential to aggravate spinal trauma. The neck should be in a neutral position and protected with a well-fitting cervical collar.

If the victim has ineffective respiration or apnea, ventilatory support must be initiated immediately. Mouth-to-mouth or mouth-to-nose breathing by trained bystanders often restores spontaneous ventilation and is preferable to manual methods of artificial respiration. Positive-pressure bag-mask ventilation with high inspired oxygen concentration should be substituted as soon as possible in patients with respiratory insufficiency. Supplemental oxygen should be administered uniformly regardless of the patient's condition.

If apnea, cyanosis, hypoventilation, or labored respiration persists, endotracheal intubation should be performed by trained personnel as soon as possible. Endotracheal intubation is also indicated to protect the airway in patients with depressed mental status or hemodynamic instability. Hypercapnia and hypoxia must be corrected to optimize the chances of recovery.

Heart rate and rhythm, blood pressure, temperature, and end-organ perfusion require quick assessment: slow capillary refill, cool extremities, and altered mental status are potential indicators of shock. Electrocardiographic monitoring assists with the diagnosis and treatment of arrhythmias.

Intravenous fluid administration is often required to improve perfusion. Two large-bore intravenous catheters or a central venous line should be established as soon as possible. Non–dextrose-containing, isotonic fluid (lactated Ringer's solution or normal saline) is usually given as a bolus to augment preload.

In children with cardiac arrest after submersion, electrical defibrillation or cardioversion is often urgently necessary for children with ventricular fibrillation or ventricular tachycardia. Catecholamine infusions may be required to support myocardial function and blood pressure. In severely hypothermic patients, the restoration of normal sinus rhythm and adequate perfusion is difficult until core body temperature is at least partially corrected.

Attention to hypothermia in the field is of great importance, both to initiate rewarming measures and to prevent the consequences of deeper hypothermia. All hypothermic victims should have damp clothes removed, the skin dried, warm blankets applied, and a warm environmental temperature provided as soon as possible. If available, both warmed intravenous fluids (40–43°C) and humidified oxygen (42–46°C) should be used. Patients with severe hypothermia (core temperature < 30°C) require active internal warming measures provided as soon as possible.

Hospital-Based Evaluation and Treatment. At a minimum, monitoring of vital signs (especially temperature and respiratory rate), careful examination, chest radiography, and assessment of oxygenation by arterial blood gas or oximetry should be performed on all submersion victims. Even children who initially appear unaffected after a significant submersion need to be carefully observed for at least 8–12 hr.

Neurologic Management. The most effective neurointensive care in near-drowning is the rapid restoration of adequate oxygenation, ventilation, and perfusion. Otherwise, present neurologic management entails avoiding exacerbation of central nervous system injury. Ongoing close monitoring is necessary.

Other Management Issues. Some submersion victims may have traumatic injury, especially if they were participating in water sports such as boating, diving, or surfing. A high index of suspicion is required. Spinal precautions should be maintained in victims with altered mental status and suspected traumatic injury.

PROGNOSIS. Approximately 80% of pediatric submersion victims survive, and 92% of survivors make a complete recovery. In those children requiring tertiary intensive care, just over half survive neurologically intact, but 13–35% die and 7–27% survive with severe brain damage.

CHAPTER 59

Burn Injuries
(Nelson Textbook, Chapter 70)

Burns are a leading cause of unintentional death in children, second only to motor vehicular accidents.

ACUTE CARE, RESUSCITATION, AND ASSESSMENT

INDICATIONS FOR ADMISSION. Burns covering more than 10–15% of total body surface area (BSA), burns associated with smoke inhalation, burns resulting from high-tension electrical injuries, and burns associated with suspected child abuse or neglect should be treated as emergencies and the child hospitalized. Small first- and second-degree burns of the hands, feet, face, perineum, and joint surfaces also require admission if close follow-up care is difficult to provide. Children who have been in enclosed-space fires and those who have face and neck burns should be hospitalized for at least 24 hr of observation.

FIRST AID MEASURES. Acute care should include the following:

1. Extinguish flames by rolling on the ground; cover the child with a blanket, coat, or carpet.

2. After determining that the airway is patent, remove smoldering clothing or clothing saturated with hot liquid. Jewelry, particularly rings and bracelets, should be removed or cut away to prevent constriction and vascular compromise during the edema phase in the first 24–72 hr post burn.

3. In cases of chemical injury, brush off any remaining chemical if powdered or solid; then use copious irrigation or wash the affected area with water. Call Poison Control for the neutralizing agent to treat a chemical ingestion.

4. Cover the burned area with clean, dry sheeting and apply cold (not iced) wet compresses to small injuries. Significant large burn surface area injury (>15–20% BSA) decreases body temperature control and contraindicates the use of cold compress dressings.

5. If the burn is caused by hot tar, use mineral oil to remove the tar.

EMERGENCY CARE. Life support measures should include the following:

1. Rapidly review the cardiovascular and pulmonary status and document pre-existing or physiologic lesions (asthma, congenital heart disease, renal or hepatic disease).

2. Ensure and maintain an adequate airway and provide humidified oxygen by mask or nasotracheal intubation. If hypoxia or carbon monoxide poisoning is suspected, 100% oxygen should be used.

3. Children with burns greater than 15% of BSA require intravenous fluid resuscitation to maintain adequate perfusion. All inhalation injuries, regardless of the extent of BSA burn, require venous access to control fluid intake. All high-tension and electrical injuries require venous access to ensure forced alkaline diuresis in case of muscle injury and myoglobinuria. Lactated Ringer's solution, 10–20 mL/kg/hr (normal saline may be used if Ringer's lactate is not available) is infused until proper fluid replacement can be calculated. Consultation with a specialized burn unit should be made to coordinate fluid therapy, type of fluid, preferred formula for calculation, and preferences for use of colloid agents, particularly if transfer to a burn center is anticipated.

4. Evaluate the child for associated injuries, which are common in patients with a history of high-tension electrical burn, especially if there has been a fall from a height.

5. Children with burns greater than 15% BSA should not

receive oral fluids (initially), because they may develop ileus. These children require insertion of a nasogastric tube in the emergency department to prevent aspiration.

6. A Foley catheter should be inserted to monitor urine output in all children who require intravenous fluid resuscitation.

7. All wounds should be wrapped with sterile towels until a decision is made about whether to treat the victim on an outpatient basis or to refer the victim to an appropriate facility for treatment.

CLASSIFICATION OF BURNS. *First-degree burns* involve only the epidermis and are characterized by swelling, erythema, and pain (similar to a mild sunburn). Tissue damage is usually minimal, and there is no blistering. Pain resolves in 48–72 hr.

A *second-degree burn* involves injury to the entire epidermis and a variable portion of the dermal layer (vesicle and blister formation are characteristic of second-degree burns). A superficial second-degree burn is extremely painful because a large number of remaining viable nerve endings are exposed. Superficial second-degree burns heal in 7–14 days as the epithelium regenerates in the absence of infection. *Midlevel* to *deep* second-degree burns also heal spontaneously if wounds are kept clean and free of infection. Fluid losses and metabolic effects of deep dermal (second-degree) burns are essentially the same as those of third-degree burns.

Full-thickness or *third-degree* burns involve destruction of the entire epidermis and dermis, leaving no residual epidermis cells to repopulate the damaged area. The wound cannot epithelialize and can heal only by wound contraction or skin grafting.

ESTIMATION OF BODY SURFACE AREA OF BURN. Appropriate burn charts for different childhood age groups should be used to accurately estimate the extent of BSA burned. The volume of fluid needed in resuscitation is calculated from the estimation of the extent and depth of burn surface.

TREATMENT

OUTPATIENT MANAGEMENT OF MINOR BURNS. First- and second-degree burns less than 10% BSA may be treated on an outpatient basis unless there is inadequate family support or there are issues of child neglect or abuse. Blisters should be left intact and dressed with silver sulfadiazine cream (Silvadene). Dressings should be changed twice daily, after the wound is washed with lukewarm water to remove any cream left from the previous application.

FLUID RESUSCITATION. For most children the Parkland formula is an appropriate starting guideline for fluid resuscitation (4 mL Ringer's lactate/kg body weight/% BSA burned). One half of the fluid is given over the first 8 hr calculated from the time of onset of injury. The remaining half is given at an even rate over the next 16 hr. The rate of infusion is adjusted according to the patient's response to therapy.

During the second 24 hr after the burn, patients will begin to reabsorb edema fluid and to diurese. One half of the first day's fluid requirement is infused as lactated Ringer's solution in 5% dextrose. Children younger than age 5 yr may require the addition of 5% dextrose in the first 24 hr of resuscitation. Controversy exists as to whether colloid should be provided in the early period of burn resuscitation.

Oral supplementation may start as early as 48 hr after the burn. Milk formula, artificial feedings, homogenized milk, or soy-based products can be given by bolus or constant infusion through a nasogastric or small bowel feeding tube. As oral fluids are tolerated, intravenous fluids are decreased proportionately.

Five percent albumin infusions may be used to maintain the serum albumin levels at a desired 2 g/dL. Packed red cell infusion is recommended if the hematocrit falls below 24% (hemoglobin < 8 g/dL). Sodium supplementation may be required for children having burns greater than 20% BSA, if 0.5% silver nitrate solution is used as the topical antibacterial burn dressing.

PREVENTION OF INFECTION. Controversy exists over the prophylactic use of penicillin for all acute hospitalized burn patients and the periodic replacement of central venous catheters.

NUTRITIONAL SUPPORT. Supporting the increased energy requirements of a burn is a high priority. The burn injury produces a hypermetabolic response characterized by both protein and fat catabolism. The objective of caloric supplementation programs is to maintain body weight and decrease metabolic demands.

TOPICAL THERAPY. Topical therapy is widely used and is effective against most burn pathogens. A number of agents (0.5% silver nitrate, sulfacetamide acetate, silver sulfadiazine cream) are available, and preferences vary among burn units.

INHALATIONAL INJURY. Evaluation aims at early identification of inhalational airway injuries. These may occur from (1) direct heat (greater problems occur in steam burns), (2) acute asphyxia, (3) carbon monoxide poisoning, and (4) toxic fumes, including cyanides from combustible plastics.

The pulmonary complications of burns and inhalation can be divided into three syndromes with distinct clinical manifestations and temporal patterns: (1) Early carbon monoxide poisoning, airway obstruction, and pulmonary edema are major concerns. (2) The acute respiratory distress syndrome (ARDS) usually becomes clinically evident later, at 24–48 hr, although it can occur even later. (3) Late complications (days to weeks) include pneumonia and pulmonary emboli. Inhalation injury should be assessed by evidence of obvious injury (swelling or carbonaceous material in nasal passages) and laboratory determination of carboxyhemoglobin and arterial blood gases. Treatment is initially focused on establishing and maintaining a patent airway through prompt and early nasotracheal intubation and adequate ventilation and oxygenation. Aggressive pulmonary toilet and chest physiotherapy are necessary in prolonged nasotracheal intubation or tracheotomy.

PAIN RELIEF AND PSYCHOLOGIC ADJUSTMENT. It is important to provide adequate analgesia, anxiolytics, and psychologic support to reduce early metabolic stress, decrease the potential for post-traumatic stress syndrome, and allow future stabilization and rehabilitation. Patients and family require team support to work through a grieving process and accept long-term changes in appearance.

CHAPTER 60

Cold Injuries
(Nelson Textbook, Chapter 71)

Cold injury may produce either local tissue damage, with the injury pattern depending on exposure to damp cold (frostnip, immersion foot or trench foot), dry cold (which leads to local frostbite), or generalized systemic effects (hypothermia).

CLINICAL MANIFESTATIONS

Frostnip. This results in the presence of firm, cold white areas on the face, ears, or extremities. Blistering and peeling may occur over the next 24–72 hr, occasionally leaving mild increased hypersensitivity to cold for some days or weeks. Treatment consists of warming the area with an unaffected hand or warm object before the lesion reaches a stage of stinging or aching and before numbness supervenes.

Immersion Foot (Trench Foot). This occurs in cold weather when the feet remain in damp or wet, poorly ventilated boots. The feet become cold, numb, pale, edematous, and clammy. Tissue maceration and infection are likely, and prolonged autonomic disturbance is common. The treatment is largely prophylactic and consists of using well-fitting, insulated, waterproof, nonconstricting footwear. The disturbance in skin integrity is managed by keeping the affected area dry and well ventilated and preventing or treating infection.

Frostbite. With frostbite, initial stinging or aching of the skin progresses to cold, hard, white anesthetic and numb areas. On rewarming, the area becomes blotchy, itchy, and often red, swollen, and painful. *Treatment* consists of warming the damaged area. It is important not to cause further damage by attempting to rub the area with ice or snow; initial warming as in frostnip may be tried.

Hypothermia. Immersion and wet wind chill rapidly produce hypothermia. As the core temperature of the body falls, an insidious onset of extreme lethargy, fatigue, incoordination, and apathy follows, followed by mental confusion, clumsiness, irritability, hallucinations, and finally bradycardia. The decrease in rectal temperature to less than 34°C (93°F) is the most helpful diagnostic feature.

Prevention is a high priority. Treatment at the scene aims at prevention of further heat loss and early transport to adequate shelter. Dry clothing should be provided as soon as practical, and transport should be undertaken if the victim has a pulse. If no pulse is detected at the initial review, cardiopulmonary resuscitation is indicated. On arrival at a treatment center, inhalation of warm, moist air or oxygen, heating pads, or thermal blankets should be used while a warming bath of 45–48°C (113–118°F) is prepared. Monitoring of serum chemistry values and an electrocardiogram are necessary until the core temperature rises above 35°C and can be stabilized.

CHAPTER 61

Anesthesia and Perioperative Care
(Nelson Textbook, Chapter 73)

PREOPERATIVE ASSESSMENT

All infants and children scheduled for surgery should be evaluated preoperatively both to screen for conditions that may require specific treatment or optimization of therapy (e.g., evaluation of anemia, adjustment of asthma medications) and to counsel patients and parents about the expected course of anesthesia and surgery. The cornerstone of assessment is a systematic history and detailed physical examination with emphasis on airway anatomy and cardiorespiratory status.

FASTING GUIDELINES (NPO ORDERS). Preoperative fasting is advised because anesthetic induction involves loss of airway reflexes that prevent aspiration of regurgitated gastric contents (Table 61–1).

AN ACCEPTABLE HEMATOCRIT. A hematocrit of 28% lies within the normal range for infants at 3 mo of age. In many patients with chronic renal insufficiency or hematologic disorders, it may be appropriate to administer anesthesia with a substantially lower hematocrit.

SURGICAL TIMING AND EVALUATION OF ANESTHETIC RISK. The proper timing of surgery in infants depends on both anesthetic risks and effects of timing on surgical outcome. Infants remain at greater risk than older children. Emergency surgery is more risky than

TABLE 61-1 Fasting Guidelines*

Clear fluids	2 hr
Breast milk	4 hr
Infant formula	6 hr
Solids (light meal)	6 hr
Solids (fatty meal)	8 hr

*These are general guidelines and may not reflect local hospital policies.
Data from a report of a Task Force on Practice Guidelines of the American Society of Anesthesiologists, 1998. Available from the ASA website at www.asahg.org.

elective surgery. Formerly preterm infants up to perhaps 60 wk after conception are at risk for periodic breathing, apnea, and bradycardia after general anesthesia or sedation.

LATEX ALLERGY. Intraoperative allergic reactions to latex antigens have been described with increasing frequency during the past decade. In response to this problem, many hospitals have made nonlatex gloves routinely available.

PREANESTHETIC PREPARATION AND PREMEDICATION

For most children, the primary purpose of premedication is to diminish the fear and anxiety associated with separation from parents and with other aspects of anesthetic induction, such as fear of the mask. Premedication should not substitute for efforts to make the experience of induction as atraumatic as possible.

ANESTHETIC INDUCTION

Before proceeding with an operation, it is important to correct dehydration, decrease excessive fever, correct acid-base balance, and restore a depleted blood volume. Choice of anesthetic induction technique is dictated by specific patient risks and disease status in certain circumstances.

INTRAOPERATIVE MANAGEMENT

Anesthesia can be maintained by either intravenous agents or inhalation anesthetics or by a combination of both. Airway maintenance by mask is useful for many short and elective operations. Tracheal intubation is indicated in the following: (1) operations of the head and neck; (2) thoracic, abdominal, and cranial procedures; (3) operations in the prone position; and (4) most emergency procedures, because there is uncertainty about the contents of the stomach. In younger infants, especially those younger than 6 mo, airway maintenance and adequacy of respiratory effort are more problematic and tracheal intubation is widely preferred for all but the briefest operations.

Pediatricians should become familiar with safe dosing guidelines for local anesthetics in children: 5 mg/kg (7 mg/kg with epinephrine) for lidocaine and 2 mg/kg (2.5 mg/kg with epinephrine) for bupivacaine.

FLUID THERAPY. For all but the most superficial operations, children should receive intravenous cannulation, both as a port of access for medications and as a means for replacing fluid deficits and providing maintenance requirements.

THERMOREGULATION. Thermoregulation is impaired during general or major regional anesthesia, and young infants are particularly susceptible to hypothermia or hyperthermia in the operating room. Continuous monitoring of body temperature is essential during general anesthesia.

POSTANESTHETIC RECOVERY

Recovery room facilities and nursing care must be available to provide constant surveillance of airway patency, adequate ventilation, and circulatory stability. Common sequelae of general anesthesia in infants and children include postanesthetic excitement, vomiting, and pain.

ANESTHESIA AND CONSCIOUS SEDATION AWAY FROM THE OPERATING ROOM

Common diagnostic and therapeutic procedures include bone marrow aspiration and biopsy, radiologic imaging, radiation therapy, and endoscopic procedures. Sedation and anesthesia in these settings can be of great benefit in reducing children's distress and improving ease of conduct of the procedure. The American Academy of Pediatrics has promoted monitoring standards to reduce the risks of conscious sedation outside the operating room.

CHAPTER 62

Pain Management in Children
(Nelson Textbook, Chapter 74)

CLINICAL ASSESSMENT OF PAIN. Whenever feasible, pain is best assessed by asking children about the character, location, quality, and intensity of their pain. For the most part, patients should be believed, and self-report is the most useful guide to assessment. For infants and preverbal children, parents, pediatricians, nurses, and other caregivers are constantly challenged to interpret whether the distressed behaviors of the children represent pain, fear, hunger, or a range of other perceptions or emotions.

Investigators have devised a range of behavioral distress scales for infants and younger children, mostly emphasizing facial expressions, crying, and body movement. Facial expression measures appear to be most useful and specific in neonates. Autonomic signs, including tachycardia and hypertension, can indicate pain, but these signs may be nonspecific and may reflect a range of other processes unrelated to pain, including fever, hypoxemia, and cardiac or renal dysfunction.

NONPHARMACOLOGIC APPROACHES TO MANAGEMENT OF PAIN. Various nonpharmacologic methods can be used to relieve pain, fear, and anxiety, including relaxation training, guided imagery, self-hypnosis, and a range of physical therapeutic methods.

ACETAMINOPHEN, ASPIRIN, AND NONSTEROIDAL ANTI-INFLAMMATORY DRUGS (Table 62–1). Acetaminophen and nonsteroidal anti-inflammatory drugs (NSAIDs) have replaced aspirin as the most commonly used antipyretics and oral nonopioid analgesics.

OPIOIDS. These are used to treat various types of acute and chronic pain in infants and children. Opioids are most frequently administered for moderate and severe pain (Table 62–2).

LOCAL ANESTHETICS. Local anesthetics are widely used in children for topical application, cutaneous infiltration, peripheral nerve block, and intraspinal punctures. In general, local anesthetics can be used with excellent safety and effectiveness. Topical local anesthetic preparations have diverse uses in reducing pain, such as for suturing lacerations, intravenous catheter placements, lumbar punctures, and accessing indwelling central ports. Application of tetracaine, epinephrine, and cocaine (TAC) results in good anesthesia for suturing wounds. It should not be used on mucous membranes. Cocaine is not essential; combinations of tetracaine with phenylephrine or lidocaine-epinephrine-tetracaine are equally effective. EMLA is a topical eutectic mixture of lidocaine and prilocaine that is used to anesthetize intact skin and is commonly applied for venipuncture, lumbar puncture, and other needle procedures. EMLA is safe for use in neonates.

Lidocaine is the most commonly used local anesthetic for cutaneous infiltration. Maximum safe doses of lidocaine are 5 mg/kg without epinephrine and 6 mg/kg with epinephrine. Concentrated solutions (e.g., 2%) should be avoided, because solutions as dilute as 0.3% are equally effective as 1–2% solutions and the dilute solutions permit larger doses.

MANAGEMENT OF BRIEF DIAGNOSTIC AND THERAPEUTIC PROCEDURES. Procedures such as endoscopy, bone marrow aspiration and biopsy, or radiologic imaging procedures may require either analgesia to make the procedure more comfortable, anxiolysis to make the procedure less terrifying, or sedation to permit a child to lie motionless for imaging studies or radiation therapy. The term *conscious sedation* refers to a condition in which a patient is sleepy, comfortable, and more cooperative but maintains protective airway and ventilatory reflexes. The term *deep sedation* refers to a state of unarousability to voice and greater suppression of reflex

TABLE 62–1 Commonly Used Nonopioid Medications

Drug	Dosing Guidelines	Comments
Acetaminophen	10–15 mg/kg PO q 4h 20–30 mg/kg PR q 4 h Maximum daily dosing: 90 mg/kg/24 hr (children) 60 mg/kg/24 hr (infants) 30–45 mg/kg/24 hr (neonates)	No anti-inflammatory action No antiplatelet or gastric effects Toxic dosing can produce hepatic failure
Aspirin	10–15 mg/kg PO q 4 h Maximum daily dosing: 120 mg/kg/24 hr (children)	Anti-inflammatory effects Prolonged antiplatelet effects Can cause gastritis
Ibuprofen	8–10 mg/kg PO q 6 hr	Anti-inflammatory effects Reversible antiplatelet effects Can cause gastritis Extensive pediatric safety experience
Naprosyn	5–7 mg/kg PO q 8–12 hr	Anti-inflammatory effects Reversible antiplatelet effects Can cause gastritis More prolonged duration than that of ibuprofen
Ketorolac	0.25–0.5 mg/kg IV q 6 hr, to a maximum of 5 days	Anti-inflammatory effects Reversible antiplatelet effects Can cause gastritis Useful for short-term situations when oral dosing is not feasible
Choline magnesium salicylate	10–20 mg/kg PO q 8–12 hr	Weak anti-inflammatory effects Lower risk of bleeding and gastritis than with conventional NSAIDs
Nortriptyline, amitriptyline	Begin at 0.1–0.2 mg/kg PO q 24 hr, advance as needed or tolerated to 1.5 mg/kg/24 hr; some patients require a portion of the dose, e.g., 25%, in the morning, others remain at q hr dosing	Useful for neuropathic pain Rare risk of dysrhythmias; should screen for rhythm disturbances Side effects include dry mouth, sedation, constipation, urinary retention, orthostatic hypotension, palpitations

TABLE 62–2 Analgesic Initial Dosage Guidelines*

Drug	Equianalgesic Doses		Usual Starting IV or SC Doses and Intervals		Parenteral/Oral Dose Ratio	Using Starting Oral Doses and Intervals	
	Parenteral	Oral	Child <50 kg	Child >50 kg		Child <50 kg	Child >50 kg
Codeine	N/R	200 mg	N/R	N/R	1:2	0.5–1 mg/kg q 3–4 hr	30–60 mg q 3–4 hr
Morphine	10 mg	30 mg	Bolus: 0.1 mg/kg q 2–4 hr; Infusion: 0.03 mg/kg/hr	Bolus: 5–8 mg q 2–4 hr; Infusion: 1.5 mg/hr	1:3	Immediate release: 0.3 mg/kg q 3–4 hr; Sustained release: 20–35 kg: 10–15 mg q 8–12 hr; 35–50 kg: 15–30 mg q 8–12 hr	Immediate release: 15–20 mg q 3–4 hr; Sustained release: 30–45 mg q 8–12 hr
Oxycodone	N/A	30 mg	N/A	N/A	N/A	0.1–0.2 mg/kg q 3–4 hr	5–10 mg q 3–4 hr
Methadone†	10 mg	20 mg	Bolus: 0.1 mg/kg q 4–8 hr	Bolus: 5–8 mg q 4–8 hr	1:2	0.2 mg/kg q 4–8 hr	10 mg q 4–8 hr
Fentanyl	100 µg (0.1 mg)	N/A	Bolus: 0.5–1 µg/kg q 1–2 hr; Infusion: 0.5–1.5 µg/kg/hr	Bolus: 25–50 µg q 1–2 hr; Infusion: 25–75 µg/hr	N/A	N/A	N/A
Hydromorphone	1.5–2 mg	6–8 mg	Bolus: 0.02 mg/kg q 2–4 hr; Infusion: 0.006 mg/kg/hr	Bolus: 1 mg q 2–4 hr; Infusion: 0.3 mg/hr	1:4	0.04–0.08 mg/kg q 3–4 hr	2–4 mg q 3–4 hr
Meperidine (pethidine)‡	75 mg	300 mg	Bolus: 0.8–1 mg/kg q 2–3 hr	Bolus: 50–75 mg q 2–3 hr	1:4	2–3 mg/kg q 3–4 hr	100–150 mg q 3–4 hr

*Doses refer to patients >6 mo of age. In infants <6 mo, initial doses/kg should begin at roughly 25% of the doses/kg recommended here. All doses are approximate and should be adjusted according to clinical circumstances.

†Methadone requires additional vigilance, because it can accumulate and produce delayed sedation. If sedation occurs, doses should be withheld until sedation resolves. Thereafter, doses should be substantially reduced and/or the dosing interval should be extended to 8–12 hr.

‡Meperidine should generally be avoided if other opioids are available, especially with chronic use, because its metabolite can cause seizures.

N/A = not applicable; N/R = not recommended.

TABLE 62–3 Drugs Used for Conscious Sedation in Children

Drug	Suggested Starting Dose(s)	Comments
Midazolam	0.05 mg/kg incremental doses IV q 5–10 min up to 3–5 doses (to a maximum incremental dose of 1 mg) 0.1–0.2 mg/kg IM (maximum dose 10 mg) 0.3–0.6 mg/kg PO (maximum dose 20 mg)	Good anxiolytic Flumazenil is a reversal agent Dose more cautiously when combined with opioids
Fentanyl	0.5 µg/kg increments q 5 min up to 3–5 doses	Rapid infusion of large doses can produce chest wall rigidity Respiratory depression is amplified by co-administration of sedatives
Pentobarbital	1 mg/kg increments IV q 10 min up to 3 doses 2–4 mg/kg IM 4–6 mg/kg PO	Good sedative, no analgesia Used primarily for radiologic procedures Occasionally produces prolonged sedation
Chloral hydrate	25–100 mg/kg PO or PR 30–40 min before the procedure 0.2–0.5 mg/kg increments q 10 min × 3	Higher incidence of failed sedation with 25–50 mg/kg
Ketamine	1–2 mg/kg IM	Co-administration of midazolam or other benzodiazepines is recommended to reduce the risk of dysphoria or bad dreams Use should be restricted to cases managed by physicians with extensive airway expertise

responses. To ensure that patients receive optimal, safe care, it is recommended that hospitals develop conscious sedation guidelines, such as those established by the American Academy of Pediatrics. These guidelines should include recommendations for withholding feeding before procedures, drug dosages (Table 62–3), strategies to achieve patient comfort, necessary monitoring, required resuscitation equipment, and a quality improvement program for tracking outcomes and ensuring efficacy and safety.

PART 9

Genetics and Metabolic Diseases

CHAPTER 63

Molecular Diagnosis of Genetic Diseases and Patterns

(Nelson Textbook, Chapters 75, 76, and 77)

GENETIC ABNORMALITIES. Genetic abnormalities are a common cause of disease, handicap, and death among infants and children. Genetic disease accounts for the primary diagnosis of 11–16% of patients admitted to the pediatric units of teaching hospitals.

DIAGNOSIS. The most striking advantage of the diagnosis of genetic disease through the molecular genetic approach is that a gene can be identified through examination of the DNA from almost any cell of a patient. Diagnosis of a genetic disorder can be accomplished by either the direct approach—a gene is examined for mutations associated with a disease—or the indirect approach, generally applied before a gene has been fully characterized—a "disease" gene is followed within a family by its linkage with defined sequences that are co-inherited with high probability.

THE NATURE OF MUTATIONS. Human genetics deals with the variations between individuals. These variations are reflections of differences that exist at the DNA level. Variations that have an impact on the functioning of the gene are usually referred to as mutations. Other variations that do not have an impact on the health or functioning of an organism are called polymorphisms; the dilemma often arises during molecular investigations in deciding whether a newly observed change is a mutation or a harmless polymorphism. Mutations may arise in somatic cells as well as in germ cells, but only those changes present in the germ cells will be heritable.

Mutations result from a change of a single base-pair of DNA (substitution), from the loss or addition of DNA (deletions, insertions, duplications, expansions), and from rearrangements (inversions and translocations). The effects of mutations depend on the alteration in the amount or structure of the protein that is formed and whether the change occurs in domains of the protein crucial to its normal functioning.

PATTERNS OF INHERITANCE

Each single mutant gene exhibits one of the four patterns of mendelian inheritance: autosomal recessive, autosomal dominant, X-linked recessive, or X-linked dominant. This method of grouping genetic diseases is often helpful in understanding the clinical presentation of a disorder.

AUTOSOMAL RECESSIVE INHERITANCE. The pedigree illustrating this pattern of inheritance shows the following characteristics: the child of two heterozygous parents has a 25% chance of being homozygous. Males and females are affected with equal frequency; the affected individuals are almost always born in only one generation of a family; the children of the affected (homozygous) person are all heterozygotes; and the children of a homozygote can be affected only if the spouse is a heterozygote.

AUTOSOMAL DOMINANT INHERITANCE. In this pedigree both males and females are affected, transmission occurs from one parent to child, and the responsible mutant gene can arise by spontaneous mutation of a gene.

X-LINKED RECESSIVE INHERITANCE. In this pedigree only males are clinically affected; affected males are related through carrier females; all daughters of affected males are carriers of the mutant gene; and affected males do not have affected sons but may have affected grandsons born to carrier females. The female carrier has a 50% chance of giving her chromosome that bears the mutant gene to each of her children. In other words, each daughter of a carrier has a 50% chance of being a carrier, and each son has a 50% chance of inheriting the mutant gene and having the disease that it causes. Therefore, in each pregnancy the female carrier has a 25% chance of having an affected son.

X-LINKED DOMINANT INHERITANCE. Very few X-linked dominant genes have been identified in humans. Both males and females are affected, but males are often more severely affected; the disorder is transmitted from generation to generation; and all daughters of an affected father will be affected but none of his sons.

MULTIFACTORIAL INHERITANCE. The term *multifactorial inheritance* refers to the process in which either continuously variable (quantitative) traits (such as height or blood pressure) or a disease state is the result of additive and interactive effects of one or more genes plus environmental factors. The estimate of the contribution of genes to such a trait or disorder is termed the *heritability*. These disorders include most of the common malformations (neural tube defects, cleft lip and palate, congenital dislocation of the hip) and common multifactorial diseases of adulthood (schizophrenia, essential hypertension, coronary heart disease, diabetes mellitus) and childhood (allergic diseases, some types of hyperlipidemia).

ATYPICAL PATTERNS OF INHERITANCE. There is a growing appreciation that genetic disorders are sometimes inherited in ways that do not follow the usual patterns of dominant, recessive, X-linked, or multifactorial inheritance. These atypical patterns of inheritance sometimes involve specific diseases and in other instances can apply to virtually any hereditary disorder.

CHAPTER 64

Chromosomal Clinical Abnormalities

(Nelson Textbook, Chapters 78, 79, and 80)

Chromosomal anomalies occur in 0.4% of live births. They are an important cause of mental retardation and congenital anomalies.

ABNORMALITIES OF CHROMOSOME NUMBER

ANEUPLOIDY AND POLYPLOIDY. When a human cell has 23 chromosomes, it is referred to as a haploid cell (the number of chromosomes in an ova or sperm). Any number of chromosomes that is an exact multiple of the haploid number (e.g., 46, 69, 92 in humans) is referred to as euploid. Euploid cells with more than the normal diploid number of 46 chromosomes are called polyploid cells. Polyploid conceptions are usually not viable. However, they may be present in mosaic (more than one cell line) forms, which allow survival. Cells deviating from the multiples of the haploid number are called *aneuploid* (i.e., not euploid), indicating a missing or extra chromosome.

TRISOMIES. The most common abnormalities of chromosome number are trisomies. These occur when there are three representatives of a particular chromosome instead of the usual two. Trisomy may be present in all cells or may occur in mosaic form. Most individuals with trisomies exhibit a consistent and specific phenotype depending on the chromosome involved (Table 64–1).

Translocation Down Syndrome. Approximately 4% of Down syndrome individuals have a translocation involving chromosome 21. Translocations account for 9% of the children with Down syndrome born to mothers younger than 30 yr of age. Parents who are carriers of a translocation involving chromosome 21 produce three types of viable offspring: normal phenotype and karyotype, a phenotypically normal translocation carrier, and the translocation trisomy 21. The majority of translocations that give rise to Down syndrome are fusions at the centromere between chromosomes 13, 14, 15, or 21 t(21q21q). The phenotype in

TABLE 64–1 Chromosomal Trisomies and Their Clinical Findings

Syndrome	Incidence	Clinical Manifestations
Trisomy 13, Patau syndrome	1/10,000 births	Cleft lip often midline; flexed fingers with polydactyly; ocular hypotelorism, bulbous nose; low-set malformed ears; small abnormal skull; cerebral malformation, especially holoprosencephaly; microphthalmia; cardiac malformations; scalp defects; hypoplastic or absent ribs; visceral and genital anomalies
Trisomy 18, Edwards syndrome	1/6,000 births	Low birth weight, closed fists with index finger overlapping the 3rd digit and the 5th digit overlapping the 4th, narrow hips with limited abduction, short sternum, rocker-bottom feet, microcephaly, prominent occiput, micrognathia, cardiac and renal malformations and mental retardation; 95% of cases are lethal in the 1st yr
Trisomy 21, Down syndrome	1/600–800 births	Hypotonia, flat face, upward and slanted palpebral fissures and epicanthic folds, speckled irises (Brushfield spots); varying degrees of mental and growth retardation; dysplasia of the pelvis, cardiac malformations, and simian crease; short, broad hands, hypoplasia of middle phalanx of 5th finger, intestinal atresia, and high arched palate; 5% of patients with Down syndrome are the result of a translocation—t(14q21q), t(15q21q), and t(13q21q)—in which the phenotype is the same as trisomy 21 Down syndrome
Trisomy 8, mosaicism	1/20,000 births	Long face, high prominent forehead, wide upturned nose, thick everted lower lip, microretrognathia, low-set ears, high arched, sometimes cleft palate. Osteoarticular anomalies are common; moderate mental retardation.

translocation Down syndrome is not distinguishable from regular trisomy 21 Down syndrome.

ABNORMALITIES OF CHROMOSOME STRUCTURE

DELETION. Deletions occur when a piece of chromosome is missing. The most commonly observed deletions in humans are associated with well-described phenotypes. *Microdeletions* are defined as small chromosome deletions that are detectable only in high-quality (pro) metaphase preparations.

TRANSLOCATIONS. Translocations involve the transfer of chromosomal material from one chromosome to another.

SEX CHROMOSOME ANOMALIES

TURNER SYNDROME. The chromosomal finding in Turner syndrome is the loss of part or all of one of the sex chromosomes. Half the affected individuals have 45,X in their lymphocyte studies. The other half have a variety of abnormalities of one of their sex chromosomes and may be mosaic. The phenotype in Turner syndrome is female and is characterized by short stature and underdeveloped gonads.

KLINEFELTER SYNDROME. These individuals have a male karyotype with an extra X chromosome, 47,XXY, and the phenotype is male. Individuals with Klinefelter syndrome are usually relatively tall. They may have gynecomastia, and secondary sex development may be delayed. They usually have azoospermia and small testes and are infertile.

FRAGILE SITES

Fragile sites are defined as regions of chromosomes that show a tendency to separation, breakage, or attenuation under particular growth conditions. Numerous fragile sites have been identified.

FRAGILE X SYNDROME. The fragile site located on the distal long arm of chromosome X at Xq27.3 has been associated with the fragile X syndrome, which is the most common form of mental retardation in males. The main clinical manifestations of fragile X syndrome in affected males are mental retardation; macroorchidism; large size; characteristic facial features, including long face, prominent jaw, and large prominent ears; and stereotyped behavior and speech. Females affected with fragile X syndrome show varying degrees of mental retardation. The inheritance of fragile X is different from the usual single gene inheritance patterns. It involves an area of the gene with CGG/CCG repeats (triplet repeats). The fragile X syndrome is due to the allelic expansion, which interferes with gene function. The number of copies seen in disorders associated with allelic expansion may be related to the age at onset and severity of the disease.

CHROMOSOMAL BREAKAGE SYNDROMES

There are a number of recessive disorders that are associated with breakage or rearrangement of chromosomes, or both. The breaks may be spontaneous, or they can be induced by a variety of environmental agents and different techniques. Chromatid breaks are found in Fanconi anemia, Nijmegen syndrome, Bloom syndrome, and Werner syndrome.

MOSAICISM

Mosaicism is the term used to describe an individual who has two different cell lines derived from a single zygote (fertilized egg).

UNIPARENTAL DISOMY

Uniparental disomy (UPD) is the term used when both chromosomes of a pair of chromosomes in a person with a normal number of chromosomes have been inherited from only one parent. Uniparental isodisomy means that the two chromosomes are identical, whereas uniparental heterodisomy means that the two chromosomes are different members of a pair, both of which were inherited from one parent. If the offspring of a carrier parent has isodisomy for a chromosome with an abnormal gene, the abnormal gene will be present in two copies and the phenotype will be that of the autosomal recessive disorder; however, this occurs when only one parent is actually a carrier of the recessive disorder. The autosomal recessive disorders spinal muscular atrophy, cystic fibrosis, cartilage-hair hypoplasia, α- and β-thalassemias, and Bloom syndrome have been reported to have occurred because of uniparental disomy.

CHAPTER 65

An Approach to Inborn Errors
(Nelson Textbook, Chapter 81)

Many childhood conditions are caused by gene mutations that encode specific proteins. These mutations can result in the alteration of primary protein structure or the amount of protein synthesized. The functional ability of protein, whether it is an enzyme, receptor, transport vehicle, membrane, or structural element, may be relatively or seriously compromised. These hereditary biochemical disorders are collectively termed *inborn errors of metabolism.*

Children with inborn errors of metabolism may present with one or more of a large variety of signs and symptoms. These may include metabolic acidosis, persistent vomiting, failure to thrive, developmental delay, elevated blood or urine levels of a particular metabolite (an amino acid or ammonia), a peculiar odor, or physical changes such as hepatomegaly. Diagnosis is facilitated by considering those presenting in the neonatal period separately from children presenting later in life.

NEONATAL PERIOD. Inborn errors of metabolism causing clinical manifestations in the neonatal period are usually severe and are often lethal if proper therapy is not promptly initiated. Clinical findings are usually nonspecific and similar to those seen in infants with sepsis.

Infants with metabolic disorders are usually normal at birth; however, signs and symptoms such as lethargy, poor feeding, convulsions, and vomiting may develop as early as a few hours after birth. A history of clinical deterioration in a previously normal neonate should suggest an inborn error of metabolism. A history of consanguinity and/or death in the neonatal period in the immediate family should increase suspicion of this diagnosis. Some of these disorders have a high incidence in specific population groups.

Physical examination usually reveals nonspecific findings, with most signs related to the central nervous system. Hepatomegaly, however, is a common finding in a variety of inborn errors of metabolism. Occasionally, an unusual odor may offer an invaluable aid to the diagnosis.

Diagnosis usually requires a variety of specific laboratory studies. Measuring serum concentrations of ammonia, bicarbonate, and pH is often very helpful in differentiating major causes of metabolic disorders. Elevation of the blood ammonia level is usually due to defects in urea cycle enzymes. These infants with elevated blood ammonia levels commonly have normal serum pH and bicarbonate. Elevation of serum ammonia level, however, has also been observed in some infants with certain organic acidemias. These infants are severely acidotic because of accumulation of organic acids in body fluids.

When blood ammonia, pH, and bicarbonate values are normal, other aminoacidopathies (e.g., hyperglycinemia) or galactosemia should be considered.

CHILDREN AFTER THE NEONATAL PERIOD. Most inborn errors of metabolism that cause symptoms in the first few days of life exhibit milder variant forms that have a more insidious onset. These forms may escape detection during the neonatal period, and the diagnosis may be delayed for months or even years. The early clinical manifestations in children with these forms are commonly nonspecific and may be attributed to perinatal insults.

Clinical manifestations, such as mental retardation, motor deficits, and convulsions are the most constant findings in these children. There may be an episodic or intermittent pattern with episodes of acute clinical manifestations separated by periods of seemingly disease-free states. The episodes are usually triggered by a stress or a nonspecific insult such as an infection.

DEFECTS IN METABOLISM OF AMINO ACIDS
(Nelson Textbook, Chapter 81)

Only a few representative diseases are presented as examples.

Phenylalanine

CLASSIC PHENYLKETONURIA (PKU). This form of the disorder is caused by the complete or near-complete deficiency of phenylalanine hydroxylase.

Clinical Manifestations. The affected infant is normal at birth. Mental retardation may develop gradually and may not be evident for a few months. It has been estimated that an untreated infant loses about 50 points in IQ by the end of the first yr of life (4 IQ points/mo). Mental retardation is usually severe, and most patients require institutional care. Vomiting, sometimes severe enough to be misdiagnosed as pyloric stenosis, may be an early symptom. Older untreated children become hyperactive with purposeless movements, rhythmic rocking, and athetosis.

On physical examination these infants are blonder than unaffected siblings; they have fair skin and blue eyes. Some may have a seborrheic or eczematoid rash, which is usually mild and disappears as the child grows older. These children have an unpleasant odor of phenylacetic acid, which has been described as musty or mousey. There are no consistent findings on neurologic examination. However, most infants are hypertonic with hyperactive deep tendon reflexes.

Diagnosis. The diagnosis depends on measuring blood levels of phenylalanine.

Treatment. The goal of therapy is to reduce phenylalanine and its metabolites in body fluids to prevent or minimize brain damage. This can be achieved by instituting a diet low in phenylalanine. The optimum serum level to be maintained probably lies between 3 mg/dL (0.18 mM) and 15 mg/dL (0.9 mM). Because phenylalanine is not synthesized in the body, "overtreatment," particularly in rapidly growing infants, may lead to phenylalanine deficiency, manifested by lethargy, anorexia, anemia, rashes, diarrhea, and even death.

HYPERPHENYLALANINEMIA DUE TO DEFICIENCY OF COFACTOR TETRAHYDROBIOPTERIN (BH$_4$) ("MALIGNANT" HYPERPHENYLALANINEMIA). In about 2% of infants with hyperphenylalaninemia, the defect resides in one of the enzymes necessary for production or recycling of the cofactor BH$_4$.

Clinical Manifestations. These signs and symptoms are similar and usually indistinguishable from those of classic PKU. These patients are identified during screening programs for PKU because of evidence of hyperphenylalaninemia, but neurologic manifestations, such as a loss of head control, hypertonia, drooling, swallowing difficulties, and myoclonic seizures, develop after 3 mo of age despite adequate dietary therapy.

Treatment. The long-term efficacy of various therapies is unknown.

BENIGN HYPERPHENYLALANINEMIA. Infants with hyperphenylalaninemia are occasionally identified as those whose blood levels of phenylalanine are only slightly elevated. These infants are asymptomatic and may develop normally without special dietary treatment.

Tyrosine

TYROSINEMIA TYPE I (TYROSINOSIS; HEREDITARY TYROSINEMIA, HEPATO-RENAL TYROSINEMIA). In this condition, caused by a deficiency of the enzyme fumarylacetoacetate hydrolyase, a moderate elevation of serum tyrosine is associated with severe involvement of the liver, kidney, and central nervous system. These findings are thought to be due to an accumulation of intermediate metabolites of tyrosine in the body, especially succinylacetone.

Clinical Manifestations. The affected infant may become symptomatic as early as 2 wk of age or may remain seemingly healthy during the 1st yr of life. The earlier the presentation, the poorer the prognosis. The major organs affected are the liver, peripheral nerves, and kidneys. An acute hepatic crisis commonly heralds the onset of the disease and is precipitated by an intercurrent illness that produces a catabolic state. Fever, irritability, vomiting, hemorrhage (melena, hematemesis, hematuria), hepatomegaly, jaundice, elevated levels of serum transaminases, and hypoglycemia are common. An odor resembling boiled cabbage may be present.

Diagnosis is established by measurement of fumarylacetoacetate hydrolyase activity in liver biopsy specimens or fibroblast cultured cells.

Treatment. A diet low in tyrosine, phenylalanine, and methionine may result in some clinical improvement in some patients. However, in most patients the progression of the disease cannot be halted by diet alone. Inhibition of the enzyme 4-hydroxyphenylpyruvate dioxygenase by 2-(nitro-4 trifluoro-methyl-benzoyl)-1-3-cyclohexanedione (NTBC) has been shown to cause significant improvement in clinical and biochemical findings. The long-term effect of this treatment, however, has not yet been determined. Liver transplantation, especially if performed early in the course of the disease, remains the most effective therapy.

Methionine

HOMOCYSTINURIA (HOMOCYSTINEMIA). Three major forms of homocystinemia and homocystinuria have been identified.

Homocystinuria Due to Cystathionine Synthase Deficiency (Homocystinuria Type I, Classic Homocystinuria). This is the most common inborn error of methionine metabolism. About 40% of affected patients respond to high doses of vitamin B_6 and usually have milder clinical manifestations than those who are unresponsive to vitamin B_6 therapy. These patients possess some residual enzyme activity.

Infants with this disorder are normal at birth. Clinical manifestations during infancy are nonspecific and may include failure to thrive and developmental delay. The diagnosis is usually made after 3 yr of age, when subluxation of the ocular lens (ectopia lentis) occurs. This causes severe myopia and iridodonesis (quivering of the iris). Progressive mental retardation is common. Psychiatric and behavioral disorders have been observed in more than 50% of affected patients. Affected individuals with homocystinuria manifest skeletal abnormalities resembling those of Marfan syndrome.

Treatment with high doses of vitamin B_6 (200–1000 mg/24 hr) causes dramatic improvement in patients who are responsive to this therapy, but some patients may not respond because of folate depletion; therefore, a patient should not be considered unresponsive to vitamin B_6 until folic acid (1–5 mg/ 24 hr) has been added to the treatment regimen. Restriction of methionine intake in conjunction with cysteine supplementation is recommended for all patients regardless of their response to vitamin B_6.

Homocystinuria Due to Defects in Methylcobalamin Formation (Homocystinuria Type II). There are at least five distinct defects in the intracellular metabolism of cobalamin that may interfere with the formation of methylcobalamin. The clinical manifestations are similar in patients with all of these defects. Vomiting, poor feeding, lethargy, hypotonia, and developmental delay may occur in the first few months of life. Treatment with vitamin B_{12} in the form of hydroxycobalamin (1–2 mg/24 hr) is used to correct the clinical and biochemical findings.

Homocystinuria Due to Deficiency of Methylenetetrahydrofolate Reductase (Homocystinuria Type III). The severity of the enzyme defect and of the clinical manifestations varies considerably in different families. Complete absence of enzyme activity results in neonatal apneic episodes and myoclonic seizures that may lead rapidly to coma and death. Partial deficiency may result in a more chronic clinical picture, manifested by mental retardation, convulsions, microcephaly, and spasticity. Early treatment with betaine seems to have the most beneficial effect.

Cysteine/Cystine

SULFITE OXIDASE DEFICIENCY (MOLYBDENUM COFACTOR DEFICIENCY). Most patients who were originally diagnosed as having sulfite oxidase deficiency have proved to have molybdenum cofactor deficiency. Both deficiencies produce identical clinical manifestations. Refusal to feed, vomiting, severe intractable seizures (tonic, clonic, and myoclonic), and severe developmental delay may develop within a few weeks after birth. Bilateral dislocation of ocular lenses is a common finding in patients who survive the neonatal period.

Tryptophan

HARTNUP DISORDER. In this autosomal recessive disorder, there is a single defect in the transport of monoamino-monocarboxylic amino acids (neutral amino acids) by the intestinal mucosa and renal tubules. The major clinical manifestation in the rare symptomatic patient is cutaneous photosensitivity. The skin becomes rough and red after moderate exposure to the sun, and with greater exposure a pellagra-like rash may develop. Some patients may have intermittent ataxia with or without the rash. Identification of asymptomatic children with Hartnup defect suggests that it can be a benign disorder. Treatment with nicotinic acid or nicotinamide (50–300 g/24 hr) and a high-protein diet have resulted in a favorable response in symptomatic patients.

Valine, Leucine, Isoleucine, and Related Organic Acidemias

The early steps in the degradation of these three essential amino acids, the branched-chain amino acids, are similar. Only one enzyme system (branched-chain α-ketoacid dehydrogenase) is involved in the decarboxylation of their three ketoacid derivatives. The intermediate metabolites are all organic acids, and deficiency of any of the degradative enzymes, except for the transaminases, causes acidosis; in such instances, the organic acids before the enzymatic block accumulate in body fluids and are excreted in the urine. These disorders cause severe metabolic acidosis, which usually occurs during the first few days of life. Although most of the clinical findings are nonspecific, some manifestations may provide important clues to the nature of the enzyme deficiency. Definitive diagnosis is usually established by identifying and measuring specific organic acids in body fluids, especially urine, and by the enzyme assay.

MAPLE SYRUP URINE DISEASE (MSUD). Based on clinical and biochemical findings, five phenotypes of MSUD have been identified.

Classic MSUD. This form has the most severe clinical manifestations. Affected infants who are normal at birth develop poor feeding and vomiting during the 1st wk of life; lethargy and coma ensue within a few days. Physical examination reveals hypertonicity and muscular rigidity with severe opisthotonos. Periods of hypertonicity may alternate with bouts of flaccidity. Neurologic findings are often mistaken for generalized sepsis and meningitis. Convulsions occur in most infants, and hypoglycemia is common. However, in contrast to most hypoglycemic states, correcting the blood glucose concentration does not improve the clinical condition. Routine laboratory studies are usually unremarkable, except for severe metabolic acidosis. Death usually occurs in untreated patients within the first few weeks or months of life.

Diagnosis is often suspected because of the peculiar odor of maple syrup found in urine, sweat, and cerumen. It is usually confirmed by amino acid analysis showing marked elevations in plasma levels of leucine, isoleucine, valine, and alloisoleucine, and depression of alanine.

Treatment of the acute state is aimed at quick removal of the branched-chain amino acids and their metabolites from the tissues and body fluids. Peritoneal dialysis is the most effective mode of therapy and should be promptly instituted. Treatment after recovery from the acute state requires a low branched-chain amino acid diet. The long-term prognosis of affected children remains guarded.

Glycine

HYPERGLYCINEMIA. Elevated levels of glycine in body fluids occur in patients having propionic acidemia and methylmalonic acidemia. These disorders have been collectively referred to as *ketotic hyperglycinemia* because episodes of severe acidosis and ketosis occur. The pathogenesis of hyperglycinemia in these disorders is not fully understood, but inhibition of the glycine cleavage enzyme system by the various organic acids has been shown to occur in some of the affected patients. The term *nonketotic hyperglycinemia* is reserved for the clinical condition caused by the genetic deficiency of the glycine cleavage enzyme system. In this condition hyperglycinemia is present without ketosis.

NONKETOTIC HYPERGLYCINEMIA (NKH). Four forms of NKH have been identified: neonatal, infantile, late onset, and transient.

Neonatal NKH. This is the most common form of NKH. Clinical manifestations develop during the first few days of life (between 6 hr to 8 days after birth). Poor feeding, failure to suck, lethargy, and profound hypotonia may progress rapidly to a deep coma, apnea, and death. Convulsions, especially myoclonic seizures and hiccups, are common. About 30% of affected infants die despite supportive therapy. Those who survive develop profound psychomotor retardation and intractable seizure disorders (myoclonic and/or grand mal seizures).

Infantile NKH. These previously normal infants develop signs and symptoms of neonatal NKH (see earlier) after 6 mo of age. Seizures are the common presenting signs. This condition appears to be a milder form; infants usually survive, and mental retardation is not as profound as in the neonatal form.

Serine

3-PHOSPHOGLYCERATE DEHYDROGENASE DEFICIENCY. Severe mental retardation, seizures, hypertonia, and microcephaly develop shortly after birth. The administration of serine normalizes the serine levels in the blood and in the cerebrospinal fluid and controls seizures.

Proline and Hydroxyproline

PROLIDASE DEFICIENCY. The clinical manifestations of this rare condition and the age at onset are quite variable. Skin lesions (recurrent ulcers, fine purpuric rash, crusting erythematous dermatitis), mental and motor deficits, susceptibility to infections, and joint laxity are major findings. Oral supplementation with proline, ascorbic acid, and manganese and the topical use of proline and glycine result in an improvement in leg ulcers.

Glutamic Acid

GLUTATHIONE SYNTHETASE DEFICIENCY. Two forms of this condition have been reported.

Glutathione Synthetase Deficiency, Severe Form (Pyroglutamic Acidemia, 5-Oxoprolinuria). Chronic metabolic acidosis and mild to moderate hemolytic anemia, which become manifest in the first few days of life, are cardinal findings in this rare autosomal recessive disorder. Life-threatening metabolic acidosis may occur after a surgical procedure or intercurrent infection. Treatment is mainly directed toward correcting the acidosis, avoiding drugs and oxidants that may cause hemolysis, and preventing stressful states.

Glutathione Synthetase Deficiency, Mild Form. These patients have mild hemolytic anemia and jaundice without 5-oxoprolinuria and acidosis. The enzyme deficiency is limited to the red blood cells.

Urea Cycle and Hyperammonemia

In addition to genetic defects of the urea cycle enzymes, a marked increase in plasma level of ammonia is also observed in other inborn errors of metabolism.

CLINICAL MANIFESTATIONS. In the neonatal period, symptoms and signs are mostly related to brain dysfunction and are similar regardless of the cause of the hyperammonemia. In general, the affected infant is normal at birth but becomes symptomatic after a few days of protein feeding. Refusal to eat, vomiting, tachypnea, and lethargy quickly progress to a deep coma. Convulsions are common. Physical examination may reveal hepatomegaly in addition to the neurologic signs of deep coma. In infants and older children, acute hyperammonemia is manifested by vomiting and neurologic abnormalities such as ataxia, mental confusion, agitation, irritability, and combativeness. These manifestations may alternate with periods of lethargy and somnolence that may progress to coma.

Routine laboratory studies show no specific findings when hyperammonemia is due to defects of the urea cycle enzymes.

DIAGNOSIS. The plasma ammonia concentration in the ill infant is usually above 200 μM (normal values <35 μM).

TREATMENT. Acute hyperammonemia should be treated promptly and vigorously. The goal of therapy is to remove ammonia from the body and provide adequate calories and essential amino acids to halt further breakdown of endogenous proteins. Because ammonia is poorly cleared by the kidneys, its removal from the body must be expedited by formation of compounds with a high renal clearance. Each mole of benzoate removes 1 mole of ammonia as glycine. One mole of phenylacetate removes 2 moles of ammonia as glutamine from the body. Arginine administration is effective in the treatment of hyperammonemia that is due to the defects of the urea cycle (except in patients with arginase deficiency) because it supplies the urea cycle with ornithine and *N*-acetylglutamate. Benzoate, phenylacetate, and arginine may be administered together for maximal therapeutic effect.

Histidine

HISTIDINEMIA. This disorder is due to a deficiency of histidase, which normally converts histidine to urocanic acid. Clinical manifestations include impaired speech, growth retardation, or mental retardation. However, the relationship of these findings to histidinemia remains unclear; routine amino acid screening has uncovered a significant number of asymptomatic subjects with histidinemia. Treatment with a diet low in histidine has produced excellent biochemical control. However, no clinical improvement in symptomatic patients has been observed.

Lysine

GLUTARIC ACIDURIA TYPE I. Glutaric aciduria type I, a disorder caused by a deficiency of glutaryl CoA dehydrogenase, should be differentiated from glutaric aciduria type II, a distinct clinical and biochemical disorder caused by defects in the electron transport system.

Clinical Manifestations. Affected patients with glutaric aciduria type I may develop normally up to 2 yr of life. The hallmark of the disease is a progressive dystonia and dyskinesia (choreoathetoic movements). Symptoms of hypotonia, choreoathetosis, seizures, generalized rigidity, opisthotonos, and dystonia may occur suddenly after a minor infection. In other patients, these signs and symptoms may develop gradually during the first few years of life. Acute episodes of vomiting, ketosis, seizures, and coma with hepatomegaly, hyperammonemia, ketosis, and elevation of serum transaminase values, a combination of symptoms that resembles Reye syndrome, may occur during an intercurrent infection or stress. Death usually occurs in the first decade of life during one of these episodes.

Laboratory Findings. During acute episodes, mild to moderate metabolic acidosis and ketosis may occur. High concentrations of glutaric acid are usually found in urine and blood.

Treatment. A low-protein diet (especially a diet restricted in lysine and tryptophan) and high doses (200–300 mg/24 hr) of riboflavin (the coenzyme for glutaryl CoA dehydrogenase) and carnitine (50–100 mg/kg/24 hr) have resulted in a dramatic decrease in the levels of glutaric acid in body fluids, but the clinical effect has been variable.

Aspartic Acid

CANAVAN DISEASE. Canavan disease, an autosomal recessive disorder characterized by spongy degeneration of the white matter of the brain, leads to a severe form of leukodystrophy.

Clinical Manifestations. The severity of Canavan disease covers a wide spectrum. Infants usually appear normal at birth and may not manifest symptoms of the disease until 3–6 mo of age, when they develop progressive macrocephaly, severe hypotonia, and persistent head lag. As the infant grows older, delayed milestones become evident. These children become hyperreflexic and hypertonic, and joint stiffness may be encountered because of disuse. Seizures and optic atrophy develop as they grow older. Most patients die in the first decade of life; however, with improved nursing care, they may survive through the second decade.

Diagnosis. Computed tomography and magnetic resonance imaging reveal diffuse white matter degeneration, primarily in the cerebral hemispheres, with less involvement in the cerebellum and brain stem. Definitive diagnosis can be established by finding elevated amounts of *N*-acetylaspartic acid in the urine or blood.

DEFECTS IN METABOLISM OF LIPIDS
(Nelson Textbook, Chapter 83)

A few representative diseases are presented as examples.

Disorders of Mitochondrial Fatty Acid Oxidation

Genetic defects have been recognized in nearly all the steps in the fatty acid oxidation path. All these disorders are recessively inherited. Clinical manifestations are fairly similar among the disorders. The most common presentation is an acute attack of life-threatening coma and hypoglycemia induced by a period of fasting. Other manifestations frequently include chronic cardiomyopathy and muscle weakness or, more rarely, acute rhabdomyolysis. Because the defects can be asymptomatic except during fasting stress, attacks of illness may be misdiagnosed as Reye syndrome or sudden infant death syndrome. Fatty acid oxidation disorders are easily overlooked because the only specific clue to the diagnosis may be the finding of inappropriately low concentrations of urinary ketones in an infant who has hypoglycemia. In a similar manner, genetic defects in ketone utilization may be overlooked because ketosis is an expected finding with fasting hypoglycemia.

Defects in the β-Oxidation Cycle

MEDIUM-CHAIN ACYL-COA DEHYDROGENASE DEFICIENCY

Clinical Manifestations. Affected patients usually present in the first 2–3 yr of life with episodes of acute illness triggered by prolonged fasting for more than 12–16 hr. Signs and symptoms include vomiting and lethargy, which rapidly progress to coma or seizures and cardiorespiratory collapse. The liver may be slightly enlarged with fat deposition. Attacks are rare until the infant is beyond the first few months of life.

Laboratory Findings. During acute attacks of illness, hypoglycemia is usually present. Plasma and urinary ketone concentrations are inappropriately low (hypoketotic hypoglycemia). Because of the absence of ketones, there is little or no acidemia. Plasma and tissue concentrations of total carnitine are reduced to 25–50% of normal, and the fraction of total carnitine esterified is increased. This pattern of *secondary carnitine deficiency* is seen in almost all the fatty acid oxidation defects. Diagnosis can be made by demonstrating abnormal metabolites in plasma (octanoylcarnitine) or urine (glycine conjugates of hexanoate and phenylpropionate), or by showing deficiency of the enzyme in cultured fibroblasts.

Treatment. Acute illnesses should be promptly treated with intravenous fluids containing 10% dextrose. Chronic therapy consists of ensuring that exposure to starvation stress is eliminated.

Defects in the Carnitine Cycle

PLASMA MEMBRANE CARNITINE TRANSPORT DEFECT (PRIMARY CARNITINE DEFICIENCY).

The most common presentation is progressive cardiomyopathy with or without skeletal muscle weakness that begins at 2–4 yr of age. Diagnosis of the carnitine transporter defect is aided by the fact that patients have extremely reduced carnitine levels in plasma and muscle to 1–2% of normal. Treatment of this disorder with pharmacologic doses of oral carnitine is highly effective in correcting the cardiomyopathy and muscle weakness as well as any impairment in fasting ketogenesis.

Defects in Electron Transfer Pathway

ELECTRON TRANSFER FLAVOPROTEIN (ETF) AND ELECTRON TRANSFER FLAVOPROTEIN DEHYDROGENASE (ETF-DH) DEFICIENCIES (GLUTARIC ACIDURIA TYPE 2, MULTIPLE ACYL-COA DEHYDROGENATION DEFICIENCIES).

Deficiencies of ETF or ETF-DH produce illness that combines the features of impaired fatty acid oxidation and impaired oxidation of several of the amino acids, such as leucine and lysine. Complete deficiencies of either enzyme are associated with severe illness in the newborn period, characterized by acidosis, hypoglycemia, coma, hypotonia, and cardiomyopathy. Some affected neonates have had facial dysmorphia and polycystic kidneys. Diagnosis can be made from the urinary organic acid profile. Most severely affected infants have not survived the neonatal period.

Disorders of Very Long Chain Fatty Acids

Peroxisomal Disorders

The peroxisomal diseases are genetically determined disorders due to either the failure to form or maintain the peroxisome or a defect in the function of a single enzyme that is normally located in this organelle. These disorders cause serious disability in childhood and occur more frequently and present a wider range of phenotype than has been recognized in the past.

ETIOLOGY. Peroxisomal disorders are subdivided into two major categories (Table 65–1). In category A (import disorders), the basic defect is the failure to import one or more proteins into the organelle. Category B includes disorders with defects that affect a single peroxisomal protein.

CLINICAL MANIFESTATIONS

Disorders of Peroxisome Biogenesis Group A. Zellweger syndrome, neonatal adrenoleukodystrophy (ALD), and infantile Refsum disease represent a continuum, with the Zellweger syndrome the most severe and infantile Refsum disease the least severe.

Newborns with Zellweger syndrome show striking and consistent abnormalities that are easily recognized. Of central diagnostic importance are the typical facial appearance (high forehead, non-

---

TABLE 65–1 Classification of Peroxisomal Disorders

A: *Disorders of peroxisome import*	B: *Defects of single peroxisomal enzyme*
A1: Zellweger syndrome	B1: X-linked adrenoleukodystrophy
A2: Neonatal adrenoleukodystrophy	B2: Acyl-CoA oxidase deficiency
A3: Infantile Refsum disease	B3: Bifunctional enzyme deficiency
A4: Rhizomelic chondrodysplasia punctata	B4: Peroxisomal thiolase deficiency
	B5: DHAP acyltransferase deficiency
	B6: Alkyl DHAP synthase deficiency
	B7: Classic Refsum disease
	B8: Mevalonic aciduria
	B9: Glutaric aciduria type III
	B10: Hyperoxaluria type I
	B11: Acatalasemia

slanting palpebral fissures, hypoplastic supraorbital ridges, and epicanthal folds), severe weakness and hypotonia, neonatal seizures, and eye abnormalities (cataracts, glaucoma, corneal clouding, Brushfield spots, pigmentary retinopathy, and optic nerve dysplasia).

Patients with neonatal ALD show fewer and occasionally no dysmorphic features. Neonatal seizures occur frequently. Some degree of psychomotor development is present; function remains in the severely or profoundly retarded range and may regress after 3–5 yr of age. Enlarged liver and impaired liver function, pigmentary degeneration of the retina, and severely impaired hearing are almost always present.

Patients with *infantile Refsum disease* have survived to the 2nd decade or longer. They are able to walk, although gait may be ataxic and broad-based. Cognitive function is in the severely retarded range. All have sensorineural hearing loss and pigmentary degeneration of the retina. They have moderately dysmorphic features that may include epicanthal folds, a flat bridge of the nose, and low-set ears. Early hypotonia and enlarged liver with impaired function are common.

Rhizomelic Chondrodysplasia Punctata. Rhizomelic chondrodysplasia punctata (RCDP) is characterized by the presence of stippled foci of calcification within the hyaline cartilage and is associated with dwarfing, cataracts (72%), and multiple malformations due to contractures.

TREATMENT. The most effective therapy is the dietary treatment of classic Refsum disease with a phytanic acid–restricted diet. For patients with the somewhat milder variants of the peroxisome-important disorders, considerable success has been achieved with multidisciplinary early intervention, including physical and occupational therapy, hearing aids, alternative communication, nutrition, and support for the parents.

Adrenoleukodystrophy (X-Linked)

CLINICAL MANIFESTATIONS. There are seven relatively distinct phenotypes, three of which present in childhood. In all the phenotypes, development is usually normal during the first 3–4 yr.

In the *childhood cerebral* form of ALD, symptoms are first noted most commonly between the ages of 4 and 8 yr and at 3 yr at the earliest. The most common initial manifestations are hyperactivity and worsening school performance in a child who had previously been a good student. Auditory discrimination is often impaired. Other initial symptoms are disturbances of vision, ataxia, poor handwriting, seizures, and strabismus. Seizures occur in nearly all patients and may represent the first manifestation of the disease. Cerebral childhood ALD tends to progress rapidly with increasing spasticity and paralysis, visual and hearing loss, and loss of ability to speak or swallow.

Adolescent ALD designates patients who experience neurologic symptoms between the ages of 10 and 21 yr. The manifestations resemble those of childhood cerebral ALD except that progression is slower.

TREATMENT. Corticosteroid replacement for adrenal insufficiency or adrenocortical hypofunction is effective. ALD patients require the establishment of a comprehensive management program and partnership among the family, physician, visiting nursing staff, school authorities, and counselors.

Disorders of Lipoprotein Metabolism and Transport

A few representative diseases are presented as examples.

Epidemiology of Blood Lipids and Cardiovascular Disease

Although there are no data directly linking cholesterol levels in children with adult heart disease, most of the evidence suggest that such an association exists. There is a consensus that children with cholesterol levels greater than the 75th percentile should be considered hypercholesterolemic and potentially at risk for adult heart disease.

Treatment of Hyperlipidemia

DIETARY MANAGEMENT OF HYPERLIPIDEMIA. For hypercholesterolemic children (average LDL cholesterol > 110 mg/dL) older than 2 yr, dietary modification is the best initial intervention. Their daily food intake should provide no more than 30% of total calories as fat (approximately equally distributed among saturated, monounsaturated, and polyunsaturated fats), and no more than 100 mg cholesterol/1000 calories (maximum 300 mg/24 hr) in such a modification program. This has become commonly referred to as the prudent, or Step I American Heart Association, diet.

DRUG THERAPY. The Expert Panel on Treatment of Hyperlipidemia in Children recommended that drug therapy be considered in children aged 10 yr and older if, after an adequate trial (6 mo–1 yr) of diet therapy:

1. LDL cholesterol remains greater than 190 mg/dL.
2. LDL cholesterol remains greater than 160 mg/dL and
   a. There is a positive family history of premature CHD (before 55 yr of age), or
   b. Two or more other risk factors are present in the child or adolescent after vigorous attempts have been made to control these risk factors (diabetes, hypertension, smoking, low high-density lipoprotein cholesterol, severe obesity, physical inactivity).

Primary (Genetic) Dyslipidemias

Disorders Associated with Hypercholesterolemia and Normal Triglycerides (<100 mg/dL)

FAMILIAL HYPERCHOLESTEROLEMIA (FH). FH is caused by mutations in the low-density lipoprotein (LDL) receptor, which prevent its synthesis, reduce its appearance on the cell surface, or impair its ability to bind and internalize LDL. Elevated LDL cholesterol levels lead to the major complication of this condition: premature atherosclerotic cardiovascular disease.

HETEROZYGOUS FAMILIAL HYPERCHOLESTEROLEMIA. It is characterized by elevated total and LDL cholesterol levels with normal triglycerides and a family history of hypercholesterolemia or premature cardiovascular disease. The finding of tendon xanthomas is virtually diagnostic of FH, although absence of xanthomas does not exclude the diagnosis, especially in children with heterozygous FH in whom xanthomas are rare. Treatment should be initiated with a step I diet and followed by the step II diet if needed. Dietary therapy can help reduce the LDL cholesterol but rarely normalizes it. Thus, most heterozygous FH patients eventually require lipid-lowering drug therapy.

HOMOZYGOUS FAMILIAL HYPERCHOLESTEROLEMIA. Homozygous FH is caused by the inheritance of two mutant LDL receptor alleles that result in the production of little or no LDL receptors and a severe defect in the catabolism of LDL. Patients with homozygous FH often present in childhood with cutaneous xanthomas on the hands, wrists, elbows, knees, heels, or buttocks. The absence of xanthomas in children does not exclude the diagnosis. The current treatment of choice for homozygous FH is LDL apheresis, which can promote regression of xanthomas and retard progression of atherosclerosis. The age at which LDL apheresis should be initiated is uncertain.

Disorders Associated with Hypercholesterolemia and Moderately Elevated Triglyceride Levels (100–1000 mg/dL)

FAMILIAL COMBINED HYPERLIPIDEMIA (FCHL). FCHL generally presents in adulthood but can be identified in children. The risk of premature heart disease for persons with FCHL is high despite the fact that lipid levels in affected individuals may be only moderately elevated. Children in these families should therefore be identified, and initial dietary treatment should be aimed at controlling the hypercholesterolemia and hypertriglyceridemia using the step I or step II diet. When dietary modification alone does not achieve desired results, drug therapy may be considered.

Disorders Associated with Hypercholesterolemia and Severely Elevated Triglycerides (>1000 mg/dL)

FAMILIAL CHYLOMICRONEMIA SYNDROME: LIPOPROTEIN LIPASE DEFICIENCY AND APOLIPOPROTEIN C-II DEFICIENCY. The familial chylomicronemia syndrome is characterized by presentation in childhood with acute pancreatitis in the setting of triglyceride levels greater than 1000 mg/dL. Recurrent abdominal pain is a common historical feature. The mainstay of treatment for familial chylomicronemia syndrome is restriction of total dietary fat. If dietary fat restriction alone is not successful, some patients may respond to a cautious trial of fish oils.

Conditions Associated with Low Cholesterol Levels

ABETALIPOPROTEINEMIA. The most prominent and debilitating clinical manifestations of abetalipoproteinemia are neurologic and usually begin in the 2nd decade. The first sign of disease is usually the loss of deep tendon reflexes, followed by decreased distal lower extremity vibratory and proprioceptive senses and cerebellar signs such as dysmetria, ataxia, and spastic gait. The majority of the clinical symptoms of abetalipoproteinemia are the result of defects in absorption and transport of fat-soluble vitamins. Most of the major clinical symptoms, especially those of the nervous system and retina, are primarily due to vitamin E deficiency.

Lipidoses

Lipid storage disorders are diverse diseases that are related by their molecular pathology. In each, there is an inherited deficiency of a lysosomal hydrolase leading to the lysosomal accumulation of the enzyme's specific sphingolipid substrate. Progressive lysosomal accumulation of glycosphingolipids in the central nervous system leads to neurodegeneration, whereas storage in visceral cells can lead to organomegaly, skeletal abnormalities, pulmonary infiltration, and other manifestations. The biochemical basis of lipid storage disorders is well characterized, including the determination of each of the enzymatic activities and the various storage products. A few representative diseases are presented as examples.

GM₁ GANGLIOSIDOSIS. The clinical manifestations of the infantile form of GM_1 gangliosidosis (type 1 disease) may be evident in the newborn as hepatosplenomegaly, edema, and skin eruptions. It most frequently presents within the first 6 mo of life as developmental arrest followed by progressive psychomotor retardation and the onset of tonic-clonic seizures. A typical facies characterized by low-set ears, frontal bossing, a depressed nasal bridge, and abnormally long philtrum is also evident; up to 50% of patients have a macular cherry-red spot. By the end of the 1st yr of life, most patients are blind and deaf, with severe neurologic impairment characterized by decerebrate rigidity. Death usually occurs by 3 to 4 yr. The juvenile-onset form of GM_1 gangliosidosis (type 2) is clinically distinct, with a variable age at onset. Affected patients present primarily with neurologic symptoms, including ataxia, dysarthria, mental retardation, and spasticity. There is no specific treatment for either form of GM$_1$ gangliosidosis.

THE GM$_2$ GANGLIOSIDOSES. The GM$_2$ gangliosidoses include Tay-Sachs disease and Sandhoff disease. Patients with clinical manifestations of the infantile form of Tay-Sachs disease present in infancy with loss of motor skills, increased startle reaction, and the presence of macular pallor and cherry-red spot on retinoscopy. Affected infants usually develop normally until about 5 mo of age when decreased eye contact and an exaggerated startle response to noise are noted. Macrocephaly, not associated with hydrocephalus, may develop. In the 2nd yr of life, seizures requiring anticonvulsant therapy develop. Neurodegeneration is relentless, with death occurring by the age of 4 or 5 yr. The juvenile-onset form initially presents as ataxia and dysarthria; it is not associated with a macular cherry-red spot. There is no treatment available for Tay-Sachs disease or Sandhoff disease.

GAUCHER DISEASE. Clinical manifestations of Gaucher disease type 1 have a variable age at onset, from early childhood to late adulthood, with most symptomatic patients presenting by adolescence. At presentation, patients may have easy bruisability due to thrombocytopenia, chronic fatigue secondary to anemia, hepatomegaly with or without elevated liver function test results, splenomegaly, and bone pain. Treatment of patients with Gaucher disease is primarily symptomatic, including administration of blood transfusions for anemia, partial or total splenectomy for severe mechanical pulmonary compromise or hypersplenism, analgesics for bone pain, and orthopedic procedures for joint replacement in those patients with severe bony involvement.

NIEMANN-PICK DISEASE (NPD). The original description of NPD referred to what is now known as type A NPD, a fatal disorder of infancy characterized by failure to thrive, hepatosplenomegaly, and a rapidly progressive neurodegenerative course that leads to death by 2–3 yr of age. Currently, a total of six subtypes of NPD have been described, including type B, which is a non-neuronopathic form that presents with hepatosplenomegaly, and other, rarer forms that result from cholesterol metabolism defects. Currently there is no specific treatment for NPD.

Mucolipidoses

I-cell disease (mucolipidosis II, ML-II) and pseudo-Hurler polydystrophy (mucolipidosis III, ML-III) are biochemically related, rare autosomal recessive disorders that share some clinical features with Hurler syndrome.

I-CELL DISEASE. Some patients have clinical features evident at birth, including coarse facial features, craniofacial abnormalities, restricted joint movement, and hypotonia. Nonimmune hydrops may be present in the fetus. The remainder of patients present in the 1st yr with severe psychomotor retardation, coarse facial features, and skeletal manifestations that include kyphoscoliosis and a lumbar gibbus. Progressive, severe psychomotor retardation leads to death in early childhood. No treatment is available.

DEFECTS IN METABOLISM OF CARBOHYDRATES

Defects in glycogen metabolism typically cause an accumulation of glycogen in the tissues, hence the name *glycogen storage disease* (Table 65–2). Defects in gluconeogenesis or the glycolytic pathway, including galactose and fructose metabolism, do not result in an accumulation of glycogen. The defects in pyruvate metabolism in the pathway of the conversion of pyruvate to carbon dioxide and water via mitochondrial oxidative phosphorylation are often associated with lactic acidosis and tissue glycogen accumulation.

Mucopolysaccharidoses

Mucopolysaccharidoses (MPSs) are inheritable disorders caused by a deficiency of lysosomal enzymes needed for the degradation of glycosaminoglycans (GAGs, also known by the older term *mucopolysaccharides*). These storage diseases comprise a heterogeneous group of disorders characterized by the intralysosomal accumulation of GAGs, excessive urinary excretion of GAGs, progressive mental and physical deterioration, and, in severe forms, premature death. Each type has a specific lysosomal enzyme deficiency with a characteristic degree of organ involvement and rate of deterioration. No definitive therapy is available for patients with an MPS disorder. Bone marrow transplantation has resulted in significant clinical improvement of somatic disease in MPS I and increased long-term survival. Resolution or improvements have been noted in hepatosplenomegaly, joint stiffness, facial appearance, obstructive sleep apnea, heart disease, communicating hydrocephalus, and hearing loss. The skeletal and ocular anomalies are not corrected. The neuropsychologic outcomes of MPS have varied widely after bone marrow transplantation.

DISORDERS OF PURINE AND PYRIMIDINE METABOLISM

The inherited disorders of purine and pyrimidine metabolism cover a broad spectrum of illnesses with various presentations. These include hyperuricemia, acute renal failure, gout, unexplained neurologic deficits (seizures, muscle weakness, choreoathetoid and dystonic movements), developmental disability, mental retardation, compulsive self-injury and aggression, autistic-like behavior, unexplained anemia, failure to thrive, susceptibility to recurrent infection (immune deficiency), and deafness.

Inborn errors in the *synthesis* of purine nucleotides include (1)

TABLE 65-2 Features of the Disorders of Carbohydrate Metabolism

Disorders (Type/Common Name)	Basic Defects	Clinical Presentation	Comments
Liver Glycogenoses			
Ia/Von Gierke	Glucose-6-phosphatase	Growth retardation, hepatomegaly, hypoglycemia; elevated blood lactate, cholesterol, triglyceride, and uric acid levels	Common, severe hypoglycemia
Ib	Glucose-6-phosphate translocase	Same as type Ia, with additional findings of neutropenia and impaired neutrophil function	10% of type Ia
II/Pompe			
Infantile	Acid maltase (acid α-glucosidase)	Cardiomegaly, hypotonia, hepatomegaly; onset: birth–6 mo	Common, cardiorespiratory failure leading to death by age 2 yr
Juvenile	Acid maltase (acid α-glucosidase)	Myopathy, variable cardiomyopathy; onset: childhood	Residual enzyme activity
Adult	Acid maltase (acid α-glucosidase)	Myopathy, respiratory insufficiency; onset: adulthood	Residual enzyme activity
IIIa/Cori or Forbes	Liver and muscle debrancher deficiency (amylo, 1,6 glucosidase)	Childhood: hepatomegaly, growth retardation, muscle weakness, hypoglycemia, hyperlipidemia, elevated transaminase levels; liver symptoms improve with age	Common, intermediate severity of hypoglycemia
IIIb	Liver debrancher deficiency; normal muscle enzyme activity	Liver symptoms same as in type IIIa; no muscle symptoms	15% of type III
IV/Andersen	Branching enzyme	Failure to thrive, hypotonia, hepatomegaly, splenomegaly, progressive cirrhosis (death usually before 5th yr), elevated transaminase levels	Rare neuromuscular variants exist
VI/Hers	Liver phosphorylase	Hepatomegaly, mild hypoglycemia, hyperlipidemia, and ketosis	Rare, benign glycogenosis

Table continued on following page

221

TABLE 65-2 Features of the Disorders of Carbohydrate Metabolism *Continued*

Disorders (Type/Common Name)	Basic Defects	Clinical Presentation	Comments
Liver Glycogenoses Continued			
Phosphorylase kinase deficiency	Phosphorylase kinase	Hepatomegaly, mild hypoglycemia, hyperlipidemia, and ketosis	Common, benign glycogenosis
Glycogen synthetase deficiency	Glycogen synthetase	Early morning drowsiness and fatigue, fasting hypoglycemia, and ketosis	Decreased liver glycogen store
Fanconi-Bickel syndrome	Glucose transporter-2 (GLUT-2)	Failure to thrive, rickets, hepatorenomegaly, proximal renal tubular dysfunction, impaired glucose and galactose utilization	GLUT-2 expressed in liver, kidney, pancreas, and intestine
Muscle Glycogenoses			
V/McArdle	Myophosphorylase	Exercise intolerance, muscle cramps, increased fatigability	Common, male predominance
VII/Tarui	Phosphofructokinase	Exercise intolerance, muscle cramps, hemolytic anemia, myoglobinuria	Prevalent in Japanese and Ashkenazi Jews
Phosphoglycerate kinase deficiency	Phosphoglycerate kinase	As with type V	Rare, X-linked
Phosphoglycerate mutase deficiency	M subunit of phosphoglycerate mutase	As with type V	Rare, majority of patients are African-American
Lactate dehydrogenase deficiency	M subunit of lactate dehydrogenase	As with type V	Rare
Galactose Disorders			
Galactosemia with transferase deficiency	Galactose-1-phosphate uridyltransferase	Vomiting, hepatomegaly, cataracts, aminoaciduria, failure to thrive	African-American patients tend to have milder symptoms
Galactokinase deficiency	Galactokinase	Cataracts	Benign
Generalized uridine diphosphate galactose 4-epimerase deficiency	Uridine diphosphate galactose 4-epimerase	Similar to transferase deficiency with additional findings of hypotonia and nerve deafness	A benign variant exists

222

Fructose Disorders

Essential fructosuria	Fructokinase	Urine reducing substance	Benign
Hereditary fructose intolerance	Fructose 1-phosphate aldolase	Acute: vomiting, sweating, lethargy Chronic: failure to thrive, hepatic failure	Prognosis good with fructose restriction

Disorders of Gluconeogenesis

Fructose 1,6-diphosphatase deficiency	Fructose 1,6-diphosphatase	Episodic hypoglycemia, apnea, acidosis	Good prognosis, avoid fasting
Phosphoenolpyruvate carboxykinase deficiency	Phosphoenolpyruvate carboxykinase	Hypoglycemia, hepatomegaly, hypotonia, failure to thrive	Rare

Disorders of Pyruvate Metabolism

Pyruvate dehydrogenase complex defect	Pyruvate dehydrogenase	Severe fatal neonatal to mild late onset, lactic acidosis, psychomotor retardation, and failure to thrive	Most commonly due to E1 α-subunit defect X-linked
Pyruvate carboxylase deficiency	Pyruvate carboxylase	Same as above	Rare, autosomal recessive
Respiratory chain defects (oxidative phosphorylation disease)	Complex I to V, many mitochondrial DNA mutations	Heterogeneous with multisystem involvement	Mitochondrial inheritance

Other Carbohydrate Disorders

Pentosuria	L-Xylulose reductase	Urine reducing substance	Benign

TABLE 65–3 Manifestations of Hypoglycemia in Childhood

Features Associated with Activation of Autonomic Nervous System and Epinephrine Release*	Features Associated with Cerebral Glucopenia
Anxiety†	Headache†
Perspiration†	Mental confusion†
Palpitation (tachycardia)†	Visual disturbances ($\downarrow$ acuity, diplopia)†
Pallor	Organic personality changes†
Tremulousness	Inability to concentrate†
Weakness	Dysarthria
Hunger	Staring
Nausea	Seizures
Emesis	Ataxia, incoordination
Angina (with normal coronary arteries)	Somnolence, lethargy
	Coma
	Stroke, hemiplegia, aphasia
	Paresthesias
	Dizziness
	Amnesia
	Decerebrate or decorticate posture

*Some of these features will be attenuated if the patient is receiving β-adrenergic blocking agents.
†Common.

phosphoribosylpyrophosphate synthetase superactivity and (2) adenylosuccinase deficiency. Disorders resulting from abnormalities in purine *catabolism* include (3) muscle adenosine monophosphate (AMP) deaminase deficiency, (4) adenosine deaminase deficiency, (5) purine nucleoside phosphorylase deficiency, and (6) xanthine oxidase deficiency. Disorders resulting from the purine *salvage* pathway include (7) hypoxanthine-guanine phosphoribosyltransferase (HPRT) deficiency and (8) adenine phosphoribosyltransferase (APRT) deficiency.

Inborn errors of pyrimidine metabolism include (1) hereditary orotic aciduria (uridine monophosphate synthase deficiency), (2) dihydropyrimidine dehydrogenase deficiency, (3) dihydropyrimidinase deficiency, and (4) pyrimidine 5'-nucleotidase deficiency.

THE PORPHYRIAS

The porphyrias are inherited and acquired disorders resulting from a partial or nearly complete deficiency of the enzymes of the heme biosynthetic pathway. Abnormally elevated levels of porphyrins or their precursors, or both, are produced, accumulate in tissues, and are excreted in urine and stool. Acute hepatic porphyrias are characterized by acute episodes of neurologic disturbances and by an overproduction of porphyrin precursors,

TABLE 65–4 Classification of Hypoglycemia in Infants and Children

Neonatal—Transient Hypoglycemia

Associated with inadequate substrate or enzyme function
    Prematurity
    Small for gestational age (SGA)
    Smaller of twins
    Infants with severe respiratory distress
    Infant of toxemic mother
Associated with hyperinsulinemia
    Infants of diabetic mothers
    Infants with erythroblastosis fetalis
    Perinatal asphyxia—SGA

Neonatal—Infantile or Childhood Persistent Hypoglycemia

Hyperinsulinemic states
Persistent hyperinsulinemic hypoglycemia of infancy
    Autosomal recessive (SUR and $K_{IR}6.2$ mutations)*
    Autosomal dominant
    Glucokinase activating mutation
    Glutamate dehydrogenase activating mutation
    Sporadic
    β-cell hyperplasia
    β-cell adenoma
    Beckwith-Wiedemann syndrome
    Leucine sensitivity
    Falciparum malaria
Hormone deficiency
    Panhypopituitarism
    Isolated growth hormone deficiency
    ACTH deficiency
    Addison disease
    Glucagon deficiency
    Epinephrine deficiency
Substrate limited
    Ketotic hypoglycemia
    Branched-chain ketonuria (maple syrup urine disease)
Glycogen storage disease
    Glucose-6-phosphatase deficiency
    Amylo-1,6-glucosidase deficiency
    Liver phosphorylase deficiency
    Glycogen synthetase deficiency
Disorders of gluconeogenesis
    Acute alcohol intoxication
    Hyperglycinemia, carnitine deficiency
    Salicylate intoxication
    Fructose-1,6-diphosphatase deficiency
    Pyruvate carboxylase deficiency
    Phosphoenol pyruvate carboxykinase (PEPCK deficiency)
Other enzyme defects
    Galactosemia: galactose-1-phosphate uridyl transferase deficiency
    Fructose intolerance: fructose-1-phosphate aldolase deficiency
Disorders of fat (alternate fuel) metabolism
    Primary carnitine deficiency
    Secondary carnitine deficiency
    Carnitine palmitoyl transferase deficiency
    Long-, medium-, short-chain fatty acid acyl-CoA dehydrogenase deficiency

Table continued on following page

TABLE 65–4 Classification of Hypoglycemia in Infants and Children
Continued

Other Etiologies

Poisoning—drugs
  Salicylates
  Alcohol
  Oral hypoglycemic agents
  Insulin
  Propranolol
  Pentamidine
  Quinine
  Disopyramide
  Ackee fruit (unripe)—hypoglycin
  Vacor (rat poison)
  Trimethoprim-sulfamethoxazole (with renal failure)
Liver disease
  Reye syndrome
  Hepatitis
  Cirrhosis
  Hepatoma
Amino acid and organic acid disorders
  Maple syrup urine disease
  Propionic acidemia
  Methylmalonic acidemia
  Tyrosinosis
  Glutaric aciduria
  3-Hydroxy-3-methylglutaric aciduria
Systemic disorders
  Sepsis
  Carcinoma/sarcoma (secreting—insulin-like growth factor II)
  Heart failure
  Malnutrition
  Malabsorption
  Anti-insulin receptor antibodies
  Anti-insulin antibodies
  Neonatal hyperviscosity
  Renal failure
  Diarrhea
  Burns
  Shock
  Postsurgical
  Pseudohypoglycemia (leukocytosis, polycythemia)
  Excessive insulin therapy of insulin-dependent diabetes mellitus
  Factitious

*SUR = sulfonylurea receptor; $K_{IR}6.2$ = inward rectifying potassium channel (see text for details).

Adapted from Sperling M, Chernausek S: Nelson's Essentials of Pediatrics. Philadelphia, WB Saunders, 1990, p 617.

whereas cutaneous porphyrias are characterized by cutaneous photosensitivity and by an excessive production of porphyrins.

HYPOGLYCEMIA

Any value of blood glucose less than 40 mg/dL in neonates should be viewed with suspicion and vigorously treated. This is particularly applicable after the initial 2–3 hr of life, when glucose normally has reached its nadir; subsequently, blood glucose levels begin to rise and achieve values of 50 mg/dL or higher after 12–24 hr. In older infants and children, a blood glucose concentration of less than 40 mg/dL (10–15% higher for serum or plasma) represents hypoglycemia. The major long-term sequelae of severe, prolonged hypoglycemia are mental retardation, recurrent seizure activity, or both.

CLINICAL MANIFESTATIONS. Clinical features generally fall into two categories (Table 65–3). Although these classic symptoms occur in older children, the symptoms of hypoglycemia in infants may be more subtle and include cyanosis, apnea, hypothermia, hypotonia, poor feeding, lethargy, and seizures. Occasionally, hypoglycemia may be asymptomatic in the immediate newborn period. In childhood, hypoglycemia may present as behavior problems, inattention, ravenous appetite, or seizures.

CLASSIFICATION OF HYPOGLYCEMIA IN INFANTS AND CHILDREN. Classification is based on knowledge of the control of glucose homeostasis in infants and children (Table 65–4).

TREATMENT. The prevention of hypoglycemia and its resultant effects on central nervous system development are important in the newborn period. Treatment of acute neonatal or infant hypoglycemia includes intravenous administration of 2 mL/kg of $D_{10}W$, followed by a continuous infusion of glucose at 6–8 mg/kg/min, adjusting the rate to maintain blood glucose levels in the normal range. For neonates with hyperinsulinemia not associated with maternal diabetes, subtotal pancreatectomy may be needed, unless hypoglycemia can be readily controlled with somatostatin analogs or diazoxide. The management of persistent neonatal or infantile hypoglycemia includes increasing the rate of intravenous glucose infusion to 8–15 mg/kg/min or more, if needed. This may require a central venous catheter to administer a hypertonic 15–20% glucose solution. In addition, intramuscular or intravenous hydrocortisone, 5 mg/kg/24 hr given in divided doses every 8 hr, or oral prednisone, 1-2 mg/kg/24 hr given in divided doses every 6–12 hr, and intramuscular growth hormone, 1 mg/24 hr, may be added if hypoglycemia is unresponsive to intravenous glucose.

PART 10

The Fetus and the Neonatal Infant

Noninfectious Disorders

CHAPTER 66

Overview of Mortality and Morbidity
(Nelson Textbook, Chapter 89)

Although the neonatal period is considered to be the first 4 wk of life after birth, both fetal and extrauterine life form a continuum during which human growth and development are affected by genetic, socioeconomic, and environmental factors. *Neonatal mortality* is highest during the first 24 hr of life and overall accounts for about 65% of deaths before age 1 yr. *Perinatal mortality* designates fetal and neonatal deaths influenced by prenatal conditions and circumstances surrounding delivery (Table 66–1). It is often defined as deaths of fetuses and infants from the 20th wk of gestational life through the 28th day after birth. *Infant mortality rates* (deaths occurring from birth–12 mo/1000 live births) vary by country; in 1996, they were lowest in Singapore and Japan (3.8/1000 births); moderate in the United States (7.3/1000); and highest in developing countries (30–150/1000). The number of low-birth-weight (LBW) infants is a major determinant of both the neonatal and infant mortality rates and, together with lethal congenital anomalies, contributes significantly to childhood morbidity. *The LBW rate* (infants weighing 2500 g or less at birth each year) in the United States increased from 6.6% to 7.5% between

TABLE 66–1 Major Causes of Perinatal Mortality

Fetal	Preterm	Full Term
Placental insufficiency	Severe immaturity	Congenital abnormalities
Intrauterine infection	Respiratory distress syndrome	Birth asphyxia, trauma
Severe congenital malformations	Intraventricular hemorrhage	Infection
Umbilical cord accident	Congenital anomalies	Meconium aspiration pneumonia
Abruptio placentae	Infection	Persistent pulmonary hypertension
Hydrops fetalis	Necrotizing enterocolitis	
	Chronic lung disease	

1981 and 1997, whereas the very-low-birth-weight (VLBW) rate (infants weighing 1500 g or less at birth) has been 1.1–1.4% of all births. The LBW and VLBW rates and the infant mortality rates are 2 times higher in black infants than in white infants.

Postneonatal mortality refers to deaths between 28 days and 1 yr of life. Historically, these infant deaths were due to causes outside the neonatal period, such as sudden infant death syndrome, infections (respiratory, enteric), and trauma. With the advent of modern neonatal care, many VLBW infants who would have died in the 1st mo of life now survive the neonatal period only to succumb to the sequelae.

CHAPTER 67

The Newborn Infant

(Nelson Textbook, Chapter 90)

ROUTINE DELIVERY ROOM CARE

Low-risk infants should be placed head downward immediately after delivery to clear the mouth, pharynx, and nose of fluid, mucus, blood, and amniotic debris by gravity; gentle suction with a bulb syringe or soft rubber catheter may also be helpful in removing this material. Wiping the palate and pharynx with gauze may lead to abrasions and the development of thrush, pterygoid ulcers (Bednar aphthae), or, rarely, tooth bud infection. Their stomachs should be emptied by gastric tube to prevent aspiration of gastric contents. If infants appear to be in satisfactory condition, they may be given directly to their mothers for immediate bonding and nursing. If there is a concern about respiratory distress, they should be placed under a warmer, with the head dependent. Infants who fail to initiate respiration should receive prompt resuscitation and close observation subsequently.

The *Apgar score* is a practical method of systematically assessing newborns immediately after birth to help identify infants requiring resuscitation (Table 67–1). A low score does not necessarily signify fetal hypoxia-acidosis; additional factors may reduce the score. The 1-min Apgar score may signal the need for immediate resuscitation, and the 5-, 10-, 15-, and 20-min scores may indicate the probability of successfully resuscitating an infant. Apgar scores of 0–3 at 20 min predict high mortality and morbidity.

MAINTENANCE OF BODY HEAT. Under the usual delivery room conditions (20–25°C), an infant's skin temperature falls, resulting usually in a cumulative loss of 2–3°C in deep body temperature. Term infants exposed to cold after birth may develop metabolic acidosis, hypoxemia, hypoglycemia, and increased renal excretion

TABLE 67–1 Apgar Evaluation of the Newborn Infant

Sign	0	1	2
Heart rate	Absent	Below 100	Over 100
Respiratory effort	Absent	Slow, irregular	Good, crying
Muscle tone	Limp	Some flexion of extremities	Active motion
Response to catheter in nostril (tested after oropharynx is clear)	No response	Grimace	Cough or sneeze
Color	Blue, pale	Body pink, extremities blue	Completely pink

Sixty sec after the complete birth of the infant (disregarding the cord and placenta), the 5 objective signs above are evaluated, and each is given a score of 0, 1, or 2. A total score of 10 indicates an infant in the best possible condition. An infant with a score of 0–3 requires immediate resuscitation.
Modified from Apgar V, James LS: Further observations on the newborn scoring system. Am J Dis Child 104:419, 1962.

of water and solutes owing to their efforts to compensate for heat loss. Hypoglycemic or hypoxic infants cannot increase their oxygen consumption when exposed to a cold environment, and their central temperature decreases. Therefore, it is desirable to ensure that infants are dried and either wrapped in blankets or placed under a warmer while having skin-to-skin contact with the mother. Because carrying out resuscitative measures on a covered infant or one enclosed in an incubator is difficult, a radiant heat source should be used to receive the newborn immediately after delivery.

ANTISEPTIC SKIN AND CORD CARE. To reduce the incidence of skin and periumbilical colonization with pathogenic bacteria and infections (omphalitis), the entire skin and cord should be cleansed, once an infant's temperature has stabilized, with sterile cotton soaked in warm water or a mild, nonmedicated soap solution. Infants may be rinsed with water at body temperature if care is taken to avoid chilling. They are then dried and wrapped in sterile blankets and taken to the nursery. To reduce colonization with *Staphylococcus aureus* and other pathogenic bacteria, the umbilical cord may be treated daily with triple dye, a bactericidal agent, or bacitracin. Alternatively, chlorhexidine washing may be used. Nursery personnel should use chlorhexidine or iodophor-containing antiseptic soaps for routine hand washing before caring for each infant. Rigidly enforcing hand-to-elbow washing for 2 min in the initial wash and 15–30 sec in the second wash is essential for staff and visitors entering the nursery. Shorter but equally thorough washes between handling infants should also be required.

OTHER MEASURES. The eyes of all infants must be protected against gonococcal infection by instilling 1% silver nitrate drops; erythromycin (0.5%) and tetracycline (1.0%) sterile ophthalmic ointments are alternative measures.

Although hemorrhage in newborns can be due to factors other than vitamin K deficiency, an intramuscular injection of 1 mg of water-soluble vitamin K_1 (phytonadione) is recommended for all infants immediately after birth to prevent hemorrhagic disease of the newborn.

Neonatal screening is available for various genetic, metabolic, hematologic, and endocrine diseases. All infants should be screened with otoacoustic emission hearing testing.

NURSERY CARE

Non–high-risk healthy infants may be taken to the "regular" newborn nursery or placed in the mother's room if the hospital has rooming-in.

The bassinet, preferably of clear plastic to allow for easy visibility and care, should be cleaned frequently. All professional care should be given in the bassinet, including the physical examination, clothing changes, temperature taking, skin cleansing, and other procedures that if performed elsewhere would establish a common contact point and possibly provide a channel for cross infection. The clothing and bedding should be minimal, only those needed for an infant's comfort; the nursery temperature should be kept at approximately 24°C (75°F). The infant's temperature should be taken by axillary measurement; although the interval between temperature taking depends on many circumstances, it need not be shorter than 4 hr during the first 2–3 days and 8 hr thereafter. Axillary temperatures of 36.4–37.0°C (97.0–98.5°F) are within normal limits. Weighing at birth and daily thereafter is sufficient. Healthy infants should be placed supine to reduce the risk of sudden infant death syndrome.

TABLE 67–2 Drugs and Breast-Feeding

Contraindicated	Avoid or Give with Great Caution	Probably Safe But Give with Caution
Antineoplastic agents	Amiodarone	Acetaminophen
Amphetamines	Anthroquinones	Acyclovir
Bromocriptine	(laxatives)	Aldomet
Clemastine	Aspirin (salicylates)	Anesthetics
Cimetidine	Atropine	Antibiotics (not tetracycline)
Chloramphenicol	Birth control pills	Antithyroid (not methimazole)
Cocaine	Bromides	Antihistamines*
Cyclophosphamide	Calciferol	Antiepileptics
Cyclosporine	Cascara	Antihypertensive/cardiovascular
Diethylstilbestrol	Danthron	Bishydroxycoumarin
Doxorubicin	Dihydrotachysterol	Chlorpromazine*
Ergots	Estrogens	Codeine*
Gold salts	Ethanol	Digoxin
Heroin	Metoclopramide	Diuretics
Immunosuppressants	Metronidazole	Fluoxetine
Iodides	Narcotics	Furosemide
Lithium	Phenobarbital*	Haloperidol*
Meprobamate	Primidone	Hydralazine
Methimazole	Psychotropic drugs	Indomethacin, other nonsteroidal
Methylamphetamine	Reserpine	antiinflammatory drugs
Nicotine (smoking)	Salicylazosulfapyridine	Methadone*
Phencyclidine (PCP)	(sulfasalazine)	Muscle relaxants
Phenindione		Phenytoin
Radiopharmaceuticals		Prednisone
Tetracycline		Propranolol
Thiouracil		Propylthiouracil
		Quinolones
		Sedatives*
		Theophylline
		Vitamins
		Warfarin

*Watch for sedation.

Vernix is spontaneously shed within 2–3 days, much of it adhering to the clothing, which should be completely changed daily. The diaper should be checked before and after feeding and when the infant cries; it should be changed when wet or soiled. Meconium or feces should be cleansed from the buttocks with sterile cotton moistened with sterile water. The foreskin of the male infant should not be retracted. Circumcision is an elective procedure.

Early discharge (<48 hr) or very early discharge (<24 hr) may increase the risk of rehospitalization for hyperbilirubinemia, sepsis, failure to thrive, dehydration, and missed congenital anomalies. Early discharge requires careful ambulatory follow-up at home (visiting nurse) or in the office within 48 hr.

DRUGS AND BREAST FEEDING. Maternal medications may affect the production and safety of breast milk (Table 67–2).

CHAPTER 68

High-Risk Pregnancies
(Nelson Textbook, Chapters 91 and 92)

Pregnancies in which factors exist that increase the likelihood of abortion, fetal death, premature delivery, intrauterine growth retardation (IUGR), fetal or neonatal disease, congenital malformations, mental retardation, or other handicaps are called high-risk pregnancies (Table 68–1). Based on their history, 10–20% of pregnant patients can be identified as high risk; less than half of all perinatal mortality and morbidity is associated with these pregnancies. Although assessing antepartum risk is important in reducing perinatal mortality and morbidity, some women become at high risk only during labor and delivery; therefore, careful monitoring is critical throughout the intrapartum course

GENETIC FACTORS. The occurrence of chromosomal abnormalities, congenital anomalies, inborn errors of metabolism, mental retardation, or any familial disease in blood relatives increases the risk of the same condition in the infant.

MATERNAL FACTORS. Both teenage pregnancies and those among women older than 40 yr, particularly primiparous women, carry an increased risk for IUGR, fetal distress, and intrauterine death. Maternal illness, multiple pregnancies (particularly those involving monochorionic twinning), infections, and certain drugs increase the risk for the fetus. Preterm birth is common among high-risk pregnancies. Factors associated with prematurity are noted in Table 68–1.

Polyhydramnios and oligohydramnios indicate high-risk pregnancies. A volume estimated at greater than 2000 mL in the 3rd

TABLE 68–1 Factors Associated with High-Risk Pregnancy

Economic	*Reproductive*
Poverty	Prior cesarean section
Unemployment	Prior infertility
Uninsured, underinsured health insurance	Prolonged gestation
Poor access to prenatal care	Prolonged labor
	Prior infant with cerebral palsy, mental retardation, birth trauma, congenital anomalies
Cultural-Behavioral	Abnormal lie (breech)
Low educational status	Multiple gestation
Poor health care attitudes	Premature rupture of membranes
No care or inadequate prenatal care	Infections (systemic, amniotic, extra-amniotic, cervical)
Cigarette, alcohol, drug abuse	Pre-eclampsia or eclampsia
Age < 16 or > 35 yr	Uterine bleeding (abruptio placentae, placenta previa)
Unmarried	
Short interpregnancy interval	Parity (0 or more than 5)
Lack of support group (husband, family, religion)	Uterine or cervical anomalies
	Fetal disease
Stress (physical, psychologic)	Abnormal fetal growth
Black race	Idiopathic premature labor
	Iatrogenic prematurity
Biologic-Genetic	High or low levels of maternal serum α-fetoprotein
Previous low-birth-weight infant	***Medical***
Low maternal weight at her birth	Diabetes mellitus
Low weight for height	Hypertension
Poor weight gain during pregnancy	Congenital heart disease
	Autoimmune disease
Short stature	Sickle cell anemia
Poor nutrition	TORCH infection
Inbreeding (autosomal recessive?)	Intercurrent surgery or trauma
	Sexually transmitted diseases
Intergenerational effects	Maternal hypercoagulable states
Hereditary diseases (inborn error of metabolism)	

trimester constitutes polyhydramnios, and a volume estimated at less than 500 mL indicates oligohydramnios.

FETAL GROWTH AND MATURITY

Ultrasonography of the fetus is both safe and accurate. The most accurate assessment of gestational age is by a 1st trimester ultrasound measurement of crown-rump length. The biparietal diameter is used to assess gestational age beginning in the 2nd trimester. Through 34 wk the biparietal diameter accurately estimates gestation to within plus or minus 10 days. Later in gestation, the accuracy falls to plus or minus 3 wk.

FETAL DISTRESS

Fetal compromise may occur during the antepartum or intrapartum periods. Fetal compromise may be asymptomatic in the antenatal period. Antepartum fetal surveillance is warranted for women at increased risk for fetal distress, including those with a history of stillbirth, IUGR, oligohydramnios or polyhydramnios, multiple gestation, Rhesus sensitization, hypertensive disorders, diabetes mellitus or other chronic maternal disease, decreased fetal movement, and post-term pregnancy. The predominant cause of antepartum fetal distress is uteroplacental insufficiency. Fetal distress may be manifested as IUGR, fetal hypoxia, increased vascular resistance in fetal blood vessels, and, when severe, mixed respiratory and metabolic (lactic) acidosis. The goals of antepartum fetal surveillance are to prevent intrauterine fetal demise, to prevent hypoxic brain injury, and to prolong gestation in women at risk for preterm delivery, when this is safe, or to deliver a fetus when it is in jeopardy. The most commonly used tests are the nonstress test (NST), the contraction stress test (CST), and the biophysical profile (BPP). Fetal distress during labor may be detected by monitoring fetal heart rate, uterine pressure, and fetal scalp blood pH.

MATERNAL DISEASE AND THE FETUS

INFECTIOUS DISEASES. Almost any maternal infection with severe systemic manifestations may result in miscarriage, stillbirth, or premature labor. Regardless of the severity of the maternal infection, certain agents frequently infect a fetus, with serious sequelae. Such fetuses are frequently small for gestational age. Some infections, such as rubella, may also produce congenital malformations if they occur during the period of organogenesis.

NONINFECTIOUS DISEASES. Maternal diabetes may result in organomegaly, hypertrophy and hyperplasia of the beta cells of the fetal pancreas, and metabolic derangements in the neonate. A high incidence of intrauterine death occurs after the 36th wk of gestation in unmonitored and poorly controlled mothers. Eclampsia/pre-eclampsia of pregnancy, chronic hypertension, and renal disease result in small fetal size for gestational age, prematurity, and intrauterine death. Uncontrolled maternal hypothyroidism or hyperthyroidism is responsible for relative infertility, a tendency to abort, premature labor, and fetal death. Maternal immunologic diseases, such as idiopathic thrombocytopenic purpura, systemic lupus, myasthenia gravis, and Graves disease frequently result in a transient illness in the newborn.

MATERNAL MEDICATION AND THE FETUS

The effects of drugs taken by the mother vary considerably, especially in relation to the time in pregnancy when they are taken. Miscarriage or congenital malformations result from maternal ingestion of teratogenic drugs during the period of organogenesis. Maternal medications taken later, particularly during the last few weeks of gestation or during labor, tend to affect the function of specific organs or enzyme systems, adversely affecting the neonate rather than the fetus. Individual genetic makeup may determine susceptibility to some drugs. In addition, the effects of drugs may be evident immediately in the delivery room or may be delayed.

IDENTIFICATION OF FETAL DISEASE

Diagnostic procedures are used to identify fetal diseases when abortion is being considered, when direct fetal treatment is possible, or when a decision is made to deliver a viable but premature infant to avoid intrauterine fetal demise. Fetal assessment is also indicated in a broader context when the family, medical, or reproductive history of the mother suggests the presence of a high-risk pregnancy or a high-risk fetus.

Various methods are used for identifying fetal disease. Fetal ultrasonographic imaging may detect fetal growth abnormalities or fetal malformations. Amniocentesis, the transabdominal withdrawal of amniotic fluid during pregnancy for diagnostic purposes, is frequently done to determine the timing of the delivery of fetuses with erythroblastosis fetalis or the need for a fetal transfusion. It is also done for genetic indications, usually between the 15th and 16th gestational weeks, with results available within 1–2 wk. Analysis of amniotic fluid may also help in identifying neural tube defects (elevation of α-fetoprotein), adrenogenital syndrome (elevation of 17-ketosteroids and pregnanetriol), and thyroid dysfunction. Chorionic villus biopsy (transvaginal or transabdominal) performed in the 1st trimester provides fetal cells but may pose a slightly increased risk for fetal loss or limb reduction defects.

The best available chemical indices of fetal maturity are provided by determinations of amniotic fluid creatinine and lecithin, which reflect the maturity of the fetal kidneys and lungs, respectively. A determination of saturated phosphatidylcholine (L) or phosphatidylglycerol (PG) concentrations in amniotic fluid may be more specific and sensitive predictors of pulmonary maturity.

Cordocentesis, or percutaneous umbilical blood sampling, is used to diagnose fetal hematologic abnormalities, genetic disorders, infections, and fetal acidosis. Under direct ultrasonographic visualization, a long needle is passed into the umbilical vein at its entrance to the placenta or fetal abdominal wall. Blood may be withdrawn to determine fetal hemoglobin, platelet concentration, lymphocyte DNA, or Pa_{O_2}, pH, P_{CO_2}, and lactate levels.

TREATMENT AND PREVENTION OF FETAL DISEASE

The incidence of sensitization of Rh-negative women by Rh-positive fetuses has been reduced by prophylactic administration of Rh(D) immunoglobulin to mothers early in pregnancy and after each delivery or abortion, thus reducing the frequency of hemolytic disease in their subsequent offspring. Fetal erythroblastosis may now be accurately diagnosed by amniotic fluid analysis and treated with intrauterine intraperitoneal or intravenous transfusions of packed Rh-negative blood cells to maintain the fetus until it is mature enough to have a reasonable chance of survival. Pharmacologic approaches to fetal immaturity (e.g., administration of corticosteroids to the mother to accelerate fetal lung maturation and to decrease the incidence of respiratory distress syndrome in prematurely delivered infants) are successful. Management of definitively diagnosed fetal genetic disease or congenital anomalies consists of parental counseling or abortion; rarely, high-dose vitamin therapy for a responsive inborn error of metabolism (e.g., biotin-dependent disorders) or fetal transfusion (with red blood cells or platelets) may be indicated. Fetal surgery remains an experimental approach to therapy.

TERATOGENS

Although only a relatively few agents teratogenic in humans are recognized, new agents continue to be identified. Overall, only 10% of anomalies are due to recognizable teratogens. Reduced enzyme activity of the folate methylation pathway, particularly the formation of 5-methyltetrahydrofolate, may be responsible for neural tube or other birth defects. Folate supplementation for all pregnant women during organogenesis may overcome this genetic enzyme defect, thus reducing the incidence of neural tube defects.

CHAPTER 69

The High-Risk Infant
(Nelson Textbook, Chapter 93)

Infants particularly at risk during the neonatal period should be identified as early as possible to decrease neonatal morbidity and mortality. The term *high-risk infant* designates an infant who should be under close observation by experienced physicians and nurses. Approximately 9% of all births require special or neonatal intensive care. Infants in the high-risk category are listed in Table 69–1.

Examination of a fresh placenta, cord, and membranes may

TABLE 69–1 High-Risk Infants

Demographic Social Factors

Maternal age < 16 or > 40 yr
Illicit drug, alcohol, cigarette use
Poverty
Unmarried
Emotional or physical stress

Past Medical History

Genetic disorders
Diabetes mellitus
Hypertension
Asymptomatic bacteriuria
Rheumatologic illness (SLE)
Long-term medication

Prior Pregnancy

Intrauterine fetal demise
Neonatal death
Prematurity
Intrauterine growth retardation
Congenital malformation
Incompetent cervix
Blood group sensitization, neonatal jaundice
Neonatal thrombocytopenia
Hydrops
Inborn errors of metabolism

Present Pregnancy

Vaginal bleeding (abruptio placentae, placenta previa)
Sexually transmitted diseases (colonization: herpes simplex, group B *Streptococcus*),
    chlamydia, syphilis, hepatitis B
Multiple gestation
Pre-eclampsia
Premature rupture of membranes
Short interpregnancy time
Polyoligohydramnios
Acute medical or surgical illness
Inadequate prenatal care
Familial or acquired hypercoagulable states

Labor and Delivery

Premature labor (< 37 wk)
Post dates (> 42 wk)
Fetal distress
Immature L/S ratio: absent phosphatidylglycerol
Breech presentation
Meconium-stained fluid
Nuchal cord
Cesarean section
Forceps delivery
Apgar score < 4 at 1 min

Neonate

Birth weight < 2500 or > 4000 g
Birth before 37 or after 42 wk of gestation
SGA, LGA growth status
Tachypnea, cyanosis
Congenital malformation
Pallor, plethora, petechiae

SLE = Systemic lupus erythematosus; SGA = small for gestational age; LGA = large for gestational age; L/S = lecithin/sphingomyelin.

alert the physician to newborns at high risk. Fetal blood loss may be indicated by placental pallor, retroplacental hematoma, and tears of a velamentous cord or of chorionic blood vessels supplying succenturiate lobes. Placental edema and subsequent deficiency of immunoglobulin G in newborns may be associated with fetofetal transfusion syndrome, hydrops fetalis, congenital nephrosis, or hepatic disease. Amnion nodosum (granules on the amnion) and oligohydramnios are associated with pulmonary hypoplasia and renal agenesis, whereas small whitish nodules on the cord suggest a candidal infection.

Meconium staining suggests asphyxia and the risk of pneumonia, and opacity of the fetal placental surface suggests infection. Single umbilical arteries are associated with an increased incidence of congenital abnormalities.

MULTIPLE PREGNANCIES

INCIDENCE. Although the incidence of spontaneous multifetal gestation is stable, the overall incidence is increasing, owing to the treatment of infertility with ovarian stimulants (clomiphene, gonadotropins) and in vitro fertilization. Twins represent about 2.5% of births but 20% of very-low-birth-weight (VLBW) infants.

Problems of twin gestation include polyhydramnios, hyperemesis gravidarum, pre-eclampsia, prolonged rupture of membranes, vasa previa, velamentous insertion of the umbilical cord, abnormal presentations (breech), and premature labor. Compared with the first-born twin, the second, or B, twin is at increased risk for respiratory distress syndrome and asphyxia. Twins are at risk for intrauterine growth retardation (IUGR), twin-twin transfusion, and congenital anomalies that occur predominantly in monozygotic twins.

Placental vascular anastomoses occur with high frequency only in monochorionic twins. In the fetal transfusion syndrome, an artery from one twin acutely or chronically delivers blood that is drained into the vein of the other. The latter becomes plethoric and large, and the former is anemic and small. Treatment of this highly lethal problem includes maternal digoxin, reductive amniocentesis for polyhydramnios, selective twin termination, or neodymium:yttrium-aluminum-garnet laser or fetoscopic ablation of the anastomosis.

PREMATURITY AND IUGR

DEFINITIONS. Liveborn infants delivered before 37 wk from the first day of the last menstrual period are termed *premature*. The term *premature* is also often used to denote immaturity. Infants of extremely-low-birth-weight (ELBW) are less than 1000 g. Historically, prematurity was defined by a birth weight of 2500 g or less, but today infants who weigh 2500 g or less at birth, low-birth-weight (LBW) infants, are considered to be premature with a shortened gestational period, to have IUGR for their gestational age (also referred to as small for gestational age [SGA]), or both. Prematurity and IUGR are associated with increased neonatal morbidity and mortality.

VERY-LOW-BIRTH-WEIGHT INFANTS. VLBW infants account for over 50% of neonatal deaths and 50% of handicapped infants; their survival is directly related to birth weight, with approximately 20% of those between 500 and 600 g and 85–90% of those between 1250 and 1500 g surviving. Compared with term infants, VLBW neonates have a higher incidence of rehospitalization during the 1st yr of life for sequelae of prematurity, infections, neurologic sequelae, and psychosocial disorders.

FACTORS RELATED TO PREMATURE BIRTH AND LOW BIRTH WEIGHT. A strong positive correlation exists between both premature birth and IUGR and low socioeconomic status. Families of low socioeconomic status have relatively high incidences of maternal undernutrition, anemia, and illness; inadequate prenatal care; drug addiction; obstetric complications; and maternal histories of reproductive inefficiency (relative infertility, abortions, stillbirths, premature or LBW infants). Other associated factors such as single-parent families, teenage pregnancies, close spacing of pregnancies, and mothers who have borne more than 4 previous children are also encountered more frequently. Overt or symptomatic bacterial infection of the amniotic fluid and membranes (chorioamnionitis) also may initiate preterm labor.

IUGR is associated with medical conditions that interfere with the circulation and efficiency of the placenta, with the development or growth of the fetus, or with the general health and nutrition of the mother. Many factors are common to both prematurely born and LBW infants with IUGR.

ASSESSMENT OF GESTATIONAL AGE AT BIRTH. Compared with a premature infant of appropriate weight, an infant with IUGR has a reduced birth weight and may appear to have a disproportionately larger head relative to body size; infants in both groups lack subcutaneous fat. In general, neurologic maturity (e.g., nerve conduction velocity) correlates with gestational age despite reduced fetal weight. Physical signs may be useful in estimating gestational age at birth.

SPECTRUM OF DISEASE IN LBW INFANTS. Immaturity tends to increase the severity but reduce the distinctiveness of the clinical manifestations of most neonatal diseases. Immature organ function, complications of therapy, and the specific disorders that caused the premature onset of labor contribute to neonatal morbidity and mortality associated with premature, LBW infants (Table 69–2).

NURSERY CARE. At birth, the measures needed for clearing the airway, initiating breathing, caring for the cord and eyes, and

TABLE 69–2   Neonatal Problems Associated with Premature Infants

Respiratory

Respiratory distress syndrome—RDS (hyaline membrane disease—HMD)*
Chronic lung disease (bronchopulmonary dysplasia—BPD)*
Pneumothorax, pneumomediastinum; interstitial emphysema
Congenital pneumonia
Pulmonary hypoplasia
Pulmonary hemorrhage
Apnea*

Cardiovascular

Patent ductus arteriosus—PDA*
Hypotension
Hypertension
Bradycardia (with apnea)*
Congenital malformations

Hematologic

Anemia (early or late onset)
Hyperbilirubinemia—indirect*
Subcutaneous, organ (liver, adrenal) hemorrhage*
Disseminated intravascular coagulopathy
Vitamin K deficiency
Hydrops—immune or nonimmune

Gastrointestinal

Poor gastrointestinal function—poor motility*
Necrotizing enterocolitis
Hyperbilirubinemia—direct
Congenital anomalies producing polyhydramnios

Metabolic-Endocrine

Hypocalcemia*
Hypoglycemia*
Hyperglycemia*
Late metabolic acidosis
Hypothermia*
Euthyroid but low T_4 status

Central Nervous System

Intraventricular hemorrhage*
Periventricular leukomalacia
Hypoxic-ischemic encephalopathy
Seizures
Retinopathy of prematurity
Deafness
Hypotonia*
Congenital malformations
Kernicterus (bilirubin encephalopathy)
Drug (narcotic) withdrawal

Renal

Hyponatremia*
Hypernatremia*
Hyperkalemia*
Renal tubular acidosis
Renal glycosuria
Edema

Other

Infections* (congenital, perinatal, nosocomial; bacterial, viral, fungal, protozoal)

*Common.

administering vitamin K are the same in immature infants as in those of normal weight and maturity. Special care is required to maintain a patent airway and avoid potential aspiration of gastric contents. Additional considerations are the need for (1) incubator care and heart rate and respiration monitoring, (2) oxygen therapy, and (3) special attention to the details of feeding. Safeguards against infection can never be relaxed.

Incubator Care. Modern incubators conserve body heat through provision of a warm atmospheric environment and standard conditions of humidity. They also may reduce atmospheric contamination if they are scrupulously cleaned. The survival of LBW and sick infants is greater when they are cared for at or near their neutral thermal environment. Maintaining a relative humidity of 40–60% aids in stabilizing body temperature by reducing heat loss at lower environmental temperatures; by preventing drying and irritation of the lining of respiratory passages, especially during administration of oxygen and after or during endotracheal intubation (usually 100% humidity); and by thinning viscid secretions and reducing insensible water loss from the lungs. Administering oxygen to reduce the risk of injury from hypoxia and circulatory insufficiency must be balanced against the risks of hyperoxia to the eyes (retinopathy of prematurity) and oxygen injury to the lungs.

Feeding. The method of feeding each LBW infant should be individualized. It is important to avoid fatigue and the aspiration of food by regurgitation or by the feeding process. No feeding method averts these problems unless the person feeding the infant has been well trained in the method. Oral feedings (nipple) should not be initiated or should be discontinued in infants having respiratory distress, hypoxia, circulatory insufficiency, excessive secretions, gagging, sepsis, central nervous system depression, immaturity, or signs of serious illness. These infants require parenteral or gavage feedings to supply calories, fluid, and electrolytes. The main principle in feeding premature infants is to proceed cautiously and gradually. Careful early feeding of glucose or formula tends to reduce the risk of hypoglycemia, dehydration, and hyperbilirubinemia without the additional risk of aspiration, provided the presence of respiratory distress or other disorders does not present an indication for withholding oral feedings and administering electrolytes, fluids, and calories intravenously.

Water intake in term infants is usually begun at 60–70 mL/ kg on day 1 and increased to 100–120 mL/kg by days 2–3. Smaller, more premature infants may need to be started with 70–100 mL/ kg on day 1 and advanced to 150 mL/kg or more by days 3–4. Fluid volumes should be titrated individually, although it is unusual to exceed 150 mL/kg/24 hr.

PREVENTION OF INFECTION. Premature infants have an increased susceptibility to infection, which requires nursery personnel to wash rigorously hand to elbow before and after handling each infant, take measures to reduce contamination of food and objects coming in contact with the infant, prevent air contamination, avoid overcrowding, and limit direct and indirect contacts with themselves and other infants. No one with an infection should be permitted into the nursery.

PROGNOSIS. There is now a 95% or greater chance of survival for infants born weighing 1501–2500 g, but those weighing less still have a significantly higher mortality. Intensive care has extended the period during which a VLBW infant is likely to die of complications of perinatal disease, such as chronic lung disease, necrotizing enterocolitis, or secondary infection.

DISCHARGE FROM HOSPITAL. Before discharge, a premature infant should be taking all nutrition by nipple, either bottle or breast. Growth should be occurring at steady increments of 10–30 g/24 hr. Temperature should be stabilized in an open crib. There should have been no recent apnea or bradycardia, and parenteral drug administration should have been discontinued or converted to oral dosing. Infants previously treated with oxygen should have an eye examination to determine the presence, stage, or absence of retinopathy of prematurity. All LBW infants should have a hearing test.

POST-TERM INFANTS

Post-term infants are those born after 42 wk of gestation, calculated from the mother's last menstrual period, regardless of weight at birth. This designation is often used synonymously with the term *postmature* for infants whose gestation exceeds the normal 280 days by 7 days or more. The cause of post-term birth or postmaturity is unknown.

CLINICAL MANIFESTATIONS. Post-term infants may be clinically indistinguishable from term infants, but some have received the designation "postmature" because their appearance and behavior suggest those of an infant 1–3 wk of age. These post-term, postmature infants are often of increased birth weight and characterized by the absence of lanugo, decreased or absent vernix caseosa, long nails, abundant scalp hair, white parchment-like or desquamating skin, and increased alertness. If placental insufficiency occurs, the amniotic fluid and fetus may be meconium stained and abnormal fetal heart rates may be observed; the infant may have growth retardation. Although this syndrome is frequently confused with postmaturity, only about 20% of infants with placental insufficiency syndrome are post term. The majority of those affected are term and preterm infants, particularly those SGA who are infants of toxemic mothers, older primigravidas, and women with chronic hypertension.

Those infants born post term in association with presumed

placental insufficiency may have various physical signs: desquamation, long nails, abundant hair, pale skin, alert faces, and loose skin, especially around the thighs and buttocks, giving them the appearance of having recently lost weight; meconium-stained nails, skin, vernix, umbilical cord, and placental membranes.

TREATMENT. Careful obstetric monitoring usually provides a rational basis for choosing a course of nonintervention, induction of labor, or cesarean section. Meconium aspiration pneumonia or hypoxic encephalopathy is treated symptomatically.

LARGE FOR GESTATIONAL AGE

Neonatal mortality rates decrease with increasing birth weight until approximately 4000 g, after which mortality increases. These oversized infants are usually born at term, but preterm infants with weights high for gestational age also have a significantly higher mortality than infants of the same size born at term; maternal diabetes and obesity are predisposing factors. Infants who are very large, regardless of their gestational age, have a higher incidence of birth injuries, such as cervical and brachial plexus injuries, phrenic nerve damage with paralysis of the diaphragm, fractured clavicles, cephalhematomas, subdural hematomas, and ecchymoses of the head and face. The incidence of congenital anomalies, particularly congenital heart disease, is also higher than in term infants of normal weight. Intellectual and developmental retardation is statistically more common in high-birth-weight term and preterm infants than in infants of appropriate weight for gestational age.

CHAPTER 70

Clinical Manifestations of Diseases in the Newborn Period

(Nelson Textbook, Chapter 94)

Recognizing disease in newborns depends on knowledge about the disorder and evaluation of a limited number of relatively nonspecific clinical signs and symptoms.

Central cyanosis has respiratory, cardiac, central nervous system (CNS), hematologic, or metabolic causes (Table 70–1). Respiratory insufficiency may be due to pulmonary conditions or may be secondary to CNS depression due to drugs, intracranial hemorrhage, or anoxia. Cyanosis persisting for several days, unaccompanied by obvious signs of respiratory difficulty, suggests cyanotic congenital heart disease or methemoglobinemia. Episodes of cya-

TABLE 70–1   Differential Diagnosis of Cyanosis in the Newborn

Central or Peripheral Nervous System Hypoventilation
Birth asphyxia
Intracranial hypertension, hemorrhage
Oversedation (direct or through maternal route)
Diaphragm palsy
Neuromuscular diseases
Seizures

Respiratory Disease

Upper Airway
Choanal atresia/stenosis
Pierre Robin syndrome
Intrinsic airway obstruction (laryngeal/bronchial/tracheal stenosis)
Extrinsic airway obstruction (bronchogenic cyst, duplication cyst, vascular compression)

Lower Airway
Respiratory distress syndrome
Transient tachypnea
Meconium aspiration
Pneumonia (sepsis)
Pneumothorax
Congenital diaphragmatic hernia
Pulmonary hypoplasia
Persistent fetal circulation (persistent pulmonary hypertension of newborn)

Cardiac Right-to-Left Shunt

Abnormal Connections (Pulmonary Blood Flow Normal or Increased)
Transposition of the great vessels
Total anomalous pulmonary venous return
Truncus arteriosus
Hypoplastic left heart syndrome
Single ventricle or tricuspid atresia with large ventricular septal defect without pulmonic stenosis

Obstructed Pulmonary Blood Flow (Pulmonary Blood Flow Decreased)
Pulmonic atresia with intact ventricular septum
Tetralogy of Fallot
Critical pulmonic stenosis with patent foramen ovale or atrial septal defect
Tricuspid atresia
Single ventricle with pulmonic stenosis
Ebstein malformation of the tricuspid valve
Persistent fetal circulation (persistent pulmonary hypertension of newborn)

Methemoglobinemia
Congenital (hemoglobin M, methemoglobin reductase deficiency)
Acquired (e.g., nitrates, nitrites)

Inadequate Ambient O_2 or Less O_2 Delivered Than Expected (Rare)
Disconnection of O_2 supply to nasal cannula, head hood
Connection of air, rather than O_2, to a mechanical ventilator

Spurious/Artifactual
Oximeter artifact (poor contact between probe and skin, poor pulse searching)
Arterial blood gas artifact (contamination with venous blood)

Other
Hypoglycemia
Adrenogenital syndrome
Polycythemia
Blood loss

From Smith F: Cyanosis. *In:* Kliegman R, Nieder M, Super D (eds): Practical Strategies in Pediatric Diagnosis and Therapy. Philadelphia, WB Saunders, 1996.

nosis also may be the presenting sign of hypoglycemia, bacteremia, meningitis, shock, or pulmonary hypertension.

Pallor, in addition to anemia or acute hemorrhage, should suggest hypoxia, asphyxia, hypoglycemia, sepsis, shock, or adrenal failure.

Hypotension in term infants suggests shock due to hypovolemia, the systemic inflammatory response syndrome, cardiac dysfunction, pneumothorax, pneumopericardium, pericardial effusion, or metabolic disorders. Hypotension is a common problem in sick very-low-birth-weight infants and may be due to any of the problems noted in a term infant.

Convulsions usually point to a disorder of the CNS and suggest hypoxic-ischemic encephalopathy resulting from asphyxia, intracranial hemorrhage, cerebral anomaly, subdural effusion, meningitis, hypocalcemia, hypoglycemia, infarction, benign familial seizures, and, rarely, pyridoxine dependence, hyponatremia, hypernatremia, inborn errors of metabolism, or drug withdrawal.

Lethargy may be a manifestation of infection, asphyxia, hypoglycemia, hypercarbia, sedation from maternal analgesia or anesthesia, cerebral defect, and of almost any severe disease including inborn errors of metabolism.

Irritability may be a sign of discomfort accompanying intra-abdominal conditions, meningeal irritation, drug withdrawal, infections, congenital glaucoma, or any condition producing pain.

Hyperactivity, especially of the premature infant, may be a sign of hypoxia, pneumothorax, emphysema, hypoglycemia, hypocalcemia, CNS damage, drug withdrawal, thyrotoxicosis, bronchospasm, esophageal reflux, or discomfort due to a cold environment.

Failure to feed well is seen in most sick newborns and should always occasion a careful search for infection, central or peripheral nervous system disorder, intestinal obstruction, and other abnormal conditions.

Fever may be the result of too high an environmental temperature due to weather, overheated nurseries or incubators, or too many clothes or bedclothes. It is also noted in "dehydration fever" of newborns. If these causes of fever can be eliminated, then serious infection must be considered, although such infections often occur without provoking a febrile response in newborns. An unexplained *fall in body temperature* may accompany infection or other serious disturbances of the circulation or CNS.

Periods of *apnea*, particularly in premature infants, may be associated with various disturbances.

Jaundice during the first 24 hr of life should be considered to be due to erythroblastosis fetalis until proven otherwise. Septicemia and intrauterine infections should also be considered.

Jaundice after the first 24 hr may be "physiologic" or may be due to septicemia, hemolytic anemia, galactosemia, hepatitis, congenital atresia of the bile ducts, inspissated bile syndrome after erythroblastosis fetalis, syphilis, herpes simplex, or congenital infections.

Vomiting during the 1st day of life suggests obstruction in the upper digestive tract or increased intracranial pressure. Vomiting also may be a nonspecific symptom of an illness such as septicemia. It is a common manifestation of overfeeding or inexperienced feeding technique, pyloric stenosis, milk allergy, duodenal ulcer, stress ulcer, or adrenal insufficiency.

Diarrhea may be a symptom of overfeeding (especially high caloric-density formula), acute gastroenteritis, or malabsorption or a nonspecific symptom of infection.

Abdominal distention, usually a sign of intestinal obstruction or an intra-abdominal mass, may also be seen in infants with enteritis, necrotizing enterocolitis, ileus accompanying sepsis, respiratory distress, ascites, or hypokalemia.

Failure to move an extremity (pseudoparalysis) or part of it suggests fracture, dislocation, or nerve injury. It is also seen in osteomyelitis and other infections.

CONGENITAL ANOMALIES

Congenital anomalies are a major cause of stillbirths and neonatal deaths but are perhaps even more important as causes of physical defects and metabolic disorders. Early recognition of anomalies is important for planning care.

CHAPTER 71

Birth Injury

(Nelson Textbook, Chapter 95)

The term *birth injury* is used to denote avoidable and unavoidable mechanical and hypoxic-ischemic injury incurred by an infant during labor and delivery. The incidence of birth injuries has been estimated at 2–7/1000 live births.

CRANIAL INJURIES

Caput succedaneum is a diffuse, sometimes ecchymotic, edematous swelling of the soft tissues of the scalp involving the portion presenting during vertex delivery. It may extend across the midline and across suture lines. The edema disappears within the first few days of life. No specific treatment is needed, but if there are extensive ecchymoses, phototherapy for hyperbilirubinemia may be indicated. *Molding* of the head and overriding of the parietal bones are frequently associated with caput succedaneum and become more evident after the caput has receded but disappear during the first weeks of life.

Erythema, abrasions, ecchymoses, and *subcutaneous fat necrosis* of facial or scalp soft tissues may be seen after forceps- or vacuum-assisted deliveries.

Subconjunctival and retinal hemorrhages are frequent, and *petechiae* of the skin of the head and neck are common. Parents should be assured that they are temporary and the result of *normal* hazards of delivery.

Cephalohematoma is a subperiosteal hemorrhage, hence always limited to the surface of one cranial bone. There is no discoloration of the overlying scalp, and swelling is usually not visible until several hours after birth. An underlying skull fracture, usually linear and not depressed, is occasionally associated with cephalohematoma. Cephalohematomas require no treatment, although phototherapy may be necessary to ameliorate hyperbilirubinemia.

Fractures of the skull may occur as a result of pressure from forceps or from the maternal symphysis pubis, sacral promontory, or ischial spines. Linear fractures, the most common, cause no symptoms and require no treatment. Depressed fractures are usually indentations of the calvarium similar to a dent in a Ping-Pong ball; it is advisable to elevate severe depressions to prevent cortical injury from sustained pressure. Fracture of the occipital bone with separation of the basal and squamous portions almost invariably causes fatal hemorrhage.

INTRACRANIAL-INTRAVENTRICULAR HEMORRHAGE

ETIOLOGY AND EPIDEMIOLOGY. Intracranial hemorrhage may result from trauma or asphyxia and, rarely, from a primary hemorrhagic disturbance or congenital vascular anomaly. Intracranial hemorrhages often involve the ventricles (intraventricular hemorrhage [IVH]) of premature infants delivered spontaneously without apparent trauma. IVH in premature infants occurs in the gelatinous subependymal germinal matrix. Predisposing factors or events for IVH include prematurity, respiratory distress syndrome (RDS), hypoxic-ischemic or hypotensive injury, reperfusion of damaged vessels, increased or decreased cerebral blood flow, reduced vascular integrity, increased venous pressure, pneumothorax, hypervolemia, and hypertension. Similar injurious factors (hypoxic-ischemic-hypotensive) or venous obstruction from an IVH may produce periventricular hemorrhage/necrosis (echodensities) due to hemorrhagic infarction. Periventricular leukomalacia is a common associated cystic finding.

CLINICAL MANIFESTATIONS. The incidence of IVH increases with decreasing birth weight. IVH is rarely present at birth; however, 80–90% of cases occur between birth and the 3rd day of life and 50% occur on the 1st day. The most common symptoms are diminished or absent Moro reflex, poor muscle tone, lethargy, apnea, and somnolence. Premature infants with IVH often have a precipitous deterioration on the 2nd or 3rd day of life. Periods of apnea, pallor, or cyanosis; failure to suck well; abnormal eye signs; a high-pitched, shrill cry; muscular twitchings, convulsions, decreased muscle tone, or paralyses; metabolic acidosis; shock; and a decreased hematocrit or its failure to increase after transfusion may be the first indications. The fontanel may be tense and bulging. Severe neurologic depression progresses to coma after more severe IVH, with associated hemorrhage in the cerebral cortex and ventricular dilation. In some cases (grade I, II) there may be no clinical manifestations.

Periventricular leukomalacia is usually asymptomatic until the neurologic sequelae of white matter necrosis become apparent in later infancy as spastic diplegia.

DIAGNOSIS. Intracranial hemorrhage is diagnosed on the basis of the history, clinical manifestations, transfontanel cranial ultrasonography or computed tomography, and knowledge of the birth-weight–specific risks of the type of hemorrhage. The diagnosis of *subdural hemorrhage* in a large-for-gestational-age term infant with cephalopelvic disproportion may be delayed 1 mo until the chronic subdural fluid volume expands, producing megalocephaly, frontal bossing, a bulging fontanel, seizures, and anemia.

TREATMENT. IVH associated with hypoxic-ischemic encephalopathy is frequently associated with multiple organ system dysfunction. Seizures are treated with anticonvulsant drugs, anemia-shock requires transfusion with packed red blood cell or fresh frozen plasma, and acidosis is treated with judicious and slow administration of 1–2 mEq/kg sodium bicarbonate. Neurosurgical placement of an external ventriculostomy catheter may be needed in the early stage of uncontrolled symptomatic hydrocephalus. Symptomatic subdural hemorrhage in large term infants should be treated by removing the subdural fluid collection.

SPINE AND SPINAL CORD

Strong traction exerted when the spine is hyperextended or when the direction of pull is lateral, or forceful longitudinal traction on the trunk while the head is still firmly engaged in the pelvis, especially when combined with flexion and torsion of the vertical axis, may produce fracture and separation of the vertebrae. Hemorrhage and edema may produce neurologic signs that are indistinguishable from those of transection except that they may not be permanent. Areflexia, loss of sensation, and complete paralysis of voluntary motion occur below the level of injury. If the injury is severe, the infant, who from birth may be in poor condition owing to respiratory depression, shock, or hypothermia, may deteriorate rapidly to death within several hours before neurologic signs are obvious. Alternatively, the course may be protracted, with symptoms and signs appearing at birth or later in the 1st wk; immobility, flaccidity, and associated brachial plexus injuries may not be recognized for several days. Treatment of the survivors is supportive.

PERIPHERAL NERVE INJURIES

BRACHIAL PALSY. Injury to the brachial plexus may cause paralysis of the upper arm with or without paralysis of the forearm or hand or, more commonly, paralysis of the entire arm. In *Erb-Duchenne paralysis,* the injury is limited to the 5th and 6th cervical nerves. The infant loses the power to abduct the arm from the shoulder, to rotate the arm externally, and to supinate the forearm. The characteristic position consists of adduction and internal rotation of the arm with pronation of the forearm. *Klumpke's paralysis* is a rarer form of brachial palsy; injury to the 7th and 8th cervical nerves and the 1st thoracic nerve produces a paralyzed hand and ipsilateral ptosis and miosis (Homer syndrome) if the sympathetic fibers of the 1st thoracic root are also injured. Treatment consists of partial immobilization and appropriate positioning to prevent development of contractures. If the paralysis persists without improvement for 3–6 mo, neuroplasty, neurolysis, end-to-end anastomosis, or nerve grafting offers hope for partial recovery.

PHRENIC NERVE PARALYSIS. Phrenic nerve injury (3rd, 4th, 5th cervical nerves) with diaphragmatic paralysis must be considered when cyanosis and irregular and labored respirations develop. There is no specific treatment; infants should be placed on the involved side and given oxygen if necessary. Recovery usually occurs spontaneously by 1–3 mo; rarely, surgical plication of the diaphragm may be indicated.

FACIAL NERVE PALSY. Facial palsy usually is a peripheral paralysis that results from pressure over the facial nerve in utero, from efforts during labor, or from forceps use during delivery. Peripheral paralysis is flaccid and, when complete, involves the entire side of the face, including the forehead. When the infant cries, there is movement only on the nonparalyzed side of the face, and the mouth is drawn to that side. On the affected side the forehead is smooth, the eye cannot be closed, the nasolabial fold is absent, and the corner of the mouth droops.

VISCERA

The liver is the only internal organ other than the brain that is injured with any frequency during birth. The damage usually results from pressure on the liver during delivery of the head in breech presentations. Hepatic rupture may result in the formation of a subcapsular hematoma, which may tamponade further bleeding. Infants usually appear normal for the first 1–3 days. Nonspecific signs related to loss of blood into the hematoma may appear early and include poor feeding, listlessness, pallor, jaundice, tachypnea, and tachycardia. A mass may be palpable in the right upper quadrant; the abdomen may appear blue. The hematoma may be large enough to cause anemia. Shock and death may occur if the hematoma breaks through the capsule into the peritoneal cavity, reducing pressure and allowing fresh hemorrhage. Surgical repair of a laceration may be required.

Rupture of the spleen may occur alone or in association with rupture of the liver. The causes, complications, treatment, and prevention are similar.

FRACTURES

CLAVICLE. This bone is fractured during labor and delivery more frequently than any other bone. The infant characteristically does not move the arm freely on the affected side; crepitus and bony irregularity may be palpated, and discoloration is occasionally visible over the fracture site. The Moro reflex is absent on the affected side, and there is spasm of the sternocleidomastoid muscle with obliteration of the supraclavicular depression at the site of the fracture. In greenstick fractures there may be no limitation of movement, and the Moro reflex may be present. Treatment, if any, consists of immobilization of the arm and shoulder on the affected side.

HYPOXIA-ISCHEMIA

Hypoxic-ischemic encephalopathy is an important cause of permanent damage to central nervous system cells, which may result in neonatal death or which may be manifested later as cerebral palsy or mental deficiency.

CLINICAL MANIFESTATIONS. The signs of hypoxia in a fetus are usually noted a few minutes to a few days before delivery. The fetal heart rate slows, and the beat-to-beat variability declines. Continuous heart rate recording may reveal a variable or late (type II dips) deceleration, pattern and fetal scalp blood analysis may show a pH less than 7.20.

At delivery, the presence of yellow, meconium-stained amniotic fluid is evidence that fetal distress has occurred. At birth, these infants are frequently depressed and fail to breathe spontaneously. During the ensuing hours, they may remain hypotonic or change from hypotonia to extreme hypertonia, or their tone may appear normal (Table 71–1). Pallor, cyanosis, apnea, slow heart rate, and unresponsiveness to stimulation also are signs of hypoxic-ischemic encephalopathy. Although most often a result of the hypoxic-ischemic encephalopathy, seizures in asphyxiated newborns may also be due to hypocalcemia and hypoglycemia.

TABLE 71-1 Hypoxic-Ischemic Encephalopathy in Term Infants

Signs	Stage 1	Stage 2	Stage 3
Level of consciousness	Hyperalert	Lethargic	Stuporous, coma
Muscle tone	Normal	Hypotonic	Flaccid
Posture	Normal	Flexion	Decerebrate
Tendon reflexes/clonus	Hyperactive	Hyperactive	Absent
Myoclonus	Present	Present	Absent
Moro reflex	Strong	Weak	Absent
Pupils	Mydriasis	Miosis	Unequal, poor light reflex
Seizures	None	Common	Decerebration
Electroencephalographic	Normal	Low voltage changing to seizure activity	Burst suppression to isoelectric
Duration	<24 hr if progresses; otherwise, may remain normal	24 hr to 14 days	Days to weeks
Outcome	Good	Variable	Death, severe deficits

Modified from Sarnat H, Sarnat M: Neonatal encephalopathy following fetal distress: A clinical and electroencephalographic study. Arch Neurol 33:696, 1976. Copyright 1976, American Medical Association.

In addition to central nervous system dysfunction, congestive heart failure and cardiogenic shock, persistent pulmonary hypertension (persistent fetal circulation), respiratory distress syndrome, gastrointestinal perforation, hematuria, and acute tubular necrosis are associated with perinatal asphyxia.

TREATMENT. Therapy is supportive and directed at the organ system manifestations. There is no established effective treatment for the brain tissue injury.

CHAPTER 72

Delivery Room Emergencies
(Nelson Textbook, Chapter 96)

The most common and important emergency related to newborns in the delivery room is the failure to initiate and maintain respirations. Less frequent but of major importance are shock, severe anemia, plethora, convulsions, and management of life-threatening congenital malformations.

RESPIRATORY DISTRESS AND FAILURE. Disorders of respiration in newborns can be categorized as either central nervous system (CNS) failure, representing depression or failure of the respiratory center, or peripheral respiratory difficulty, indicating interference with the alveolar exchange of oxygen and carbon dioxide. Cyanosis occurs in both groups. The respiratory problems encountered in the delivery room are most frequently those of airway obstruction and of depression of the CNS (maternal medications, asphyxia), with the absence of adequate respiratory effort.

Respiratory distress in the presence of good respiratory effort should lead to an immediate consideration of peripheral causes; *it is an indication for a radiographic examination of the chest*, if this is at all possible.

If respiratory movements are made with the mouth closed but the infant fails to move air in and out of the lungs, bilateral choanal atresia or other obstruction of the upper respiratory tract should be suspected. The mouth should be opened, and the mouth and posterior pharynx should be cleared of secretions by gene suction. An oropharyngeal airway should be inserted, and the source of the obstruction should be sought immediately. If effective respiratory flow is not produced by opening the infant's mouth and clearing the airway, laryngoscopy is indicated. With obstructive malformations of the mandible, epiglottis, larynx, or trachea, an endotracheal tube should be inserted; prolonged endotracheal intubation or tracheostomy may be required. Respiratory failure due to depression or injury of the CNS may require continuous artificial ventilation with a face mask and bag or through an endotracheal tube.

FAILURE TO INITIATE OR SUSTAIN RESPIRATION. This usually originates in the CNS as a result of asphyxia; immaturity in itself is seldom a causative factor except in infants weighing less than 1000 g.

Narcosis results from heavy doses of morphine, meperidine (Demerol), fentanyl, barbiturates, or tranquilizers administered to the mother shortly before delivery or from maternal anesthesia, given during the second stage of labor. Infants are cyanotic and hypotonic at birth and slow to cry or breathe; when respiration is established, it is extremely slow.

Narcosis should be avoided by using appropriate analgesic and anesthetic practices. Treatment includes initial physical stimulation and securing a patent airway. If effective ventilation is not initiated, artificial breathing with a mask and bag must be instituted. At the same time, if depression is due to morphine or its derivatives, naloxone (Narcan), 0.1 mg/kg, should be given by intravenous, subcutaneous, intratracheal, or intramuscular routes and repeated two to three times if needed.

RESUSCITATION. The *goals* of neonatal resuscitation are to prevent the morbidity and mortality associated with hypoxic-ischemic tissue (brain, heart, kidney) injury and to re-establish adequate spontaneous respiration and cardiac output. The steps in neonatal resuscitation follow the ABCs: A = anticipate and establish a patent airway by suctioning and, if necessary, perform endotracheal intubation; B = initiate breathing using tactile stimulation or positive-pressure ventilation with a bag and mask or through an endotracheal tube; and C = maintain the circulation with chest compression and medications, if needed.

If there are no respirations or if the heart rate is below 100 beats/min, positive-pressure ventilation with 100% oxygen is given through a tightly fitted face mask and bag for 15–30 sec. Although the first breath may require pressures as low as 15–20 cm H_2O, pressures as high as 30–40 cm HO may be needed. Subsequent breaths are given at a rate of 40–60 breaths/min, with pressures of 15–20 cm H_2O. Noncompliant stiff lungs due to hyaline membrane disease, congenital pneumonia, or meconium aspiration need higher pressures (20–40 cm H_2O). Successful ventilation is determined by good chest rise, symmetric breath sounds, improved pink color, heart rate greater than 100 beats/min, spontaneous respirations, and improved tone.

If the heart rate does not improve after 15–30 sec with bag and mask (or endotracheal) ventilation and remains below 60 beats/min or if the rate is less than 80 beats/min and not rising, ventilation is continued and chest compression with two fingers is initiated over the lower third of the sternum at a rate of 120/min. The ratio of compressions to ventilation is 3:1.

Medications should be administered when the heart rate is less than 80 beats/min after 30 sec of combined ventilation and chest compressions or during asystole. The umbilical vein usually can be readily cannulated and should be used for immediate administration of medications, glucose, and volume expanders during neonatal resuscitation. Epinephrine (0.1–0.3 mL/kg of a 1:10,000 solution, intravenous or intratracheal) is given for asystole or for failure to respond to 30 sec of combined resuscitation. The dose may be repeated every 5 min. If there is no response, some authorities recommend using 5 to 10 times the standard dose of epinephrine. Ten to 20 mL/kg of volume expanders (normal saline, blood, Ringer's lactate, 5% albumin) should be given for hypovolemia, pallor, electrical-mechanical dissociation (weak pulses with normal heart rate), history of blood loss, suspicion of septic shock, hypotension, or poor response to resuscitation. Sodium bicarbonate (1–2 mEq/kg, 0.5 mEq/mL of a 4.2% solution) should be given slowly (1 mEq/kg/min) if there is a documented metabolic acidosis and the resuscitation is prolonged. Sodium bicarbonate should be given after effective ventilation has been established

Severe asphyxia also may depress myocardial function, causing cardiogenic shock despite recovery of heart and respiratory rates. Dopamine or dobutamine administered as a continuous infusion (5–20 μg/kg/min) and volume expanders should be started after the initial resuscitation effort to improve cardiac output in an infant with poor peripheral perfusion, weak pulses, hypotension, tachycardia, and poor urine output. Epinephrine (0.1–1.0 μg/kg/min) may be indicated for infants in severe shock who do not respond to dopamine or dobutamine. Less severe degrees of asphyxia can usually be managed by brief periods of bag and mask ventilation of 100% oxygen. Chest compression and medications are not needed for most neonates who have mild to moderate birth depression.

CHAPTER 73

Respiratory Tract Disorders
(Nelson Textbook, Chapter 97)

Disturbances of respiration in the immediate postnatal period may have originated in utero, in the delivery room, or in the nursery. A wide variety of pathologic lesions may be responsible for one or more of the signs of respiratory distress; cyanosis is common, and if respiratory embarrassment is severe, pallor may also be present. It is occasionally difficult to distinguish cardiovascular from respiratory disturbances on the basis of clinical signs alone. Any sign of postnatal respiratory distress is an indication for a radiograph of the chest.

BREATHING PATTERNS IN NEWBORNS. During sleep in the first months of life, normal full-term infants may have infrequent episodes when regular breathing is interrupted with short pauses. This *periodic breathing* pattern, shifting from a regular rhythmicity to cyclic brief episodes of intermittent apnea, is more common in premature infants, who may have apneic pauses of 5–10 sec followed by a burst of rapid respirations at a rate of 50–60/min for 10–15 sec. They rarely have an associated change in color or heart rate, and it often stops without apparent reason. Periodic breathing persists intermittently, usually until premature infants are about 36 wk of gestational age.

APNEA

Periodic breathing must be distinguished from prolonged apneic pauses, because the latter may be associated with serious illnesses. Apnea is due to many primary diseases that affect neonates (Table 73–1). *Idiopathic apnea of prematurity* occurs in the absence of identifiable predisposing diseases. Apnea is a disorder of respiratory control and may be obstructive, central, or mixed. The most common pattern of idiopathic apnea among preterm neonates

---

TABLE 73–1 Potential Causes of Neonatal Apnea and Bradycardia

Central Nervous System

Intraventricular hemorrhage, drugs, seizures, hypoxic injury, herniation, neuromuscular disorders, Leigh syndrome, brain stem infarction or anomalies (e.g., olivopontocerebellar atrophy), following general anesthesia

Respiratory

Pneumonia, obstructive airway lesions, upper airway collapse, atelectasis, extreme prematurity (<1000 g), laryngeal reflex, phrenic nerve paralysis, severe hyaline membrane disease, pneumothorax, hypoxia

Infectious

Sepsis, necrotizing enterocolitis, meningitis (bacterial, fungal, viral), respiratory syncytial virus

Gastrointestinal

Oral feeding, bowel movement, gastroesophageal reflux, esophagitis, intestinal perforation

Metabolic

↓ Glucose, ↓ calcium, ↓ ↑ sodium, ↑ ammonia, ↑ organic acids, ↑ ambient temperature, hypothermia

Cardiovascular

Hypotension, hypertension, heart failure, anemia, hypovolemia, vagal tone

Other

Immaturity of respiratory center, sleep state

has a mixed etiology (50–75%), with obstructive apnea preceding (usually) or following central apnea. Short apneas are usually central, whereas prolonged apneas are often mixed.

CLINICAL MANIFESTATIONS. The incidence of idiopathic apnea of prematurity varies inversely with gestational age. In preterm infants, it is rare on the 1st day of life; apnea immediately after birth signifies another illness. The onset of idiopathic apnea occurs on the 2nd–7th day of life. The onset of apnea in a previously well premature neonate after the 2nd wk of life or in a term infant at any time is a critical event that warrants immediate investigation. In preterm infants, serious apnea is defined as cessation of breathing for longer than 20 sec or any duration if accompanied by cyanosis and sinus bradycardia.

TREATMENT. Infants at risk for apnea should be monitored with apnea monitors. *Gentle cutaneous stimulation* is often adequate therapy for neonatal infants having mild and intermittent episodes. Infants having recurrent and prolonged apnea require immediate *bag and mask ventilation. Oxygen* should be administered to treat hypoxia. Apnea of prematurity not due to a precipitating identifiable cause should be treated with *theophylline* or *caffeine*. Transfusion of packed red blood cells also may reduce the incidence of idiopathic apnea among severely anemic infants. *Nasal continuous positive airway pressure* (CPAP, 3–5 cm H_2O) is effective therapy for mixed or obstructive apneas.

HYALINE MEMBRANE DISEASE (RESPIRATORY DISTRESS SYNDROME)

INCIDENCE. HMD occurs primarily in premature infants; incidence is inversely proportional to the gestational age and birth weight.

ETIOLOGY. Surfactant deficiency (decreased production and secretion) is the primary cause of HMD.

CLINICAL MANIFESTATIONS. Signs of HMD usually appear within minutes of birth, although they may not be recognized for several hours in larger premature infants until rapid, shallow respirations have increased to 60 breaths/min or greater. The late onset of tachypnea should suggest other conditions. Characteristically, tachypnea, prominent (often audible) grunting, intercostal and subcostal retractions, nasal flaring, and duskiness are noted. Cyanosis increases and is often relatively unresponsive to oxygen administration. Breath sounds may be normal or diminished, with a harsh tubular quality; and on deep inspiration, fine rales may be heard, especially over the lung bases posteriorly. The natural course is characterized by progressive worsening of cyanosis and dyspnea. If the condition is inadequately treated, blood pressure and body temperature may fall; fatigue, cyanosis, and pallor increase, and grunting decreases or disappears as the condition worsens. Apnea and irregular respirations occur as infants tire and are ominous signs requiring immediate intervention. Patients may also have a mixed respiratory-metabolic acidosis, edema, ileus, and oliguria. Signs of asphyxia secondary to apnea or partial respiratory failure occur when there is rapid progression of the disease. In most cases, the symptoms and signs may reach a peak within 3 days, after which improvement is gradual.

DIAGNOSIS. The clinical course, radiograph of the chest, and blood gas and acid-base values help to establish the clinical diagnosis. Radiographically, the lungs may have a characteristic but not pathognomonic appearance, which includes a fine reticular granularity of the parenchyma and air bronchograms that are often more prominent early in the left lower lobes.

PREVENTION. Most important is prevention of prematurity, including avoidance of unnecessary or poorly timed cesarean section, appropriate management of high-risk pregnancy and labor, and prediction and possible in utero acceleration of pulmonary immaturity. Administration of *dexamethasone* or *betamethasone* to women 48 hr before delivery of fetuses between 24 and 34 wk of gestation significantly reduces the incidence and the mortality and morbidity of HMD.

TREATMENT. Early supportive care of low-birth-weight infants, especially treatment of acidosis, hypoxia, hypotension, and hypothermia, appears to lessen the severity of HMD. Arterial catheterization is frequently necessary. Treatment of these infants is best carried out in a specially staffed and equipped hospital unit, the neonatal intensive care unit (NICU). To avoid chilling and to minimize oxygen consumption, infants should be placed in an Isolette and core temperature maintained between 36.5°C and 37°C. Calories and fluids should be provided intravenously. Warm humidified oxygen should be provided at a concentration sufficient initially to keep arterial levels between 55 and 70 mm Hg (>90% saturation). If the Pao_2 cannot be maintained above 50 mm Hg at inspired oxygen concentrations of 60% or greater, applying CPAP at a pressure of 6–10 cm H_2O by nasal prongs is indicated. If an infant on CPAP cannot maintain an arterial oxygen tension above 50 mm Hg while breathing 70–100% oxygen, assisted ventilation is required.

Multidose endotracheal instillation of *exogenous surfactant* to low-birth-weight infants requiring 30% oxygen and mechanical ventilation for the treatment (*rescue therapy*) of respiratory distress syndrome has dramatically improved survival and reduced the incidence of pulmonary air leaks but has not consistently reduced the incidence of chronic lung disease (CLD). Treatment (rescue) is initiated as soon as possible in the first 24 hr of life; therapy is given via the endotracheal tube every 6–12 hr for a total of 2–4 doses, depending on the preparation.

Metabolic acidosis in HMD may be a result of perinatal asphyxia and hypotension and is often encountered when an infant has required resuscitation. Sodium bicarbonate, 1–2 mEq/kg, may be administered for treatment over a 10- to 15-min period through a peripheral vein with the acid-base determination repeated within 30 min, or it may be administered over several hours. Periodic monitoring of Pao_2 and $Paco_2$ and of pH is an important part of the management; if assisted ventilation is being used, this monitoring is essential. Blood should be obtained from the umbilical or peripheral artery.

Because of the difficulty of distinguishing group B streptococcal or other infections from HMD, routinely administering antibacterial agents is indicated until the results of blood cultures are available.

COMPLICATIONS OF HMD AND INTENSIVE CARE. The most serious complications of *tracheal intubation* are asphyxia from obstruction of the tube, cardiac arrest during intubation or suctioning, and subsequent development of subglottic stenosis. The risks of *umbilical arterial catheterization* include vascular embolization, thrombosis, spasm, and perforation; ischemic or chemical necrosis of abdominal viscera; infection; accidental hemorrhage; and impaired circulation to a leg, with subsequent gangrene. *Extrapulmonary extravasation* of air is another frequent complication of the management of HMD. There may be clinically significant shunting through a patent ductus arteriosus in some neonates with HMD. Most infants respond to general supportive measures, including diuretics and fluid restriction. In patients in whom spontaneous closure does not occur and in whom there is progressive deterioration despite supportive and cardiotonic treatment, intravenous indomethacin, 0.2 mg/kg at 12- to 24-hr intervals for 3 doses, may induce pharmacologic closure.

CLD, previously called bronchopulmonary dysplasia, is a result of lung injury in infants requiring mechanical ventilation and supplemental oxygen. CLD is present if the neonate is oxygen dependent at 36 wk after conception. The occurrence of CLD is inversely related to gestational age. Instead of showing improvement on the 3rd–4th day, consistent with the natural course of respiratory distress syndrome, some infants radiographically show a worsening of their pulmonary condition. Respiratory distress persists and is characterized by hypoxia, hypercarbia, oxygen dependence, and, in severe cases, the development of right-sided heart failure. The chest radiograph is described as gradually changing from a picture of almost complete opacification with air bronchogram and interstitial emphysema to one of small, round, lucent areas alternating with areas of irregular density resembling a sponge. Most surviving neonates with persistent radiographic changes recover by 6–12 mo, but some require prolonged hospitalization and may have respiratory symptoms persisting through childhood (bronchospasm). Right-sided heart failure and viral necrotizing bronchiolitis are major causes of death in infancy.

The treatment of CLD includes nutritional support, fluid restriction, drug therapy, maintenance of adequate oxygenation, and prompt treatment of infection. Growth must be monitored because recovery is dependent on the growth of lung tissue and remodeling of the pulmonary vascular bed.

Patients with CLD often go home on oxygen, diuretics, and bronchodilator therapy. Prevention of sleep-associated hypoxia improves growth, as does a hypercaloric formula.

TRANSIENT TACHYPNEA OF THE NEWBORN

Transient tachypnea, occasionally called respiratory distress syndrome type II, usually follows uneventful normal preterm or term vaginal delivery or cesarean delivery. It may be characterized by the early onset of tachypnea, sometimes with retractions, or expiratory grunting and, occasionally, cyanosis that is relieved by minimal oxygen (<40%). Patients usually recover rapidly within 3 days, although they may rarely appear severely ill and have a more protracted course.

ASPIRATION OF FOREIGN MATERIAL (FETAL ASPIRATION SYNDROME: ASPIRATION PNEUMONIA)

During prolonged labors and difficult deliveries, infants often initiate vigorous respiratory movements in utero because of interference with the supply of oxygen through the placenta. Under such circumstances, the infant may aspirate amniotic fluid containing vernix caseosa, epithelial cells, meconium, or material from the birth canal, which may block the smallest airways and interfere with alveolar exchange of oxygen and carbon dioxide. Pulmonary aspiration may also occur in newborns because of tracheoesophageal fistula, esophageal and duodenal obstructions, gastroesophageal reflux, improper feeding practices, and administration of depressant medicines.

The contents of the stomach should be aspirated through a soft catheter just before operation or other procedures that require anesthesia or significantly disturb an infant. Once aspiration has occurred, treatment consists of general and respiratory support and treatment of pneumonia.

MECONIUM ASPIRATION

CLINICAL MANIFESTATIONS. Either in utero or more often with the first breath, thick, particulate meconium is aspirated into the lungs. The resulting small airway obstruction may produce respiratory distress within the first hours, with tachypnea, retraction, grunting, and cyanosis in severely affected infants. Partial obstruction of some airways may lead to pneumothorax or pneumomediastinum, or both. Overdistention of the chest may be prominent. The condition usually improves within 72 hr, but when its course requires assisted ventilation, it may be severe and its potential for mortality high. Tachypnea may persist for many days or even several weeks.

PREVENTION. The risk of meconium aspiration may be decreased by paying careful attention to fetal distress and initiating prompt delivery in the presence of fetal acidosis, late decelerations, or poor beat-to-beat variability.

TREATMENT. In the absence of fetal distress, a vigorous infant (Apgar score of 8 or more) can be born through thin meconium and may not require treatment. Depressed infants and possibly those delivered through thick particulate (pea soup) meconium-stained fluid (particularly those who did not undergo DeLee suctioning) should undergo endotracheal intubation, and suction should be applied directly to the endotracheal tube to remove meconium from the airway. Treatment of meconium aspiration pneumonia includes supportive care and standard management for respiratory distress.

PERSISTENT PULMONARY HYPERTENSION OF THE NEWBORN (PPHN)

PPHN occurs in term and post-term infants after birth asphyxia, meconium aspiration pneumonia, group B streptococcal sepsis, HMD, hypoglycemia, polycythemia, and pulmonary hypoplasia due to diaphragmatic hernia, amniotic fluid leak, oligohydramnios, or pleural effusions. It is often idiopathic.

CLINICAL MANIFESTATIONS. Infants become ill in the delivery room or within the first 12 hr of life. PPHN due to polycythemia, idiopathic causes, hypoglycemia, or asphyxia may result in severe cyanosis with tachypnea, although there may initially be minimal signs of respiratory distress. Infants who have PPHN associated with meconium aspiration, group B streptococcal pneumonia, diaphragmatic hernia, or pulmonary hypoplasia usually have cyanosis, grunting, flaring, retractions, tachycardia, and shock.

DIAGNOSIS. Hypoxia is universal and is unresponsive to 100% oxygen given by oxygen hood but may respond transiently to hyperoxic hyperventilation administered after endotracheal intubation or application of a bag and mask. Real-time echocardiography combined with Doppler flow studies demonstrates right-to-left shunting across a patent foramen ovale and a ductus arteriosus.

TREATMENT. Therapy is directed toward correcting any predisposing disease (hypoglycemia, polycythemia) and improving poor tissue oxygenation. Initial management includes oxygen administration and correction of acidosis, hypotension, and hypercarbia.

Persistent hypoxia should be managed with intubation and mechanical ventilation.

Exogenous surfactant therapy has been beneficial in some patients. Inhaled nitric oxide (iNO), a potent and selective pulmonary vasodilator (equivalent to endothelium-derived relaxation factor), when given in 10–20 ppm (occasionally 60–80 ppm), has improved oxygenation in patients with PPHN and reduced the need for extracorporeal membrane oxygenation (ECMO).

Extracorporeal Membrane Oxygenation. In 5–10% of patients with PPHN (approximately 1:4000 births) there is a poor response to 100% oxygen, mechanical ventilation, and drugs. ECMO has been used to treat carefully selected severely ill infants. ECMO is a form of cardiopulmonary bypass that augments systemic perfusion and provides gas exchange. Most experience has been with venoarterial bypass, which requires placement of large catheters in the right internal jugular vein and carotid artery and may necessitate carotid artery ligation.

EXTRAPULMONARY EXTRAVASATION OF AIR (PNEUMOTHORAX, PNEUMOMEDIASTINUM, AND PULMONARY INTERSTITIAL EMPHYSEMA)

Asymptomatic pneumothorax, usually unilateral, is estimated to occur in 1–2% of all newborns; symptomatic pneumothorax and pneumomediastinum are less common. Pneumothorax is more common in males than in females and in term and post-term infants than in premature ones. The incidence is increased among infants with lung disease, such as meconium aspiration and HMD; in those who have had vigorous resuscitation or are receiving assisted ventilation, especially if high inspiratory pressure or a continuous elevation of end-expiratory pressure is used; and in infants with urinary tract anomalies.

CLINICAL MANIFESTATIONS. The physical findings of *asymptomatic pneumothorax* are hyperresonance and diminished breath sounds over the involved side of the chest with or without tachypnea.

Symptomatic pneumothorax is characterized by respiratory distress, which varies from only an increased respiratory rate to severe dyspnea, tachypnea, and cyanosis. Irritability and restlessness or apnea may be the earliest signs. The onset is usually sudden but may be gradual; an infant may rapidly become critically ill. The chest may appear asymmetric with increased anteroposterior diameter and bulging of the intercostal spaces on the affected side, and there may be hyperresonance and diminished or absent breath sounds. The heart is displaced toward the unaffected side, and the diaphragm is displaced downward, as is the liver with right-sided pneumothorax. Because both sides are affected in approximately 10% of patients, symmetry of findings does not rule out pneumothorax. In tension pneumothorax there may be signs of shock, and the apex of the heart is pushed away from the affected side.

Pneumomediastinum occurs in at least 25% of patients with pneumothorax and is usually asymptomatic. The degree of respiratory distress depends on the amount of trapped air. If it is great, there is bulging of the midthoracic area, the neck veins are distended, and the blood pressure is low. Although few clinical signs may exist, subcutaneous emphysema in newborns is almost pathognomonic of pneumomediastinum.

Pulmonary interstitial emphysema (PIE) may precede the development of a pneumothorax or may occur independently, resulting in increasing respiratory distress due to decreased compliance, hypercarbia, and hypoxia. Progressive enlargement of blebs or air may result in cystic dilatations and respiratory deterioration resembling pneumothorax. Avoidance of high inspiratory or mean ventilatory pressures may prevent the development of PIE.

DIAGNOSIS. Pneumothorax and pneumomediastinum should be suspected in any newborn who shows signs of respiratory distress or who displays restlessness or irritability or has a sudden change in condition. The diagnosis is established radiographically.

Pneumopericardium may be asymptomatic, requiring only general supportive treatment, but usually presents as sudden shock with tachycardia, muffled heart sounds, and poor pulses suggesting tamponade, which requires prompt evacuation of entrapped air. Pneumoperitoneum from air dissecting through the diaphragmatic apertures during mechanical ventilation may also be confused with perforation of an abdominal organ.

TREATMENT. Without a continued air leak, asymptomatic and mildly symptomatic small pneumothoraces require only close observation. Frequent small feedings may prevent gastric dilatation and minimize crying, which can further compromise ventilation and worsen the pneumothorax. Breathing 100% oxygen accelerates the resorption of free pleural air into the blood. With severe respiratory or circulatory embarrassment, emergency needle aspiration is indicated. Either immediately or after needle aspiration, a chest tube should be inserted and attached to underwater-seal drainage. Severe localized interstitial emphysema may respond to selective bronchial intubation.

PULMONARY HEMORRHAGE

The cause of massive pulmonary hemorrhage is usually not identified; the incidence is increased in association with acute pulmonary infection, severe asphyxia, HMD, surfactant therapy, assisted ventilation, congenital heart disease, erythroblastosis fetalis, hemorrhagic disease of the newborn, kernicterus, inborn errors of ammonia metabolism, and cold injury. Treatment includes blood replacement, positive end-expiratory pressure, suctioning to clear the airway, and intratracheal administration of epinephrine.

CHAPTER 74

Digestive System Disorders

(Nelson Textbook, Chapter 98)

VOMITING. Infants may vomit mucus (occasionally blood streaked) in the first few hours after birth. This vomiting rarely persists after the first few feedings; it may be due to irritation of the gastric mucosa by material swallowed during delivery. If the vomiting is protracted, gastric lavage with physiologic saline solution may relieve it.

Bile-stained emesis suggests intestinal obstruction beyond the duodenum, but it may also be idiopathic. Abdominal radiographs (kidney-ureter-bladder [KUB] and cross-table lateral views) should be performed in neonates with persistent emesis and in all infants with bile-stained emesis to detect air-fluid levels, distended bowel loops, characteristic patterns of obstruction (double-bubble: duodenal atresia), and pneumoperitoneum (intestinal perforation). Vomiting from esophageal obstruction occurs with the first feeding. The diagnosis of esophageal atresia can be suspected if there is unusual drooling from the mouth and if resistance is encountered in an attempt to pass a catheter into the stomach.

Vomiting due to *obstruction of the small intestine* usually begins on the 1st day of life and is frequent, persistent, usually nonprojectile, copious, and, unless the obstruction is above the ampulla of Vater, bile-stained; it is associated with abdominal distention, visible deep peristaltic waves, and reduced or absent bowel movements. Malrotation with obstruction from midgut volvulus is an acute emergency that must be considered. Upright radiographic films of the abdomen show the distribution of air in the intestine and often aid in locating the site of the obstruction; malrotation may be identified by contrast studies.

MECONIUM PLUGS. Lower colonic or anorectal plugs with a lower than normal water content may cause intestinal obstruction. Meconium plugs are associated with small left colon syndrome in the infant of a diabetic mother, cystic fibrosis, rectal aganglionosis, maternal drug abuse, and magnesium sulfate therapy for preeclampsia. The plug may be evacuated by irrigating it with isotonic sodium chloride solution.

MECONIUM ILEUS IN CYSTIC FIBROSIS

In a newborn, impaction of meconium causes intestinal obstructions often associated with cystic fibrosis. Abdominal distention is prominent, and persistent vomiting soon occurs. Infrequently, one or more inspissated meconium stools may be passed shortly after birth. Treatment is by high Gastrografin enema. If treatment is unsuccessful or if there is reason to suspect a perforation of the bowel wall, laparotomy is performed.

MECONIUM PERITONITIS. Perforation of the intestine may occur in utero or shortly after birth.

Such perforations occur most often as a complication of meconium ileus in infants with cystic fibrosis, but the perforation occasionally is due to a meconium plug or intestinal obstruction of another cause. Treatment consists primarily of elimination of the intestinal obstruction and drainage of the peritoneal cavity.

NEONATAL NECROTIZING ENTEROCOLITIS

This serious disease of the newborn is of unknown cause and is characterized by various degrees of mucosal or transmural necrosis of the intestine.

CLINICAL MANIFESTATIONS. Onset usually occurs in the first 2 wk but can be as late as 3 mo of age in very-low-birth-weight infants. The first signs are abdominal distention with gastric retention. Manifestations usually develop after the onset of enteric feedings. Obvious bloody stools are seen in 25% of patients. The onset is often insidious, and sepsis may be suspected before an intestinal lesion is noted. There is a wide spectrum of illness from mild with only guaiac-positive stools to severe with peritonitis, bowel perforation, systemic inflammatory response syndrome, shock, and death. Progression may be rapid, but it is unusual for the disease to progress from mild to severe after 72 hr.

DIAGNOSIS. Plain abdominal radiographs may demonstrate pneumatosis intestinalis, a finding that is diagnostic of necrotizing enterocolitis in a newborn.

TREATMENT. Intensive therapy is advisable for suspected as well as diagnosed cases. Cessation of feeding, nasogastric decompression, and intravenous fluids with careful attention to respiratory status, coagulation profile, and acid-base and electrolyte balance are very important. Once blood cultures are taken, systemic antibiotics (usually ampicillin or an anti-*Pseudomonas* penicillin [e.g., ticarcillin] with an aminoglycoside [e.g., gentamicin]) should be started. If hypotension develops, resuscitation with crystalloid, blood, plasma, and dopamine is essential. A surgeon should be consulted early in the course of treatment. Evidence of perforation is usually an indication for resection of necrotic bowel.

JAUNDICE AND HYPERBILIRUBINEMIA IN THE NEWBORN

Hyperbilirubinemia is a common and in most cases benign problem in neonates. Nonetheless, untreated severe, indirect hyperbilirubinemia is potentially neurotoxic, and conjugated direct hyperbilirubinemia often signifies a serious illness.

The color usually results from accumulation in the skin of unconjugated, nonpolar, lipid-soluble bilirubin pigment (indirect-reacting) formed from hemoglobin. It may also be due in part to deposition of the pigment after it has been converted in the liver to the polar, water-soluble ester glucuronide of bilirubin (direct-reacting). The unconjugated form is neurotoxic for infants at certain concentrations and under various conditions.

CLINICAL MANIFESTATIONS. Jaundice may be present at birth or may appear at any time during the neonatal period, depending on the cause. Jaundice usually begins on the face and, as the serum level increases, progresses to the abdomen and then the feet. Jaundice to the midabdomen, signs or symptoms, high-risk factors that suggest nonphysiologic jaundice, or hemolysis must be evaluated further. Jaundice resulting from deposition of indirect bilirubin in the skin tends to appear bright yellow or orange; jaundice of the obstructive type (direct bilirubin) appears greenish or muddy yellow. This difference is usually apparent only in severe jaundice. Affected infants may be lethargic and may feed poorly. Signs of kernicterus rarely appear on the first day of jaundice.

DIFFERENTIAL DIAGNOSIS. Jaundice, consisting of indirect or direct bilirubin, that is present at birth or appears within the first 24 hr of life requires immediate attention and may be due to erythroblastosis fetalis, concealed hemorrhage, sepsis, cytomegalic inclusion disease, rubella, or congenital toxoplasmosis. Hemolysis is suggested by a rapid rise of serum bilirubin (>0.5 mg/dL/hr), anemia, pallor, reticulocytosis, hepatosplenomegaly, and a positive family history. Jaundice that first appears on the 2nd or 3rd day is usually "physiologic" but may represent a more severe form. Familial nonhemolytic icterus (Crigler-Najjar syndrome) and early-onset breast-feeding jaundice are seen initially on the 2nd or 3rd day. *Jaundice appearing after the 3rd day and within the 1st wk should suggest bacterial sepsis or urinary tract infections*; it may be due to other infections, notably syphilis, toxoplasmosis, cytomegalovirus, or enterovirus. Jaundice secondary to extensive ecchymosis or hematoma may occur during the 1st day or later, especially in premature infants. Polycythemia may lead to early jaundice.

Jaundice that is noted initially after the 1st wk of life suggests breast milk jaundice, septicemia, congenital atresia of the bile ducts, hepatitis, galactosemia, hypothyroidism, cystic fibrosis, paucity of bile ducts, congenital hemolytic anemia (spherocytosis), or possibly the crises of other hemolytic anemias (such as pyruvate kinase and other glycolytic enzyme deficiencies or hereditary nonspherocytic anemia), or hemolytic anemia due to drugs (as in congenital deficiencies of the enzymes glucose-6-

phosphate dehydrogenase, glutathione synthetase, reductase, or peroxidase).

Persistent jaundice during the 1st mo of life suggests the inspissated bile syndrome (which may follow hemolytic disease of the newborn), hyperalimentation-associated cholestasis, hepatitis, cytomegalic inclusion disease, syphilis, toxoplasmosis, familial nonhemolytic icterus, congenital atresia of the bile ducts, or galactosemia. Rarely, physiologic jaundice may be prolonged for several weeks, as in infants with hypothyroidism or pyloric stenosis.

Low-risk jaundiced infants who are full term and asymptomatic may be evaluated by monitoring serum total bilirubin levels. Regardless of the gestational age or time of appearance of jaundice, significant hyperbilirubinemia and all patients with symptoms or signs require a complete diagnostic evaluation, which should include determination of the direct and indirect bilirubin fractions, hemoglobin, reticulocyte count, blood type, Coombs test, and an examination of the peripheral blood smear.

PHYSIOLOGIC JAUNDICE (ICTERUS NEONATORUM). Under normal circumstances, the level of indirect-reacting bilirubin in umbilical cord serum is 1–3 mg/dL and rises at a rate of less than 5 mg/dL/ 24 hr; thus, jaundice becomes visible on the 2nd–3rd day, usually peaking between the 2nd and 4th days at 5–6 mg/dL and decreasing to below 2 mg/dL between the 5th and 7th days of life. Jaundice associated with these changes is designated "physiologic" and is believed to be the result of increased bilirubin production after breakdown of fetal red blood cells combined with transient limitation in the conjugation of bilirubin by the liver.

Overall, 6–7% of full-term infants have indirect bilirubin levels greater than 12.9 mg/dL and less than 3% have levels greater than 15 mg/dL. Risk factors for indirect hyperbilirubinemia include maternal diabetes, race (Chinese, Japanese, Korean, and Native American), prematurity, drugs (vitamin K_3, novobiocin), altitude, polycythemia, male sex, trisomy 21, cutaneous bruising, cephalohematoma, oxytocin induction, breast-feeding, weight loss (dehydration or caloric deprivation), delayed bowel movement, and a sibling who had physiologic jaundice. Infants without these variables rarely develop indirect bilirubin levels above 12 mg/dL, whereas infants with several risks are more likely to have higher bilirubin levels. Indirect bilirubin levels in full-term infants decline to adult levels (1 mg/dL) by 10–14 days of life.

The ability to predict which neonatal infants are at risk for exaggerated physiologic jaundice can be based on hour-specific bilirubin levels in the first 24–72 hr of life.

Among premature infants, the rise in serum bilirubin tends to be the same as or a little slower than that in term infants but is of longer duration, which generally results in higher levels, the peak being reached between the 4th and 7th days. Peak levels of

8–12 mg/dL usually are not reached until the 5th–7th day, and jaundice is infrequently observed after the 10th day.

The diagnosis of physiologic jaundice in term or preterm infants can be established only by precluding known causes of jaundice on the basis of the history and clinical and laboratory findings. In general, a search to determine the cause of jaundice should be made if (1) it appears in the first 24–36 hr of life; (2) serum bilirubin is rising at a rate greater than 5 mg/dL/24 hr; (3) serum bilirubin is greater than 12 mg/dL in full-term (especially in the absence of risk factors) or 10–14 mg/dL in preterm infants; (4) jaundice persists after 10–14 days of life; or (5) direct-reacting bilirubin is greater than 2 mg/dL at any time.

PATHOLOGIC HYPERBILIRUBINEMIA. Jaundice and its underlying hyperbilirubinemia are considered pathologic if their time of appearance, duration, or pattern of serially determined serum bilirubin concentrations varies significantly from that of physiologic jaundice; or if the course is compatible with physiologic jaundice but other reasons exist to suspect that the infant is at special risk from the neurotoxicity of unconjugated bilirubin. The risk of hyperbilirubinemia is related to the development of kernicterus (bilirubin encephalopathy) at high indirect serum bilirubin levels.

JAUNDICE ASSOCIATED WITH BREAST-FEEDING. An estimated 2% of breast-fed term infants develop significant elevations in unconjugated bilirubin (breast milk jaundice) after the 7th day of life, reaching maximum concentrations as high as 10–30 mg/dL during the 2nd–3rd wk. If breast-feeding is continued, the hyperbilirubinemia gradually decreases and then may persist for 3–10 wk at lower levels. If nursing is discontinued, the serum bilirubin level falls rapidly, usually reaching normal levels within a few days. Cessation of breast-feeding for 1–2 days and substitution of formula for breast milk results in a rapid decline in serum bilirubin, after which nursing can be resumed without a return of the hyperbilirubinemia to its previously high levels. If indicated, phototherapy may be of benefit. These infants have no other sign of illness; nonetheless, kernicterus has been reported.

This syndrome should be distinguished from an early-onset accentuated unconjugated hyperbilirubinemia (breast-feeding jaundice) in the 1st wk of life, when breast-fed infants have higher bilirubin levels than formula-fed infants. This observation may be due to decreased milk intake with dehydration or reduced caloric intake.

KERNICTERUS

Kernicterus is a neurologic syndrome resulting from the deposition of unconjugated bilirubin in brain cells. The precise blood level above which indirect-reacting bilirubin or free bilirubin will be toxic for an individual infant is unpredictable, but kernicterus is rare in healthy term infants and in the absence of hemolysis if the serum level is under 25 mg/dL. The duration of exposure necessary to produce toxic effects is also unknown.

CLINICAL MANIFESTATIONS. Signs and symptoms of kernicterus usually appear 2–5 days after birth in term infants and as late as the 7th day in premature ones, but hyperbilirubinemia may lead to the syndrome at any time during the neonatal period. The early signs may be subtle and indistinguishable from those of sepsis, asphyxia, hypoglycemia, intracranial hemorrhage, and other acute systemic illnesses in a neonatal infant. Lethargy, poor feeding, and loss of the Moro reflex are common initial signs. Subsequently, the infant may appear gravely ill and prostrated, with diminished tendon reflexes and respiratory distress. Opisthotonos, with a bulging fontanel, twitching of face or limbs, and a shrill high-pitched cry may follow. In advanced cases, convulsions and spasm occur, with the infant stiffly extending his or her arms in inward rotation with fists clenched. Rigidity is rare at this late stage.

Many infants who progress to these severe neurologic signs die; the survivors are usually seriously damaged but may appear to recover and for 2–3 mo show few abnormalities. Later in the 1st yr of life, opisthotonos, muscle rigidity, irregular movements, and convulsions tend to recur. In the 2nd yr, opisthotonos and seizures abate but irregular, involuntary movements, muscle rigidity, or, in some infants, hypotonia increases steadily. By age 3 yr, the complete neurologic syndrome is often apparent, consisting of bilateral choreoathetosis with involuntary muscle spasm, extrapyramidal signs, seizures, mental deficiency, dysarthric speech, high-frequency hearing loss, squinting, and defective upward movement of the eyes. In mildly affected infants, the syndrome may be characterized only by mild to moderate neuromuscular incoordination, partial deafness, or "minimal brain dysfunction," occurring singly or in combination; these problems may be inapparent until the child enters school.

TREATMENT OF HYPERBILIRUBINEMIA. Regardless of cause, the goal of therapy is to prevent the concentration of indirect-reacting bilirubin in the blood from reaching levels at which neurotoxicity may occur; it is recommended that phototherapy and, if unsuccessful, exchange transfusion be used to keep the maximum total serum bilirubin below the levels indicated in Tables 74–1 (for preterm) and 74–2 (for healthy term infants without hemolysis). When identified, the underlying cause of the icterus should be treated (e.g., antibiotics for septicemia). Physiologic factors that increase the risk of neurologic damage should also be treated (e.g., correction of acidosis).

Phototherapy. Clinical jaundice and indirect hyperbilirubinemia are reduced on exposure to a high intensity of light in the visible spectrum. Bilirubin absorbs light maximally in the blue range

TABLE 74–1 Suggested Maximum Indirect Serum Bilirubin Concentrations (mg/dL) in Preterm Infants

Birth Weight (g)	Uncomplicated	Complicated*
<1000	12–13	10–12
1000–1250	12–14	10–12
1251–1499	14–16	12–14
1500–1999	16–20	15–17
2000–2500	20–22	18–20

*Complications include perinatal asphyxia, acidosis, hypoxia, hypothermia, hypoalbuminemia, meningitis, intraventricular hemorrhage, hemolysis, hypoglycemia, or signs of kernicterus.

Phototherapy is usually started at 50–70% of the maximum indirect level. If values greatly exceed this level, if phototherapy is unsuccessful in reducing the maximum bilirubin level, or if there are signs of kernicterus, exchange transfusion is indicated.

TABLE 74–2 Approach to Indirect Hyperbilirubinemia in Healthy Term Infants without Hemolysis*

	Treatment Strategies		
Age (hr)	Phototherapy	Intensive Phototherapy and Preparation for Exchange Transfusion †	Exchange Transfusion if Phototherapy Fails ‡
<24	§	§	§
24–48‖	≥15–18	≥25	≥20
49–72	≥18–20	≥30	≥25
>72	≥20	≥30	≥25
>2 wk	¶	¶	¶

*With hemolysis, exchange transfusion is initiated with an indirect bilirubin value of ≥20, at any age.

The precise level of unconjugated bilirubin among healthy breast-fed term infants who require therapy is unknown. Treatment options include continued breast-feeding and initiation of phototherapy, or interrupted breast-feeding (use formula as substitute) with or without phototherapy.

If there are any signs of kernicterus during the evaluation or treatment as suggested anywhere in the table or at any level of bilirubin, an emergent exchange transfusion must be performed.

†If the initial bilirubin on presentation is high, intense phototherapy should be initiated and preparation made for exchange transfusion. If the phototherapy fails to reduce the bilirubin level to the levels noted on the column to the right, initiate exchange transfusion.

‡Intensive phototherapy should be initiated for bilirubin levels in this column and usually reduces serum bilirubin levels 1–2 mg/dL in 4–6 hr; this is often associated with administration of intravenous fluids at 1–1.5 times maintenance; oral alimentation should also continue.

§Jaundice in the 1st 24 hr of life is not seen in "healthy" infants.

‖Hyperbilirubinemia of this degree within 48 hr of birth is unusual and should suggest hemolysis, concealed hemorrhage, or causes of conjugated (direct) hyperbilirubinemia.

¶Jaundice suddenly appearing in the 2nd wk of life or continuing beyond the 2nd wk of life with significant hyperbilirubinemia levels to warrant therapy should be investigated in detail, because it most probably is due to a serious underlying cause such as biliary atresia, galactosemia, hypothyroidism, or neonatal hepatitis.

(from 420–470 nm). The use of phototherapy has decreased the need for exchange transfusion in term and preterm infants with hemolytic and nonhemolytic jaundice. Phototherapy may be initiated at the bilirubin levels noted in Tables 74–1 and 74–2.

Complications of phototherapy include loose stools, erythematous macular rashes, a purpuric rash associated with transient porphyrinemia, overheating and dehydration (increased insensible water loss, diarrhea), chilling from exposure of the infant, and bronze baby syndrome. Phototherapy is contraindicated in the presence of porphyria. The term *bronze baby syndrome* refers to a dark grayish-brown discoloration of the skin sometimes noted in infants undergoing phototherapy.

Exchange Transfusion. This widely accepted treatment should be repeated as frequently as necessary to keep indirect bilirubin levels in the serum under those noted in Tables 74–1 and 74–2. Appearance of clinical signs suggesting kernicterus is an indication for exchange transfusion at any level of serum bilirubin.

CHAPTER 75

Blood Disorders

(Nelson Textbook, Chapter 99)

ANEMIA IN THE NEWBORN

Hemoglobin increases with advancing gestational age: at term, cord blood hemoglobin is 16.8 g/dL (14–20 g/dL); hemoglobin levels in very-low-birth-weight (VLBW) infants are 1–2 g/dL below those at term. Determinations of less than the normal range for birth weight and postnatal age are defined as anemia. A "physiologic" decrease in hemoglobin content is noticed at 8–12 wk in term infants (hemoglobin 11 g/dL) and at about 6 wk in premature infants (7–10 g/dL).

Anemia at birth is manifested by pallor, heart failure, or shock. It may be due to acute or chronic blood loss, hemolysis, or underproduction of erythrocytes. It is usually caused by hemolytic disease of the newborn but may also be a result of tearing or cutting of the umbilical cord during delivery, abnormal cord insertions, communicating placental vessels, placenta previa or abruptio, nuchal cord, incision into the placenta, internal hemorrhage (liver, spleen, or intracranial), α-thalassemia, congenital parvovirus infection or hypoplastic anemias, and twin-twin transfusion in monozygotic twins with arteriovenous placental connections.

Anemia appearing in the first few days after birth is also most frequently a result of hemolytic disease of the newborn. Other causes are hemorrhagic disease of the newborn, bleeding from an improperly tied or clamped umbilical cord, large cephalohematoma, intracranial hemorrhage, or subcapsular bleeding from rupture of the liver, spleen, adrenals, or kidneys. Rapid decreases in hemoglobin or hematocrit values during the first few days of life may be the initial clue to these conditions.

Later in the neonatal period, delayed anemia from hemolytic disease of the newborn, with or without exchange transfusion or phototherapy, may be seen.

Anemia of prematurity occurs in low-birth-weight (LBW) infants 1–3 mo after birth, is associated with hemoglobin levels below 7–10 g/dL, and presents as pallor, apnea, poor weight gain, decreased activity, tachypnea, tachycardia, and feeding problems. Repeated phlebotomy for blood tests, shortened red blood cell (RBC) survival, rapid growth, and the physiologic effects of the transition from fetal (low Pao_2 and hemoglobin saturation) to neonatal life (high Pao_2 and hemoglobin saturation) contribute to anemia of prematurity.

Treatment of neonatal anemia by blood transfusion depends on the severity of symptoms, the hemoglobin level, and the presence of co-morbid diseases (chronic lung disease, cyanotic congenital heart disease, hyaline membrane disease) that interfere with oxygen delivery. Treatment with blood should be balanced by concern about transfusion-acquired infection.

HEMOLYTIC DISEASE OF THE NEWBORN (ERYTHROBLASTOSIS FETALIS)

Erythroblastosis fetalis results from transplacental passage of maternal antibody active against RBC antigens of the infant, leading to an increased rate of RBC destruction. Significant disease is associated primarily with the D antigen of the Rh group and with incompatibility of ABO factors.

HEMOLYTIC DISEASE OF THE NEWBORN DUE TO RH INCOMPATIBILITY

CLINICAL MANIFESTATIONS. A wide spectrum of hemolytic disease occurs in affected infants born to sensitized mothers, depending on the nature of the individual immune response. The severity of the disease may range from only laboratory evidence of mild hemolysis (15% of cases) to severe anemia with compensatory hyperplasia of erythropoietic tissue, leading to massive enlargement of the liver and spleen. When the compensatory capacity of the hematopoietic system is exceeded, profound anemia results in pallor, signs of cardiac decompensation (cardiomegaly, respiratory distress), massive anasarca, and circulatory collapse. This clinical picture of excessive abnormal fluid in two or more fetal compartments (skin, pleura, pericardium, placenta, peritoneum, amniotic fluid), termed *hydrops fetalis,* frequently results in death in utero or shortly after birth. The severity of hydrops is related to the level of anemia and the degree of reduction in serum albumin (oncotic pressure), which is due in part to hepatic dysfunction. Alternatively, heart failure may increase right-sided heart pressures, with the development of edema and ascites.

Jaundice may be absent at birth because of placental clearance of lipid-soluble unconjugated bilirubin, but in severe cases bilirubin pigments stain the amniotic fluid, cord, and vernix caseosa yellow. Icterus is generally evident on the 1st day of life because the infant's bilirubin-conjugating and excretory systems are unable to cope with the load resulting from massive hemolysis. Indirect-reacting bilirubin therefore accumulates postnatally and may rapidly reach extremely high levels, which represent a significant risk of bilirubin encephalopathy.

Infants born after intrauterine transfusion for prenatally diagnosed erythroblastosis may be severely affected, because the indications for the transfusion are evidence of already severe disease in utero (e.g., hydrops, fetal anemia). Such infants usually have very high (but extremely variable) cord levels of bilirubin.

LABORATORY DATA. Before treatment, the direct Coombs test result is usually positive. Anemia is usual. The blood smear usually shows polychromasia and a marked increase in nucleated RBCs. The reticulocyte count is increased. The cord bilirubin is usually between 3 and 5 mg/dL (51–86 μmol/L); there may be a substantial elevation of direct-reacting (conjugated) bilirubin. The indirect-reacting bilirubin rises rapidly to high levels in the first 6 hr of life.

DIAGNOSIS. The definitive diagnosis of erythroblastosis fetalis requires demonstration of blood group incompatibility and of corresponding antibody bound to the infant's RBCs.

Antenatal Diagnosis. In Rh-negative women, a history of previous transfusions, abortion, or pregnancy should suggest the possibility of sensitization. Expectant parents' blood types should be tested for potential incompatibility, and the maternal titer of IgG antibodies to D should be assayed at 12–16, 28–32, and 36 wk.

Assessment of the fetus may require information obtained from ultrasonography, amniocentesis, and percutaneous umbilical cord blood sampling. Hemolysis of fetal RBCs produces hyperbilirubinemia before the onset of severe anemia. Bilirubin is cleared by the placenta, but a significant proportion enters the amniotic fluid and can be measured by spectrophotometry.

Postnatal Diagnosis. Immediately after the birth of any infant to an Rh-negative woman, blood from the umbilical cord or from the infant should be examined for ABO blood group, Rh type, hematocrit and hemoglobin, and reaction of the direct Coombs test. If the Coombs test result is positive, baseline serum bilirubin level should be measured, and a commercially available RBC panel should be used to identify RBC antibodies that are present in the mother's serum, both tests being done not only to establish the diagnosis but also to ensure the selection of the most compatible blood for exchange transfusion should it be necessary.

TREATMENT. The main goals of therapy are (1) to prevent intrauterine or extrauterine death from severe anemia and hypoxia and (2) to avoid neurotoxicity from hyperbilirubinemia.

Treatment of the Unborn Infant. Survival of a severely affected fetus has been improved by the use of ultrasonographic and amniotic fluid analysis to identify the need for in utero transfusion. Intrauterine transfusion into the fetal peritoneal cavity is being replaced by direct intravascular transfusion of packed RBCs. Hydrops or fetal anemia (hematocrit <30%) is an indication for umbilical vein transfusion in infants with pulmonary immaturity.

Treatment of the Liveborn Infant. The birth should be attended by the physician who will care for the affected infant afterward. Fresh, low-titer, group O, Rh-negative blood, cross-matched against the maternal serum, should be immediately available. If clinical signs of severe hemolytic anemia (pallor, hepatosplenomegaly, edema, petechiae, or ascites) are evident at birth, immediate resuscitation and supportive therapy, temperature stabilization, and monitoring before proceeding with exchange transfusion may save some severely affected infants.

Exchange Transfusion. When an infant's clinical condition at birth does not require an immediate full or partial exchange transfusion, the decision to perform one should be based on a judgment that there is a high risk of rapid development of a dangerous degree of anemia or of hyperbilirubinemia. The hemoglobin, hematocrit, and serum bilirubin levels should be measured at 4- to 6-hr intervals at first, with extension to longer intervals if and as the rate of change diminishes. The decision to perform an exchange transfusion is based on the likelihood that the trend of bilirubin levels plotted against hours of age indicates that the serum bilirubin will reach the level indicated in Table 74–1 and in term infants with levels greater than 20 mg/dL, above which there is an increased risk of kernicterus. Careful monitoring of the serum bilirubin level is essential until a falling trend has been demonstrated in the absence of phototherapy.

Late Complications. Infants who have hemolytic disease or who have had an exchange or an intrauterine transfusion must be observed carefully for the development of anemia and cholestasis. Treatment with supplemental iron, erythropoietin, or blood transfusion may be indicated.

Prevention of Rh Sensitization. The risk of initial sensitization of Rh-negative mothers has been reduced from between 10% and 20% to less than 1% by intramuscular injection of 300 µg of human anti-D globulin (1 mL of RhoGAM) within 72 hr of delivery of an ectopic pregnancy, abdominal trauma in pregnancy, amniocentesis, chorionic villus biopsy, or abortion.

HEMOLYTIC DISEASE OF THE NEWBORN DUE TO A AND B INCOMPATIBILITY

Major blood group incompatibility between mother and fetus usually results in milder disease than does Rh incompatibility.

CLINICAL MANIFESTATIONS. The infant is not generally affected at birth; pallor is not present, and hydrops fetalis is extremely rare. The liver and spleen are not greatly enlarged, if at all. Jaundice usually appears during the first 24 hr. Rarely, it may become severe, and symptoms and signs of kernicterus develop rapidly.

DIAGNOSIS. A presumptive diagnosis is based on the presence of ABO incompatibility, a weakly to moderately positive direct Coombs test result, and spherocytes in the blood smear, which may at times suggest the presence of hereditary spherocytosis.

TREATMENT. Phototherapy may be effective in lowering serum bilirubin levels. Otherwise, treatment is directed at correcting dangerous degrees of anemia or hyperbilirubinemia by exchange transfusions with type O blood of the same Rh type as the infant. The indications for this procedure are similar to those previously described for hemolytic disease due to Rh incompatibility.

PLETHORA IN THE NEWBORN (POLYCYTHEMIA)

Plethora, a ruddy, deep red-purple appearance associated with a high hematocrit, is often due to polycythemia, defined as a central hematocrit of 65% or higher. Clinical manifestations include anorexia, lethargy, tachypnea, respiratory distress, feeding disturbances, hyperbilirubinemia, hypoglycemia, and thrombocytopenia. Severe complications include seizures, pulmonary hypertension, necrotizing enterocolitis, and renal failure. Many affected infants are asymptomatic. The treatment of symptomatic plethora of newborns is phlebotomy and replacement with saline or, less often, albumin. A partial exchange transfusion to reduce the hematocrit to 50% is a technically simpler and therapeutically more effective approach.

HEMORRHAGE IN THE NEWBORN

HEMORRHAGIC DISEASE OF THE NEWBORN. A moderate decrease of factors II, VII, IX, and X normally occurs in all newborns by 48–72 hr after birth, with a gradual return to birth levels by 7–10 days of age. This transient deficiency of vitamin K-dependent factors probably is due to lack of free vitamin K in the mother and absence in the infant of bacterial intestinal flora normally responsible for synthesis of vitamin K. Rarely, among term infants and more frequently among premature infants there is an accentuation and prolongation of this deficiency between the 2nd and 7th days of life, resulting in spontaneous and prolonged bleeding.

Hemorrhagic disease of the newborn resulting from severe transient deficiencies of vitamin K–dependent factors is characterized by bleeding that tends to be gastrointestinal, nasal, subgaleal, intracranial, or a result of circumcision. Mild bleeding may occur before serious intracranial hemorrhage. The prothrombin time, blood coagulation time, and partial thromboplastin time are prolonged, and the levels of prothrombin and factors VII, IX, and X are significantly decreased.

Administering 1 mg of natural oil-soluble vitamin K intramuscularly (phylloquinone) at the time of birth prevents the fall in vitamin K–dependent factors in full-term infants but is not uniformly effective in the prophylaxis of hemorrhagic disease of the newborn in premature infants. The disease may be effectively treated with a slow intravenous infusion of 1–5 mg of vitamin K, with improvement of coagulation defects and cessation of bleeding within a few hours. However, serious bleeding, particularly in premature infants or those with liver disease, may require a transfusion of fresh frozen plasma or whole blood.

CHAPTER 76

The Umbilicus
(Nelson Textbook, Chapter 101)

UMBILICAL CORD. The cord contains the two umbilical arteries, the vein, the rudimentary allantois, the remnant of the omphalomesenteric duct, and a gelatinous substance called Wharton jelly. When the cord sloughs after birth, portions of these structures remain in the base. The blood vessels are functionally closed but are patent anatomically for 10–20 days. The umbilical cord usually sloughs within 2 wk. *Delayed separation of the cord*, after more than 1 mo, has been associated with neutrophil chemotactic defects and overwhelming bacterial infection. Approximately one third of infants with a single umbilical artery have congenital abnormalities.

CONGENITAL OMPHALOCELE. An omphalocele is a herniation or protrusion of abdominal contents into the base of the umbilical cord. In contrast to the more common umbilical hernia, the sac is covered with peritoneum without overlying skin. Immediate surgical repair, before infection has taken place and before the tissues have been damaged by drying (saline-soaked sterile dressings should be applied immediately) or by rupture of the sac, is essential for survival.

HEMORRHAGE. Hemorrhage from the umbilical cord may be due to trauma, inadequate ligation of the cord, or failure of normal thrombus formation. It may also indicate hemorrhagic disease of the newborn or other coagulopathies, septicemia, or local infection. The infant should be observed frequently during the first few days of life so that if hemorrhage does occur, it will be detected promptly.

INFECTIONS. Inflammation in the umbilical region, which may be caused by any of the pyogenic bacteria, is especially serious because of the danger of hematogenous spread or extension to the liver or peritoneum. Daily baths or daily application of triple dye to the umbilical stump and surrounding skin may reduce the incidence of umbilical infection. *Treatment* includes prompt antibacterial therapy and, if there is abscess formation, surgical incision and drainage.

UMBILICAL HERNIA. Often associated with diastasis recti, umbilical hernia is due to an imperfect closure or weakness of the umbilical ring. Common especially in low-birth-weight, female, and black infants, it appears as a soft swelling covered by skin that protrudes during crying, coughing, or straining and can be reduced easily through the fibrous ring at the umbilicus. The hernia consists of omentum or portions of the small intestine. The size of the defect varies from less than 1 cm in diameter to as much as 5 cm, but large ones are rare. Most umbilical hernias that appear before the age of 6 mo disappear spontaneously by 1 yr of age. Even large hernias (5–6 cm in all dimensions) have been known to disappear spontaneously by 5–6 yr of age. Surgery is not advised unless the hernia persists to the age of 3–4 yr, causes symptoms, becomes strangulated, or becomes progressively larger after the age of 1–2 yr.

CHAPTER 77

Metabolic Disturbances

(Nelson Textbook, Chapter 102)

HYPERTHERMIA IN THE NEWBORN (TRANSITORY FEVER OF THE NEWBORN; DEHYDRATION FEVER)

Elevations of temperature (38–39°C or 100–103°F) are occasionally noted on the 2nd–3rd day of life in infants whose clinical course has been otherwise satisfactory. This disturbance is especially likely to occur in breast-fed infants whose intake of fluid has been particularly low or in infants exposed to high environmental temperatures, either in an incubator or in a bassinet near a radiator or in the sun. The apparent vigor of the infant contrasts to the usual appearance of "being sick" in the presence of infection.

Administering oral or parenteral fluids or lowering the environmental temperature leads to prompt reduction of the fever and alleviation of symptoms.

NEONATAL COLD INJURY

Neonatal cold injury usually occurs among infants in inadequately heated homes during damp cold spells when the outside temperature is in the freezing range. The presenting features are apathy, refusal of food, oliguria, and coldness to touch. The body temperature is usually between 29.5°C and 35°C (85–95°F), and immobility, edema, and redness of the extremities, especially of the hands, feet, and face, are observed. Bradycardia and apnea may also occur. The facial erythema frequently gives a false impression of health, delaying recognition that the infant is ill. Local hardening over areas of edema may lead to confusion with scleredema. Rhinitis is common, as are serious metabolic disturbances, particularly hypoglycemia and acidosis. Hemorrhagic manifestations are frequent; massive pulmonary hemorrhage is a common finding at autopsy. Treatment consists of warming and paying scrupulous attention to recognizing and correcting hypotension and metabolic imbalances, particularly hypoglycemia. Prevention consists of providing adequate environmental heat.

SUBSTANCE ABUSE AND WITHDRAWALS

Physiologic addiction to narcotics or toxic effects occur in most infants born to actively addicted mothers, because opiates cross the placenta. Withdrawal may be manifested even before birth by increased activity of the fetus when the mother feels the need for the drug or develops withdrawal symptoms. Pregnancy in women who use illegal drugs or alcohol is, by definition, a high risk.

Heroin addiction results in a 50% incidence of low-birth-weight infants, half of whom are small for gestational age. Clinical manifestations of withdrawal occur in 50–75% of infants, usually beginning within the first 48 hr, depending on the daily maternal dose (<6 mg/24 hr is associated with no or mild symptoms); duration of addiction (>1 yr has a >70% incidence of withdrawal); and time of last maternal dose (there is a higher incidence if the last dose was taken within 24 hr of birth). Symptoms rarely appear as late as 4–6 wk of age. Tremors and hyperirritability are the most prominent symptoms. The tremors may be fine or jittery and indistinguishable from those of hypoglycemia but are more often coarse, "flapping," and bilateral; the limbs are often rigid, hyperreflexic, and resistant to flexion and extension. Irritability and hyperactivity are generally marked and may lead to skin abrasions. Other signs include wakefulness, hyperacusis, hypertonicity, tachypnea, diarrhea, vomiting, high-pitched cry, fist sucking, poor feeding (disorganized sucking), and fever.

Methadone addiction is associated with severe withdrawal symptoms, the incidence varying from 20–90%. The average birth weight of infants of mothers taking methadone is higher than that of infants of heroin-addicted mothers; the clinical manifestations are similar except that the former group has a higher incidence of seizures (10–20%) and of late onset (2–6 wk of age) of symptoms and signs.

Cocaine abuse among pregnant women is common, but withdrawal in their infants is unusual; pregnancy may be complicated by premature labor, abruptio placentae, and fetal asphyxia. Infants may have intrauterine growth retardation, microcephaly, intracranial hemorrhage, possible anomalies of the gastrointestinal and renal tracts, sudden infant death syndrome (SIDS), and neurobehavioral deficits characterized by rigidity, impaired state regulation, developmental delay, and learning disabilities. Family disorganization, child abuse, neglect, and the acquired immunodeficiency syndrome are common in these families.

Treatment of heroin and methadone withdrawals has been successful using various combinations of narcotics, sedatives, and hypnotics. Therapy is indicated for seizures, for diarrhea, or for such irritability that normal sleep and feeding patterns are disturbed and weight gain is poor. Phenobarbital, 5–10 mg/kg/24 hr in 3–4 divided doses, can effectively reduce irritability and prevent seizures. Paregoric at a beginning dose of 0.05–0.1 mL/kg is given every 3–4 hr and increased by 0.05 mL every 4 hr if necessary, depending on the size and response of the infant.

FETAL ALCOHOL SYNDROME. High levels of alcohol ingestion during pregnancy can be damaging to embryonic and fetal development. A specific pattern of malformation identified as the fetal alcohol syndrome has been documented. The characteristics of the fetal alcohol syndrome include (1) prenatal onset and persistence of growth deficiency for length, weight, and head circumference; (2) facial abnormalities, including short palpebral fissures, epicanthal folds, maxillary hypoplasia, micrognathia, and thin upper lip; (3) cardiac defects, primarily septal defects; (4) minor joint and limb abnormalities, including some restriction of movement and altered palmar crease patterns; and (5) delayed development and mental deficiency varying from borderline to severe. Fetal alcohol syndrome is a common cause of mental retardation. No specific therapy exists.

CHAPTER 78

The Endocrine System
(Nelson Textbook, Chapter 103)

Primary hypothyroidism occurs in approximately 1/4000 births. Because most of these infants are asymptomatic at birth, all states screen for this serious and treatable disease. Thyroid deficiency may also be apparent at birth in genetically determined *cretinism* or in infants of mothers treated with thiouracil or its derivatives during pregnancy. Constipation, prolonged jaundice, goiter, lethargy, or poor peripheral circulation as shown by persistently mottled skin or cold extremities should suggest cretinism. Early diagnosis and treatment of congenital deficiency of thyroid hormone improves intellectual outcome and is facilitated by screening all newborns for this deficiency.

Temporary *hyperthyroidism* may occur at birth in the infants of mothers with hyperthyroidism or of those who have been receiving thyroid medication.

Transient *hypoparathyroidism* may be manifested as tetany of the newborn.

Adrenocortical hyperplasia is suggested by vomiting, diarrhea, dehydration, hyperkalemia, hyponatremia, shock, or clitoral enlargement. Because the condition is genetically determined, newborn siblings of patients with the salt-losing variety of adrenocortical hyperplasia should be closely observed for manifestations of adrenal insufficiency. Screening is also possible for this disorder.

INFANTS OF DIABETIC MOTHERS

Control of diabetes mellitus with insulin has led to improved outcome for diabetic women who bear children. Fetal loss throughout pregnancy is associated with poorly controlled maternal diabetes (especially ketoacidosis). The neonatal mortality rate is over five times that of infants of nondiabetic mothers and is higher at all gestational ages and in every birth weight for gestational age category.

CLINICAL MANIFESTATIONS. The infants of diabetic and gestational diabetic mothers often bear a surprising resemblance to each other. They tend to be large and plump as a result of increased body fat and enlarged viscera, with puffy, plethoric fades resembling those of patients who have been receiving a corticosteroid. These infants may, however, also be of normal or low birth weight, particularly if they are delivered before term or if there is associated maternal vascular disease. The infants tend to be jumpy, tremulous, and hyperexcitable during the first 3 days of life, although hypotonia, lethargy, and poor sucking also may occur. They may have any of the diverse manifestations of hypoglycemia. Early appearance of these signs is more likely to be related to hypoglycemia, and later appearance is related to hypocalcemia; these abnormalities also may occur together.

Twenty-five to 50 percent of infants of diabetic mothers and 15–25% of infants of mothers with gestational diabetes develop hypoglycemia, but only a small percentage of these infants become symptomatic. The probability of an infant's developing hypoglycemia increases and the glucose levels are likely to be lower at higher cord or maternal fasting blood glucose levels. The nadir in an infant's blood glucose concentration is usually reached between 1 and 3 hr; spontaneous recovery may begin by 4–6 hr.

Many infants of diabetic mothers develop tachypnea during the first 5 days of life, which may be a transient manifestation of hypoglycemia, hypothermia, polycythemia, cardiac failure, transient tachypnea, or cerebral edema due to birth trauma or asphyxia. A greater incidence of respiratory distress syndrome appears in infants of diabetic mothers than in infants of normal mothers born at comparable gestational age.

Cardiomegaly is common (30%), and heart failure occurs in 5–10% of infants of diabetic mothers. Asymmetric septal hypertrophy may occur. Birth trauma is also common, owing to fetal macrosomia. There is also an increased incidence of hyperbilirubinemia, polycythemia, and renal vein thrombosis; the latter should be suspected in the presence of a flank mass, hematuria, and thrombocytopenia. The incidence of congenital anomalies is increased threefold in infants of diabetic mothers. These infants may also develop abdominal distention caused by a transient delay in the development of the left side of the colon, the *small left colon syndrome.*

TREATMENT. Treatment of these infants should be initiated before birth by frequent prenatal evaluation of all pregnant women with overt or gestational diabetes, by evaluation of fetal maturity, by biophysical profile, by Doppler velocimetry, and by planning delivery of these infants in hospitals where expert obstetric and pediatric care is continuously available. Periconception glucose control reduces the risk of anomalies, and glucose control during labor reduces the incidence of neonatal hypoglycemia. Regardless of size, all infants of diabetic mothers should initially receive intensive observation and care. Asymptomatic infants should have a blood glucose determination within 1 hr of birth and then every hour for the next 6–8 hr; if the infant is clinically well and normoglycemic, oral or gavage feedings with breast milk or formula should be started as soon as possible and continued at 3-hr intervals. If any question arises about an infant's ability to tolerate oral feeding, the feeding should be discontinued and glucose given by peripheral intravenous infusion at a rate of 4–8 mg/kg/min. Hypoglycemia should be treated, even in asymptomatic infants, with intravenous infusions of glucose sufficient to keep the blood levels well above this level.

HYPOGLYCEMIA

Hypoglycemia is present when serum glucose levels are significantly lower than the range among postnatal age-matched normal infants. Although hypoglycemia may also be defined as the presence of neurologic (lethargy, coma, apnea, seizures) or sympathomimetic (pallor, palpitations, diaphoresis) manifestations that respond to glucose, many neonates with low serum glucose levels are asymptomatic, whereas normoglycemic infants may have nonspecific signs of hypoglycemia.

Early feeding decreases the incidence, whereas prematurity, hypothermia, hypoxia, maternal diabetes, maternal glucose infusion in labor, and intrauterine growth retardation increase the incidence of hypoglycemia. Serum glucose levels decline after birth until 1–3 hr of age, when levels spontaneously increase in normal infants. In healthy term infants, serum glucose values are rarely less than 35 mg/dL (1.9 mmol/L) between 1 and 3 hr of life, less than 40 mg/dL (2.2 mmol/L) from 3–24 hr, and less than 45 mg/dL (2.5 mmol/L) after 24 hr.

Both premature and full-term infants are at risk for serious neurodevelopmental deficits from equally low glucose levels. This risk is related to the depth and duration of the hypoglycemia.

Four pathophysiologic groups of neonatal infants are at high risk of developing hypoglycemia:

1. Infants of mothers with diabetes mellitus or gestational diabetes and infants with severe erythroblastosis fetalis, insulinomas, leucine sensitivity with hyperammonemia, familial or sporadic hyperinsulinemia, Beckwith syndrome, and panhypopituitarism have hyperinsulinism.

2. Infants with intrauterine growth retardation or those who are preterm may have experienced intrauterine malnutrition resulting in reduced hepatic glycogen stores and total body fat; the smaller of discordant twins (especially if discordant by 25% or more in weight with a weight of <2.0 kg), polycythemic infants, infants of toxemic mothers, and infants with placental abnormalities are particularly vulnerable.

3. Very immature or severely ill infants may develop hypoglycemia owing to increased metabolic needs disproportionate to substrate stores and calories supplied; low-birth-weight infants with respiratory distress syndrome, perinatal asphyxia, polycythemia, hypothermia, and systemic infections, as well as infants in heart failure with cyanotic congenital heart disease, are at increased risk. Interruption of intravenous infusions may also result in precipitous onset of hypoglycemia.

4. Rare infants with genetic or primary metabolic defects, such

as galactosemia, glycogen storage disease, fructose intolerance, propionic acidemia, methylmalonic acidemia, tyrosinemia, maple syrup urine disease, and long- or medium-chain acyl-CoA dehydrogenase deficiency, are also susceptible.

CLINICAL MANIFESTATIONS. The incidence of symptomatic hypoglycemia is highest in small-for-gestational-age infants. These infants usually fall into category two or three of the earlier pathophysiologic groupings, and some are referred to as having *transient symptomatic idiopathic neonatal hypoglycemia.* The onset of symptoms varies from a few hours to a week after birth. In approximate order of frequency there are jitteriness or tremors, apathy, episodes of cyanosis, convulsions, intermittent apneic spells or tachypnea, weak or high-pitched cry, limpness or lethargy, difficulty in feeding, and eye rolling. Episodes of sweating, sudden pallor, hypothermia, and cardiac arrest and failure also occur. It is critical to measure serum glucose levels and to determine whether they disappear with the administration of sufficient glucose to raise the blood sugar to normal levels; if they do not, other diagnoses must be considered.

TREATMENT. When symptoms other than seizures are present, an intravenous bolus of 200 mg/kg (2 mL/kg) of 10% glucose is effective in elevating the blood glucose concentration. In the presence of convulsions, 4 mL/kg of 10% glucose as a bolus injection is indicated. After initial therapy, a glucose infusion should be given at 8 mg/kg/min. If hypoglycemia recurs, the infusion rate should be increased until 15–20% glucose is used. If intravenous infusions of 20% glucose are inadequate to eliminate symptoms and maintain constant normal serum glucose concentrations, hyperinsulinemia is probably present and diazoxide should be administered.

HYPOGLYCEMIA WITH MACROGLOSSIA (BECKWITH SYNDROME)

Beckwith described a syndrome of intractable neonatal hypoglycemia occurring in infants with macroglossia, large size, visceromegaly, mild microcephaly, omphalocele, facial nevus flammeus, a characteristic earlobe crease, increased risk of tumors (Wilms, hepatoblastoma, gonadoblastoma), and renal medullary dysplasia. The prognosis is poor.

Infections in Neonatal Infants

CHAPTER 79

Pathogenesis and Epidemiology

(Nelson Textbook, Chapter 105)

Infections are a frequent and important cause of morbidity and mortality in the neonatal period.

ETIOLOGY

A number of agents may infect newborns in utero, intrapartum, or post partum. Prenatal infections that are known to be transmitted transplacentally include syphilis, rubella, toxoplasmosis, tuberculosis, and those caused by *Borrelia burgdorferi*, cytomegalovirus (CMV), parvovirus B19, hepatitis B virus, herpes simplex virus, human immunodeficiency virus, varicella-zoster, *Listeria monocytogenes*, and *Trypanosoma cruzi*.

Any microorganism inhabiting the vagina or lower gastrointestinal tract may cause intrapartum and postpartum infection. The most common bacteria are group B streptococci, enteric organisms, gonococci, and chlamydiae. The more common viruses include herpes simplex virus and enteroviruses. Community-acquired pathogens, such as *Streptococcus pneumoniae*, may also cause infection in newborns after discharge from the hospital.

The list of organisms causing nosocomial infections is long. The common causes are coagulase-negative staphylococci, gram-negative bacilli *(Klebsiella pneumoniae, Escherichia coli, Salmonella, Campylobacter, Enterobacter, Citrobacter, Pseudomonas aeruginosa, Serratia)*, enterococci, *Staphylococcus aureus*, and *Candida*. Viruses contributing to nosocomial neonatal infections include enteroviruses, CMV, hepatitis A, adenoviruses, influenza, respiratory syncytial virus, rhinovirus, parainfluenza, herpes simplex virus, and rotavirus.

Congenital pneumonia may be caused by CMV, rubella virus, and *Treponema pallidum* and less commonly by the other agents producing transplacental infection. Microorganisms causing pneumonia acquired in the perinatal period include group B streptococci, gram-negative enteric aerobes, *Listeria monocytogenes*, genital *Mycoplasma, Chlamydia trachomatis*, CMV, herpes simplex virus, and *Candida* species.

EPIDEMIOLOGY

PREMATURITY. The most important neonatal factor predisposing to infection is prematurity or low birth weight; these infants have a 3- to 10-fold higher incidence of infection and sepsis than do full-term, normal birth-weight infants.

CHORIOAMNIONITIS. Attack rates of neonatal infection increase significantly in the presence of chorioamnionitis, diagnosed by amniotic fluid analysis or histologically. Clinical signs of chorioamnionitis include intrapartum fever (>38°C), maternal leukocytosis (white blood cells >18,000), and uterine tenderness.

EARLY-ONSET AND LATE-ONSET INFECTIONS. Neonatal infections are those presenting during the first 28 days of life; however, similar infections may occur in older infants, particularly premature infants, during the first 6 mo of life. These are referred to as late-onset infections.

NOSOCOMIAL NURSERY INFECTION. Neonatal infections acquired in the hospital are nosocomial. Maternally acquired infections usually appear within the first 48 hr of life. Thus, presentation 48 hr after admission to the nursery is generally used as a criterion for nosocomial infection in a newborn. Nosocomial infections are relatively uncommon in normal full-term infants. In contrast, the rates of nosocomial infections among low-birth-weight infants in neonatal intensive care units are higher than in any other site in the hospital.

Multiple risk factors influence the probability of nosocomial infection in the neonatal intensive care unit. These include low birth weight, length of stay, invasive procedures, indwelling vascular catheters, ventricular shunts, endotracheal tubes, alterations in the skin and mucous membrane barriers, and frequent use of broad-spectrum antibiotics.

PATHOGENESIS

Newborns may be infected at different times via three different routes: in utero (transplacental), intrapartum (ascending), and post partum (nosocomial or community). In most cases, intrauterine infection is a result of clinical or subclinical maternal infection with transplacental transmission to the fetus. Infection acquired in utero may result in resorption of the embryo, abortion, stillbirth, congenital malformation, intrauterine growth retardation, premature birth, acute disease in the neonatal period, or asymptomatic persistent infection with neurologic sequelae later in life. In some cases, there are no apparent effects on the newborn. Maternal infection is a necessary prerequisite for transplacental infections.

Perinatal infections are acquired just before or during delivery, with vertical transmission of the microorganism from mother to newborn. The *amniotic infection syndrome* refers to microbial invasion of amniotic fluid, usually as a result of prolonged rupture of the chorioamniotic membrane.

Resuscitation at birth, particularly if it involves endotracheal intubation, insertion of an umbilical vessel catheter, or both, is associated with an increased risk of bacterial infection. Postnatal infection also may be transmitted by direct contact from various human sources, such as the mother, family contacts, and hospital personnel; from breast milk (human immunodeficiency virus, CMV); or from inanimate sources, such as contaminated equipment.

CHAPTER 80

Clinical Syndromes
(Nelson Textbook, Chapter 106)

CLINICAL MANIFESTATIONS OF NEONATAL INFECTIONS

Infection in newborns may be limited to a single organ or may involve many organs (focal or systemic). The absence of clinical signs at the time of the initial physical examination does not preclude infection. Some infections may be asymptomatic and remain asymptomatic. Early manifestations of infection may be subtle and nonspecific. Nonspecific clinical manifestations of neonatal infections are listed in Table 80–1.

FEVER. Only about 50% of infected newborns have a temperature greater than 37.8°C (axillary), and fever in newborns does

TABLE 80–1 Presenting Signs and Symptoms of Infection in Newborns

General	*Cardiovascular System*
Fever, temperature instability	Pallor; mottling; cold, clammy skin
"Not doing well"	Tachycardia
Poor feeding	Hypotension
Edema	Bradycardia
Gastrointestinal System	*Central Nervous System*
Abdominal distention	Irritability, lethargy
Vomiting	Tremors, seizures
Diarrhea	Hyporeflexia, hypotonia
Hepatomegaly	Abnormal Moro reflex
Respiratory System	Irregular respirations
Apnea, dyspnea	Full fontanel
Tachypnea, retraction	High-pitched cry
Flaring, grunting	*Hematologic System*
Cyanosis	Jaundice
Renal System	Splenomegaly
Oliguria	Pallor
	Petechiae, purpura
	Bleeding

not always signify infection. In premature infants, the normal body temperature is lower, and hypothermia or temperature instability is more likely to accompany infection, but some degree of temperature instability is not unusual in low-birth-weight infants.

RASH. Cutaneous manifestations of infection include impetigo, cellulitis, mastitis, omphalitis, and subcutaneous abscesses. *Ecthyma gangrenosum* is indicative of pseudomonal infection. The presence of small salmon-pink papules suggests *Listeria monocytogenes* infection.

OMPHALITIS. This is a unique neonatal infection resulting from inadequate care of the umbilical cord. The umbilical stump is colonized by bacteria from the maternal genital tract and the environment. Omphalitis may spread to the abdominal wall, leading to fasciitis or to the umbilical or portal vessels, the liver, and peritoneum, often resulting in sepsis.

TETANUS. Neonatal tetanus is a major cause of death in Southeast Asia, Africa, and the eastern Mediterranean region; it usually results from unhygienic birth and management of the umbilical cord. The onset is usually at 3–14 days, marked by poor sucking and irritability. With the more specific signs of trismus, difficulty swallowing, spasms, and opisthotonos, diagnosis is relatively simple. Treatment includes neutralization of toxin with human tetanus immunoglobulin, omphalectomy to remove the site of production of toxin, antimicrobial therapy, and management of seizures and respirations.

PNEUMONIA. Early signs and symptoms of pneumonia often are nonspecific, including poor feeding, lethargy, irritability, poor color, alteration in temperature, abdominal distention, and the overall impression that the infant is doing less well than previously. Cough indicates an abnormality, often infection, of the lower respiratory tract. As the degree of respiratory compromise increases, tachypnea, tachycardia, flaring of alae nasi, grunting, retractions, cyanosis, apnea, and progressive respiratory failure may ensue.

The physical signs of pneumonia, such as dullness to percussion, change in breath sounds, and the presence of rales or rhonchi, are very difficult to appreciate in a neonate. Radiographs of the chest may reveal new infiltrates or an effusion, but if the neonate has underlying hyaline membrane disease or bronchopulmonary dysplasia, it usually is not possible to determine whether the radiographic changes represent a new process or worsening of the underlying process. The progression of neonatal pneumonia can be variable.

SEPSIS. *Neonatal sepsis, sepsis neonatorum,* and *neonatal septicemia* are terms that have been used to describe the systemic response to infection in newborns. There is little agreement on the proper use of the term, that is, whether it should be restricted to bacterial infections, positive blood cultures, or severity of illness. Criteria for neonatal sepsis should include documentation of infection in a newborn with a serious systemic illness in which noninfectious explanations for the abnormal pathophysiologic state are excluded or unlikely.

In patients with multisystem involvement or when the cardiorespiratory signs are consistent with severe illness, *sepsis* should be considered. The initial presentation may be limited to only one system, such as apnea, tachypnea with retractions, or tachycardia, but a full clinical and laboratory evaluation usually reveals other abnormalities. Infants with suspected sepsis should be evaluated for multiorgan system disease. Metabolic acidosis is common. Hypoxemia and carbon dioxide retention may be associated with adult and congenital respiratory distress syndrome or pneumonia.

Late manifestations of sepsis include signs of cerebral edema or thromboses; respiratory failure as a result of acute respiratory distress syndrome; pulmonary hypertension; cardiac failure; renal failure; hepatocellular disease with hyperbilirubinemia and elevated enzymes, prolonged prothrombin time and partial thromboplastin time; septic shock; adrenal hemorrhage with adrenal insufficiency; bone marrow failure (thrombocytopenia, neutropenia, anemia); and disseminated intravascular coagulation.

DIAGNOSIS

The differential diagnosis in symptomatic newborns with primary respiratory disorders, cardiac disease, central nervous system (CNS) injury, anemia, and metabolic abnormalities usually includes infection. The newborn may have been exposed to a central or peripheral intravenous line, umbilical or Foley catheter, endotracheal tube, peritoneal dialysis, or surgical procedure. The maternal history may provide important information about maternal infection, exposure to infection in a sexual partner, maternal immunity (natural or acquired), maternal colonization, and obstetric risk factors (prematurity, prolonged ruptured membranes, maternal chorioamnionitis). Serologic screening tests may have been performed for *Treponema pallidum*, rubella, and hepatitis B virus. Maternal cultures may have been taken for *Neisseria gonorrhoeae*, group B streptococci, herpes simplex virus (HSV), or *Chlamydia*.

If there is a high likelihood of maternal infection with a known teratogenic agent, fetal ultrasound examination is strongly recommended. If the serologic studies of the mother point to a specific pathogen, it is sometimes possible to culture the organism from amniotic fluid. Polymerase chain reaction is particularly helpful to diagnose human immunodeficiency virus (HIV) infection in cordocentesis samples and in blood samples taken from the newborn.

Neonatal infections due to toxoplasmosis, rubella, cytomegalovirus (CMV), HSV, and syphilis present a diagnostic dilemma because (1) their clinical features overlap and may initially be indistinguishable, (2) disease may be inapparent, (3) maternal infection is often asymptomatic, (4) special laboratory studies may be needed, and (5) specific treatment for toxoplasmosis, syphilis, and HSV infection is predicated on an accurate diagnosis and may reduce significant long-term morbidity. Common shared features that should suggest the diagnosis of an intrauterine infection include prematurity, intrauterine growth retardation, hematologic involvement (anemia, neutropenia, thrombocytopenia, petechiae, purpura), ocular signs (chorioretinitis, cataracts, keratoconjunctivitis, glaucoma, microphthalmia), CNS signs (microcephaly, hydrocephaly, intracranial calcifications), and other organ system involvement (pneumonia, myocarditis, nephritis, hepatitis with hepatosplenomegaly, jaundice) or nonimmune hydrops.

Physical examination shortly after birth can identify a *congenital infection*, either acute or chronic. Chronic signs include microcephaly, hydrocephaly, intracranial calcification, retinitis, hepatomegaly, lymphadenopathy, and splenomegaly, implicating infection through the transplacental route. Acute congenital infection usually presents as a serious illness in an infant with low Apgar scores, CNS depression, and respiratory insufficiency. When the clinical presentation suggests an acute infection and the focus is unclear, additional studies should be performed. These include, in addition to blood cultures, a lumbar puncture, urine examination and culture, gastric aspirate for Gram stain and culture, and a chest radiograph. Urine should be collected by catheterization or suprapubic aspiration.

Diagnostic evaluations may be indicated for asymptomatic infants because of maternal chorioamnionitis. The probability of neonatal infection and subsequent neonatal sepsis correlates with the degree of prematurity and bacterial contamination of amniotic fluid. In an asymptomatic term infant whose mother has chorioamnionitis, two blood cultures should be obtained and a gastric aspirate should be examined to confirm the maternal diagnosis and identify presumptively the organisms by Gram stain. Presumptive treatment should be initiated.

The diagnosis of pneumonia in a neonate usually is presumptive; microbiologic proof of infection generally is lacking because lung tissue is not easily cultured. The differential diagnosis of pneumonitis in neonates is broad and includes hyaline membrane disease, meconium aspiration syndrome, transient tachypnea of the newborn, diaphragmatic hernia, congenital heart disease, persistent fetal circulation, and chronic lung disease.

The diagnosis of meningitis is confirmed by examination of the cerebrospinal fluid (CSF) and identification of a bacterium, virus, or fungus by culture or antigen detection. Blood culture and complete blood cell count are part of the initial evaluation because 70–85% of neonates with meningitis have positive results of a blood culture. The incidence of positive blood cultures is highest with early-onset sepsis and meningitis. Infants with bacteremia should have a CSF examination and culture.

Lumbar puncture may be deferred in a severely ill infant if the lumbar puncture would further compromise respiratory status. In these situations, blood culture and antigen detection assays should be performed and treatment initiated for presumed meningitis until a lumbar puncture can be safely performed.

Normal, uninfected infants from birth–4 wk may have elevated CSF protein levels = 84 ± 45 mg/dL, glucose = 46 ± 10, and elevated CSF leukocyte counts = 11 ± 10 with the 90th percentile = 22. The percent of polymorphonuclear leukocytes = 2.2 ± 3.8, with 90th percentile = 6. The upper limit of absolute neutrophil count = 3/mm^3. Preterm infants may develop elevated CSF protein levels and leukocyte counts and hypoglycorrhachia after intraventricular hemorrhage. Many nonpyogenic congenital infections also can produce asymptomatic alterations of CSF protein and leukocytes (toxoplasmosis, CMV, syphilis, HIV).

The Gram stain of CSF yields a positive result in the majority of patients with bacterial meningitis. The leukocyte count is usually elevated, with a predominance of neutrophils (>70–90%); the number is often greater than 1000 but may be less than 100 in infants with neutropenia or early in the disease. Microorganisms are recovered from most patients who have not been pretreated with antibiotics. Bacteria have also been isolated from CSF that did not have an abnormal number of cells (<25) or an abnormal protein level (<200 mg/dL).

LABORATORY FINDINGS

The acronym *TORCH* refers to toxoplasmosis, other agents, rubella, CMV, and HSV. It was modified to *STORCH* to include syphilis. Although the term may be helpful in remembering some of the etiologic agents of neonatal infections, the TORCH battery of serologic tests has a poor diagnostic yield, and the appropriate diagnostic studies should be selected for each etiologic agent under consideration. CMV and HSV require cultural methods.

Identification of a bacterial or fungal infection may be made by isolating the etiologic agent from a body fluid that is normally sterile (blood, CSF, urine, joint fluid), by demonstrating endotoxin or bacterial antigen in a body fluid (CSF, urine, or serum), or by demonstrating infection in the placenta or at autopsy. It is preferable to obtain two specimens for blood culture by venipuncture from different sites to avoid confusion caused by skin contamination. Samples should be obtained from an umbilical catheter only at the time of initial insertion.

The total white blood cell count and differential and the ratio of immature to total neutrophils provide immediately predictive information when compared with age standards. Neutropenia is more common than neutrophilia in severe neonatal sepsis, but neutropenia also occurs in association with maternal hypertension, pre-eclampsia, intrauterine growth retardation, neonatal sensitization, necrotizing enterocolitis, periventricular hemorrhage, seizures, surgery, and possibly hemolysis.

TREATMENT

Once bacterial infection has been suspected and appropriate cultures have been obtained, intravenous or intramuscular antibiotic therapy should be instituted immediately. Initial empirical treatment of early-onset and late-onset community-acquired bacterial infections should consist of ampicillin and an aminoglycoside (usually gentamicin). Nosocomial infections acquired in a neonatal intensive care unit are more likely to be caused by staphylococci, various Enterobacteriaceae, *Pseudomonas,* or *Candida.* Thus, an antistaphylococcal drug, nafcillin for *Staphylococcus aureus* or vancomycin for coagulase-negative staphylococci, should be substituted for ampicillin. A history of recent antimicrobial therapy or the presence of antibiotic-resistant infections in the neonatal intensive care unit suggests the need for a different aminoglycoside agent (amikacin), and vancomycin is used for methicillin-resistant staphylococci. When the history or the presence of necrotic skin lesions suggests *Pseudomonas* infection, initial therapy should be ticarcillin or carbenicillin and gentamicin. Doses of the commonly used antibiotics are provided in Table 80–2. Once the pathogen has been identified and the antibiotic sensitivities determined, the most appropriate drugs should be selected.

Therapy for most infections should be continued for a total of 7–10 days or for at least 5–7 days after a clinical response has occurred. The course of treatment for meningitis caused by group B streptococci is usually for 14 days and for a minimum of 14 days after sterilization of the CSF in gram-negative meningitis. A blood culture taken 24–48 hr after initiation of therapy should yield negative results.

Antimicrobial therapy is often begun presumptively on the basis of nonspecific clinical findings, and cultures are subsequently sterile. The use of antifungal therapy should be considered in very-low-birth-weight infants who have mucosal colonization with C. *albicans* and who are at high risk for invasive disease.

Because a negative blood culture result does not preclude bacterial infection, the clinician must decide whether an infection is

TABLE 80–2 Dosages of Antibiotics Commonly Prescribed for Newborns

Antibiotics	Routes	Weight <1200 g Age 0–4 wk	Weight 1200–2000 g Age 0–7 days	Weight 1200–2000 g >7 days	Weight >2000 g Age 0–7 days	Weight >2000 g >7 days
			Dosages (mg/kg) and Intervals of Administration			
Amikacin*	IV, IM	7.5 q18–24h	7.5 q12–18h	7.5 q8–12h	10 q12h	10 q8h
Ampicillin	IV, IM					
Meningitis		50 q12h	50 q12h	50 q8h	50 q8h	50 q6h
Other diseases		25 q12h	25 q12h	25 q8h	25 q8h	25 q6h
Aztreonam	IV, IM	30 q12h	30 q12h	30 q8h	30 q8h	30 q6h
Cefazolin	IV, IM	20 q12h	20 q12h	20 q12h	20 q12h	20 q8h
Cefotaxime	IV, IM	50 q12h	50 q12h	50 q8h	50 q12h	50 q8h
Ceftazidime	IV, IM	50 q12h	50 q12h	50 q8h	50 q8h	50 q8h
Ceftriaxone	IV, IM	50 q24h	50 q24h	50 q24h	50 q24h	75 q24h
Cephalothin	IV	20 q12h	20 q12h	20 q8h	20 q8h	20 q6h
Chloramphenicol†	IV, PO	25 q24h	25 q24h	25 q24h	25 q24h	25 q12h
Clindamycin	IV, IM, PO	5 q12h	5 q12h	5 q8h	5 q8h	5 q6h
Erythromycin	PO	10 q12h	10 q12h	10 q8h	10 q12h	10 q8h
Gentamicin	IV, IM	2.5 q18–24h	2.5 q12–18h	2.5 q8h	2.5 q12h	2.5 q8h
Imipenem	IV, IM	20 q18–24h	20 q12h	20 q12h	20 q12h	20 q8h
Kanamycin	IV, IM	7.5 q18–24h	7.5 q12–18h	7.5 q8–12h	10 q12h	10 q8h

Drug	Route					
Methicillin	IV, IM					
Meningitis		50 q12h	50 q12h	50 q8h	50 q8h	50 q6h
Other diseases		25 q12h	25 q12h	25 q8h	25 q8h	25 q6h
Metronidazole	IV, PO	7.5 q48h	7.5 q12h	7.5 q12h	7.5 q12h	15 q12h
Mezlocillin	IV, IM	75 q12h	75 q12h	75 q8h	75 q12h	75 q8h
Nafcillin	IV	25 q12h	25 q12h	25 q8h	25 q8h	25 q6h
Netilmicin‡	IV, IM	2.5 q18–24h	2.5 q12–18h	2.5 q8–12h	2.5 q12h	2.5 q8h
Oxacillin	IV, IM	25 q12h	25 q12h	30 q8h	25 q8h	25 q6h
Penicillin G	IV					
Meningitis		50,000 U q12h	50,000 U q12h	75,000 U q8h	50,000 U q8h	50,000 U q6h
Other diseases		25,000 U q12h	25,000 U q12h	25,000 U q8h	25,000 U q8h	25,000 U q6h
Penicillin G	IM					
Benzathine		50,000 U (one dose)	50,000 U (one dose)	50,000 U (one dose)	50,000 U (one dose)	50,000 U (one dose)
Procaine		50,000 U q24h	50,000 U q24h	50,000 U q24h	50,000 U q24h	50,000 U q24h
Ticarcillin	IV, IM	75 q12h	75 q12h	75 q8h	75 q8h	75 q6h
Tobramycin*	IV, IM	2.5 q18–24h	2.5 q12–18h	2.5 q8–12h	2.5 q12h	2.5 q8h
Vancomycin§	IV	15 q24h	10 q12–18h	15 q8–12h	15 q12h	15 q8h

*Aminoglycoside levels should be monitored if therapy continues >3 days. Optimal peak levels 6–8 μg/mL, trough < 2 μg/mL.
†Serum levels are highly variable. Chloramphenicol should be given to newborns only if serum levels can be monitored.
‡0.5 mg/kg/24 hr can increase to 1 mg/kg/24 hr if needed or give every other day. Treat for cumulative dose of 10–30 mg/kg.
§Because of variable pharmacokinetics, vancomycin levels should be monitored if therapy continues >3 days. Optimal peak levels 20–30 μg/mL, trough < 10 μg/mL.
Recommendations for infants weighing <1000 g based on Prober et al: Pediatr Infect Dis J 9:111, 1990.
Adapted from Nelson JD: Pocketbook of Pediatric Antimicrobial Therapy, 12th ed. Baltimore, Williams & Wilkins, 1997.

likely and antibiotics should be continued. With another explanation for the clinical findings and normal laboratory data (neutrophils, erythrocyte sedimentation rate, C-reactive protein, interleukin-6), infection is unlikely and antibiotics may be discontinued.

Treatment of newborns whose mothers received antibiotics during labor should be individualized. If in utero infection is likely, then treatment of the infant should be continued until there is evidence that there was no infection (the infant remains asymptomatic for 24–72 hr) or there is clinical and laboratory evidence of recovery.

For *pneumonia* presenting in the first 7–10 days of life a combination of ampicillin and an aminoglycoside or cefotaxime is appropriate. Nosocomial pneumonia, generally manifested after this time, can be treated empirically with methicillin or vancomycin and a third-generation cephalosporin.

Presumptive antimicrobial therapy of *bacterial meningitis* should include ampicillin in maximum doses and cefotaxime or ampicillin and gentamicin unless staphylococci are the likely cause, which is an indication for vancomycin. Susceptibility testing of gram-negative enteric organisms is important because resistance to cephalosporins and aminoglycosides occurs.

Meningitis due to group B streptococci usually responds within 24–48 hr and should be treated for 14–21 days. Gram-negative bacilli may continue to grow from repeated CSF samples for 72–96 hr after therapy despite the use of appropriate antibiotics. Treatment of gram-negative meningitis should be continued for 21 days or for at least 14 days after sterilization of the CSF, whichever is longer. Meningitis due to *Pseudomonas aeruginosa* infection should be treated with ceftazidime. Metronidazole is the treatment of choice for infection caused by *Bacteroides fragilis*.

Treatment of *sepsis* may be divided into antimicrobial therapy for the suspected or known pathogen and supportive care. Fluids, electrolytes, and glucose levels should be monitored carefully with correction of hypovolemia, hyponatremia, hypocalcemia, and hypoglycemia and limitation of fluids if there is inappropriate antidiuretic hormone secretion. Shock, hypoxia, and metabolic acidosis should be identified and managed with inotropic agents, fluid resuscitation, and mechanical ventilation. Adequate oxygenation of tissues should be maintained; ventilatory support is frequently necessary for respiratory failure caused by congenital pneumonia, persistent fetal circulation, or acute respiratory distress syndrome (shock lung). Disseminated intravascular coagulation may complicate neonatal septicemia and may be treated by management of the primary sepsis. However, if bleeding occurs, disseminated intravascular coagulation may be treated with fresh frozen plasma, platelet transfusions, or whole blood.

PART 11

Special Health Problems During Adolescence

CHAPTER 81

The Epidemiology of Adolescent Disease
(Nelson Textbook, Chapters 107 and 108)

Behavioral and psychosocial risks, including injuries, account for a substantial proportion of both the utilization of health care services by adolescents and the causes of morbidity and mortality. The health conditions having the greatest impact on the status of adolescent health are early unintended pregnancy, sexually transmitted diseases, mental disorders, injuries, and substance use and abuse. Health destructive behavior, such as cigarette and marijuana smoking and the abuse of alcohol and recreational drugs (often in combination with driving), continues to present a serious problem for adolescents. Automobile and motorcycle accidents are the leading causes of adolescent morbidity and mortality. Homicides are the second leading cause of death for all adolescents and the most common cause of death for black males. Firearm deaths and injuries are a major contributor to these events. Certain chronic diseases affecting adults have their origins during adolescence. Heart disease, diabetes, and respiratory conditions related to smoking are most common. Health education and promotion as well as disease prevention should be the focus of every visit with a teenager (Table 81–1).

LEGAL ISSUES

In the United States, the right of a minor to consent to treatment without parental knowledge is governed by state laws. Minors are also exempt from the requirement of parental consent for medical treatment under the following circumstances:

1. *Emancipated minors.* These are children who live away from home, are no longer subject to parental control, are economically self-supporting, are married, or are members of the military.

2. *Emergencies.* In a medical emergency a minor may be treated without consent of parents if, in the physician's judgment, the delay resulting from attempts to contact parents would jeopardize the life or health of the minor.

3. *Mature minor rule.* An emerging trend in the law is the recognition that many minors are sufficiently mature to under-

TABLE 81–1 Supervision Guidelines

Source	American Academy of Pediatrics
Periodicity	*Annually*
Anticipatory Guidance	
Parenting	X
Adolescent development	X
Safety practices	X
Diet and fitness	X
Healthy lifestyles	X
Oral health	X
Screening History	
Tobacco use	X
Alcohol and drug use	X
Sexual behavior	X
School performance	X
Depression/suicide risk	X
Eating disorders	X
Learning problems	
Abuse	X
Physical Assessment with Specific Recommendations	
Hypertension	X*
Obesity	X*
Breast cancer (self-examination)	X
Comprehensive examination	X
Scoliosis	X
Tests	
Hyperlipidemia	X
Tuberculin	X†,‡
Vision	X
Anemia	X
Gonococcus, chlamydia, syphilis§	X
Genital warts (HPV)§	
Human immunodeficiency virus infection	X
Cervical cancer‖	X
Immunizations	
MMR	X
dT	X
Hepatitis B	X

*Recommends obtaining and plotting measures only.
†Under specific conditions.
‡At least one during adolescence (14–16 year old).
§For adolescents who are sexually active.
‖For adolescent girls who are sexually active or ≥18 yr old.

stand the nature of their illness and the potential risks and benefits of proposed therapy and, therefore, should receive such treatment on their own consent.

CHAPTER 82

Depression

(Nelson Textbook, Chapter 109)

Changes in mood are part of the normative developmental
"adjustment" to changes in body, roles, and relationships in adolescence. The challenge for a pediatrician is to distinguish between
these normative variations and disorders requiring mental health
intervention.

EPIDEMIOLOGY. Depression is two to three times higher in postpubertal girls than in postpubertal boys. The lifetime prevalence of
major depression is similar to adults and ranges between 15%
and 20%.

ETIOLOGY. There appears to be an interactive effect of genetics
and environment in major depressive disorders, with studies in
adults suggesting individuals with a high genetic risk may be
more vulnerable to adverse environmental stressors when compared with those with low genetic risk.

CLINICAL MANIFESTATIONS. An adolescent who presents with
school failure or another behavioral disorder may have an underlying depressive issue. The characteristics of a sadness problem
encompass (1) depressed or irritable mood, (2) diminished interest or pleasure, (3) weight loss or gain or failure to make expected
weight gains, (4) insomnia or hypersomnia, (5) psychomotor
agitation or retardation, (6) fatigue or energy loss, (7) feelings of
worthlessness or excessive or inappropriate guilt, and (8) diminished ability to think or concentrate. The quality of these symptoms is less intense with a sadness problem, as compared with
major depression, and the impact on the adolescent's functioning
is mild. When these symptoms occur daily for a period of 2 wk or
longer, with or without recurrent thoughts of death and suicidal
ideation, the diagnosis falls into the realm of a major depressive
disorder. When these symptoms occur within 3 mo of an identifiable stressor, the presentation is considered an adjustment disorder with depressed mood.

OFFICE SCREENING FOR DEPRESSION. The screening for depressive
symptoms is recommended as a component of the routine health
maintenance assessment for an adolescent. Although the diagnosis of the full depressive disorder is based on interviewing the
adolescent and obtaining observational data from parents or primary caretakers, alertness during a medical evaluation can raise
suspicion early in the course of the disorder.

TREATMENT. There are several therapeutic modalities for the treatment of depression, including individual and group therapy, family intervention, and others, along with, or independent of, psychopharmacologic treatment. The role of the pediatrician relative to the timing of a referral to a mental health professional is determined by his or her training and experience in managing mental health problems.

CHAPTER 83

Suicide
(Nelson Textbook, Chapter 110)

The recognition of risk factors for suicidal behavior is an important aspect in the prevention efforts directed toward adolescents, particularly those with mood disorder. Suicide is the third leading cause of death for all adolescents and young adults 15–24 yr old; it is the second leading cause of death for white males.

CLINICAL MANIFESTATIONS. Suicidal ideation alone is not necessarily a risk factor for suicidal behavior. As many as 12–25% of older children and adolescents express some form of suicidal ideation. The risk should be taken much more seriously when the ideation is accompanied by a specific plan. Psychologic autopsies after successful suicides have also uncovered the frequent occurrence of a stressful event, such as a disciplinary crisis, disappointment, or rejection, immediately preceding the suicide.

TREATMENT. Consultation with a skilled psychiatrist is essential in the assessment of every teenager who attempts suicide. When the three most serious risk factors—prior suicide attempt, mood disorder, and substance abuse—are present, there is no proof that hospitalization prevents repeated attempts and the ultimate completion of suicide. However, a hospitalization may assist in resolution of an existing conflict and provide a secure setting in which the patient can have underlying problems addressed.

CHAPTER 84

Violent Behavior
(Nelson Textbook, Chapter 111)

Interpersonal and community violence, physical abuse, and domestic violence lead to significant rates of injury and death for specific age, gender, and racial sectors of the population in the United States. Youth and minority populations are disproportionately affected.

EPIDEMIOLOGY. In 1993–1994, the United States led the industrialized world in the number of youth deaths due to firearms, both homicide and unintentional firearm deaths. From 1983–1993, the firearm homicide rate more than tripled from 5 to 18/100,000.

CLINICAL MANIFESTATIONS. There are several clinical entities directly associated with violent behavior that require recognition and intervention. The most common behavioral diagnoses associated with aggressive behavior in adolescents are mental retardation, learning disabilities, moderately severe language disorders, and mental disorders such as attention deficit hyperactivity, mood, anxiety, and personality disorders. Inability to master prosocial skills such as the establishment and maintenance of positive family and peer relations and the resolution of conflict may put adolescents with these disorders at higher risk for physical violence and other risky behaviors. Conduct disorder and oppositional defiant disorder are specific psychiatric diagnoses whose definitions are associated with violent behavior. They occur comorbidly with other disorders such as attention deficit hyperactivity disorder and increase an adolescent's vulnerability for juvenile delinquency, substance use or abuse, sexual promiscuity, adult criminal behavior, incarceration, and antisocial personality disorder. Victims as well as witnesses of violence are at risk for posttraumatic stress disorder.

TREATMENT. In the instance of acute injury secondary to violent assault, the treatment plan should follow standards established by the American Academy of Pediatrics model protocol, which includes, but is not limited to, the stabilization of the injury, evaluation and treatment of the injury, evaluation of the assault circumstance, psychologic evaluation of the functioning of the victim through to the rehabilitation of the injury, and outpatient follow-up of the behavioral and physical sequelae.

CHAPTER 85

Anorexia Nervosa and Bulimia

(Nelson Textbook, Chapter 112)

EPIDEMIOLOGY. The incidence of anorexia nervosa (AN) and bulimia has increased over the past 2 decades. It is estimated that 1 in every 100 females, 16–18 yr old, has anorexia nervosa.

DIAGNOSIS. *The Diagnostic and Statistical Manual of Mental Disorders (DSM-IV)* criteria for the diagnosis of AN include (1) intense fear of becoming obese, which does not diminish as weight loss progresses; (2) disturbance in the way in which one's body weight, size, or shape is experienced (e.g., claiming to "feel fat" even when one is emaciated or believing that one area of the body is "too fat" even when obviously underweight); (3) refusal to maintain body weight over a minimal normal weight for age and height (e.g., weight loss leading to maintenance of body weight 15% below expected, failure to make expected weight gain during period of growth leading to body weight 15% less than that expected); and (4) in females, absence of at least three consecutive menstrual cycles when otherwise expected to occur (primary or secondary amenorrhea).

The *DSM-IV* separates *bulimia* from AN as a diagnostic entity, defining bulimia as (1) recurrent episodes of binge eating (rapid consumption of a large amount of food in a discrete period of time, usually less than 2 hr); (2) during the eating binges, a fear of not being able to stop eating; (3) regular engagement in self-induced vomiting, use of laxatives, or rigorous dieting or fasting to counteract the effects of binge eating; (4) a minimum average of two binge-eating episodes per week for at least 3 mo; and (5) self-evaluation unduly influenced by body weight and shape. The disturbance does not occur exclusively during episodes of AN.

CLINICAL MANIFESTATIONS. AN and bulimia are associated with disturbances in almost every organ system, although it is uncertain which may be primary and which is the result of severe malnutrition. The death rate in AN is approximately 10% and is usually caused by severe electrolyte disturbance, cardiac arrhythmia, or congestive heart failure in the recovery phase. Bradycardia and postural hypotension are common, with pulse rates as low as 20 beats/min. Both improve with nutritional therapy. A variety of electrocardiographic abnormalities is common, including low voltage, T-wave inversion and flattening, and ST segment depression, as well as supraventricular and ventricular dysrhythmias, some preceded by a prolonged QT_c interval.

Sleep disturbances occur in some anorexics and include a short rapid eye movement latency time, similar to that often found in depressed patients. Problems of thermal regulation, particularly hypothermia, are common. Hypothermia also occurs in some bulimics of normal weight. Disorders of the hypothalamic-pituitary-ovarian axis are manifested as amenorrhea.

Neuropsychologic effects of AN include impairment of concentration and problem solving, as well as attentional-perceptual motor function. Bone marrow hypoplasia is common in AN, with leukopenia, anemia, and (rarely) thrombocytopenia. Low erythrocyte sedimentation rates are common. Constipation is a common complication of motility problems in AN, as is esophagitis in those who vomit. Electrolyte imbalance results from vomiting, "waterloading" (a practice of surreptitiously drinking large amounts of water to achieve an agreed-upon weight gain), or abuse of diuretics or laxatives.

TREATMENT. Most of the regimens in current use combine psychotherapy (individual and family), behavior modification techniques, and nutritional rehabilitation. Pharmacologic therapy (primarily with antidepressant medications) appears to be helpful for that subset of depressed patients with eating disorders.

CHAPTER 86

Substance Abuse
(Nelson Textbook, Chapter 113)

Developmental considerations are probably most important for this age group. Substance use for most teenagers is not an issue of psychopathology but of the influence on normal functioning. Drug use in younger, less-experienced adolescents can act as a substitute for developing age-appropriate coping strategies and enhance vulnerability to poor decision-making. When drug use begins to negatively alter functioning in older adolescents at school and in the family, and risk-taking behavior is seen, intervention is warranted. Serious drug use is not an isolated phenomenon. It is a part of a complex set of family and individual issues that should be addressed in a comprehensive fashion. Specific historical questions can assist in determining the severity of the drug problem through a rating system as depicted in Table 86–1.

CLINICAL MANIFESTATIONS. Although manifestations vary by the specific substance of use, adolescents who use drugs often present in an office setting with no obvious physical findings. An adolescent presenting to an emergency setting with an impaired sensorium as part of a toxic syndrome should be evaluated for substance use as a part of the differential diagnosis, again accompanied by appropriate screening and physical examination (Table 86–2).

ALCOHOL. Alcohol use among adolescents has increased during the past decade and poses a threat to the normal functioning of the teenager as well as to the lives of those potentially jeopardized by drunken drivers.

CLINICAL MANIFESTATIONS. Alcohol acts primarily as a central nervous system (CNS) depressant. It produces euphoria, grogginess, talkativeness, and impaired short-term memory, and it increases the pain threshold. Alcohol's ability to produce vasodilation and hypothermia is also centrally mediated. At very high serum levels, respiratory depression occurs. The gastrointestinal complications of alcohol use can occur from a single large ingestion. The most common is acute erosive gastritis, which is manifested by epigastric pain, anorexia, vomiting, and guaiac-positive stools.

TREATMENT. The usual mechanism of death from the alcohol overdose syndrome is respiratory depression, and artificial venti-

TABLE 86-1 Assessing the Seriousness of Adolescent Drug Abuse

Variable	0	+1	+2
Age (yr)	>15 yr	<15 yr	
Sex	Male	Female	
Family history of drug abuse		Yes	
Setting of drug use	In group		Alone
Affect before drug use	Happy	Always poor	Sad
School performance	Good, improving		Recently poor
Use before driving	None		Yes
History of accidents	None		Yes
Time of week	Weekend	Weekdays	
Time of day		After school	Before school
Type of drug	Marijuana, beer, wine	Hallucinogens, amphetamines	Whiskey, opiates, cocaine, barbiturates

Total score: 0–3 less worrisome, 3–8 serious, 8–18 very serious.

TABLE 86–2 The Most Common Toxic Syndromes

Anticholinergic Syndromes

Common Signs

Delirium with mumbling speech, tachycardia, dry, flushed skin, dilated pupils, myoclonus, slightly elevated temperature, urinary retention, and decreased bowel sounds. Seizures and dysrhythmias may occur in severe cases.

Common Causes

Antihistamines, antiparkinsonian medication, atropine, scopolamine, amantadine, antipsychotic agents, antidepressant agents, antispasmodic agents, mydriatic agents, skeletal muscle relaxants, and many plants (notably jimson weed and *Amanita muscaria*).

Sympathomimetic Syndromes

Common Signs

Delusions, paranoia, tachycardia (or bradycardia if the drug is a pure α-adrenergic agonist), hypertension, hyperpyrexia, diaphoresis, piloerection, mydriasis, and hyperreflexia. Seizures, hypotension, and dysrhythmias may occur in severe cases.

Common Causes

Cocaine, amphetamine, methamphetamine (and its derivatives 3,4-methylenedioxyamphetamine, 3,4-methylenedioxymethamphetamine, and 2,5-dimethoxy-4-bromoamphetamine), and over-the-counter decongestants (phenylpropanolamine, ephedrine, and pseudoephedrine). In caffeine and theophylline overdoses, similar findings, except for the organic psychiatric signs, result from catecholamine release.

Opiate, Sedative, or Ethanol Intoxication

Common Signs

Coma, respiratory depression, miosis, hypotension, bradycardia, hypothermia, pulmonary edema, decreased bowel sounds, hyporeflexia, and needle marks. Seizures may occur after overdoses of some narcotics, notably propoxyphene.

Common Causes

Narcotics, barbiturates, benzodiazepines, ethchlorvynol, glutethimide, methyprylon, methaqualone, meprobamate, ethanol, clonidine, and guanabenz.

Cholinergic Syndromes

Common Signs

Confusion, central nervous system depression, weakness, salivation, lacrimation, urinary and fecal incontinence, gastrointestinal cramping, emesis, diaphoresis, muscle fasciculations, pulmonary edema, miosis, bradycardia or tachycardia, and seizures.

Common Causes

Organophosphate and carbamate insecticides, physostigmine, edrophonium, and some mushrooms.

From Kulig K: Initial management of ingestions of toxic substances. N Engl J Med 326:1678, 1992.

latory support must be provided. Dialysis should be considered when the blood level is higher than 400 mg/dL.

MARIJUANA

CLINICAL MANIFESTATIONS. In addition to the "desired" effects of elation and euphoria, marijuana may cause impairment of short-term memory, poor performance of tasks requiring divided attention (e.g., those involved in driving), loss of critical judgment, and distortion of time perception. Visual hallucinations and perceived body distortions occur rarely, but there may be "flashbacks" or recall of frightening hallucinations experienced under marijuana's influence that usually occur during stress or with fever.

Temperature may be lowered. Tachycardia is apparent within 20 min of smoking marijuana and is followed 30 min later by transient systolic and diastolic hypertension, which disappears by 3 hr. Certain drugs may interact with marijuana to potentiate sedation (i.e., alcohol, diazepam), potentiate stimulation (i.e., cocaine, amphetamines), or be antagonistic (i.e., propranolol, phenytoin).

VOLATILE SUBSTANCES

The most popular inhalants among adolescents are glue, gasoline, and volatile nitrites.

CLINICAL MANIFESTATIONS. The major effects of inhalants are psychoactive. Toluene, the main ingredient in airplane glue and some rubber cements, causes relaxation and pleasant hallucinations for up to 2 hr. Tolerance and physical dependence may occur. Gasoline, a popular inhalant among rural adolescents and Native American youth, contains a complex mixture of organic solvents. Euphoria is followed by violent excitement, and coma may result from prolonged or rapid inhalation. Volatile nitrites, such as amyl nitrite, butyl nitrite, and related compounds marketed as room deodorizers, are used as euphoriants, enhancers of musical appreciation, and aphrodisiacs among older adolescents and young adults. They may result in headaches, syncope, and lightheadedness; profound hypotension and cutaneous flushing followed by vasoconstriction and tachycardia; transiently inverted T waves and depressed ST segments on electrocardiography; methemoglobinemia; increased bronchial irritation; and increased intraocular pressure.

TREATMENT. Treatment is generally supportive and directed toward control of arrhythmia and stabilization of respirations and circulation. Withdrawal symptoms do not usually occur.

HALLUCINOGENS

Lysergic Acid Diethylamide (LSD)

LSD's high potency allows effective doses to be applied to objects as small as postage stamps and paper blotters. It is rapidly absorbed from the gastrointestinal tract. The onset of action can be between 30 and 60 min, and it peaks between 2 and 4 hr. By 10–12 hr, an individual returns to the predrug state.

CLINICAL MANIFESTATIONS. The common somatic symptoms are dizziness, dilated pupils, nausea, flushing, elevated temperature, and tachycardia. The sensation of synesthesia or "seeing" smells and "hearing" colors has been reported with LSD use. Delusional ideation, body distortion, and suspiciousness to the point of toxic psychosis are the more serious of the psychic symptoms.

TREATMENT. An individual is considered to have a "bad trip" when the setting causes the user to become terrified or panicked. These episodes should be treated by removing the individual from the aggravating situation or setting and attempting to re-establish contact with reality through calm verbal interaction. Any physical complication such as hyperthermia, seizure, or hypertension should be treated supportively. "Flashbacks" or LSD-induced states after the drug has worn off and tolerance to the effects of the drug are additional complications of its use. LSD use has not been associated with a withdrawal syndrome.

Methylenedioxymethamphetamine (MDMA, Ecstasy)

CLINICAL MANIFESTATIONS. Euphoria, a heightened sensual awareness, and increased psychic and emotional energy are the observed acute effects of MDMA. Nausea, jaw clenching, teeth grinding, and blurred vision are somatic symptoms, whereas anxiety, panic attacks, and psychosis are the adverse psychic outcomes. There are no specific treatment regimens recommended for acute toxicity.

Phencyclidine (PCP)

CLINICAL MANIFESTATIONS. The clinical manifestations are dose related. Euphoria, nystagmus, ataxia, and emotional lability occur within 2–3 min after smoking 1–5 mg and last for hours. Hallucination may involve bizarre distortions of body image that often precipitate panic reactions. With doses of 5–15 mg, a toxic psychosis may occur, with disorientation, hypersalivation, and abusive language lasting for more than 1 hr. After oral ingestion of 15 mg or more, the patient usually becomes comatose within 30–60 min, with alternating periods of wakefulness, with dystonic posturing, muscular rigidity, or myoclonic jerks. Hypotension, generalized seizures, and cardiac arrhythmias commonly occur with plasma concentrations from 40–200 mg/dL. Death has been reported during psychotic delirium, from hypertension, hypotension, hypothermia, seizures, and trauma. The coma of PCP may be distinguished from that of the opiates by the absence of respiratory depression; the presence of muscle rigidity, hyperreflexia, and nystagmus; and the lack of response to naloxone.

TREATMENT. Management of the PCP-intoxicated patient includes placement in a darkened, quiet room on a floor pad, safe from injury. Diazepam, in a dose of 10–20 mg orally or 10 mg intramuscularly every 4 hr, may be helpful if the patient is agitated and not comatose. Supportive therapy of the comatose patient is indicated with particular attention to hydration, which may be compromised by PCP-induced diuresis.

COCAINE

Crack cocaine, the highly addictive form of cocaine that can be smoked, has increased availability and severity of cocaine use in the presence of a decrease in use in the overall population.

CLINICAL MANIFESTATIONS. Cocaine produces euphoria, increased motor activity, decreased fatigability, and occasionally paranoid ideation. Its sympathomimetic properties are responsible for pupillary dilatation, tachycardia, hypertension, and hyperthermia. Binge patterns of use are common. Neurologic effects such as dizziness, paresthesias, and seizures can occur. Lethal effects are possible. Although addiction and tolerance develop in the chronic user, withdrawal symptoms on its discontinuation have not been reported. Pregnant adolescents who use cocaine place their fetus at risk for premature delivery, complications of low birth weight, and possibly congenital malformations and developmental disorders.

TREATMENT. Intensive supportive therapy is directed at the clinical manifestations of acute intoxication.

AMPHETAMINES

CLINICAL MANIFESTATIONS. High doses produce slowing of cardiac conduction in the face of ventricular irritability. Hypertensive and hyperpyrexic episodes can occur as can seizures. Binge effects result in the development of psychotic ideation with the potential for sudden violence. Cerebrovascular damage and psychosis can result from chronic use. There is a withdrawal syndrome associated with amphetamine use. The early phase is characterized as a "crash" phase with depression, agitation, anergia, and desire for more of the drug. Loss of physical and mental energy, limited interest in the environment, and anhedonia mark the intermediate phase. In the final phase, drug craving returns, often triggered by particular situations or objects.

TREATMENT. Agitation and delusional behaviors can be treated with haloperidol or droperidol. Phenothiazines are contraindicated and may cause a rapid drop in blood pressure or seizure activity. Other supportive treatment consists of a cooling blanket for hyperthermia and treatment of the hypertension and arrhythmias, which may respond to sedation with lorazepam (Ativan) or diazepam (Valium).

OPIATES

CLINICAL MANIFESTATIONS. The clinical manifestations are determined by the pharmacologic effects of heroin or its adulterants, combined with the conditions and the route of administration. The cerebral effects include euphoria, diminution in pain, and pinpoint pupils. An effect on the hypothalamus is suggested by the lowering of body temperature. Respiratory depression is mediated centrally. Pulmonary edema is common in death from the overdose syndrome. The most common dermatologic lesions are the "tracks," the hypertrophic linear scars that follow the course of large veins. Abscesses secondary to nonsterile techniques of drug administration are commonly found. Constipation results from decreased smooth muscle propulsive contractions and increased anal sphincter tone. Hepatic enzyme activities are frequently elevated in heroin users, the majority of whom have serologic evidence suggesting viral infection with hepatitis B. Infection with human immunodeficiency virus is another complication of needle use.

Withdrawal. After a period of 8 hr or more without heroin, the addicted individual undergoes, during a period of 24–36 hr, a series of physiologic disturbances referred to collectively as "withdrawal" or the *abstinence syndrome*. The earliest sign is yawning, followed by lacrimation, mydriasis, insomnia, "goose flesh," cramping of the voluntary musculature, hyperactive bowel sounds and diarrhea, tachycardia, and systolic hypertension. The occurrence of grand mal seizures is rare in adolescent addicts. A short course of diazepam is effective and safe treatment for heroin detoxification. An alternative for detoxification is treatment with methadone.

Overdose Syndrome. The overdose syndrome is an acute reaction after the administration of an opiate. It is the leading cause of death among drug users. The clinical signs include stupor or coma, seizures, miotic pupils (unless severe anoxia has occurred), respiratory depression, cyanosis, and pulmonary edema. Diagnosis of opiate toxicity is facilitated by intravenous administration of the opiate antagonist naloxone, 0.01 mg/kg (a vial of 0.4 mg usually suffices for an adolescent), which causes dilation of pupils constricted by the opiate. Treatment consists of maintaining adequate oxygenation and continued administration of naloxone every 5 min, when necessary.

ANABOLIC STEROIDS

CLINICAL MANIFESTATIONS. The most immediate effect for all users of anabolic steroids is increasing acneiform lesions. Other dermatologic manifestations include linear keloids, stria, oily hair, and hirsutism. Males can experience gynecomastia, breast pain, testicular atrophy, and azoospermia. Women experience more irreversible side effects, such as breast atrophy, clitoral enlargement, and menstrual abnormalities. Serious psychologic effects also have been reported from the use of high doses of these agents (often 100 times the therapeutic doses), including uncontrollable rage, depression, mania, mood fluctuations, and alterations in libido. Abnormalities of the liver can be acute, such as hepatitis and hepatomegaly, or more long-term, such as the increased risk of hepatocellular carcinoma. The early adolescent is at risk for growth retardation because of the possibility of accelerating epiphyseal closure.

CHAPTER 87

The Breast

(Nelson Textbook, Chapter 115)

NORMAL VARIANTS. Minor breast asymmetry is common in adult females and sexually mature adolescent females. Other conditions that rarely occur but should be ruled out include Poland syndrome and unilateral breast aplasia, hypoplasia, or hypertrophy. Poland syndrome is marked by a hypoplastic breast nipple and areola with hypoplastic ipsilateral chest wall structures. Unilateral or bilateral juvenile (virginal) hypertrophy occurs with specific histopathologic changes but without any known cause. The enlargement may be mild and cause back pain and postural problems or severe enough to be associated with tissue and skin necrosis. Accessory breast tissue can also occur in males and females. This lesion can consist of a supernumerary nipple or breast tissue, or both, and usually occurs along both milk lines of the thorax and the abdomen. Reconstructive surgical repair is indicated in severe breast asymmetry but is recommended after sex maturity rating 5 has been reached.

FEMALE DISORDERS

MASSES. The most common adolescent breast disorder is a mass, the majority of which are benign cysts or fibroadenomas. Persistence of the mass or its enlargement over three menstrual cycles is an indication for surgical consultation. When multiple small masses are palpable, associated with pain or tenderness and varying with the stage of the menstrual cycle, they are most often fibrocystic lesions. The use of combination oral contraceptives of low progesterone potency may be beneficial. A biopsy is rarely indicated with this presentation. The fibroadenoma tends not to vary in size during the menstrual cycle, often distinguishing it from a cyst. Carcinoma of the breast in the adolescent is rare.

NIPPLE DISCHARGE. Nipple discharge in adolescents is usually due to local stimulation; use of medications, including oral contraceptives; and pregnancy. Benign conditions are associated with a milky, sticky, thick discharge; infection is associated with a purulent discharge; and intraductal papilloma and cancer are associated with a serous, serosanguineous, or bloody discharge.

MALE DISORDERS

Gynecomastia occurs in approximately one third of normal males during early to mid puberty and often causes concern that may not be openly voiced. The response should be factual information and reassurance of its usually transient nature. Other conditions associated with nonpubertal gynecomastia are secondary to endocrine disorders, neoplasms, chronic disease, trauma, and myriad medications as well as to drugs of abuse.

CHAPTER 88

Menstrual Problems

(Nelson Textbook, Chapter 117)

Some variety of menstrual dysfunction occurs in about 50% of adolescent females. Most of the problems are minor; however, severe dysmenorrhea or prolonged menstrual bleeding can be debilitating to a teenager.

NORMAL MENSTRUATION

In a large office-based study in the United States, 35% of white girls and 62% of African-American girls had initiated menses between ages 12 and 13 yr. The age of menarche in Tanner's English series ranges from ages 9–16 yr, with a mean age of 13.46 yr. Menarche usually occurs about 2.3 yr after the initiation of puberty, with a range of 1–3 yr, and becomes regular after 2–2.5 yr. The length of the menstrual cycle from the first day of menses of one cycle to the first day of the next cycle can range from 21–45 days, although the average is about 28 days. The length of blood flow ranges from 2–7 days, with an average of 3–5 days.

AMENORRHEA

CLINICAL MANIFESTATIONS. Amenorrhea, or absence of menses, may be primary or secondary. The diagnosis of primary amenorrhea assumes that the patient has passed the age at which menarche normally occurs, from 10–16 yr. Accordingly, the determination of primary amenorrhea should first be based on an assessment of the patient's stage of pubertal development. If the patient has not entered puberty by the expected time or if pubertal development is completed without the onset of menses, she should be thoroughly evaluated, even if her chronologic age is within the normal range. The distinguishing characteristic of the clinical presentation of amenorrhea is the presence or absence of virilization. Clinical features such as clitoromegaly, hirsutism, or excessive acne are associated with adrenal or ovarian disease. Other clinical presentations such as slender or obese body habitus or short stature also are characteristic of syndromes associated with amenorrhea.

The first consideration in the adolescent who presents with secondary amenorrhea is pregnancy. This possibility also exists, albeit rarely, as a cause of primary amenorrhea, if fertilization of the first released ovum occurred before menses.

DIFFERENTIAL DIAGNOSIS. In *primary amenorrhea*, chromosomal or congenital abnormalities, such as gonadal dysgenesis, the triple X syndrome, isochromosomal abnormalities, testicular feminization syndrome, and, rarely, true hermaphroditism, should be considered in addition to the conditions that cause secondary amenorrhea. When primary amenorrhea occurs with advanced pubertal development, a structural anomaly of the müllerian duct system should be suspected. Imperforate hymen is most common and is associated with recurrent (monthly) abdominal pain and, after some time has passed, a midline lower abdominal mass, the blood-filled vagina, or hematocolpos. Diagnosis is made by inspection of the introitus, revealing a bulging hymen with bluish discoloration. If the obstruction is at the level of the cervix, the blood-filled uterus (hematometrium) is apparent on bimanual examination or ultrasonography.

Primary or secondary amenorrhea may also be caused by chronic illness, particularly that associated with malnutrition or tissue hypoxia, such as diabetes mellitus, inflammatory bowel disease, cystic fibrosis, or cyanotic congenital heart disease. A central nervous system tumor, most commonly a craniopharyngioma, may present as amenorrhea. Abnormalities of the thyroid gland, typically hyperthyroidism, may first be suspected by delayed sexual maturation or amenorrhea, even in the absence of other signs and symptoms.

LABORATORY FINDINGS. The pregnancy test, preferably a qualitative serum (3-subunit human chorionic gonadotropin [hCG]), is the key laboratory test to perform in the evaluation of secondary amenorrhea regardless of the history or sexual activity given by the patient or signs of virilization. The next step for laboratory determinations is performed according to the individual's response to an initial progesterone challenge or after the findings of the vaginal smear for estrogen.

TREATMENT. Determination of the cause of amenorrhea may permit the initiation of corrective intervention. When the disorder is not amenable to remediation, consideration should be given to establishing regular pseudomenses to allow the adolescent to feel like her peers.

ABNORMAL UTERINE BLEEDING

DIFFERENTIAL DIAGNOSIS. Most abnormal vaginal bleeding in adolescents results from anovulatory cycles, normally occurring in the 1st yr of menarche. This is called *dysfunctional uterine bleeding;* this term is used when no demonstrable organic lesion is identified to account for the abnormal bleeding. Organic lesions are found in about 9% of young women aged 10–20 yr, the most common including ectopic pregnancy, threatened abortion, endometritis, and hormonal contraceptives

LABORATORY FINDINGS. The hemoglobin and hematocrit from a complete blood cell count are the most important elements in the initial evaluation. The secondary evaluation should include liver and thyroid function studies, prothrombin time, partial thromboplastin time, and bleeding time.

TREATMENT. In mild cases, iron supplementation is recommended, and the patient should keep a menstrual calendar to follow the subsequent flow patterns. With moderate disturbances, cycling with oral contraceptives, barring any contraindications, should be considered along with monitoring the iron status. Severe bleeding, not requiring hospitalization, can usually be stopped with hormonal therapy, either (1) medroxyprogesterone acetate (Provera) 10 mg/24 hr for 10–14 days; (2) conjugated estrogen (Premarin) 2.5 mg four times a day for 21 days, plus Provera on days 17–21; or (3) a combination oral contraceptive (OC) using two to four pills a days until the bleeding stops, then one pill/day for the remainder of the cycle. Once a patient is hospitalized, Premarin, 20–40 mg every 4 hr up to 24 hr given intravenously, is required.

DYSMENORRHEA

Painful menstrual cramps are experienced by nearly two thirds of postmenarcheal teenagers in the United States. Primary dysmenorrhea is characterized by the absence of any specific pelvic pathologic condition and is the more commonly occurring form. Prostaglandins F_2 and E_2, produced by the endometrium, stimulate the myometrium to contract, producing pain. Secondary dysmenorrhea results from an underlying structural abnormality of the cervix or uterus, a foreign body such as an intrauterine device, endometriosis, or endometritis.

A pelvic examination must be performed to exclude the causes of secondary dysmenorrhea; and if none is found, a diagnosis of primary dysmenorrhea should be considered. Adolescents suffering from dysmenorrhea have high levels of prostaglandins F_2 and E_2 and experience symptomatic relief when prostaglandin synthetase inhibitors are administered.

CHAPTER 89

Contraception

(Nelson Textbook, Chapter 117)

Adolescents bear a disproportionate risk for the adverse consequences of sexual activity, sexually transmitted diseases (STDs), and early unintended pregnancy. They should be encouraged to postpone sexual involvement; however, contraceptive counseling and services should be offered to adolescents who are sexually active.

BARRIER METHODS

CONDOMS. This method prevents sperm from being deposited in the vagina. There are no major side effects associated with the use of a condom. Its effectiveness in preventing pregnancy is low, however, with 15 pregnancies occurring/100 woman-years of use by adult women in the United States. The main advantages of condoms are their low price, availability without prescription, little need for advance planning, and, most important for this age group, their effectiveness in preventing transmission of STDs, including human immunodeficiency virus infection. A female condom is now available over the counter in single-size disposable units.

DIAPHRAGM AND CERVICAL CAP. These methods have few side effects but are much less likely to be used by teenagers.

SPERMICIDES

A variety of agents containing the spermicide nonoxynol-9 are available as foams, jellies, creams, films, or effervescent vaginal suppositories. They must be placed in the vaginal cavity shortly before intercourse and reinserted before each subsequent ejaculation to be effective.

COMBINATION METHODS

The conjoint use of the condom by the male and spermicidal foam by the female adolescent is extremely effective; the failure rate is 2% (perfect use), without any of the potential side effects and complications associated with the use of other forms of contraception having comparable efficacy. This combination also prevents STDs, including human immunodeficiency virus infection.

HORMONAL METHODS

COMBINATION ORAL CONTRACEPTIVES. Oral contraceptives (OCs) are commonly referred to as "the Pill" and currently contain either 50, 35, 30, or 20 μg of estrogenic substance, typically either mestranol or ethinyl estradiol, and a progestin. The Pill is one of the most reliable contraceptive methods available, with a perfect-use pregnancy rate in the range of 0.1%/yr. Typical-use failure rates in women aged 15–19 have ranged up to 18.1%. Thrombophlebitis, hepatic adenomas, myocardial infarction, and carbohydrate intolerance are some of the more serious potential complications of exogenous estrogen use. These disorders are, however, exceedingly rare in adolescents. Major and minor contraindications to the use of estrogen-containing oral contraceptives include hepatocellular disease, migraine headaches, breast disease, and any condition in which hypercoagulability may be a problem (e.g., replaced cardiac valve, thrombophlebitis, sickle cell anemia).

ALL-PROGESTIN CONTRACEPTIVES. Progestin-only contraceptives are available for the adolescent in whom the use of estrogen is potentially deleterious. These agents ("mini-pills") are less reliable in inhibiting ovulation and are associated with a 0.5%/yr pregnancy rate (perfect use).

An injectable progestin, medroxyprogesterone (Depo-Provera, DMPA), is highly effective in birth control, with failure rates typically at 0.3–0.4%. This substance needs to be administered only once every 3 mo and is completely reversible in its anovulatory action.

A long-acting progestational agent, levonorgestrel (Norplant), is contained in six small Silastic tubes that are implanted subcutaneously. The contraceptive potency remains for 5 yr. This method is the most effective of all reversible birth control methods available, with a typical 1st-yr failure rate for all women at 0.09% and 5-yr failure rates at 0.9–1.1%.

EMERGENCY CONTRACEPTION

Outside the United States, several agents are used for emergency contraception: oral high-dose estrogens, high-dose combination estrogen-progestins, high-dose progestins, danazol, mifepristone, and the postcoital insertion of a copper intrauterine device (IUD). The Yuzpe method is most commonly used in the United States, consisting of combination pills totaling 200 μg of ethinyl estradiol and 2.0 mg of norgestrel or 1.0 mg levonorgestrel.

INTRAUTERINE DEVICES

IUDs are small, flexible, plastic objects introduced into the uterine cavity through the cervix. They are effective in preventing pregnancy in 97–99% of women.

CHAPTER 90

Pregnancy
(Nelson Textbook, Chapter 118)

Sexual activity at an early age coupled with nonuse or improper use of contraceptives contributes to a disproportionately high rate of teenage pregnancy in the United States when compared with other industrialized nations.

CLINICAL MANIFESTATIONS. Adolescents may experience the traditional symptoms of pregnancy, that is, morning sickness, swollen tender breasts, weight gain, and amenorrhea; however, the presentation is often more vague. Headache, fatigue, abdominal pain, and scanty or irregular menses are common presenting symptoms. Denial of sexual activity and menstrual irregularity should not preclude the diagnosis in the presence of other clinical or historical information. Pregnancy is still the most common diagnosis when an adolescent presents with secondary amenorrhea.

DIAGNOSIS. On physical examination, the findings of an enlarged uterus, cervical cyanosis (Chadwick sign), or a soft cervix (Goodell sign) are highly suggestive of an intrauterine pregnancy. A confirmatory pregnancy test is recommended. The most commonly used method is a qualitative measurement of the beta subunit for human chorionic gonadotropin (hCG) by blood or urine. The results are positive in 98% of women within 7 days after implantation. The most sensitive test is a quantitative β-hCG radioimmunoassay in which results are reliable within 7 days after fertilization.

TREATMENT. Confidentiality and privacy are key components of counseling the adolescent in whom pregnancy is suspected. The younger the adolescent, the greater should be the concern that the sexual activity may have been coercive. If the adolescent's pregnancy test result is negative, it is prudent to repeat the test in 2 wk. If the adolescent is pregnant, the options available to manage the pregnancy should be presented and discussed in the context of her family, as well as individual, situation. Adolescents should be encouraged to include parents fully in the discussion of their options.

CHAPTER 91

Sexually Transmitted Diseases

(Nelson Textbook, Chapter 119)

The behavioral and physiologic characteristics of adolescence predispose sexually active adolescents to the increased acquisition and adverse consequences of sexually transmitted diseases (STDs).

CLINICAL MANIFESTATIONS. STD syndromes are generally characterized by the location of the manifestation (vaginitis) or the type of lesion (genital ulcer). In addition, certain constellations of presenting symptoms suggest the inclusion of a possible STD in the differential diagnosis (Table 91–1).

Urethritis. Urethritis is an inflammation of the urethra classically presenting as a urethral discharge or dysuria, or both. Urgency, frequency of urination, erythema of the urethral meatus, and scrotal pain are less common clinical presentations. Asymptomatic or minimally symptomatic presentations are common in males.

TABLE 91–1 Sexually Transmitted Disease Clinical Syndromes

Sexually Transmitted Disease Syndromes

Urethritis
Epididymitis
Vaginitis (vulvitis)
Cervicitis
Pelvic inflammatory disease
Genital ulcer disease
Genital lesions and ectoparasites

Conditions Suggestive of Sexually Transmitted Disease

Lower abdominal pain (female)
Scrotal swelling and pain
Arthritis
Exanthem, alopecia
Pharyngitis
Conjunctivitis
Hepatitis, perihepatitis
Local and generalized lymphadenitis
Proctitis

From Morse SA, Moreland AA, Holmes KK: Atlas of Sexually Transmitted Diseases and AIDS, 2nd ed. London, Mosby-Wolfe, 1996.

Chlamydia trachomatis and Neisseria gonorrhoeae are the most common pathogens.

Epididymitis. The inflammation of the epididymis in adolescent males, unlike that in adult males, is most often associated with an STD. The same pathogens associated with urethritis are prevalent. The presentation of scrotal swelling and tenderness, associated with the history of a spontaneously resolving urethral discharge, constitute the presumptive diagnosis of epididymitis. Males who practice insertive anal intercourse are also vulnerable to *Escherichia coli* infection.

Vaginitis (Vulvitis). Vaginitis is a superficial infection of the vaginal mucosa frequently presenting as a vaginal discharge, with or without vulvar involvement. Pruritus and the presence of an odor help differentiate the cause of the infection. Colonization without infection, as in bacterial vaginosis, can also present as a vaginal discharge. Trichomoniasis and candidiasis, together with bacterial vaginosis, are the predominant diseases associated with vaginal discharge.

Cervicitis. The inflammatory process in cervicitis involves the deeper structures in the mucous membrane of the cervix uteri. Vaginal discharge can be a manifestation of cervicitis if the cervical discharge is profuse. Less subtle clinical manifestations of cervicitis are irregular or postcoital bleeding, mucopurulent discharge from the os, and a friable cervix. The pathogens associated most commonly with cervicitis are *C. trachomatis* and *N. gonorrhoeae.*

Pelvic Inflammatory Disease (PID). A spectrum of inflammatory disorders of the upper genital tract in females is encompassed under the diagnosis of PID. The spectrum includes endometritis, salpingitis, tubo-ovarian abscess, and pelvic peritonitis, usually in combination rather than as separate entities. *N. gonorrhoeae* and *C. trachomatis* predominate as the involved pathogenic organisms in younger adolescents. The clinical diagnosis of PID is based on the minimal criteria of lower abdominal tenderness, adnexal tenderness, and cervical motion tenderness in a sexually active female adolescent with no other causes for illness.

Genital Ulcer Syndromes. An ulcerative lesion in a mucosal area exposed to sexual contact is the unifying characteristic of diseases associated with these syndromes. Herpes simplex virus, *Treponema pallidum* (syphilis), and *Haemophilus ducreyi* (chancroid) are the organisms associated with genital ulcer syndromes.

Genital Lesions and Ectoparasites. Lesions that present as outgrowths on the surface of the epithelium and other limited epidermal lesions are included under this categorization of syndromes. Human papillomavirus with its association to cervical cancer causes the most concern for the long-term outcome for individuals infected during adolescence.

Human Immunodeficiency Virus Disease and Hepatitis B. HIV disease presents as an asymptomatic, unexpected occurrence in most infected adolescents.

DIAGNOSIS. Health screening guidelines recommend testing for STDs in asymptomatic patients on an annual basis.

In symptomatic patients, based on the clinical presentation, further evaluations may be needed to identify the causative agent of the syndrome accurately.

TREATMENT. The Centers for Disease Control and Prevention guidelines offer treatment options for uncomplicated urethritis, cervicitis, and vaginal discharges that reduce patient noncompliance by the use of single-dose oral medications.

PART 12

The Immunologic System and Disorders

CHAPTER 92

The Child with Suspected Immunodeficiency

(Nelson Textbook, Chapters 122 and 123)

Children with recurrent infections are among the most frequent types of patients seen by primary care physicians. Most patients with recurrent infections do not have an identifiable immunodeficiency disorder. However, primary care physicians must have a high index of suspicion if defects of the immune system are to be diagnosed early enough that appropriate treatment can be instituted before irreversible damage is done. Evaluations of immune

---

TABLE 92–1 Initial Immunologic Testing of the Child with Recurrent Infections

Complete Blood Cell Count, Manual Differential, and Erythrocyte Sedimentation Rate

Absolute lymphocyte count (normal result makes T-cell defect unlikely)
Absolute neutrophil count (normal result precludes congenital or acquired neutropenia and [usually] both forms of leukocyte adhesion deficiency, in which elevated counts are present even between infections)
Platelet count (normal result excludes Wiskott-Aldrich syndrome)
Howell-Jolly bodies (absence rules against asplenia)
Erythrocyte sedimentation rate (normal result indicates chronic bacterial or fungal infection unlikely)

Screening Tests for B-Cell Defects

IgA measurement; if abnormal, IgG and IgM measurement
Isohemagglutinins
Antibody titers to tetanus, diphtheria, *Haemophilus influenzae,* and pneumococci

Screening Tests for T-Cell Defects

Absolute lymphocyte count (normal result indicates T-cell defect unlikely)
Candida albicans intradermal skin test: 0.1 mL of a 1:1000 dilution for patients older than 6 yr, 0.1 mL of a 1:100 dilution for patients younger than 6 yr

Screening Tests for Phagocytic Cell Defects

Absolute neutrophil count
Respiratory burst assay

Screening Test for Complement Deficiency

CH_{50}

---

function should be initiated for children with clinical manifestations of a specific immune disorder or with unusual, chronic, or recurrent infections.

Familiarity with certain clinical guidelines aids in the initial selection of tests. Patients with deficiencies of antibodies, phagocytic cells, or complement have recurrent infections with encapsulated bacteria. Thus, patients with only repeated viral infections (with the exception of persistent enterovirus infections) are not as likely to have any of these disorders. Children with defects in these components of the immune system may grow and develop normally, despite their recurring infections, unless they develop bronchiectasis from repeated lower respiratory tract bacterial infections or persistent enteroviral infections of the central nervous system. By contrast, patients with deficiencies in T-cell function usually develop opportunistic infections early in life and fail to thrive.

Most immunologic defects can be excluded at minimal cost with the proper choice of screening tests (Table 92–1). Patients found to have abnormalities on any screening tests should be characterized as fully as possible before any type of immunologic treatment is begun, unless there is a life-threatening illness. If results of the initial screening including the complete blood cell count, immunoglobulin levels, and complement levels are normal, evaluations of T-cell and phagocytic cell functions may be indicated for patients with recurrent or unusual bacterial infections.

CHAPTER 93

Primary B-Cell Diseases

(Nelson Textbook, Chapter 124)

Of all of the primary immunodeficiency diseases, those affecting B-cell function are most frequent. Patients with antibody deficiency are usually recognized because they have recurrent infections with encapsulated bacteria or a history of failure responding to antibiotic treatment, but some individuals with selective IgA deficiency or infants with transient hypogammaglobulinemia may have few or no infections.

X-LINKED (BRUTON) AGAMMAGLOBULINEMIA (XLA)

CLINICAL MANIFESTATIONS. Most boys afflicted with XLA remain well during the first 6–9 mo of life by virtue of maternally transmitted IgG antibodies. Thereafter, they acquire infections with extracellular pyogenic organisms such as *Streptococcus pneumoniae* and *Haemophilus influenzae* unless given prophylactic antibiotics or immunoglobulin therapy. Viral infections are also usually handled normally, with the exceptions of hepatitis viruses and enteroviruses.

The diagnosis of XLA is suspected if serum concentrations of IgG, IgA, IgM, and IgE are far below the 95% confidence limits for appropriate age- and race-matched controls (i.e., usually <100 mg/dL total immunoglobulin) and circulating B cells are absent. Tests for natural antibodies to blood group substances and for antibodies to antigens given during standard courses of immunization are useful in distinguishing this disorder from transient hypogammaglobulinemia of infancy. Hypoplasia of adenoids, tonsils, and peripheral lymph nodes is the rule.

COMMON VARIABLE IMMUNODEFICIENCY (CVID)

CLINICAL MANIFESTATIONS. Patients with CVID often have autoantibody formation and normal-sized or enlarged tonsils and lymph nodes, and approximately 25% of patients have splenomegaly. CVID has also been associated with a spruelike syndrome, thymoma, alopecia areata, hemolytic anemia, gastric atrophy, achlorhydria, and pernicious anemia.

SELECTIVE IgA DEFICIENCY

CLINICAL MANIFESTATIONS. Infections occur predominantly in the respiratory, gastrointestinal, and urogenital tracts. Bacterial agents responsible are the same as in other antibody deficiency syndromes. Serum concentrations of other immunoglobulins are usually normal in patients with selective IgA deficiency, although IgG_2 (and other) subclass deficiency is reported. Serum antibodies to IgA are reported in as many as 44% of patients with selective IgA deficiency. If of the IgE isotype, these antibodies can cause severe or fatal anaphylactic reactions after intravenous administration of blood products containing IgA. For this reason, only five-times-washed (in 200-mL volumes) normal donor erythrocytes or blood products from other IgA absent individuals should be administered to these patients. Many intravenous immunoglobulin (IVIG) preparations contain sufficient IgA to cause anaphylactic reactions.

TRANSIENT HYPOGAMMAGLOBULINEMIA OF INFANCY

After birth, the levels of serum antibodies in an infant diminish with the decline of maternally derived antibodies, reaching a nadir at 3–4 mo of age, and then rise as an infant's own IgG production gradually increases. Extension of hypogammaglobulinemia beyond 6 mo of age is termed *transient hypogammaglobulinemia of infancy.*

IgG SUBCLASS DEFICIENCIES

Some patients have deficiencies of one or more subclasses of IgG, despite normal or elevated total IgG serum concentrations. Most patients with absent or very low concentrations of IgG_2 have IgA deficiency. IVIG should not be given to IgG subclass-deficient patients unless they are shown to have a deficiency of antibodies to a broad array of antigens.

X-LINKED LYMPHOPROLIFERATIVE DISEASE (XLP)

XLP, also referred to as Duncan disease, is an X-linked recessive trait characterized by an inadequate immune response to infection with Epstein-Barr virus (EBV). The mean age at presentation is less than 5 yr. The most common form of presentation (75%) is severe EBV infection with 80% mortality, primarily due to extensive liver necrosis. Most patients surviving the primary infection develop global cellular immune defects involving T, B, and natural killer (NK) cells; lymphomas; or hypogammaglobulinemia.

TREATMENT OF B-CELL DEFECTS

Judicious use of antibiotics and regular administration of antibodies are the only effective treatments for B-cell disorders. The most common form of replacement therapy is with IVIG. IVIG, 400 mg/kg/mo, achieves trough IgG levels close to the normal range. Systemic reactions to IVIG may occur, but rarely are these true anaphylactic reactions.

CHAPTER 94

Primary T-Cell Diseases

(Nelson Textbook, Chapter 125)

In general, patients with defects in T-cell function have infections or other clinical problems that are more severe than in patients with antibody deficiency disorders. These individuals rarely survive beyond infancy or childhood.

THYMIC HYPOPLASIA (DIGEORGE SYNDROME)

Thymic hypoplasia results from dysmorphogenesis of the 3rd and 4th pharyngeal pouches during early embryogenesis, leading to hypoplasia or aplasia of the thymus and parathyroid glands. Other structures forming at the same age are also frequently affected, resulting in anomalies of the great vessels (right-sided aortic arch), esophageal atresia, bifid uvula, congenital heart disease (atrial and ventricular septal defects), a short philtrum, hypertelorism, an antimongoloid slant to the eyes, mandibular hypoplasia, and low-set, often notched ears. The diagnosis is often first suggested by hypocalcemic seizures during the neonatal period.

CLINICAL MANIFESTATIONS. A variable degree of hypoplasia of the thymus and parathyroid glands is more frequent than total aplasia. Children with variable hypoplasia are referred to as having partial DiGeorge syndrome; they may have little trouble with infections and grow normally. Patients with complete DiGeorge syndrome resemble patients with severe combined immunodeficiency in their susceptibility to infections with low-grade or opportunistic pathogens, including fungi, viruses, and *Pneumocystis carinii*, and to graft-versus-host disease from nonirradiated blood transfusions. Concentrations of serum immunoglobulins are usually normal, but those of IgA may be diminished and those of IgE elevated. Absolute lymphocyte counts are usually only moderately low for age. The CD3-positive T-cell counts are variably decreased in number, corresponding to the degree of thymic hypoplasia, and as a result the percentage of B cells is increased.

TREATMENT. The immune deficiency in the complete DiGeorge syndrome has been corrected by thymic tissue transplants and by unfractionated HLA-identical bone marrow transplantation.

X-LINKED IMMUNODEFICIENCY WITH HYPER-IgM (HYPER IgM)

X-linked immunodeficiency with hyper-IgM, or hyper-IgM syndrome, is characterized by very low serum concentrations of IgG and IgA with a normal or, more frequently, a markedly elevated concentration of polyclonal IgM.

CLINICAL MANIFESTATIONS. Like patients with X-linked agammaglobulinemia (XLA), affected boys become symptomatic during the 1st or 2nd year of life with recurrent pyogenic infections, including otitis media, sinusitis, pneumonia, and tonsillitis. In contrast to patients with XLA, the frequent presence of lymphoid hyperplasia often leads away from a diagnosis of immunodeficiency. The frequency of autoimmune disorders is even higher than it is with other antibody-deficiency syndromes.

CHAPTER 95

Combined B- and T-Cell Diseases

(Nelson Textbook, Chapter 126)

Patients with combined B- and T-cell defects have severe, frequently opportunistic infections that lead to death in infancy or childhood without bone marrow transplantation early in life.

COMBINED IMMUNODEFICIENCY

Combined immunodeficiency (CID) is distinguished from severe immunodeficiency (SCID) by low but not absent T-cell function. Patients with CID have recurrent or chronic pulmonary infections, failure to thrive, oral or cutaneous candidiasis, chronic diarrhea, recurrent skin infections, gram-negative sepsis, urinary tract infections, or severe varicella in infancy. Neutropenia and eosinophilia are common. Serum immunoglobulins may be normal or elevated for all classes, but selective IgA deficiency, marked elevation of IgE, and elevated IgD levels occur in some cases. Although antibody-forming capacity is impaired in most patients, it is not absent.

PURINE NUCLEOSIDE PHOSPHORYLASE (PNP) DEFICIENCY

Point mutations identified in the PNP gene on chromosome 14q13.1 account for these deficiencies. In contrast to adenosine deaminase (ADA) deficiency, in this condition, serum and urinary uric acid are usually markedly deficient and no characteristic physical or skeletal abnormalities have been noted. Deaths result from generalized vaccinia, varicella, lymphosarcoma, and graft-versus-host disease. Two thirds of patients have neurologic abnormalities, and one third have autoimmune diseases. Lymphopenia is striking. Bone marrow transplantation is the only successful form of therapy.

CARTILAGE HAIR HYPOPLASIA

This unusual form of short-limbed dwarfism with frequent and severe infections occurs among the Pennsylvania Amish; non-Amish patients have been described. Features include short, pudgy hands; redundant skin; hyperextensible joints of hands and feet but an inability to extend the elbows completely; and fine, sparse, light hair and eyebrows. Severe and often fatal varicella infections, progressive vaccinia, and vaccine-associated poliomyelitis have been observed. The severity of the immunodeficiency varies.

SEVERE COMBINED IMMUNODEFICIENCY

The syndromes of SCID are caused by diverse genetic mutations that lead to absence of all adaptive immune function. Patients with this group of disorders have the most severe of all of the recognized immunodeficiencies.

CLINICAL MANIFESTATIONS. Affected infants present within the first few months of life with diarrhea, pneumonia, otitis, sepsis, and cutaneous infections. Growth may appear normal initially, but extreme wasting usually ensues after diarrhea and infections begin. Persistent infections with opportunistic organisms such as *Candida albicans, Pneumocystis carinii,* varicella, measles, parainfluenza 3, CMV, Epstein-Barr virus (EBV), and bacillus Calmette-Guérin (BCG) lead to death. Affected infants also lack the ability to reject foreign tissue and are therefore at risk for graft-versus-host disease from maternal immunocompetent T cells crossing the placenta or from T lymphocytes in nonirradiated blood products or allogeneic bone marrow. Infants with SCID have lymphopenia. Patients with ADA deficiency have the lowest absolute lymphocyte counts, usually less than 500/mm^3. Serum immunoglobulin concentrations are diminished to absent, and no antibody formation occurs after immunization. T cells are extremely low or absent in all types.

TREATMENT. This is a true pediatric emergency: unless immunologic reconstitution is achieved through bone marrow transplantation, death usually occurs in the 1st year of life and almost invariably before the end of the 2nd yr. If diagnosed at birth or within the first 3 mo of life, 95% of cases can be treated successfully with HLA-identical or T-cell–depleted haploidentical bone marrow stem cells.

X-Linked Severe Combined Immunodeficiency

X-linked SCID (XSCID) is the most common form of SCID in the United States, accounting for approximately 47% of cases. Clinically, immunologically, and histopathologically, affected individuals appear similar to those with other forms of SCID except for having uniformly low percentages of T and NK cells and an elevated percentage of B cells (T−, B+, NK−).

Autosomal Recessive SCID

ADA DEFICIENCY. An absence of the enzyme ADA is observed in approximately 15% of patients with SCID, resulting from various point and deletion mutations in the ADA gene. ADA-deficient patients usually have a much more profound lymphopenia than do infants with other types of SCID, with mean absolute lymphocyte counts of less than 500/mm^3; they rarely have elevated percentages of B or NK cells. Milder forms of this condition have been reported as leading to delayed diagnosis of immunodeficiency, even to adulthood. Other distinguishing features of ADA-deficient SCID include the presence of rib cage abnormalities similar to a rachitic rosary and numerous skeletal abnormalities of chondro-osseous dysplasia, which occur predominantly at the costochondral junctions, at the apophyses of the iliac bones, and in the vertebral bodies. ADA deficiency can be cured by HLA-identical or haploidentical T-cell–depleted bone marrow transplantation without the need for pretransplant or post-transplant chemotherapy; this remains the treatment of choice.

DEFECTIVE EXPRESSION OF MAJOR HISTOCOMPATIBILITY COMPLEX (MHC) ANTIGENS

MHC CLASS I ANTIGEN DEFICIENCY. An isolated deficiency of MHC class I antigens is rare, and the resulting immunodeficiency is much milder than in SCID, contributing to a later age at presentation. Sera from affected children contain normal quantities of MHC class I antigens and β_2-microglobulin, but MHC class I antigens are not detected on any cells in the body.

MHC CLASS II ANTIGEN DEFICIENCY. Many affected with this autosomal recessive syndrome are of North African descent. Patients present in early infancy with persistent diarrhea that is often associated with cryptosporidiosis and enteroviral infections (poliovirus, coxsackievirus). They also have an increased frequency of infections with herpesviruses and other viruses, oral candidiasis, bacterial pneumonia, *P. carinii* pneumonia, and septicemia. MHC class II–deficient patients have a very low number of CD4-positive T cells but normal or elevated numbers of CD8-positive T cells. Lymphopenia is only moderate. The MHC class II antigens HLA-DP, DQ, and DR are undetectable on blood B cells and monocytes, even though B cells are present in normal number. Patients are hypogammaglobulinemic. The thymus and other lymphoid organs are severely hypoplastic.

OMENN SYNDROME

Omenn syndrome of CID with hypereosinophilia is an autosomal recessively inherited, fatal condition characterized by profound susceptibility to infection, with T-cell infiltration of skin, intestines, liver, and spleen, leading to an exfoliative erythroderma, lymphadenopathy, hepatosplenomegaly, and intractable diarrhea. Infants so affected have a persistent leukocytosis with marked eosinophilia; elevated serum IgE; low IgG, IgA, and IgM; low or absent blood B cells; and elevated numbers of T cells but impaired T-cell function due to restricted heterogeneity of the host T-cell repertoire.

IMMUNODEFICIENCY WITH THROMBOCYTOPENIA AND ECZEMA (WISKOTT-ALDRICH SYNDROME)

Wiskott-Aldrich syndrome, an X-linked recessive syndrome, is characterized by atopic dermatitis, thrombocytopenic purpura with normal-appearing megakaryocytes but small defective platelets, and undue susceptibility to infection.

CLINICAL MANIFESTATIONS. Patients often have prolonged bleeding from the circumcision site or bloody diarrhea during infancy. The thrombocytopenia is not initially due to antiplatelet antibodies. Atopic dermatitis and recurrent infections usually develop during the 1st year of life. Infections are caused by pneumococci and other bacteria having polysaccharide capsules, resulting in otitis media, pneumonia, meningitis, or sepsis. Later, infections with agents such as *P. carinii* and the herpesviruses become more frequent. Survival beyond the teens is rare; infections, bleeding, and EBV-induced malignancy are major causes of death.

ATAXIA-TELANGIECTASIA

CLINICAL MANIFESTATIONS. The most prominent clinical features are progressive cerebellar ataxia, oculocutaneous telangiectasia, chronic sinopulmonary disease, a high incidence of malignancy, and variable humoral and cellular immunodeficiency. Ataxia typically becomes evident soon after children begin to walk and progresses until they are confined to a wheelchair, usually by the age of 10–12 yr. The telangiectasia develops between 3 and 6 yr of age.

DIAGNOSIS. The most frequent humoral immunologic abnormality is the selective absence of IgA, found in 50–80% of these patients. The thymus is very hypoplastic.

HYPERIMMUNOGLOBULINEMIA E (HYPER-IgE) SYNDROME

The hyper-IgE syndrome is a relatively rare primary immunodeficiency syndrome characterized by recurrent severe staphylococcal abscesses and markedly elevated levels of serum IgE.

CLINICAL MANIFESTATIONS. These patients have histories from infancy of staphylococcal abscesses involving the skin, lungs, joints, and other sites; persistent pneumatoceles develop as a result of their recurrent pneumonias. Laboratory features include exceptionally high serum IgE concentrations.

TREATMENT. The most effective therapy is long-term administration of therapeutic doses of a penicillinase-resistant antibiotic, adding other agents as required for specific infections. Intravenous immunoglobulin (IVIG) should be administered to antibody-deficient patients, and appropriate thoracic surgery should be provided for superinfected pneumatoceles or those persisting beyond 6 mo.

TREATMENT OF CELLULAR IMMUNODEFICIENCY

Transplantation of MHC-compatible or haploidentical (half-matched) parental bone marrow is the treatment of choice for patients with fatal T-cell or combined T- and B-cell defects. The major risk to the recipient from transplants of bone marrow is that of graft-versus-host disease.

CHAPTER 96

Disorders of Phagocyte Function

(Nelson Textbook, Chapters 127, 128, and 129)

LEUKOCYTE ADHESION DEFICIENCY

Leukocyte adhesion deficiency-1 (LAD-1) and -2 (LAD-2) are rare autosomal recessive disorders of leukocyte function. LAD-1 affects about 1 in 1 million individuals and is characterized by recurrent bacterial and fungal infections and depressed inflammatory responses despite striking blood neutrophilia.

CLINICAL MANIFESTATIONS. Patients with the severe clinical form express less than 0.3% of the normal amount of the β_2 integrins, whereas patients with the moderate phenotype may express 2–7% of the normal amount of β_2 integrin molecules. Children with severe disease present in infancy with recurrent, indolent bacterial infections of the skin, mouth, respiratory tract, lower intestinal tract, and genital mucosa. They may have a history of delayed separation of the umbilical cord, usually with associated infection of the cord stump. Skin infection may progress to large chronic ulcers with polymicrobial infection, including the presence of anaerobic organisms. The pathogens infecting patients with LAD-1 are similar to those affecting patients with severe neutropenia and include *Staphylococcus aureus* and enteric gram-negative organisms. These patients are also susceptible to fungal infections. As in profound neutropenia, the typical signs of inflammation—swelling, erythema, and warmth—may be absent. Pus does not form. Despite the paucity of neutrophils within the affected tissue, the circulating neutrophil count during infection may typically exceed 30,000/μL and can surpass 100,000/μL.

LABORATORY FINDINGS. The diagnosis of LAD-1 is made most readily by flow cytometric measurements of surface CD11b in stimulated and unstimulated neutrophils using monoclonal antibodies directed against CD11b.

TREATMENT. Treatment of LAD-1 depends on the phenotype as determined by the level of expression of functional CD11/CD18 integrins. Early allogeneic bone marrow transplantation is the treatment of choice for severe LAD-1 associated with complete absence of the CD11/CD18 integrins. Other treatment is largely supportive.

CHÉDIAK-HIGASHI SYNDROME (CHS)

CHS is a rare autosomal recessive disorder characterized by increased susceptibility to infection due to defective degranulation of neutrophils, a mild bleeding diathesis, partial oculocutaneous albinism, progressive peripheral neuropathy, and a tendency to develop a life-threatening lymphoma-like syndrome.

CLINICAL MANIFESTATIONS. Patients with CHS have light skin and silvery hair. They frequently complain of solar sensitivity and photophobia. Other signs and symptoms vary considerably, but frequent infections and neuropathy are common. The infections involve mucous membranes, skin, and the respiratory tract. The neuropathy may be sensory or motor in type, and ataxia may be a prominent feature.

LABORATORY FINDINGS. The diagnosis of CHS is established by finding large inclusions in all nucleated blood cells.

TREATMENT. High-dose ascorbic acid (200 mg/24hr for infants, 2000 mg/24 hr for adults) improves the clinical status of some children in the stable phase. The only curative therapy for the accelerated phase is bone marrow transplantation from an HLA-compatible donor or an unrelated donor compatible at the D locus. However, bone marrow transplantation does not correct or prevent the peripheral neuropathy.

MYELOPEROXIDASE DEFICIENCY

Myeloperoxidase (MPO) deficiency is a disorder of oxidative metabolism and is one of the most common inherited disorders of phagocytes. MPO deficiency usually is clinically silent. There is no specific therapy.

CHRONIC GRANULOMATOUS DISEASE

Chronic granulomatous disease (CGD) is characterized by the ability of neutrophils and monocytes to ingest but their inability to kill catalase-positive microorganisms because of a defect in the generation of microbial oxygen metabolites.

CLINICAL MANIFESTATIONS. Any patient with recurrent or unusual lymphadenitis, hepatic abscesses, osteomyelitis at multiple sites, a family history of recurrent infections, or unusual infections with catalase-positive organisms (e.g., *Staphylococcus aureus*) requires clinical evaluation for this disorder. The onset of clinical signs and symptoms may occur from early infancy to young adulthood. The attack rate and severity of infections are exceedingly variable.

TREATMENT. Marrow transplantation is the only known cure for CGD. Vigorous supportive care along with recombinant interferon-γ is used before transplantation. As part of supportive care, patients with CGD should be given daily oral trimethoprim-sulfamethoxazole for infection prophylaxis.

CHAPTER 97

Leukopenia

(Nelson Textbook, Chapter 131)

NEUTROPENIA

Neutropenia is an absolute neutrophil count (ANC = total white blood cell count/µl × percent of neutrophils and bands) more than 2 standard deviations below the normal mean. Normal neutrophil counts must be stratified for age and race. For whites, the lower limit of normal for the neutrophil count is 1500/µL; for blacks, the lower limit of normal is 1200/µL.

INFECTIOUS CAUSES. Transient neutropenia often accompanies viral infections. Neutropenia associated with common childhood viral disease occurs during the first 1–2 days of illness and may persist for 3–8 days.

DRUG-INDUCED NEUTROPENIA. Drug use remains one of the most common causes of neutropenia. Immune-mediated neutropenia usually lasts for 1 wk and is thought to arise from effects of drugs, such as propylthiouracil or penicillin, that act as haptens to stimulate antibody formation. Other drugs, including the antipsychotic drugs such as the phenothiazines, can cause neutropenia when given in toxic amounts. In contrast, idiosyncratic reactions, such as to chloramphenicol, are unpredictable with regard to dose or duration of use. The use of anticancer drugs or radiation therapy (especially therapy directed at the pelvis or sternum) is a common cause of neutropenia.

BONE MARROW REPLACEMENT. Various acquired disorders may lead to neutropenia accompanied by anemia and thrombocytopenia. The most important among these are hematologic malignancies, including leukemia and lymphoma, and metastatic solid tumors such as neuroblastoma, rhabdomyosarcoma, and Ewing sarcoma that infiltrate the bone marrow and lead to suppression of myelopoiesis.

RETICULOENDOTHELIAL SEQUESTRATION. Splenic enlargement resulting from intrinsic splenic disease, portal hypertension, or other causes of splenic hyperplasia can lead to neutropenia. The neutropenia often is mild to moderate and accompanied by a corresponding degree of thrombocytopenia and anemia, and it may be corrected by successfully treating the underlying disease.

IMMUNE NEUTROPENIA. Immune neutropenias are associated with the presence of circulating antineutrophil antibodies.

Alloimmune Neonatal Neutropenia (ANN). This form of neonatal neutropenia occurs after transplacental transfer of maternal alloantibodies directed against antigens on the infant's neutrophils, analogous to Rh hemolytic disease. Symptomatic infants may present with delayed separation of the umbilical cord, mild skin infections, fever, and pneumonia within the first 2 weeks of life.

Autoimmune Neutropenia. Autoimmune neutropenia is analogous to autoimmune hemolytic anemia and thrombocytopenia.

Neonatal Autoimmune Neutropenia. Mothers with autoimmune disease may give birth to infants who develop transient neutropenia.

INEFFECTIVE MYELOPOIESIS. Ineffective myelopoiesis may be acquired as a result of deficiency of vitamin B_{12} or folic acid. Megaloblastic pancytopenia also can result from extended use of antibiotics such as trimethoprim-sulfamethoxazole and from the use of phenytoin.

INTRINSIC DISORDERS OF PROLIFERATION AND MATURATION OF MYELOID STEM CELLS. These rare patients frequently benefit from recombinant human granulocyte colony-stimulating factor (rhG-CSF) therapy.

Cyclic Neutropenia. Cyclic neutropenia is characterized by regular, periodic oscillation in the number of peripheral neutrophils from normal to neutropenic values. The mean oscillatory period is 21 ± 3 days. During the neutropenic phase, most patients suffer from oral ulcers, fever, stomatitis, or pharyngitis, occasionally associated with lymph node enlargement.

Shwachman-Diamond Syndrome. Shwachman-Diamond syndrome is an autosomal recessive disorder characterized by digestive abnormalities and abnormally low white blood cell counts. The initial symptoms of this syndrome are usually diarrhea and failure to thrive because of insufficient absorption of nutrients.

Cartilage-Hair Hypoplasia. Cartilage-hair hypoplasia is a multisystem autosomal recessive disorder characterized by short limbs and short stature resulting from abnormal development of long bone cartilage.

CLINICAL MANIFESTATIONS. Individuals with neutrophil counts below $500/\mu L$ are at substantial risk for developing infections, primarily from their endogenous flora as well as from nosocomial organisms. The clinical presentation in most patients with profound neutropenia is temperature exceeding 101°F, cellulitis, and furunculosis. Stomatitis, gingivitis, perirectal inflammation, colitis, sinusitis, and otitis media are frequent accompaniments of profound neutropenia in children.

TREATMENT. The management of acquired transient neutropenia associated with malignancies, myelosuppressive chemotherapy, or immunosuppressive chemotherapy differs from that of congenital or chronic forms of neutropenia. In the former situation, infections sometimes are heralded only by fever, and sepsis is a major cause of death. Early recognition and treatment of infections may be lifesaving.

Therapy for severe chronic neutropenia is dictated by the clinical manifestations. Patients with benign neutropenia and no evidence of repeated bacterial infections or chronic gingivitis require no specific therapy. Superficial infections in children with mild to moderate neutropenia may be treated with appropriate oral antibiotics. However, in patients who have life-threatening infections, broad-spectrum intravenous antibiotics should be started promptly.

LYMPHOPENIA

Lymphocytopenia per se usually causes no symptoms and is often detected in the evaluation of other illnesses, particularly recurrent viral, fungal, and parasitic infections. Acquired immunodeficiency syndrome is the most common infectious disease associated with lymphocytopenia. Other viral and bacterial diseases may be associated with lymphocytopenia. Iatrogenic lymphocytopenia is caused by cytotoxic chemotherapy, radiation therapy, or long-term administration of antilymphocyte globulin.

CHAPTER 98

Leukocytosis

(Nelson Textbook, Chapter 132)

Leukocytosis is an elevation in the total white blood cell (WBC) count that is 2 standard deviations above the mean count for a particular age. A WBC count exceeding 50,000/μL is termed a *leukemoid reaction* because of the simulation of the features of leukemia. Leukemoid reactions are usually neutrophilic and are most frequently associated with septicemia and severe bacterial infections.

NEUTROPHILIA. During the first day of life, the upper limit of the normal neutrophil count ranges from 7,000–12,000/μL. Thereafter, in the 1st mo of life the neutrophil count is 1,800–5,400/μL. By 1 yr of age, the range of the neutrophil count is 1,500–8,500/μL.

Acute Acquired Neutrophilia. Neutrophilia is usually an acquired disorder and is a common finding with inflammation, infection, injury, or stress. Acute or chronic bacterial infections, trauma, and surgery are among the most common causes encountered in clinical practice.

Chronic Acquired Neutrophilia. Chronic neutrophilia is usually associated with continued stimulation of neutrophil production resulting from persistent inflammatory reactions or infections such as those occurring with tuberculosis, vasculitis, postsplenectomy states, Hodgkin disease, chronic myelogenous leukemia, chronic blood loss, and the prolonged administration of corticosteroids.

MONOCYTOSIS. Monocytosis is often a sign of an acute bacterial, viral, protozoal, or rickettsial infection. Chronic inflammatory conditions can stimulate sustained monocytosis.

LYMPHOCYTOSIS. Chronic bacterial infections such as tuberculosis and brucellosis may lead to a sustained lymphocytosis. Pertussis is accompanied by lymphocytosis. The viral diseases classically associated with lymphocytosis are infectious mononucleosis, cytomegalovirus infection, and viral hepatitis.

CHAPTER 99

Disorders of the Complement System
(Nelson Textbook, Chapter 134)

PRIMARY DEFICIENCIES OF COMPLEMENT COMPONENTS

Congenital deficiencies of all 11 proteins of the classical and membrane attack pathway and of factors D and B of the alternative pathway have been described. Most patients with primary deficiency of C1q have had systemic lupus erythematosus (SLE), an SLE-like syndrome without typical SLE serology, a chronic rash that has shown an underlying vasculitis on biopsy, or membranoproliferative glomerulonephritis (MPGN). Like individuals with C1q deficiency, patients with C1r, C1r/C1s, C4, C2, and C3 deficiencies have had a high incidence of vasculitis syndrome. More than half of the individuals reported to have congenital C5, C6, C7, or C8 deficiency have had meningococcal meningitis or extragenital gonococcal infection.

DEFICIENCIES OF PLASMA, MEMBRANE, OR SERIAL COMPLEMENT CONTROL PROTEINS

Congenital deficiencies of five plasma complement control proteins have been described. Hereditary angioedema occurs in persons born without the ability to synthesize normally functioning C1 inhibitor (C1 INH). Episodic, localized, nonpitting edema results from the vasodilatory effects of the kinin on the postcapillary venule. Swelling of the affected part progresses rapidly, without urticaria, itching, discoloration, or redness, and often without severe pain. Swelling of the intestinal wall, however, can lead to intense abdominal cramping, sometimes with vomiting or diarrhea; concurrent subcutaneous edema is often absent. Laryngeal edema can be fatal. Attacks last 2–3 days and then gradually abate. They may occur at sites of trauma, after vigorous exercise, with menses, or with emotional stress. Attacks can begin in the first 2 yr of life but are usually not severe until late childhood or adolescence.

SECONDARY DISORDERS OF COMPLEMENT

Partial deficiency of C1q has occurred in patients with severe combined immunodeficiency disease or hypogammaglobulinemia. Serum from patients with chronic MPGN contains a protein termed *nephritic factor* (NeF) that promotes activation of the alternative pathway.

Newborns are known to have mild to moderate deficiencies of all plasma components of the complement system. Patients with malnutrition or anorexia nervosa may also have significant depletion of components and functional activity of complement. Patients with sickle cell disease have normal activity of the classical pathway. Burns can induce massive activation of the complement system, especially the alternative pathway, within a few hours after injury.

TREATMENT OF DISORDERS OF THE COMPLEMENT SYSTEM

No specific therapy is available at present for genetic deficiencies of the complement system except hereditary angioedema, but much can be done to protect patients with any of these disorders from serious complications. Management of hereditary angioedema starts with avoidance of precipitating factors, usually trauma. Infusion of vapor-heated C1 INH concentrate aborts acute attacks and is safe and effective in long-term prophylaxis or in preparation for surgery or dental procedures. Adults with hereditary angioedema respond to danazol. Only supportive management is available for other primary diseases of the complement system.

CHAPTER 100

Graft-versus-Host Disease

(Nelson Textbook, Chapters 135, 136, 137, 138, 139, and 140)

Engraftment by donor lymphocytes in an immunologically compromised host (congenital or radiation- or chemotherapy-induced immune defects) can result in donor T-cell activation against host major histocompatibility complex (MHC) antigens, with resultant GVHD. Cell death results from cell-mediated cytotoxic activity (e.g., by natural killer cells) and a complex cascade of lymphokines released by activated lymphocytes (e.g., tumor necrosis factor). For this reaction to occur, the graft must contain immunocompetent cells, the host must be immunocompromised and unable to reject or mount a response to the graft, and there must be histocompatibility differences between the graft and the host. GVHD is classified as acute, occurring within the first 100 days after bone marrow transplant, or chronic, occurring after the first 100 days.

ACUTE GVHD. The acute form of GVHD (aGVHD) is characterized by erythroderma, cholestatic hepatitis, and enteritis. Typically, aGVHD presents about day 19 (median), when patients are starting to engraft. It usually starts with a pruritic macular/papular rash on the ears, palms, and soles and may progress to involve the trunk and extremities, potentially becoming a more confluent erythroderma with bulla formation and exfoliation. Fever may or may not be present. Hepatic manifestations include cholestatic jaundice with elevated values on liver function testing. The intestinal symptoms of aGVHD include crampy abdominal pain and watery diarrhea, often with blood. Prevention and treatment of GVHD require various immunosuppressive agents.

CHRONIC GVHD. Maturation of the graft may include the development of chronic GVHD (cGVHD), usually after day 100 but as early as day 60–70. cGVHD resembles a multisystem autoimmune process manifesting as Sjögren's (sicca) syndrome, systemic lupus erythematosus, and scleroderma lichen planus and as primary biliary cirrhosis. Recurrent infections (sepsis, sinusitis, pneumonia) with encapsulated bacteria and fungal and viral organisms are common and contribute significantly to transplant-related morbidity and mortality. Therapy for cGVHD consists of additional immunosuppression with agents (prednisone and cyclosporine are front-line drugs) that have the disadvantage of putting patients at risk for infectious complications.

PART 13

Allergic Disorders

CHAPTER 101

Allergy and the Immunologic Basis of Atopic Disease
(Nelson Textbook, Chapter 141)

Allergy is a specific, acquired change in host reactivity mediated by an immunologic mechanism and causing an untoward physiologic response. The terms *antigen* and *allergen* are often used interchangeably, but not all antigens are good allergens and vice versa. Most naturally occurring allergens share several common characteristics. They are protein in part, are acidic, and have molecular weights of 10,000–70,000 daltons.

The use of the term *atopy* or *atopic* in designating an allergic reaction implies a hereditary factor expressed as susceptibility to hay fever, asthma, and eczematoid dermatitis in the families of affected individuals. Although no single "atopic gene" has been discovered, atopy has been linked to certain human leukocyte antigen (HLA) histocompatibility types as well as to various chromosome loci (11q, 14, and 5q). The formation of IgE antibodies is revealed in atopic persons by "wheal and flare" reactions on skin testing with allergenic extracts. However, the capacity to form IgE antibody is not limited to atopic individuals because IgE is found in the sera and on mast cells of most normal individuals. Atopic persons, however, form IgE antibodies on exposure to common environmental substances such as pollens and mites in house dust, thus distinguishing them from nonatopic individuals.

There are three forms of humoral antibody-antigen reactions, two of which occur on the surface of cells and the third in the extracellular fluids. Of the two reactions occurring on the surface of the cells, *type 1 hypersensitivity mediated by IgE* (immediate type or anaphylactic hypersensitivity) is of greatest interest to the allergist. In this circumstance, circulating basophils and tissue mast cells, the latter strategically located around blood vessels, become "sensitized" through the binding of IgE antibodies to their surface receptors. Chemical modifications of antigens used in immunotherapy of allergic diseases suppress IgE responses. Once formed, IgE antibody becomes reversibly bound or "fixed" to surface receptors of mast cells and basophils. In nonatopic individuals, only 20–50% of the receptors are occupied by IgE molecules. In atopic individuals with high serum IgE concentrations, a larger percentage, up to almost 100%, of their basophil and mast cell receptors is occupied by IgE. Once binding of IgE occurs, the basophils and mast cells are "sensitized." The prototypic anaphylactic or IgE-mediated disease is ragweed hay fever. Others include anaphylactic reactions to insect venom, food-induced urticaria, and allergic conjunctivitis or rhinitis.

In *type II hypersensitivity (cytotoxic) interactions* between antigen and antibody at cell surfaces, IgG or IgM immunoglobulins react with antigenic determinants that either are integral parts of the cell membrane or have become adsorbed to or incorporated into the membrane. This kind of reaction activates the complement system in most instances, and the involved cell is destroyed. The *type III immunopathologic mechanism* (Arthus or immune complex) of tissue injury involving humoral antibody and antigen occurs in the extracellular spaces. At certain ratios of antigen to antibody, antigen-antibody complexes are formed that are "toxic" to tissues in which they are deposited. Toxic complex injury involves cooperation among different antibodies in the production of tissue injury. Examples of *type III reactions* include serum sickness and immune complex pericarditis or arthritis after meningococcal or *Haemophilus influenzae* infection.

In *type IV cell-mediated* or *delayed-type hypersensitivity,* pathologic changes follow interaction of antigen with specifically sensitized, thymus-derived T lymphocytes. Contact allergy (poison ivy, chemical-induced contact dermatitis) is the prototype of allergic disease mediated by delayed-type hypersensitivity.

Chapter 102

Principles of Treatment
(Nelson Textbook, Chapters 142 and 143)

Successful management of allergic disorders is based on avoidance of allergens or irritants, pharmacologic therapy, immunotherapy (hypersensitization or desensitization), and prophylaxis. When clinically relevant allergens are identified by history and judicious use of allergy skin tests, their elimination or *avoidance* is all that is needed in many cases of IgE-mediated disease.

PHARMACOLOGIC THERAPY

ADRENERGICS. These agents combine with α- and β-receptors on the surfaces of cells. With several exceptions, drugs that affect α-receptors cause physiologic responses that are excitatory (vasoconstriction), whereas drugs that influence β-receptors produce inhibitory responses (bronchodilation). β-Receptors are separated into two subclasses: β_1 and β_2; β_1-receptors have approximately equal affinity for epinephrine and norepinephrine, whereas β_2-receptors have an approximately 10-fold higher affinity for epinephrine than for norepinephrine. Agents with greater β_2-selective activity (isoetharine, metaproterenol, terbutaline, albuterol, fenoterol, bitolterol, pirbuterol, salmeterol) provide effective bronchodilation in asthma with less of the increase in heart rate than may occur with isoproterenol or epinephrine because the latter drugs stimulate both bronchial β_2-receptors and cardiac β_1-receptors, causing tachycardia. α-Adrenergic receptors have been subclassified into α_1 and α_2 subtypes; these have wide distribution and mediate different effects. Stimulation of α_1-receptors contracts vascular and airway smooth muscle.

Adrenergic drugs include catecholamines (epinephrine, isoetharine, isoproterenol, and bitolterol) and noncatecholamines (ephedrine, albuterol, metaproterenol, salmeterol, terbutaline, pirbuterol, procaterol, and fenoterol). Those of the former group are rapidly inactivated by enzymes found in the gastrointestinal tract and liver; accordingly, the use of epinephrine and isoproterenol is limited largely to injection, inhalation, and topical application to mucous membranes. Ephedrine, the oldest of the noncatecholamine sympathomimetics, has relatively weak β-stimulant activity and frequently causes adverse side effects, including increased activity, insomnia, irritability, and headache. Newer noncatecholamine adrenergic agents (metaproterenol, terbutaline, and albuterol), which may also be given orally, have a somewhat longer duration of action (up to 6 hr) than ephedrine (4 hr) and have relatively selective activity on the β_2-receptors in the airways, with less of the cardiovascular effects of isoproterenol and epinephrine, especially when delivered by inhalation.

Adverse side effects of adrenergic drugs may include skeletal muscle tremor, cardiac stimulation, worsening of hypoxemia, increased airway obstruction, headache, insomnia, irritability, nausea, vomiting, epigastric pain, flushing, hyperglycemia, hypokalemia, and tolerance (subsensitivity, refractoriness).

THEOPHYLLINE. This is a therapeutic agent for the treatment of both acute and chronic asthma. Its mode of action is uncertain. Both the therapeutic and toxic effects of theophylline are related to the serum concentration. The incidence of toxic effects increases as the serum levels rise progressively to greater than 20 µg/mL. *Measurement of serum theophylline concentration* is an important element in effective and safe use of the drug.

ANTIHISTAMINES. These drugs compete with histamine for receptors in various tissues. There are at least three histamine receptors: H_1, H_2, and H_3. In general, the H_1 antagonists are rapidly absorbed after oral administration, with onset of action within 30 min, peak plasma concentration within 1 hr, and complete absorption within 4 hr. Because antihistamines act as competitive antagonists, they are more effective in preventing than in reversing the action of histamine. To be most effective, they must be administered at doses and intervals that keep tissue histamine receptor sites saturated. In general, antihistamines are extraordinarily safe, and most are sold without prescription. In high doses or in certain sensitive patients, the anticholinergic properties of antihistamines cause undesirable adverse reactions. These include excitation, nervousness, tachycardia, palpitations, dryness of the mouth, urinary retention, and constipation. Seizures are common in antihistamine poisoning.

CROMOLYN SODIUM (DISODIUM CROMOGLYCATE). The drug is used principally in asthma but has some value in allergic rhinitis. Cromolyn appears to reduce airway hyperreactivity by a mechanism that is not yet understood, and it can prevent late-phase asthmatic responses when administered before allergen challenge.

LEUKOTRIENE INHIBITORS AND ANTAGONISTS. These agents improve pulmonary function and reduce symptoms of asthma. They afford protection against bronchoconstriction induced by exercise, cold air, platelet-activating factor, and allergens. The leukotriene antagonist *zafirlukast* can inhibit exercise-induced bronchoconstriction 2 hr after oral administration but has less protective effect at 4 hr and still less at 8 hr. *Montelukast* can inhibit exercise-induced bronchoconstriction for as long as 24 hr after oral administration.

CORTICOSTEROIDS. Corticosteroids are the most potent drugs available for treatment of allergic disorders. Some effects of prednisolone are evident within 2 hr after oral or intravenous administration (fall in peripheral eosinophils and lymphocytes); others may be delayed 6–8 hr or longer (e.g., hyperglycemia and improvement in pulmonary function in asthmatics).

Topical corticosteroids have direct local effects that include decreased inflammation, edema, mucus production, vascular permeability, and mucosal IgE levels. There is also less local accumulation of neutrophils, eosinophils, basophils, and mast cells and an attenuation of airway hyperresponsiveness. Possible complications of inhaled corticosteroids include oropharyngeal candidiasis, dysphonia, disseminated varicella, and, at high doses, suppression of the hypothalamic-pituitary-adrenal axis. Suppressive effects of corticosteroids on growth depend on dosage and duration of treatment; attainment of normal height is possible after discontinuation of corticosteroids, but prolonged administration of large doses of systemic corticosteroids can cause permanent short stature.

The short-term use of *systemic corticosteroids* in self-limited allergic conditions such as contact dermatitis due to poison ivy or occasional episodes of severe asthma is not associated with significant adverse effects. Long-term use, in contrast, especially if daily administration is required, may have substantial undesirable side effects. In children, the most common adverse effect is suppression of linear growth.

IMMUNOTHERAPY

IMMUNOLOGIC CHANGES. In the early weeks after the institution of regular injections of ragweed pollen extract, IgE antibody against ragweed pollen antigen increases; as treatment continues, however, the titer of anti-ragweed IgE antibody decreases. In untreated patients with ragweed hay fever, a rise and fall of anti-ragweed IgE occur during the year; the rise occurs with the seasonal exposure to ragweed. Injection therapy blunts this anamnestic rise.

INDICATIONS, MATERIALS, AND PROCEDURE. Immunotherapy is indicated in patients suffering from allergic rhinitis, IgE-mediated asthma, or allergy to stinging insects.

PRECAUTIONS AND ADVERSE REACTIONS. Allergenic extracts should always be administered in a physician's office, where treatment of a systemic reaction or anaphylactic shock is readily available. The patient should always remain under observation for at least 20 min after each injection because life-threatening reactions are most likely to occur within this time. Immunotherapy should not be administered during uncontrolled asthma because of diminished pulmonary reserve in the event of a systemic reaction to the allergenic extract.

CHAPTER 103

Allergic Rhinitis
(Nelson Textbook, Chapter 144)

Seasonal allergic rhinitis, seasonal pollinosis, and hay fever all describe a symptom complex that follows sensitization to windborne pollens of trees, grasses, and weeds. In *perennial allergic rhinitis* the patient has year-round symptoms. The causative agents, when they can be identified, are generally allergens to which the patient is exposed more or less continually, although exposure may vary during the year. Indoor inhalant allergens are implicated most often.

DIAGNOSIS AND CLINICAL MANIFESTATIONS. The symptoms of allergic rhinitis include sneezing, which is frequently paroxysmal; rhinorrhea, which is often watery and profuse; nasal obstruction; and itching of the nose, palate, pharynx, and ears. Itching, redness, and tearing of the eyes may also occur, causing severe discomfort.

The typical patient with allergic rhinitis presents with bilateral nasal obstruction resulting from boggy edema of the mucous membranes. Frequently, redundant mucosa is piled up on the floor of the nose. The mucous membranes are bluish and rather pale, and there is a clear mucoid nasal discharge. The child often has mannerisms caused by itching of the nose or attempts to improve the airway. The child wrinkles the nose (rabbit nose) and may rub it in characteristic ways (allergic salute). Dark circles under the eyes have been attributed to venous stasis resulting from interference with blood flow caused by edematous nasal mucous membranes. Mouth breathing is common. Fever is unusual.

The diagnosis of allergic rhinitis is substantiated by the finding of a predominance of eosinophils in a smear made of the nasal secretions. There is often a personal or family history of eczema or asthma.

TREATMENT. Treatment of either seasonal or perennial allergic rhinitis includes avoidance of exposure to suspected allergens and irritants, immunotherapy for those who cannot avoid inhalant allergens, and drug therapy.

Avoidance. It is difficult or impractical to avoid exposure to seasonal pollens, but much can be done to eliminate exposure to indoor inhalant factors such as house dust, danders, and molds.

Drug Therapy. Appropriate drugs usually relieve symptoms of allergic rhinitis. Antihistamines are useful, especially in the treatment of seasonal allergic rhinitis. Nasal itching, sneezing, and rhinorrhea are usually well controlled by antihistamine therapy, whereas nasal obstruction is relieved to a lesser degree. Nonsedating antihistamines (acrivastine, astemizole, fexofenadine, loratadine) should be used if possible. If nasal obstruction is particularly troublesome, a decongestant such as pseudoephedrine may be administered alone or in combination with an antihistamine. Insomnia and irritability are the most frequent side effects. Dosage of pseudoephedrine usually should not exceed 15 mg every 6 hr for children 2–5 yr of age, 30 mg for children 6–12 yr of age, and 60 mg every 6 hr for children older than 12 yr of age.

By far the most effective treatment of allergic rhinitis is topical use of corticosteroids. Beclomethasone, budesonide, flunisolide, fluticasone, or mometasone should be used in children whose nasal symptoms are resistant to antihistamine-decongestant therapy or as an alternative. The initial dosage is usually one to two sprays in each nostril two to three times per day. After 3–4 days, as symptoms improve, the dose and frequency of use are reduced until a minimal effective dosage is reached. Complications of topical nasal corticosteroids include local burning, irritation, and epistaxis.

CHAPTER 104

Asthma

(Nelson Textbook, Chapter 145)

Asthma is a leading cause of chronic illness in childhood. The course and severity of asthma are difficult to predict. The majority of affected children have only occasional attacks of slight to moderate severity, which are managed with relative ease. A minority experience severe, intractable asthma. The prognosis for young asthmatic children is generally good. Both prevalence and mortality from asthma have increased during the past 3 decades.

PATHOPHYSIOLOGY. Manifestations of the airway obstruction in asthma are due to bronchoconstriction, hypersecretion of mucus, mucosal edema, cellular infiltration, and desquamation of epithelial and inflammatory cells. Various allergic and nonspecific stimuli, in the presence of hyperreactive airways, initiate the bronchoconstriction and inflammatory response.

ETIOLOGY. Asthma is a complex disorder involving autonomic, immunologic, infectious, endocrine, and psychologic factors in varying degrees in different individuals.

CLINICAL MANIFESTATIONS. The onset of an asthma exacerbation may be acute or insidious. Acute episodes are most often caused by exposure to irritants such as cold air and noxious fumes (smoke, wet paint) or exposure to allergens or simple chemicals, for example, aspirin or sulfites. When airway obstruction develops rapidly in a few minutes, it is most likely due to smooth muscle spasm in large airways. Exacerbations precipitated by viral respiratory infections are slower in onset, with gradual increases in frequency and severity of cough and wheezing over a few days. Because airway patency decreases at night, many children have acute asthma at this time. The signs and symptoms of asthma include cough, which sounds tight and is nonproductive early in the course of an attack; wheezing, tachypnea, and dyspnea with prolonged expiration and use of accessory muscles of respiration; cyanosis; hyperinflation of the chest; and tachycardia and pulsus paradoxus, which may be present to varying degrees depending on the stage and severity of the attack. When the patient is in extreme respiratory distress, the cardinal sign of asthma—wheezing—may be strikingly absent.

DIAGNOSIS. Recurrent episodes of coughing and wheezing, especially if aggravated or triggered by exercise, viral infection, or inhaled allergens, are highly suggestive of asthma. However, asthma can also cause persistent coughing in children with no history of wheezing.

Laboratory Evaluation. Eosinophilia of the blood and sputum occurs with asthma. Prolonged strenuous exercise causes bronchoconstriction in virtually all asthmatic subjects when breathing dry, relatively cold air. Hyperinflation on radiographs occurs during acute asthma and may become chronic when airway obstruction is persistent.

DIFFERENTIAL DIAGNOSIS. Most children who have recurrent episodes of coughing and wheezing have asthma. Other causes of airway obstruction include congenital malformations, foreign bodies in the airway or esophagus, infectious bronchiolitis, cystic fibrosis, immunologic deficiency diseases, hypersensitivity pneumonitis, allergic bronchopulmonary aspergillosis, and a variety of rarer conditions that compromise the airway. Wheezing in the infant merits special mention because it is common and presents substantial diagnostic and therapeutic problems.

TREATMENT. Asthma therapy includes basic concepts of avoiding allergens, improving bronchodilation, and reducing mediator-induced inflammation. Systemic or topical inhaled medications are used, depending on the severity of the episode. The hyperreactivity of the asthmatic airway as an additional factor is dealt with by minimizing exposure to nonspecific irritants such as tobacco smoke, smoke from wood-burning stoves, fumes from kerosene heaters, and strong odors such as wet paint and disinfectants and by avoiding ice-cold drinks and rapid changes in temperature and humidity.

Pharmacologic therapy is the mainstay of treatment of asthma. Oxygen administered by mask or nasal prongs at 2–3 L/min is indicated in most children during acute asthma. Injection of epinephrine was the treatment of choice for acute asthma for many years, but bronchodilator aerosols are now preferable.

Inhalation of bronchodilator aerosols is rapidly effective in relieving the signs and symptoms of asthma. Despite airway obstruction, which may limit aerosol delivery to peripheral airways, aerosol therapy is probably more effective than epinephrine in reversing bronchoconstriction. Albuterol (Proventil, Ventolin) solution is safe and effective at a dose of 0.15 mg/kg (maximum 5 mg) followed by 0.05–0.15 mg/kg at intervals of 20–30 min until response is adequate. Nebulization with oxygen at 6 L/min prevents hypoxemia that might be related to the treatment. Delivery of inhaled albuterol by metered-dose inhaler, 3 to 10 puffs per dose, with a spacer such as Aerochamber, can be as effective as delivery by nebulizer, although nebulization is more effective for patients unable to coordinate inhalation sufficiently with actuation of the inhaler. If response to the β_2-agonist is not adequate, treatment with both a β_2-agonist and nebulized ipratropium bromide, 250–500 μg, may be more effective.

Theophylline should be considered for patients who have been receiving maintenance treatment with theophylline and for those unable to tolerate maximal treatment with inhaled β_2-agonists. Most acute exacerbations of asthma respond to this treatment regimen. In borderline cases, however, when the decision is made for care at home rather than in a hospital, a prescription of prednisone in decreasing doses over 5–7 days may hasten resolution of the exacerbation and causes no harm.

STATUS ASTHMATICUS. If a patient continues to have significant respiratory distress despite administration of sympathomimetic drugs with or without theophylline, the diagnosis of status asthmaticus should be considered. Status asthmaticus is a clinical diagnosis defined by increasingly severe asthma that is not responsive to drugs that are usually effective. A patient in whom the diagnosis is made should be admitted to a hospital, preferably to an intensive care unit, where the condition can be carefully monitored. The severity should be determined initially and monitored at regular intervals. An indwelling arterial catheter may be indicated. Cardiac monitoring is almost always indicated.

Patients in status asthmaticus are hypoxemic. Oxygen in carefully controlled concentrations is therefore always indicated to maintain tissue oxygenation. It may be administered effectively by nasal prongs or mask at a flow rate of 2–3 L/min. A concentration of oxygen sufficient to maintain a Pao_2 of 70–90 mm Hg or oxygen saturation greater than 92% is optimal.

Dehydration may be present owing to inadequate fluid intake, greatly increased insensible water loss as a result of tachypnea, and the diuretic effect of theophylline. Care should be taken not to overhydrate the patient.

Bronchodilator sympathomimetic aerosol therapy initiated in the emergency department should be continued. Aminophylline, 4–5 mg/kg, may be given intravenously over 20 min every 6 hr if theophylline is to be administered. It is essential to adjust the aminophylline dose by monitoring serum theophylline concentrations.

Corticosteroids, such as methylprednisolone (Solu-Medrol), 1 mg/kg every 6 hr, should be administered for the first 48 hr followed by 1–2 mg/kg/24 hr (maximum 60 mg/24 hr for a child) in two divided doses until the peak expiratory flow rate (PEFR) is 70% of the personal best or that predicted.

Treatment is guided by serial measurement of blood gases and pH every few hours or more often if indicated. If gas and pH analysis both indicate that respiratory failure is impending, an anesthesiologist should be alerted and facilities and equipment should be available for tracheal intubation and respiratory support.

DAILY MANAGEMENT OF THE ASTHMATIC CHILD. On the basis of the history, physical examination, laboratory data, pulmonary function testing, and need for medication, patients may be classified as having mild intermittent, mild persistent, moderate persistent, or severe persistent asthma.

Mild Intermittent Asthma. Children with mild intermittent asthma have exacerbations of varying frequency, up to twice each week, with decreases in PEFR of not more than 20%; they respond to bronchodilator treatment within 24–48 hr. Generally, medication is not required between exacerbations for mild asthma with symptoms less than every 2 wk, when the child is essentially free of symptoms of airway obstruction.

Mild Persistent Asthma. Symptoms more than twice each week but less often than daily indicate mild persistent asthma. Nocturnal symptoms may occur more than twice each month. The PEFR or FEV_1 is at least 80% predicted. Daily variations in PEFR may be as great as 30%. These patients usually require daily anti-inflammatory therapy, usually cromolyn or nedocromil, although inhaled corticosteroids may be more effective. Sustained-release theophylline is a less expensive alternative.

Moderate Persistent Asthma. Children with moderate persistent asthma have symptoms more frequently than those with mild disease and often have cough and mild wheezing between more severe exacerbations. Such children will generally require continuous treatment with cromolyn, nedocromil, or an inhaled corticosteroid to achieve satisfactory control of symptoms. Hyperinflation may be evident clinically and radiographically.

Severe Persistent Asthma. Children with severe persistent asthma have virtually daily wheezing and more frequent and more severe exacerbations; they require recurrent hospitalization, which is rarely required for mild or moderate asthma. They may have increased anteroposterior diameter of the chest as a result of chronic hyperinflation, evident on radiographs. Anti-inflammatory medication will be required continuously, and regimens should include regularly inhaled corticosteroids and may include systemic corticosteroids.

TREATMENT OF ACUTE ASTHMA. Children with mild asthma should receive bronchodilator medication only when symptomatic, and most exacerbations may be satisfactorily treated with adrenergic agents, preferably by aerosol (albuterol, levalbuterol, metaproterenol, terbutaline, pirbuterol, or bitolterol) or, rarely, by injection (aqueous epinephrine, terbutaline). Use of a chamber such as an AeroChamber or InspirEase enhances delivery of drug to the lower airways when a metered-dose inhaler is used by younger children who are unable to coordinate actuation of the inhaler with inhalation. When moderate or severe airway obstruction is present, nebulization with an air compressor such as the Proneb with PARI-LC jet or the DeVilbiss No. 561 Pulmo-Aide is often more effective than use of a metered-dose inhaler with a chamber.

EXERCISE-INDUCED ASTHMA. Exercise-induced asthma is most effectively prevented by inhalation of a β_2-agonist immediately before exercise. Use of a muffler or cold weather mask to warm and humidify air before inhalation also is effective. Inhaled albuterol usually affords protection for 4 hr; the effects of inhaled salmeterol (not labeled for patients younger than 12 yr by the U.S. Food and Drug Administration [FDA]) last for 12 hr.

THEOPHYLLINE. For children with persistent asthma, theophylline can be a less expensive alternative to cromolyn, nedocromil, a low-dose inhaled corticosteroid, or a long-acting inhaled β-agonist. It can be especially helpful for control of nocturnal asthma. Addition of sustained-release theophylline to low-dose inhaled corticosteroid can be as effective and less expensive than treatment with high-dose inhaled corticosteroid. If adequate control of symptoms is not achieved at the maximal doses or if adverse effects become evident, adjustment in the dosing regimen must be guided by determination of the serum theophylline concentration.

CROMOLYN AND NEDOCROMIL. Cromolyn powder inhaled four times a day from a Spinhaler or cromolyn aerosol delivered by a metered-dose inhaler or nedocromil (not FDA-labeled for patients younger than 12 yr) is useful in children with persistent asthma.

CORTICOSTEROIDS. In certain children with moderate asthma, significant flare-ups occur from time to time that may require the use of corticosteroids for a few days. Early use of corticosteroids in the child who is known to become severely ill may reduce the need for hospitalization. Early intervention with bronchodilator drugs (with or without corticosteroids, depending on the clinical setting) is important in the management of all asthmatic children, regardless of the severity of their conditions. Corticosteroids should be given in adequate doses (1–2 mg/kg/24 hr of prednisone or prednisolone in two to three doses) and should be discontinued as quickly as possible, for example, within 5–7 days; a long "weaning" period after acute asthma is unnecessary.

Inhalational corticosteroids, such as beclomethasone dipropionate (Vanceril, Beclovent), budesonide (Pulmicort), flunisolide (AeroBid), fluticasone propionate (Flovent), and triamcinolone (Azmacort), are indicated for children with moderate or severe persistent asthma. They also are appropriate for children with mild persistent asthma, especially if uncontrolled with cromolyn, nedocromil, sustained-release theophylline, or a leukotriene antagonist. Effective use of inhaled corticosteroid requires a degree of compliance by the patient not often found in children younger than 6–7 yr.

Continual treatment with an inhaled corticosteroid, nedocromil, or cromolyn is appropriate for any child with symptoms of asthma occurring as frequently as weekly except for exercise-induced asthma preventable by pretreatment with a β-agonist, cromolyn, nedocromil, theophylline, or a leukotriene antagonist.

Home monitoring of PEFR two to three times a day facilitates early detection of airway obstruction in patients with severe asthma and in patients with infrequent symptoms that may progress to severe airway obstruction.

PREVENTION OF DEATHS FROM ASTHMA. Death from childhood asthma is rare, but asthma mortality rates have been increasing. It is possible to identify many of those at greatest risk for death from their histories, for example, respiratory failure with hypercapnia, loss of consciousness caused by asthma, or psychosocial dysfunction in the patient or family. These patients require especially close monitoring and psychotherapy when indicated. Each should carry a written emergency protocol indicating current medications and recommended emergency treatment as guidance for emergency personnel who may be unfamiliar with the patient.

CHAPTER **105**

Atopic Dermatitis

(Nelson Textbook, Chapter 146)

Atopic dermatitis is an inflammatory skin disorder characterized by erythema, edema, intense pruritus, exudation, crusting, and scaling. Infants with atopic dermatitis tend to experience allergic rhinitis and asthma subsequently.

CLINICAL MANIFESTATIONS. Atopic dermatitis affects 2–10% of children and typically occurs in three stages with fairly distinctive features. The disease most often begins in infancy, usually during the first 2–3 mo of life. The onset is sometimes delayed until the 2nd or 3rd yr; 60% of patients are affected by 1 yr of age and 90% by 5 yr of age. The earliest lesions are erythematous, weepy patches on the cheeks, with subsequent extension to the remainder of the face, neck, wrists, hands, abdomen, and extensor aspects of the extremities. Involvement of flexural areas characteristically appears later but may occur as popliteal and antecubital dermatitis in early life.

Pruritus is marked; the affected infant makes incessant efforts to scratch by rubbing the face on bedclothes and against the sides of the crib. This trauma to the skin rapidly leads to weeping and crusting; secondary infection is common and may be extensive. The onset of dermatitis frequently coincides with the introduction of certain foods into the infant's diet, especially cow's milk, wheat, soy, peanuts, fish, or eggs.

Atopic dermatitis shows a tendency toward remission at 3–5 yr of age. In most cases, the disease becomes less prominent by the age of 5 yr; in some, a mild to moderate eczema may persist in the antecubital and popliteal fossae, on the wrists, behind the ears, and on the face and neck. During childhood, antecubital and popliteal involvement becomes common; extensor surfaces of the extremities may still be actively affected.

DIAGNOSIS. When pruritus is intense and the lesions characteristic, the diagnosis of atopic dermatitis may be easy. A family history of asthma, hay fever, or atopic dermatitis; the finding of elevated serum IgE concentrations and of reaginic antibodies to a variety of foods and inhalants; the presence of eosinophilia; and the demonstration of white dermographism support the diagnosis.

COMPLICATIONS. During early infancy and childhood, secondary infection of the lesions of atopic dermatitis with bacterial, fungal, or viral agents is common. Staphylococci and β-hemolytic streptococci are the bacterial agents most often recovered from infected lesions.

TREATMENT. Effective treatment of atopic dermatitis requires control of the environmental precipitants of the itch-scratch-itch cycle that perpetuate the disease, beginning with avoidance of ingestant, injectant, contactant, and atmospheric factors that can trigger itching or scratching. Extremes of temperature and humidity should be avoided. A warm climate of moderate humidity is optimal for most patients. Sweating leads to itching and aggravation of the disease. Exposure to sunlight and salt water is of benefit to many patients.

For the dry skin of atopic dermatitis, use of soaps and detergents that defat the skin should be avoided as much as possible. Bathing should be kept to a minimum. The purpose of bath oil or other creams applied to the skin is to seal water into the skin.

If a food aggravates itching, it should be excluded from the diet. Skin testing by the prick method is useful in excluding IgE-mediated food hypersensitivity.

During acute flare-ups of the disease, wet dressings (e.g., Burow's solution, 1:20) have an antipruritic and anti-inflammatory effect. Topical corticosteroid lotions or creams may be applied between changes of wet dressings. Unless scratching can be controlled, it is almost impossible to manage the disease successfully, especially during infancy and early childhood.

When infection is present (acute weeping or crusting), antibiotics should be given systemically. Erythromycin or cephalexin is a prudent choice because of frequent resistance to penicillin of the infecting *Staphylococcus aureus*.

After the acute phase has subsided, topical application of corticosteroid creams and ointments is of great value in managing the disease. Topical triamcinolone acetonide ointment, 0.1%, is often useful but is best limited to 1–3 wk at a time; after improvement, an even less potent corticosteroid should be substituted if possible. Systemic administration of corticosteroids for treatment of atopic dermatitis should be avoided except briefly in the most severely affected patients while awaiting response to other therapies.

Chapter 106

Urticaria-Angioedema

(Nelson Textbook, Chapter 147)

CLINICAL MANIFESTATIONS. Urticaria, or hives, is a common skin disorder characterized by usually well-circumscribed but sometimes coalescent, localized or generalized, erythematous, raised skin lesions (wheals or welts) of various sizes. The lesions may be intensely pruritic or itch little, if at all. The individual hive usually resolves within 48 hr, but new ones may continue to appear singly or in crops. When urticaria persists for longer than 6 wk, the condition is arbitrarily deemed chronic. Urticaria has been attributed to edema of the upper corium. In angioedema (angioneurotic edema), the deeper layers of skin or submucosa and subcutaneous or other tissues are involved; the upper respiratory tract and the gastrointestinal tract are common target organs.

TREATMENT. In most instances, urticaria is a self-limited illness requiring little treatment other than antihistamines. Hydroxyzine (Atarax), 0.5 mg/kg, is one of the most effective antihistamines for control of urticaria, but diphenhydramine (Benadryl), 1.25 mg/kg, and other antihistamines are also effective at the expense of sedation. Epinephrine 1:1,000, 0.01 mL/kg maximum of 0.3 mL, usually affords rapid relief of acute, severe urticaria.

Chapter 107

Anaphylaxis

(Nelson Textbook, Chapter 148)

Anaphylaxis is an acute, potentially life-threatening reaction caused by rapid release of mediators from mast cells and basophils that follows the interaction of allergen with specific, cell-bound IgE.

CLINICAL MANIFESTATIONS. Anaphylactic reactions are characteristically explosive, particularly when the antigen is injected. Surviving patients describe a "feeling of impending doom." The more rapidly symptoms appear after administration of the foreign material, the more serious is the reaction. Often the first symptom noted is a tingling sensation around the mouth or face, followed by a feeling of warmth, difficulty in swallowing, and tightness in the throat or chest. There may be apprehension, weakness, and diaphoresis followed by generalized pruritus. The patient becomes flushed; urticaria and angioedema then appear, along with varying degrees of hoarseness, inspiratory stridor, dysphagia, nasal congestion, itching of the eyes, sneezing, and wheezing. Abdominal cramps, diarrhea, and contractions of the uterus and other organs of smooth muscle may also occur. The patient may lose consciousness and, on examination, be hypotensive, with feeble heart sounds, bradycardia, and sometimes an arrhythmia. Cardiorespiratory arrest and death may ensue. In fatal cases, death has most often resulted from acute upper airway obstruction, although profound circulatory collapse may occur without upper airway obstruction.

Most anaphylactic reactions begin within 30 min of exposure to the allergen, especially if by injection. Signs and symptoms usually resolve within a few hours in surviving patients. Some patients experience biphasic reactions, with recurrence of signs and symptoms 1–8 hr after initial resolution in response to therapy.

Food-dependent, exercise-induced anaphylaxis occurs during exercise within 2 hr of ingestion of the food to which the patient has specific IgE (shellfish, wheat, vegetables, fruit) or after the ingestion of any food. Exercise typically is tolerated 3 hr or more after ingestion; the food has no adverse effect without subsequent exercise. Exercise-induced anaphylaxis may also occur after ingestion of aspirin or other nonsteroidal anti-inflammatory drugs.

TREATMENT. The treatment of choice is aqueous epinephrine, 1:1,000, 0.01 mL/kg (maximum 0.3 mL for a child or 0.5 mL for an adult) by intramuscular injection. If necessary, this dose may be repeated at 15-min intervals. If the reaction is to injection of an allergen extract or to a Hymenoptera sting on an extremity, one half of this dose of epinephrine may be diluted in 2 mL normal saline and infiltrated subcutaneously at the site of the injection or sting to slow absorption. A tourniquet above the site can also slow systemic distribution of the allergen. The tourniquet can be loosened after improvement or briefly at intervals of 3 min.

A persistent, serious reaction should be treated cautiously, with careful cardiac monitoring of the intravenous infusion of epinephrine at an initial infusion rate of 0.1 μg/kg/min in a child (or 2 μg/min in an adult) to sustain a systolic blood pressure of 80 mm Hg. Supplemental oxygen (100%, 4–6 L/min) is indicated. If hypotension is unresponsive to administration of epinephrine by subcutaneous injection, rapid intravenous administration of isotonic saline is indicated.

Systemic adrenocorticosteroids are appropriate after treatment of the initial manifestations of anaphylaxis, although it is uncertain whether they are helpful in preventing biphasic reactions.

CHAPTER 108

Serum Sickness
(Nelson Textbook, Chapter 149)

Serum sickness is a hypersensitivity vasculitis that follows the administration of foreign antigenic material.

CLINICAL MANIFESTATIONS. Typically, the symptoms of serum sickness begin 7–12 days after injection of the foreign material but may appear as late as 3 wk afterward. If there has been earlier exposure or previous allergic reaction to the same foreign antigen, symptoms may appear in accelerated fashion, within 1–3 days after injection, or as anaphylaxis. Fever and malaise are almost always present, as are cutaneous eruptions. Urticaria, usually generalized, is a common finding. Faint erythema with a serpiginous border at the margins of palmar or plantar skin of the hands, fingers, feet, and toes may precede the generalized cutaneous eruption. Edema, particularly around the face and neck; facial flushing; myalgia; lymphadenopathy; arthralgia or arthritis involving multiple joints (ankle, knee, wrist, fingers, toes); and gastrointestinal complaints (cramping, diarrhea, nausea) also occur. Intense pruritus accompanying the urticaria is the most distressing symptom in many patients. The site of injection of the foreign material generally becomes red and swollen, commonly 1–3 days before systemic symptoms appear. The disease generally runs a self-limited course, and the patient recovers in 7–10 days.

LABORATORY MANIFESTATIONS. The erythrocyte sedimentation rate is often increased. A sheep cell agglutinin titer of the Forssman type is usually elevated. Serum complement levels (C3 and C4) are variably depressed and may fall to low concentrations around the 10th day.

TREATMENT. Patients generally respond well to aspirin and antihistamines. When the symptoms are especially severe, corticosteroids have been used with great efficacy. High doses are given and rapidly reduced as the patient improves.

CHAPTER 109

Adverse Reactions to Drugs
(Nelson Textbook, Chapters 150 and 727)

The majority of adverse drug reactions are pharmacologic; only 6% have an allergic basis.

CLINICAL MANIFESTATIONS. Cutaneous eruptions are the most common manifestation of adverse drug reactions in children. Urticarial, exanthematous, and eczematoid eruptions predominate, but almost any morphologic condition can occur. When a child who has received prolonged antimicrobial therapy has persistent fever without other cause, drug fever should be considered. Drug fever is often suspected but rarely proved and does not generally occur as the sole manifestation of an adverse drug reaction. There may be eosinophilia, leukocytosis, and an increased erythrocyte sedimentation rate. The diagnosis is easily made when the drug is discontinued and defervescence occurs within 24–48 hr.

Diagnosis of an allergic drug reaction depends on a careful history. A definitive diagnosis of an allergic drug reaction is frequently difficult to establish. Penicillin is the only drug for which allergy skin testing is of well-established reliability in identifying anaphylactic hypersensitivity.

TREATMENT. Therapy depends on the mechanism of drug reaction and the clinical manifestations. Discontinuation of the drug is usually indicated. Under certain conditions, especially in infants and small children who experience rashes while receiving antibiotics, the circumstances may support a decision to continue administration of the drug until the cause of the rash becomes clear.

Cutaneous eruptions are the most common manifestation of drug allergy in children. The eruptions are generally self-limited and disappear when the drugs are discontinued. Treatment is therefore symptomatic. Antihistamines are most useful for urticarial rashes. Epinephrine 1:1000 in doses of 0.1–0.3 mL provides short-term relief. For a more sustained effect, a suspension of epinephrine (SusPhrine) in doses of 0.1–0.2 mL may be given subcutaneously every 6 hr. Corticosteroids are reserved for severe cases not relieved by the foregoing measures.

CHAPTER 110

Insect Allergy

(Nelson Textbook, Chapters 151 and 724)

Allergic reaction to insects can cause (1) symptoms of respiratory allergy as a result of inhalation of particulate matter of insect origin, (2) local cutaneous reactions to insect bites, and (3) anaphylactic reactions to stinging insects.

CLINICAL MANIFESTATIONS. The clinical findings in inhalant allergy caused by insects are similar to those seen with the usual inhalant allergens such as pollens. Rhinitis, conjunctivitis, and asthma have all been described.

The cutaneous reactions to biting insects are most often urticarial but may be papular, vesicular, and erythematous, particularly as the lesion progresses. Lesions that resemble typical delayed hypersensitivity reactions also occur.

Clinical reactions to stinging venomous insects range in severity from minimal pain and local erythema to life-threatening anaphylactic episodes. The usual reaction is swelling of less than 4–5 cm, lasting less than 24 hr. Large local reactions have more swelling and are of longer duration than the usual reaction. Life-threatening, immediate systemic reactions are similar to anaphylaxis (laryngeal edema, bronchospasm, hypotension, urticaria).

The diagnosis is usually easily made from the history and, in the case of biting insects, by examination of skin lesions. Papular urticaria, which is common in children, is almost always the result of insect bites, especially of mosquitoes, fleas, and bedbugs.

TREATMENT. For cutaneous reactions caused by biting insects, treatment with topical medicaments to relieve itching and local discomfort and occasionally the systemic use of an antihistamine are appropriate. In case of an anaphylactic reaction following a Hymenoptera sting, the acute treatment is essentially the same as that for anaphylaxis. Children (or their parents) who have had previous severe or anaphylactic reactions to Hymenoptera stings should be equipped with an EpiPen or EpiPen Jr., which facilitates rapid delivery of an injection of epinephrine, or with a kit that includes epinephrine for injection and an antihistamine tablet for emergency use. Patients at risk for anaphylaxis from an insect sting should also wear an identification bracelet (Medic-Alert) indicating their allergy.

CHAPTER 111

Ocular Allergies

(Nelson Textbook, Chapter 152)

Allergic reactions in the eye are known to occur on the basis of IgE-mediated allergy, as conjunctivitis in a child with ragweed hay fever, for example, or on the basis of a cell-mediated (delayed hypersensitivity) immune reaction, as in contact dermatitis of the eyelids.

EYELIDS. Eyelids are particularly prone to swelling because of their loose areolar connective tissue.

Blepharitis. This is an inflammatory eczematous reaction of the eyelid margins that may be caused by infection or allergy, or both. A chronic staphylococcal infection has been implicated as the major cause of chronic eczema of the eyelid margins. The lid margins, particularly of the lower lids, are affected by an itchy, scaly, erythematous eruption with exudate at the base of the lashes.

ALLERGIC CONJUNCTIVITIS. This frequently accompanies allergic rhinitis in patients with hay fever, especially when caused by pollens. In affected children, both eyes itch, the conjunctivae are reddened and edematous, and there may be profuse tearing. Rubbing of the eyes aggravates the condition. There is no photophobia or other signs of corneal involvement. The secretions are frequently watery but, if persistent, may appear purulent.

Atopic Keratoconjunctivitis. This condition occurs in patients with atopic dermatitis who have extreme ocular itching, red eyes, swollen and thickened eyelids, and, when the cornea is involved, photophobia.

Vernal Conjunctivitis. In the palpebral form, which is most common, the tarsal plate of the upper lid presents a characteristic "cobblestone" appearance. A thick, ropy, whitish discharge may be present over the hypertrophied, giant papillae, giving the "cobblestone" appearance. In the limbal form, the junction of the cornea and sclera is involved, with thickening and opacity of the tissue in the area. Symptoms of vernal conjunctivitis include lacrimation, extreme itching, burning, and a particularly distressing photophobia.

TREATMENT. Contact dermatitis of the lids is best managed by identification of suspected sensitizers and their elimination. A short course of topical corticosteroids is of value in managing the acute reaction.

Blepharitis is best treated by good lid hygiene, using cotton-tipped applicators and half-strength baby shampoo mixed with water to remove scales and exudate, followed by the use of antistaphylococcal ointments. If an excessive reaction to the treatment results, corticosteroids are applied topically for a few days. Because the disease tends to recur, regular lid care is indicated, often for a lifetime.

Allergic conjunctivitis in the patient with hay fever generally responds well to topical application of sympathomimetics (naphazoline or phenylephrine) in the form of eye drops. Atopic keratoconjunctivitis requires the use of topical corticosteroids, particularly if the cornea is involved. Referral to an ophthalmologist is indicated.

Vernal conjunctivitis may be treated with topical vasoconstrictors, antihistamines, cold compresses, and 0.1% lodoxamide tromethamine eye drops or, if necessary, with sparing use of corticosteroid eye drops or ointments.

CHAPTER 112

Adverse Reactions to Foods

(Nelson Textbook, Chapter 153)

The incidence of adverse reactions to foods is not known and unquestionably varies in different parts of the world. Most adverse reactions to food do not have an immunologic basis.

DIAGNOSIS. Eliminating from the diet for a period of 7–10 days a food causing difficulty should generally result in improvement in the patient's symptoms.

TREATMENT. The treatment of an adverse food reaction is directed at the clinical manifestations, which may be anaphylaxis, urticaria, diarrhea, vomiting, rhinitis, asthma, or atopic dermatitis. Offending foods should be removed from the diet.

PART 14

Rheumatic Diseases of Childhood

CHAPTER 113

Evaluation of the Patient with Suggested Rheumatic Disease

(Nelson Textbook, Chapter 154)

Rheumatic diseases result from abnormally regulated immune responses, leading to inflammation of target organs.

CLINICAL MANIFESTATIONS. The history can help distinguish rheumatic conditions from other diseases. Some symptoms and signs, although not specific, may suggest rheumatic diseases. Morning stiffness may be reported by children with juvenile rheumatoid arthritis (JRA), as well as postinfectious arthritis. Facial rashes in children with joint complaints or weakness raise the possibility of lupus or dermatomyositis. Raynaud phenomenon can be a presenting complaint of children with scleroderma and overlapping rheumatic syndromes. Weakness can be found in inflammatory myopathies, of which juvenile dermatomyositis is the most common. Fevers are commonly seen in children with rheumatic diseases; spiking fevers returning to baseline are seen in systemic JRA. Gait problems are found in children with orthopedic problems, as well as JRA.

The physical examination helps identify the organs involved, supporting a final diagnosis. Because rheumatic diseases may take time to evolve, repeated examinations are often important in detecting new manifestations. Lack of normal movement on the examination table may be a result of arthritis. Tachycardia is seen in the child with fevers of any cause or with carditis or pericarditis. Nailfold capillaroscopy can detect vasculopathy, reflecting vessel injury in dermatomyositis, scleroderma, and other rheumatic diseases. Persisting oral mucosal lesions are found in lupus. The eye can be a target in lupus, in which episcleritis may be seen, and JRA, in which posterior synechiae are a later complication of uveitis. Although persisting joint complaints suggest JRA, other rheumatic diseases, including systemic lupus erythematosus and dermatomyositis, can also present as arthritis. Erythema nodosum is sometimes the first manifestation of spondyloarthropathy.

LABORATORY FINDINGS. Certain laboratory studies screen for possible rheumatic disease and may contribute to a diagnosis. The erythrocyte sedimentation rate (ESR) is useful. A normal value does not exclude rheumatic diseases. Although transient infections can increase the ESR, elevations persisting for more than several weeks require explanation, and extensive evaluation may be necessary. Positive antinuclear antibody tests are found in children with rheumatic and other diseases. Other immunologic laboratory tests, although not diagnostic, are useful in characterizing the extent of immune activation and in monitoring response to therapy. For example, levels of total hemolytic complement (CH_{50}), C3, and C4 may be decreased in active lupus or vasculitis syndromes.

CHAPTER 114

Treatment of Rheumatic Diseases
(Nelson Textbook, Chapter 155)

The goals of treatment of rheumatic diseases are to maximize the daily functional activities of an affected child, relieve discomfort, prevent or reduce organ damage, and avoid or minimize drug toxicity. The role of the physician responsible for treating a child with a rheumatic disease includes, in addition to prescribing and monitoring medications, coordinating the efforts of the other team members and educating the child and family about the treatments and nature and expected course of the disease.

NONSTEROIDAL ANTI-INFLAMMATORY DRUGS. The NSAIDs can be prescribed to decrease inflammation in arthritis, pleuritis, pericarditis, uveitis, and some forms of vasculitis. To reduce inflammation requires regular administration of larger doses for longer periods than for analgesia alone. The most frequent toxicities with NSAIDs in children are nausea, decreased appetite, and abdominal pain. Gastritis or gastric or duodenal ulceration occurs in children less frequently than in adults. Ibuprofen has induced aseptic meningitis in patients with systemic lupus erythematosus (SLE). When used by children, naproxen is far more likely than other NSAIDs to cause a unique skin reaction called *pseudoporphyria*. The response to NSAIDs varies greatly among individual patients, but, overall, 50–60% of children with juvenile rheumatoid arthritis (JRA) experience significant improvement in their arthritis with a particular NSAID.

METHOTREXATE. This drug has a central role in the treatment of JRA and is used in approximately 60% of patients with polyarticular JRA. Methotrexate is a commonly used drug in treatment of juvenile dermatomyositis that has shown no or inadequate response to corticosteroids. About 70% of patients with dermatomyositis treated with methotrexate show improvement in the myositis. Methotrexate has also been successfully used in patients with SLE to treat arthritis, pleuritis, and, in some cases, nephritis.

CORTICOSTEROIDS. Corticosteroids are given by various routes for rheumatic diseases, including ocular, oral, intravenous, and intra-articular administration. Ocular corticosteroids are prescribed under the supervision of an ophthalmologist either as drops or injections into the soft tissue surrounding the globe (subtenon injection) for the uveitis associated with JRA. Oral corticosteroids are a cornerstone of treatment for moderate to severe SLE, dermatomyositis, and most forms of vasculitis. However, long-term oral corticosteroid use always leads to side effects. Intravenous corticosteroids have been used as alternatives to oral corticosteroids to treat the more severe, acute systemic connective tissue diseases such as SLE, dermatomyositis, and vasculitis. Intra-articular corticosteroids are prescribed with increasing frequency for children with JRA in whom one or several joints have not responded to standard parenteral drug therapy or as the initial therapy in patients with arthritis involving only one or two joints.

CHAPTER 115

Juvenile Rheumatoid Arthritis
(Nelson Textbook, Chapter 156)

Juvenile rheumatoid arthritis (JRA) is one of the most common rheumatic diseases of children and a major cause of chronic disability. It is characterized by an idiopathic synovitis of the peripheral joints, associated with soft tissue swelling and effusion.

ETIOLOGY. The etiology of the diseases classified under JRA is unknown.

EPIDEMIOLOGY. The incidence of JRA is approximately 13.9/100,000 children (15 yr of age or younger)/yr, with a prevalence of approximately 113/100,000 children.

CLINICAL MANIFESTATIONS. Initial symptoms often include morning stiffness and gelling, ease of fatigue particularly after school in the early afternoon, joint pain later in the day, and joint swelling. The involved joint is often warm, lacks full range of motion, and is occasionally painful on motion but usually not erythematous.

Oligoarthritis (pauciarticular disease) predominantly affects the joints of the lower extremities, such as the knees and ankles. Polyarthritis (polyarticular disease) is generally characterized by involvement of both large and small joints. As many as 20 to 40 separate joints are often affected, although inflammation of only five or more joints is required as a criterion for classification of this type of onset or course. Systemic-onset disease is characterized by a quotidian fever with daily temperature spikes to at least 39°C for a minimum of 2 wk. Each febrile episode is often accompanied by a characteristic faint erythematous macular rash. In addition to arthritis, patients with systemic-onset disease often have prominent visceral involvement including hepatosplenomegaly, lymphadenopathy, and serositis, such as a pericardial effusion.

DIAGNOSIS. The diagnosis of JRA is greatly aided by the American College of Rheumatology classification criteria and its subclassification of courses of disease (Table 115–1) and by the meticulous exclusion of other articular diseases. Diagnosis is based on a history compatible with inflammatory joint disease and a physical examination that confirms the presence of objective arthritis, as defined by the classification criteria. Laboratory abnormalities characteristic of inflammation (elevated erythrocyte sedimentation rate and C-reactive protein), the presence of leukocytosis, thrombocytosis, and the anemia of chronic disease support the diagnosis in the absence of results that would suggest a different disease.

Differential Diagnosis. Arthritis can be the presenting manifestation for any of the rheumatic diseases of childhood, including systemic lupus erythematosus, juvenile dermatomyositis, and the vasculitis syndromes. Diagnosis of these diseases will depend on specifically associated manifestations.

Laboratory Findings. Antinuclear antibodies are present in at least 40–85% of all children with pauciarticular or polyarticular JRA but are unusual in children with systemic-onset disease. Early radiographic changes include soft tissue swelling, osteoporosis, and periostitis about the affected joints.

TREATMENT. The long-term treatment of children with JRA is initiated and subsequently modified according to disease subtype, severity of the disease, specific manifestations of the illness, and response to therapy. A pyramid therapeutic approach should be considered; combination therapy should begin with the least toxic

TABLE 115–1   Criteria for the Classification of Juvenile Rheumatoid Arthritis

Age at onset <16 yr
Arthritis (swelling or effusion, or presence of two or more of the following signs: limitation of range of motion, tenderness or pain on motion, and increased heat) in one or more joints
Duration of disease 6 wk or longer
Onset type defined by type of disease in first 6 mo:
  Polyarthritis: 5 or more inflamed joints
  Oligoarthritis: <5 inflamed joints
  Systemic: arthritis with characteristic fever
Exclusion of other forms of juvenile arthritis

Modified from Cassidy JT, Levison JE, Bass JC, et al: A study of classification criteria for a diagnosis of juvenile rheumatoid arthritis. Arthritis Rheum 29:174, 1986.

medications, usually nonsteroidal anti-inflammatory agents, and proceeding through hydroxychloroquine, methotrexate, or possibly immunosuppressive or experimental drugs. Corticosteroids are used for management of overwhelming systemic illness, in lower doses for "bridge therapy" for the child who has not yet responded to the addition of a drug such as methotrexate, and for ophthalmic and intra-articular use. Methotrexate is considered the safest, most efficacious, and least toxic of the currently available second-line agents.

Chapter 116

Spondyloarthropathies
(Nelson Textbook, Chapter 157)

The diseases collectively referred to as spondyloarthropathies include ankylosing spondylitis, the psoriatic arthritides, arthritis accompanying inflammatory bowel diseases, and chronic reactive arthritis following enteric or genitourinary tract infections. They are characterized by inflammation of joints of the axial skeleton as well as the limbs, by the presence of enthesitis (inflammation at the sites of attachments of ligaments, tendons, fasciae, and capsules to bone), and by the absence of rheumatoid factor.

CLINICAL MANIFESTATIONS

Juvenile Ankylosing Spondylitis (JAS). Early JAS is most frequently characterized by oligoarthritis and enthesitis. Joints of the legs are more frequently affected than those of the arms, and abnormalities of the axial skeleton including sacroiliac joints are usually absent until later in the disease course. Loss of spinal flexibility may eventually be noted. Hip joint arthritis at onset is particularly suggestive of early JAS. Enthesitis, presenting as localized tenderness at characteristic locations around the foot and knee, is particularly common.

Psoriatic Arthritis. The most common pattern of psoriatic arthritis is oligoarthritis affecting large and small joints in an asymmetric pattern.

Arthritis with Inflammatory Bowel Disease. Two patterns of arthritis complicate Crohn disease and ulcerative colitis. A polyarthritis affecting large and small joints, which reflects the activity of the intestinal inflammation, is most common. Less commonly, arthritis of the sacroiliac joints and other peripheral joints (in a pattern similar to that in ankylosing spondylitis) occurs, accompanied in most instances by HLA-B27.

Reactive Arthritis. Reactive arthritis, which includes Reiter syndrome (arthritis, urethritis, and conjunctivitis), is usually preceded by gastrointestinal or genitourinary infection. The arthritis is usually oligoarticular and may be quite severe, with considerable swelling, pain, and even erythema. Joints of the lower limbs are most commonly affected.

DIAGNOSIS. The diagnosis of a spondyloarthropathy is suggested by the onset in an older child, particularly a boy, of oligoarthritis that predominantly affects the hips, knees, ankles or feet, and particularly the intertarsal joints, especially if accompanied by enthesitis. A diagnosis of ankylosing spondylitis is confirmed if there is radiographic evidence of sacroiliitis.

LABORATORY FINDINGS. Laboratory evidence of systemic inflammation is often present at the onset of disease, with elevated erythrocyte sedimentation rate and mild increase in white blood cell count and platelet count. Rheumatoid factor is absent in all children with spondyloarthropathies.

TREATMENT. The aims of therapy are to minimize pain, control inflammation, and preserve function. These are accomplished by a combination of anti-inflammatory medications, physical therapy, and psychosocial support.

CHAPTER 117

Postinfectious Arthritis and Related Conditions

(Nelson Textbook, Chapter 158)

Infections have been associated with arthritis during their course and as a postinfectious reaction observed several weeks or months afterward. *Reactive arthritis* follows an infection outside the joint, particularly involving the gastrointestinal or genitourinary tract. *Postinfectious arthritis* follows infections that are usually viral in origin and of shorter duration than reactive arthritis.

CLINICAL MANIFESTATIONS. Bacterial enteritis caused by *Shigella, Salmonella, Yersinia,* and *Campylobacter* can be followed within days to several weeks by the development of arthritis and sometimes enthesitis in a syndrome similar to spondyloarthropathy and overlapping with it. Urethritis and conjunctivitis (Reiter syndrome) will also develop occasionally. Postinfectious arthritis following less apparent illness, such as viral upper respiratory tract infections, may precede arthralgia and arthritis by 1–2 mo. Symptoms of arthralgia and joint swelling are transient, usually lasting less than 6 wk.

Certain viruses associated with arthritis may result in particular patterns of joint involvement. Rubella and hepatitis B virus typically affect the small joints, and mumps and varicella often involve large joints, in particular the knees. Parvovirus B19, responsible for erythema infectiosum (fifth disease), can infrequently cause arthralgia, symmetric joint swelling, and morning stiffness in children.

Poststreptococcal arthritis may follow infection with either group A or group G *Streptococcus*. Poststreptococcal arthritis is pauciarticular, may affect the small and large joints, and persists for months, compared with the typical course of migratory polyarthritis of rheumatic fever. The symptoms are usually mild and tend to resolve completely. *Transient synovitis* (toxic synovitis) typically affects the hip, often after a respiratory tract infection. Boys from 3–10 yr of age are most commonly affected and have complaints of pain in the hip, thigh, or knee.

DIAGNOSIS. The diagnosis of reactive postinfectious arthritis is made by exclusion after arthritis has resolved.

TREATMENT. No specific treatment is necessary for postinfectious arthritis except that directed at relief of pain and the functional limitations of arthritis.

CHAPTER 118

Systemic Lupus Erythematosus
(Nelson Textbook, Chapter 159)

Systemic lupus erythematosus (SLE, or lupus), a rheumatic disease of unknown cause, is characterized by autoantibodies directed against self-antigens and resulting inflammatory damage to target organs including the kidneys, blood cells, and the central nervous system (CNS). The natural history of SLE is unpredictable; patients may present with many years of symptoms or with acute, life-threatening disease.

ETIOLOGY. The cause and disease mechanisms of SLE remain unknown. The hallmark is autoantibody production against many self-antigens, particularly DNA, as well as other nuclear antigens, ribosomes, platelets, coagulation factors, immunoglobulin, erythrocytes, and leukocytes.

CLINICAL MANIFESTATIONS. Children most frequently present with fever, fatigue, arthralgia or arthritis, and rash. Symptoms may be intermittent or persistent.

The characteristic malar or butterfly rash includes the nasal bridge and varies from an erythematous blush to thickened epidermis to scaly patches. Rashes may be photosensitive and extend to sun-exposed areas. Mucous membrane changes from vasculitic erythema to ulcers occur particularly on palatal and nasal mucosa.

Musculoskeletal findings include arthralgia, arthritis, tendinitis, and myositis. Deforming arthritis is unusual. Avascular necrosis of bone is common and is presumed secondary to vasculopathy or corticosteroid treatment.

Serositis can affect pleural, pericardial, and peritoneal surfaces. Hepatosplenomegaly and adrenopathy are often found. Other gastrointestinal manifestations, most often resulting from vasculitis, include pain, diarrhea, infarction and melena, inflammatory bowel disease, and hepatitis.

Neurologic manifestations can involve the CNS and peripheral nervous system.

Renal disease is manifested by hypertension, peripheral edema, retinal vascular changes, and clinical manifestations in association with electrolyte abnormalities, nephrosis, or acute renal failure.

LABORATORY FINDINGS. Antinuclear antibodies (ANA) are often present in children with active SLE, and ANA testing is an excellent screening tool; however, ANA can be found without any disease or can be associated with rheumatic and other conditions. Levels of anti–double-stranded DNA, more specific for lupus, reflect the degree of disease activity. Serum levels of total hemolytic complement (CH_{50}), C3, and C4 are decreased in active disease.

TREATMENT. Patients are treated to support clinical well-being, using serologic markers of disease activity as guidelines, and to normalize serum complement levels. Corticosteroids control symptoms and autoantibody production in SLE. Treatment with corticosteroids has improved kidney disease and the rate of survival. Patients with systemic disease are often started on 1–2 mg/kg/24 hr of oral prednisone in divided doses. When complement levels rise to within the normal range, the dose is carefully tapered over 2–3 yr to the lowest effective dose.

Patients with severe disease may require cytotoxic therapy. Pulse intravenous cyclophosphamide has maintained renal function and prevented progression in patients with lupus nephritis, particularly diffuse proliferative glomerulonephritis. Cyclophosphamide has been used to treat vasculitis, pulmonary hemorrhage, and CNS disease refractory to corticosteroids. Azathioprine has been used to prevent renal disease progression.

CHAPTER 119

Juvenile Dermatomyositis

(Nelson Textbook, Chapter 160)

Juvenile dermatomyositis (JDM), the most common of the pediatric inflammatory myopathies, is a systemic vasculopathy with characteristic cutaneous findings and focal areas of myositis resulting in progressive proximal muscle weakness that is responsive to immunosuppressive therapy.

CLINICAL MANIFESTATIONS. Disease onset is often insidious; constitutional symptoms of fatigue, low-grade fever, weight loss, and irritability are common. The characteristic rash usually appears first, particularly over sun-exposed areas, followed by proximal muscle weakness after a median of 2 mo. Periorbital violaceous (heliotropic) erythema (heliotrope eyelids) may cross the nasal bridge. Periorbital and facial edema may be associated. The rash may involve the upper torso, the extensor surfaces of the arms and legs, the medial malleoli of the ankles, and the buttocks.

The onset of proximal muscle weakness is insidious and difficult to recognize. It is often detected by difficulty in climbing stairs, combing hair, or standing from a sitting position or rising unassisted from the floor without "climbing up the body" (Gowers sign). Derangement of upper airway function can be detected by hoarseness, a nasal quality to the speech, or difficulty in handling secretions. Dysphagia is a severe prognostic sign and should prompt immediate aggressive therapeutic intervention. Complaints of constipation reflect impaired gastrointestinal smooth muscle function, and abdominal pain or diarrhea may indicate occult gastrointestinal bleeding, which can progress and be life threatening. Cardiac involvement with a conduction abnormality is frequent at diagnosis.

LABORATORY FINDINGS. Elevated serum levels of muscle-derived enzymes—creatine kinase, aldolase, aspartate aminotransaminase, and lactic acid dehydrogenase—reflect the leaky muscle membranes. Antinuclear antibodies with a speckled pattern (unknown specificity) are present in more than 60% of children. Tests for antibodies to SSA, SSB, Sm, RNP, and DNA are negative.

COMPLICATIONS. Aspiration pneumonia is a frequent major complication associated with unrecognized impairment in swallowing fluids. Progressive bowel infarction can lead to perforation and death. Depression and mood swings are part of the disease spectrum of central nervous system involvement and may be accentuated by corticosteroid administration.

TREATMENT. All children with JDM should use a sunscreen (*p*-aminobenzoic acid free) that provides maximal protection (ultraviolet A and B). Vitamin D, at the dose appropriate for weight and with a diet sufficient in calcium, repairs osteopenia and decreases the frequency of bone fracture.

Children with only cutaneous findings and a negative family history of color blindness may take hydroxychloroquine (maximum dose of 2 mg/kg/24 hr), with a low daily dose of oral corticosteroids (prednisone, 0.5 mg/kg/24 hr) if needed.

With mild muscle damage, oral corticosteroids (prednisone, 1–2 mg/kg/24 hr) may suffice, with rapid normalization of the serum levels of muscle-derived enzymes. With severe disease at onset, prompt institution of high-dose intermittent intravenous methylprednisolone therapy may be lifesaving. Low-dose oral prednisone (0.5 mg/kg/24 hr) is given on days when methylprednisolone is not given intravenously.

Children with dysphagia require a soft diet, or nasogastric feedings if necessary, until treatment restores a functional, protected airway.

Chapter 120

Scleroderma

(Nelson Textbook, Chapter 161)

Scleroderma, a chronic disease of unknown cause, is characterized by fibrosis affecting the dermis and arteries of the lungs, kidneys, and gastrointestinal tract. Antinuclear antibodies (ANA) specific for topoisomerase I (SCL70) and the centromere are found in many patients.

CLINICAL MANIFESTATIONS. Raynaud phenomenon, resulting from digital arterial spasm, is often the earliest manifestation and may precede extensive skin and internal organ involvement by months or years. Induced by exposure to cold, Raynaud phenomenon affects the fingers, toes, and occasionally the ears and the tip of the nose.

Systemic Sclerosis. Systemic sclerosis often presents with a preliminary edematous phase that can last several months before chronic fibrosis develops. These early changes include puffiness around the fingers, on the dorsum of the hands, and sometimes on the face. An eventual decrease in edema is associated with tightening of the skin. Skin changes tend to spread proximally from the hands. Later, atrophic skin can become shiny and waxy in appearance. The fingers take on a tapered appearance associated with tightened skin (sclerodactyly) and eventual development of secondary and often severe flexion contractures and limitation of motion. As lesions spread proximally, flexion contractures in the elbows, hips, and knees may be associated with secondary muscle weakness and atrophy.

Pulmonary disease includes arterial and interstitial involvement and can vary from minimal disease to a progressive course that eventually results in decreased exercise tolerance, dyspnea at rest, and right-sided heart failure.

Scleroderma can also affect other organs. Renal arterial disease can cause chronic or severe episodic hypertension. Esophageal dilatation caused by fibrosis can cause dysphagia. Dilated intestinal loops can result in malabsorption and failure to thrive. Cardiac fibrosis has been associated with arrhythmias, ventricular hypertrophy, and decreased cardiac function.

Morphea and Linear Scleroderma. In localized scleroderma, the involvement is restricted to the skin; progression to systemic sclerosis is rare. In children, lesions are typically discrete and may occur anywhere on the body but particularly on the face.

TREATMENT. Although there is no specific treatment, immuno-suppressive agents, including methotrexate and corticosteroids, in the early stages of the disease may be helpful in curbing inflammation. However, corticosteroids later in the course of the disease do not appear to be effective and may exacerbate hypertension. Additional treatment includes physical and occupational therapy to improve flexion contractures and maintain muscle strength.

CHAPTER 121

Kawasaki Disease

(Nelson Textbook, Chapter 166)

Kawasaki disease (formerly known as mucocutaneous lymph node syndrome or infantile polyarteritis nodosa) is an acute febrile vasculitis of childhood.

ETIOLOGY. The cause of the illness remains unknown, but clinical and epidemiologic features strongly support an infectious origin.

EPIDEMIOLOGY. It is estimated that at least 3,000 cases are diagnosed annually in the United States. In Japan, more than 150,000 cases have been reported since the 1960s.

CLINICAL MANIFESTATIONS. Fever is generally high spiking (to 104°F or higher), remittent, and unresponsive to antibiotics. The duration of fever is generally 1–2 wk without treatment but may persist for 3–4 wk. Prolonged fever has been shown to be a risk factor for the development of coronary artery disease. The other characteristic features of the illness are bilateral bulbar conjunctival injection, usually without exudate; erythema of the oral and pharyngeal mucosa, with "strawberry" tongue and dry, cracked lips; erythema and swelling of the hands and feet; rash of various forms (maculopapular, erythema multiforme, or scarlatiniform), with accentuation in the groin area; and nonsuppurative cervical lymphadenopathy, usually unilateral, with a node size of 1.5 cm or greater in diameter. One to 3 wk after the onset of illness, periungual desquamation of the fingers and toes begins and may progress to involve the entire hand and foot. Perineal desquamation is common.

Other features include extreme irritability, especially in infants, aseptic meningitis, diarrhea, mild hepatitis, hydrops of the gallbladder, urethritis and meatitis with sterile pyuria, otitis media, and arthritis.

Cardiac involvement is the most important manifestation of Kawasaki disease. Myocarditis manifested by tachycardia and decreased ventricular function occurs in at least 50% of patients. Pericarditis with a small pericardial effusion is common during the acute illness. Coronary artery aneurysms generally develop during the 2nd–3rd wk of illness and can be detected by two-dimensional echocardiography.

DIAGNOSIS. The diagnosis of Kawasaki disease is based on demonstration of characteristic clinical signs (Table 121–1). Atypical or incomplete cases in which a patient has fever with fewer than four other features of the illness and then develops coronary artery disease have been described.

LABORATORY FINDINGS. No specific diagnostic test for the illness exists, but certain laboratory findings are characteristic. The white blood cell count is normal to elevated, with a predominance of neutrophils and immature forms. An elevated erythrocyte sedimentation rate, C-reactive protein, and other acute phase reactants are almost universally present in the acute phase of illness and may persist for 4–6 wk. Normocytic anemia is common. The platelet count is generally normal in the 1st wk of illness and rapidly rises by the 2nd–3rd wk of illness and may exceed 1 million/mm³. Antinuclear antibody and rheumatoid factor are not detectable.

TREATMENT. Patients with acute Kawasaki disease should be treated with intravenous immune globulin (IVIG) and high-dose aspirin as soon as possible after diagnosis. Treatment results in rapid defervescence and resolution of clinical signs of illness in most patients. IVIG reduces the prevalence of coronary disease from 20–25% in children treated with aspirin alone to 2–4% in those treated with IVIG and aspirin within the 1st 10 days of illness.

COMPLICATIONS AND PROGNOSIS. Recovery is complete and without apparent long-term effects for patients who do not develop coronary disease. Recurrent illness occurs in only 1–3% of cases. The

---

TABLE 121–1 Diagnostic Criteria for Kawasaki Disease

Fever lasting for at least 5 days*
Presence of at least four of the following five signs:

1. Bilateral bulbar conjunctival injection, generally nonpurulent
2. Changes in the mucosa of the oropharynx, including injected pharynx, injected and/or dry fissured lips, strawberry tongue
3. Changes of the peripheral extremities, such as edema and/or erythema of the hands or feet in the acute phase, or periungual desquamation in the subacute phase
4. Rash, primarily truncal; polymorphous but nonvesicular
5. Cervical adenopathy, ≥1.5 cm, usually unilateral lymphadenopathy

Illness not explained by other known disease process

*Experienced physicians may make the diagnosis of Kawasaki disease (and institute treatment) before the 5th day of fever in patients with classic features of the illness.

prognosis for patients with coronary abnormalities depends on the severity of coronary disease.

CHAPTER 122

Vasculitis Syndromes
(Nelson Textbook, Chapter 167)

The affected target vessels range in size from large afferent vessels in Takayasu arteritis to capillary and arteriolar occlusion characteristic of juvenile dermatomyositis. The signs and symptoms of the vasculitic syndromes are nonspecific and tend to overlap, but certain clinical features are useful in distinguishing the type of vasculature that is primarily affected. Palpable purpura suggests small vessel vasculitis located deep in the papillary dermis, whereas a circumscribed tender nodule is more likely a result of involvement of medium-sized vessels.

HENOCH-SCHÖNLEIN PURPURA (HSP)

HSP, also known as anaphylactoid purpura, is a vasculitis of small vessels. It is the most common cause of nonthrombocytopenic purpura in children.

EPIDEMIOLOGY. The cause of HSP is unknown, but it typically follows an upper respiratory tract infection.

CLINICAL MANIFESTATIONS. The disease onset may be acute, with the appearance of several manifestations simultaneously, or insidious, with sequential occurrence of symptoms over a period of weeks or months. Low-grade fever and fatigue occur in more than half of affected children.

The hallmark of the disease is the rash, beginning as pinkish maculopapules that initially blanch on pressure and progress to petechiae or purpura, characterized clinically as palpable purpura that evolve from red to purple to rusty brown before they eventually fade. The lesions tend to occur in crops, last from 3–10 days, and may appear at intervals that vary from a few days to as long as 3–4 mo. Edema occurs primarily in dependent areas (e.g., below the waist, over the buttocks [or on the back and posterior scalp in the infant]) or in areas of greater tissue distensibility, such as the eyelids, lips, scrotum, or the dorsa of the hands and feet.

Arthritis, present in more than two thirds of children with HSP, is usually localized to the knees and ankles and appears to be a concomitant of edema.

Edema and damage to the vasculature of the gastrointestinal tract may also lead to intermittent abdominal pain that is often colicky. More than half of patients have occult heme-positive stools, diarrhea (with or without blood), or hematemesis. Intussusception may occur. Renal involvement occurs in 25–50% of children, and hepatosplenomegaly and lymphadenopathy may be found during active disease.

LABORATORY FINDINGS. Routine laboratory tests are neither specific nor diagnostic.

TREATMENT. Symptomatic treatment, including adequate hydration, bland diet, and pain control with acetaminophen, is provided for self-limited complaints of arthritis, edema, fever, and malaise. Intestinal complications (e.g., hemorrhage, obstruction, and intussusception) may be life threatening and managed with corticosteroids and, when necessary, barium enema reduction or surgical reduction or resection of the intussusception. Therapy with oral or intravenous corticosteroids (1–2 mg/kg/24 hr) is often associated with dramatic improvement of both gastrointestinal and central nervous system complications. Management of renal involvement is the same as that for other forms of acute glomerulonephritis.

TAKAYASU ARTERITIS

Takayasu arteritis, or pulseless disease, is a chronic vasculitis of large vessels. Early identification and surgical excision of the predominant lesions are essential, in conjunction with institution of appropriate immunosuppressive therapy.

POLYARTERITIS NODOSA

Polyarteritis nodosa is a necrotizing vasculitis affecting small- and medium-sized arteries. Aneurysms and nodules may form at irregular intervals throughout affected arteries. The clinical presentation is variable but generally reflects the location of vessels that have become inflamed. Children may present with fever of unknown origin before other findings develop.

PART 15

Infectious Diseases

SECTION 1

General Considerations

CHAPTER 123

Fever

(Nelson Textbook, Chapters 170 and 171)

Body temperature is regulated by thermosensitive neurons located in the preoptic or anterior hypothalamus. These neurons respond to changes in blood temperature as well as to direct neural connections with cold and warm receptors located in skin and muscle. Normal body temperature varies in a regular pattern each day. This circadian temperature rhythm, or diurnal variation, results in lower body temperatures in the early morning and temperatures approximately 1°C higher in the late afternoon or early evening.

Fever is a controlled increase in body temperature over the normal values for an individual. It is regulated in the same manner as normal temperature is maintained in a cool environment, the difference being that the body's thermostat has been reset at a higher temperature. Regardless of whether fever is associated with infection, connective tissue disease, or malignancy, the thermostat is reset in response to endogenous pyrogens.

CLINICAL MANIFESTATIONS. Although fever patterns per se are not often helpful in determining a specific diagnosis, observing the clinical characteristics of fever can provide useful information. In general, a single isolated fever spike is not associated with an infectious disease. Such a spike can be attributed to the infusion of blood products, some drugs, some procedures, or manipulation of a catheter on a colonized or infected body surface. Similarly, temperatures in excess of 41°C (105.8°F) are seldom associated with an infectious cause. Causes of very high temperatures (>41°C) include central fevers (resulting from central nervous system dysfunction that involves the hypothalamus), malignant hyperthermia, malignant neuroleptic syndrome, drug fever, or heat stroke. Temperatures that are lower than normal (<36°C [96.8°F]) can be associated with overwhelming sepsis but are more commonly related to cold exposure, hypothyroidism, or overuse of antipyretics.

369

An exaggerated circadian rhythm that includes a period of normal temperatures on most days is termed *intermittent fever*; extremely wide fluctuations may be termed *septic* or *hectic fever*. A sustained fever is persistent and does not vary by more than 0.5°C/day. A remittent fever varies by more than 0.5°C during the course of a day but does not return to normal. Relapsing fevers are separated by intervals of normal temperature; tertian fevers occur on the 1st and 3rd days (*Plasmodium vivax*), and quartan fevers occur on the first and fourth days (*Plasmodium malariae*).

The relationship between a patient's pulse rate and temperature can be informative. Relative tachycardia, when the pulse rate is elevated out of proportion to the temperature, is usually due to noninfectious diseases or infectious diseases in which a toxin is responsible for the clinical manifestations. Relative bradycardia (temperature-pulse dissociation), when the pulse rate remains low in the presence of fever, suggests drug fever, typhoid fever, brucellosis, or leptospirosis. Bradycardia in the presence of fever also may be a result of a conduction defect.

TREATMENT. Fever with temperatures less than 39°C in healthy children generally do not require treatment. As temperatures become higher, patients tend to become more uncomfortable and administration of antipyretics often makes patients feel better. Other than providing symptomatic relief, antipyretic therapy does not change the course of infectious diseases in normal children. Antipyretic therapy is beneficial in high-risk patients who have chronic cardiopulmonary diseases, metabolic disorders, or neurologic diseases and in those who are at risk for febrile seizures.

Acetaminophen, aspirin, and ibuprofen are equally effective antipyretic agents. Because aspirin has been associated with Reye syndrome in children and adolescents, its use is not recommended for the treatment of fever. Acetaminophen, 10–15 mg/kg every 4 hr, is not associated with many adverse effects; however, prolonged use may produce renal injury, and massive overdose may produce hepatic failure. Ibuprofen, 5–10 mg/kg every 6–8 hr, may cause dyspepsia, gastrointestinal bleeding, reduced renal blood flow, and, rarely, aseptic meningitis, hepatic toxicity, or aplastic anemia.

DIAGNOSTIC MICROBIOLOGY

Laboratory diagnosis of infectious diseases is based on one or more of the following: (1) direct examination of specimens by microscopic or antigenic techniques, (2) isolation of microorganisms in culture, (3) serologic testing for development of antibodies (serodiagnosis), and (4) molecular genetic detection. Clinicians must select the appropriate tests and specimens and, when possible, suggest the suspected etiologic agents to the microbiologist, because this facilitates selection of the most cost-effective diagnostic approach.

<hr>

SECTION 2

Clinical Syndromes

<hr>

CHAPTER 124

<hr>

Fever Without a Focus
(Nelson Textbook, Chapter 172)

FEVER AS A MANIFESTATION OF INFECTIOUS DISEASE. Fever is a common manifestation of various infectious diseases with a wide range of severity. Benign febrile diseases in normal hosts include common viral infections (e.g., rhinitis, pharyngitis, pneumonia) and bacterial diseases (e.g., otitis media, pharyngitis, impetigo) that usually respond well to appropriate antimicrobial or supportive therapy and are not life threatening. Several bacterial infections, if untreated, may have significant morbidity or mortality; such diseases include sepsis, meningitis, pneumonia, osteoarticular infections, and pyelonephritis. There are well-defined high-risk groups that, on the basis of age, associated diseases, or immunodeficiency status, require a more extensive evaluation and, in certain situations, prompt antimicrobial therapy before a pathogen is identified (Table 124–1).

FEVER WITHOUT A FOCUS. Fever without localizing signs or symptoms is a common diagnostic dilemma for pediatricians caring for infants younger than 36 mo. Fever is usually of acute onset and is present for less than 1 wk. Infants younger than 3 mo (60 days) demonstrate a limited array of signs with infection, often making it difficult for the clinician to distinguish between serious bacterial infections and self-limited viral illnesses.

Infants Younger Than 3 Mo. Fever in an infant younger than 3 mo should always suggest the possibility of serious bacterial disease. Serious bacterial infections are present in 10–15% of infants who were born at term and were previously healthy who have rectal temperatures of 38°C (100.4°F) or greater.

Viral pathogens can be identified in 40–60% of febrile infants younger than 3 mo. In contrast to bacterial infections, which have no seasonal pattern, viral diseases have a distinct pattern: respiratory syncytial and influenza A virus infections are more

TABLE 124–1 Febrile Patients at Increased Risk for Serious Bacterial Infections

Condition	Comment
Immunocompetent Patients	
Neonates (<28 days)	Sepsis and meningitis caused by group B streptococci, *Escherichia coli*, *Listeria monocytogenes*, herpes simplex virus
Infants <3 mo	Serious bacterial disease (10–15%); bacteremia in 5% of febrile infants
Infants and children 3–36 mo	Occult bacteremia in 4%; increased risk with temperature >39°C (102.2°F) and white blood cell count >15,000/μL
Hyperpyrexia (>41°C [105.8°F])	Meningitis, bacteremia, pneumonia, heat stroke, hemorrhagic shock/encephalopathy syndrome
Fever with petechiae	Bacteremia and meningitis caused by *Neisseria meningitidis*, *Haemophilus influenzae* type b, *Streptococcus pneumoniae*
Immunocompromised Patients	
Sickle cell anemia	Pneumococcal sepsis, meningitis
Asplenia	Encapsulated bacteria
Complement/properdin deficiency	Meningococcal sepsis
Agammaglobulinemia	Bacteremia, sinopulmonary infection
Acquired immunodeficiency syndrome	*S. pneumoniae, H. influenzae* type b, *Salmonella*
Congenital heart disease	Increased risk of endocarditis
Central venous line	*Staphylococcus aureus*, coagulase-negative staphylococci, *Candida*
Malignancy	Gram-negative enteric bacteria, *S. aureus*, coagulase-negative staphylococci, *Candida*

common during the winter, whereas enterovirus infections usually occur in the summer and fall.

The approach to febrile patients younger than 3 mo should include a careful history and physical examination. Infants who are unlikely to have a serious bacterial infection are those who appear generally well; who have been previously healthy; who have no evidence of skin, soft tissue, bone, joint, or ear infection; and who have a total white blood cell (WBC) count of 5,000–15,000 cells/μL, an absolute band count of less than 1,500 cells/μL, and normal urinalysis results.

Ill-appearing (toxic) febrile infants younger than 3 mo require prompt hospitalization; cultures of blood, urine, and cerebrospinal fluid (CSF); and immediate parenteral antimicrobial therapy. ceftriaxone (50 mg/kg given once daily with normal CSF or 80 mg/kg once daily with CSF pleocytosis) or cefotaxime (50 mg/kg/dose administered every 6 hr) and ampicillin (50 mg/kg/dose given every 6 hr) (for *Listeria monocytogenes* and enterococci) are effective antimicrobial agents for the initial therapy of ill-appearing patients without focal signs. This regimen is effective against bacterial pathogens producing sepsis, urinary tract infection, and gastroenteritis. However, if meningitis caused by *Streptococcus pneumoniae* resistant to penicillin is a possibility, vancomycin (15 mg/kg/dose administered every 6 hr) should be given in addition to the ampicillin and ceftriaxone until the results of culture and susceptibility tests are known.

Occult Bacteremia in Children Age 3 mo–3 yr. Approximately 30% of febrile children 3 mo–3 yr of age have no localizing signs of infection. Occult bacteremia (bacteremia without an obvious focus of infection) due to *S. pneumoniae, Haemophilus influenzae* type b, *Neisseria meningitidis*, and *Salmonella* species occurs in approximately 4% of relatively well-appearing children between 3 and 36 mo of age with fever (rectal temperature ≥38.0°C). *S. pneumoniae* accounts for 85% of cases of occult bacteremia, with *H. influenzae* type b, *N. meningitidis*, and *Salmonella* species accounting for the remaining positive cultures. Common bacterial infections among children between 3 and 36 mo of age who do have localizing signs include otitis media, upper respiratory tract infection, pneumonia, gastroenteritis, urinary tract infection, osteomyelitis, and meningitis.

Risk factors indicating increased probability of occult bacteremia include temperature exceeding 39°C (102.2°F), total WBC count greater than 15,000/wL, or an elevated absolute neutrophil count, band count, erythrocyte sedimentation rate, or C-reactive protein value. The incidence of bacteremia among infants between 3 and 36 mo increases as the temperature and WBC count increase. However, no combination of laboratory tests or clinical assessment is completely accurate in predicting the presence of occult bacteremia. Without therapy, occult bacteremia may resolve spontaneously without sequelae, may persist, or may lead to localized infections, such as meningitis, pneumonia, cellulitis, or septic arthritis.

Treatment of toxic-appearing febrile children from 3–36 mo of age who do not have focal signs of infection includes hospitalization; cultures of blood, urine, and CSF; and prompt institution of antimicrobial therapy.

Practice guidelines published in 1993 recommended that infants 3–36 mo of age who have a temperature less than 39°C and who do not appear toxic can be observed as outpatients without performing diagnostic tests or administering antimicrobial agents. For non–toxic-appearing infants with a rectal temperature of 39°C or greater, two options are suggested: (1) obtain a blood culture and give empirical antimicrobial therapy (ceftriaxone, 50 mg/kg once daily, not to exceed 1 g) or (2) obtain a complete blood cell count, and if the WBC count is 15,000 or more cells/μL, obtain a blood culture and give empirical antimicrobial therapy.

FEVER WITH PETECHIAE. Independent of age, fever with petechiae with or without localizing signs indicates high risk for life-threatening bacterial infections such as bacteremia, sepsis, and meningitis.

FEVER IN PATIENTS WITH SICKLE CELL ANEMIA. Infection is the most common cause of death among children with sickle cell anemia. The incidence of infection is greatest among infants younger than 5 yr. Fever without a focus is a common presenting sign of sepsis or meningitis due to pneumococcus in patients with sickle cell anemia. The treatment of patients with sickle cell hemoglobinopathies requires culture of blood and, if indicated, of CSF, stool, and bone and administration of antimicrobial agents.

HYPERPYREXIA. Hyperpyrexia (temperature >41°C [105.8°F]) is uncommon. Infants and children with hyperpyrexia should be carefully evaluated, but evaluation and management need not differ from that of other children with lesser degrees of fever in excess of 39°C.

FEVER OF UNKNOWN ORIGIN (FUO). This term is reserved for children with a fever documented by a health care provider and for which the cause could not be identified after a 3-wk evaluation as an outpatient or after a 1-wk evaluation in a hospital. The principal causes of FUO in children, using more restrictive criteria, are infections and connective tissue (autoimmune or rheumatologic) diseases. Neoplastic disorders should also be seriously considered. The possibility of drug fever should be considered if a patient is receiving any drug. Most fevers of unknown or unrecognized origin result from atypical presentations of common diseases.

In the United States, the systemic infectious diseases most commonly implicated in children with FUO (by the more rigorous definition) are salmonellosis, tuberculosis, rickettsial diseases, syphilis, Lyme disease, cat-scratch disease, atypical prolonged presentations of common viral diseases, infectious mononucleosis, cytomegalovirus infection, hepatitis, coccidioidomycosis, histoplasmosis, malaria, and toxoplasmosis.

Juvenile rheumatoid arthritis and systemic lupus erythematosus are the connective tissue diseases associated most frequently with FUO.

CHAPTER 125

Sepsis and Shock

(Nelson Textbook, Chapter 173)

The recovery of bacteria in a blood culture, *bacteremia*, may be a transient phenomenon not associated with disease or may be the serious extension of an invasive bacterial infection originating elsewhere. *Sepsis* is the systemic response to infection with bacteria, viruses, fungi, protozoa, or rickettsiae. Sepsis is one of the causes of the systemic inflammatory response syndrome (SIRS), which has noninfectious causes as well. If not recognized and treated early, sepsis can progress to severe sepsis, septic shock (sepsis with hypotension), multiple organ dysfunction syndrome (MODS), and death.

EPIDEMIOLOGY. Sepsis may develop as a complication of localized community-acquired infections or may follow colonization and local mucosal invasion by virulent pathogens. Children age 3 mo–3 yr are at risk for occult bacteremia, which occasionally progresses to sepsis.

CLINICAL MANIFESTATIONS. The primary signs and symptoms of sepsis and its complications include fever, shaking chills, hyperventilation, tachycardia, hypothermia, cutaneous lesions (e.g., petechiae, ecchymoses, ecthyma gangrenosum, diffuse erythema), and changes in mental status such as confusion, agitation, anxiety, excitation, lethargy, obtundation, or coma. Secondary manifestations include hypotension, cyanosis, symmetric peripheral gangrene (purpura fulminans), oliguria or anuria, jaundice (direct hyperbilirubinemia), and signs of heart failure. There may be evidence of focal infection such as meningitis, pneumonia, arthritis, cellulitis, or pyelonephritis or of an immunocompromised status such as malignancy, T- or B-lymphocyte defects, or prior splenectomy.

LABORATORY FINDINGS. The laboratory manifestations of sepsis include positive blood cultures; Gram, Wright, methylene blue, or acridine orange stain of the buffy coat or petechial lesions demonstrating microorganisms; metabolic acidosis; thrombocytopenia; prolonged prothrombin and partial thromboplastin times; reduced serum fibrinogen levels; anemia; decreased Pao_2 and $Paco_2$; and alterations in the morphology and number of neutrophils. Elevated neutrophil count and band count (increased immature white blood cells, or "shift to the left") suggest bacterial infection, and neutropenia is an ominous sign of fulminant septic shock. Vacuolation of neutrophils, toxic granulations, and Döhle bodies are also suggestive of bacterial sepsis. Examination of the cerebrospinal fluid (CSF) may reveal neutrophils and bacteria.

TREATMENT. Specimens of blood, urine, and CSF are cultured for bacterial pathogens from patients suspected of having sepsis or septic shock. Exudates, abscesses, and cutaneous lesions should also be cultured and stained for organisms. A complete blood cell count, platelet count, prothrombin and partial thromboplastin times, fibrinogen level, arterial blood gas levels, and chest radiograph should be obtained. Affected children should be observed in an intensive care unit, where central venous pressure, continuous intra-arterial blood pressure monitoring, and cardiac output measurements are available.

Broad-spectrum bactericidal synergistic antimicrobial agents should be administered for presumed sepsis. The specific combination of antimicrobial agents depends on the presence of risk factors.

Supplemental oxygen via a high-flow nonrebreathing system should be administered during initial assessment even if oxygen saturation is normal, because oxygen delivery at the tissue level may be decreased. When possible, the airway in patients with a deteriorating clinical condition should be controlled by elective intubation rather than waiting until urgently needed.

Isotonic solutions such as normal saline and lactated Ringer solution should be given as rapid infusions of 20 mL/kg. Correction of metabolic abnormalities can also improve cardiac function. When fluid administration is unsuccessful in restoring hemodynamic stability, inotropic agents are added.

PROGNOSIS. The mortality for septic shock depends on the initial site of infection, the bacterial pathogen, the presence of MODS, and the host immune response.

Chapter 126

Central Nervous System Infections
(Nelson Textbook, Chapter 174)

Acute infection of the central nervous system (CNS) is the most common cause of fever associated with signs and symptoms of CNS disease in children. Infection may be caused by virtually any microbe, the specific pathogen being influenced by the age and immune status of the host and the epidemiology of the pathogen. In general, viral infections of the CNS are much more common than bacterial infections, which in turn are more common than fungal and parasitic infections.

Regardless of etiology, most patients with acute CNS infection have similar clinical syndromes. Common symptoms include headache, nausea, vomiting, anorexia, restlessness, and irritability. Unfortunately, most of these symptoms are quite nonspecific. Common signs of CNS infection, in addition to fever, include photophobia, neck pain and rigidity, obtundation, stupor, coma, seizures, and focal neurologic deficits. The diagnosis of diffuse

CNS infections depends on careful examination of cerebrospinal fluid (CSF) obtained by lumbar puncture (LP).

ACUTE BACTERIAL MENINGITIS BEYOND THE NEONATAL PERIOD

Bacterial meningitis is one of the most potentially serious infections in infants and older children. This infection is associated with a high rate of acute complications and risk of chronic morbidity. The pattern of bacterial meningitis and its treatment during the neonatal period (0–28 days) are generally distinct from those in older infants and children. Nonetheless, the clinical patterns of meningitis in the neonatal and postneonatal periods may overlap, especially in infants 1–2 mo old. The incidence of bacterial meningitis is sufficiently high that it should be included in the differential diagnosis of altered mental status such as lethargy or irritability or evidence of other neurologic dysfunction in febrile infants.

ETIOLOGY. During the first 2 mo of life, the bacteria that cause meningitis in normal infants reflect the maternal flora or the environment of the infant (i.e., group B *Streptococcus,* gram-negative enteric bacilli, and *Listeria monocytogenes*). In addition, meningitis in this age group may occasionally be due to *Haemophilus influenzae* (both type b and nontypable strains) and the other pathogens usually found in older patients. Bacterial meningitis in children 2 mo–12 yr of age is usually due to *Streptococcus pneumoniae, Neisseria meningitidis, or H. influenzae* type b.

CLINICAL MANIFESTATIONS. The onset of acute meningitis has two predominant patterns. The more dramatic and, fortunately, less common presentation is sudden onset with rapidly progressive manifestations of shock, purpura, and disseminated intravascular coagulation (DIC) and reduced levels of consciousness frequently resulting in death within 24 hr. More often, meningitis is preceded by several days of upper respiratory tract or gastrointestinal symptoms, followed by nonspecific signs of CNS infection such as increasing lethargy and irritability.

The signs and symptoms of meningitis are related to the nonspecific findings associated with a systemic infection and to manifestations of meningeal irritation. Nonspecific findings include fever (present in 90–95%), anorexia and poor feeding, symptoms of upper respiratory tract infection, myalgia, arthralgia, tachycardia, hypotension, and various cutaneous signs, such as petechiae, purpura, or an erythematous macular rash. Meningeal irritation is manifested as nuchal rigidity, back pain, Kernig sign (flexion of the hip 90 degrees with subsequent pain on extension of the leg), and Brudzinski sign (involuntary flexion of the knees and hips after passive flexion of the neck while supine). In some children, particularly in those younger than 12–18 mo, Kernig and Brudzinski signs may not be evident with meningitis.

Increased intracranial pressure (ICP) is suggested by headache, emesis, bulging fontanel or diastasis (widening) of the sutures, oculomotor or abducens nerve paralysis, hypertension with bradycardia, apnea or hyperventilation, decorticate or decerebrate posturing, stupor, coma, or signs of herniation. Papilledema is uncommon in uncomplicated meningitis. Focal neurologic signs usually are due to vascular occlusion. Cranial neuropathies of the ocular, oculomotor, abducens, facial, and auditory nerves also may be due to focal inflammation.

Seizures (focal or generalized) due to cerebritis, infarction, or electrolyte disturbances occur in 20–30% of patients with meningitis. Seizures that occur on presentation or within the first 4 days of onset are usually of no prognostic significance. Seizures that persist after the 4th day of illness and those that are difficult to treat are associated with a poor prognosis. Alterations of mental status and a reduced level of consciousness are common among patients with meningitis. Comatose patients have a poor prognosis.

DIAGNOSIS. The diagnosis of acute pyogenic meningitis is confirmed by analysis of the CSF, which reveals microorganisms on Gram stain and culture, a neutrophilic pleocytosis, elevated protein, and reduced glucose concentrations. LP should be performed when bacterial meningitis is suspected. Contraindications for an immediate LP include (1) evidence of increased ICP (other than a bulging fontanel); (2) severe cardiopulmonary compromise requiring prompt resuscitative measures for shock or in patients in whom positioning for the LP would further compromise cardiopulmonary function; and (3) infection of the skin overlying the site of the puncture.

Lumbar Puncture. The CSF leukocyte count in bacterial meningitis is usually elevated to greater than $1000/mm^3$ and reveals a neutrophilic predominance (75–95%). Normal healthy neonates may have as many as 30 leukocytes/mm^3, and older children without viral or bacterial meningitis may have 5 leukocytes/mm^3 in the CSF; in both age groups there is a predominance of lymphocytes or monocytes.

TREATMENT. The therapeutic approach to patients with presumed bacterial meningitis depends on the nature of the initial manifestations of the illness. A child with rapidly progressing disease of less than 24 hr duration, in the absence of increased ICP, should receive antibiotics immediately after an LP is performed. If there are signs of increased ICP or focal neurologic findings, antibiotics should be given without performing an LP and before obtaining a computed tomographic scan. Increased ICP should be treated simultaneously. Immediate treatment of associated multiple organ system failure, such as shock and adult respiratory distress syndrome, is also indicated.

Patients who have a more protracted subacute course and become ill over a 1- to 7-day period should also be evaluated for signs of increased ICP and focal neurologic deficits. Unilateral headache, papilledema, and other signs of increased ICP suggest a focal lesion such as a brain or epidural abscess or subdural empyema. Under these circumstances, antibiotic therapy should be initiated before LP and computed tomography. If no signs of increased ICP are evident, an LP should be performed.

Initial Antibiotic Therapy. The initial (empirical) choice of therapy for meningitis in immunocompetent infants and children should be based on the antibiotic susceptibilities of *S. pneumoniae, N. meningitidis, and H. influenzae* type b. Although there are substantial geographic differences in the frequency of resistance of *S. pneumoniae* to antibiotics, rates are increasing. Currently, either of the third-generation cephalosporins, cefotaxime (200 mg/kg/24 hr, given every 6 hr) or ceftriaxone (100 mg/kg/24 hr administered once per day or 50 mg/kg/dose, given every 12 hr), combined with vancomycin (60 mg/kg/24 hr, given every 6 hr) is recommended.

Duration of Antibiotic Therapy. Therapy for uncomplicated penicillin-sensitive *S. pneumoniae* meningitis should be completed with a third-generation cephalosporin or intravenous penicillin (300,000 U/kg/24 hr, given every 4–6 hr) for 10–14 days. If the isolate is resistant to penicillin and the third-generation cephalosporin, therapy should be completed with vancomycin. Intravenous penicillin (300,000 U/kg/24 hr) for 5–7 days is the treatment of choice for uncomplicated *N. meningitidis* meningitis. Uncomplicated *H. influenzae* type b meningitis should be treated for 7–10 days.

Corticosteroids. Data support the intravenous use of dexamethasone, 0.15 mg/kg/dose given every 6 hr for 2 days, in the treatment of children older than 6 wk with acute bacterial meningitis, especially for *H. influenzae* type b.

Supportive Care. Repeated medical and neurologic assessments of patients with bacterial meningitis are essential to identify early signs of cardiovascular, CNS, and metabolic complications. Pulse rate, blood pressure, and respiratory rate should be monitored frequently.

Patients should initially receive nothing by mouth. If a patient is judged to be normovolemic, with normal blood pressure, intravenous fluid administration should be restricted to one half to two thirds of maintenance, or 800–1000 mL/m^2/24 hr, until it can be established that increased ICP or syndrome of inappropriate antidiuretic hormone secretion is not present.

COMPLICATIONS. During the treatment of meningitis, complications due to CNS or systemic effects of infection are common. Neurologic complications include seizures, increased ICP, cranial nerve palsies, stroke, cerebral or cerebellar herniation, transverse myelitis, ataxia, thrombosis of dural venous sinuses, and subdural effusions.

PREVENTION. Vaccination and antibiotic prophylaxis of susceptible at-risk contacts represent the two available means of reducing the likelihood of bacterial meningitis.

Neisseria meningitidis. Chemoprophylaxis is recommended for all close contacts of patients with meningococcal meningitis regardless of age or immunization status. Close contacts should be treated with rifampin, 10 mg/kg/dose every 12 hr (maximum dose of 600 mg), for 2 days as soon as possible after identification of a case of suspected meningococcal meningitis.

Meningococcal quadrivalent vaccine against serogroups A, C, Y, and W135 is recommended for high-risk children older than 2 yr. High-risk patients include those with anatomic or functional asplenia or deficiencies of terminal complement proteins.

Haemophilus influenzae **type b.** Rifampin prophylaxis should be given to all household contacts, including adults, if any close family member younger than 48 mo has not been fully immunized or if an immunocompromised child resides in the household. The dose of rifampin is 20 mg/kg/24 hr (maximum dose of 600 mg) given once each day for 4 days. All children should be immunized with *H. influenzae* type b conjugate vaccine beginning at 2 mo of age.

Streptococcus pneumoniae. No chemoprophylaxis or vaccination is required for normal hosts who may be contacts of patients with pneumococcal meningitis. Heptavalent pneumococcal conjugate vaccine (PCV7) is recommended for use in children. The dosage depends on age and risk status.

VIRAL MENINGOENCEPHALITIS

Viral meningoencephalitis is an acute inflammatory process involving the meninges and, to a variable degree, brain tissue. These infections are relatively common and may be caused by a number of different agents. The CSF is characterized by pleocytosis and the absence of microorganisms on Gram stain and routine bacterial culture. In most instances, the infections are self-limited; in some cases, however, substantial morbidity and mortality may be observed.

EPIDEMIOLOGY. The epidemiologic pattern of viral meningoencephalitis reflects the prevalence of the enteroviruses, the primary etiology. Infection with enteroviruses is spread directly from person to person, with a usual incubation period of 4–6 days.

CLINICAL MANIFESTATIONS. The progression and ultimate severity of the clinical course are very much determined by the relative degree of meningeal and parenchymal involvement, which in turn is determined, at least in part, by the specific infectious agents. However, the clinical manifestations have a wide range of severity, even with the same etiologic agent. Some children may appear to be mildly affected initially, only to lapse into coma and die suddenly. In others, the illness may be ushered in by high fever, violent convulsions interspersed with bizarre movements, and hallucinations alternating with brief periods of clarity, but then complete recovery.

The onset of illness is generally acute, although CNS signs and symptoms often are preceded by a nonspecific acute febrile illness of a few days' duration. The presenting manifestations in older children are headache and hyperesthesia, and in infants they are irritability and lethargy. Headache is most often frontal or generalized; adolescents frequently note retrobulbar pain. Fever, nausea and vomiting, photophobia, and pain in the neck, back, and legs are common. As body temperature rises, there may be mental dullness, eventuating in stupor in combination with bizarre movements and convulsions. Focal neurologic signs may be stationary, progressive, or fluctuating. Loss of bowel and bladder control and unprovoked emotional bursts may occur.

Exanthems often precede or accompany the CNS signs, especially with echoviruses, coxsackieviruses, varicella-zoster virus, measles, and rubella. Examination often reveals nuchal rigidity without significant localizing neurologic changes, at least at the onset.

DIAGNOSIS. The diagnosis of viral encephalitis is usually made on the clinical presentation of nonspecific prodrome followed by progressive CNS symptoms. The diagnosis is supported by examination of the CSF, which usually shows a mild mononuclear predominance.

Differential Diagnosis. A number of clinical conditions that cause CNS inflammation mimic viral meningoencephalitis. The most important group of alternate infectious agents to consider is bacteria.

LABORATORY FINDINGS. The CSF contains from a few to several thousand cells per cubic millimeter. Early in the disease the cells are often polymorphonuclear; later, mononuclear cells predominate. The protein concentration in CSF tends to be normal or slightly elevated, but concentrations may be very high if brain destruction is extensive, as illustrated by herpes simplex virus encephalitis.

TREATMENT. Until a bacterial cause is excluded by culture of blood and CSF, parenteral antibiotic therapy should be administered. With the exception of the use of acyclovir for herpes simplex virus encephalitis, treatment of viral meningoencephalitis is nonspecific. Treatment of mild disease may require only symptomatic relief. Headache and hyperesthesia are treated with rest, non–aspirin-containing analgesics, and a reduction in room light, noise, and visitors. Acetaminophen is recommended for fever.

It is important to anticipate and be prepared for convulsions, cerebral edema, hyperpyrexia, inadequate respiratory exchange, disturbed fluid and electrolyte balance, aspiration and asphyxia, and cardiac or respiratory arrest of central origin. Therefore, all patients with severe encephalitis should be monitored closely.

PROGNOSIS. Supportive and rehabilitative efforts are very important after patients recover. Motor incoordination, convulsive disorders, total or partial deafness, and behavioral disturbances may appear only after an interval of time. Visual disturbances due to chorioretinopathy and perceptual amblyopia may also have a delayed appearance. Most children completely recover from viral infections of the CNS, although the prognosis depends on the severity of the clinical illness, the specific cause, and the age of the child.

PREVENTION. Widespread use of effective attenuated viral vaccines for polio, measles, mumps, rubella, and varicella has almost eliminated CNS complications from these diseases in the United States.

CHAPTER 127

Pneumonia
(Nelson Textbook, Chapter 175)

Pneumonia is an inflammation of the parenchyma of the lungs. Most cases of pneumonia are caused by microorganisms, but a number of noninfectious causes sometimes need to be considered. These noninfectious causes include but are not limited to aspiration of food or gastric acid, foreign bodies, hydrocarbons, and lipoid substances; hypersensitivity reactions; and drug- or radiation-induced pneumonitis. The most common microbiologic causes of pneumonia in normal children include respiratory viruses, *Mycoplasma pneumoniae,* and selected bacteria.

Respiratory viruses are the most common cause of pneumonia during the first several years of life. *M. pneumoniae* assumes a predominant role in the etiology of pneumonia in school-aged and older children. Although bacteria are numerically less important as causes of pneumonia, they tend to be responsible for more severe infections than those caused by the nonbacterial agents. The most common bacterial causes of pneumonia in normal children are *Streptococcus pneumoniae, S. pyogenes* (group A *Streptococcus*), and *Staphylococcus aureus.*

VIRAL PNEUMONIA

ETIOLOGY. The most common viruses causing pneumonia include respiratory syncytial virus (RSV), parainfluenza, influenza, and adenoviruses.

CLINICAL MANIFESTATIONS. Most viral pneumonias are preceded by several days of upper respiratory tract symptoms, typically rhinitis and cough. Other family members are frequently ill with similar symptoms. Although fever usually is present, temperatures are generally lower than in bacterial pneumonia. Tachypnea accompanied by intercostal, subcostal, and suprasternal retractions, nasal flaring, and use of accessory muscles is common. Severe infection may be accompanied by cyanosis and respiratory fatigue, especially in infants. Chest auscultation may reveal widespread rales and wheezing. Viral pneumonia cannot be definitely differentiated from mycoplasmal disease on clinical grounds and may, on occasion, be difficult to distinguish from bacterial pneumonia.

DIAGNOSIS. The chest radiograph is characterized by diffuse infiltrates. In some patients, transient lobar infiltrates may also be present or even dominate the picture. Hyperinflation is common. Definitive diagnosis requires isolation of a virus from a specimen obtained from the respiratory tract.

TREATMENT. Many patients are given antibiotic agents initially if bacterial pneumonia is suspected. Failure to respond to antibiotic treatment is additional evidence of a viral cause. Usually, only minimal supportive measures are required, although some patients need hospitalization for intravenous fluids, oxygen, or even assisted ventilation.

Amantadine and rimantadine are active against influenza A isolates. Treatment appears to be beneficial only if started within 48 hr of the onset of the infection. Ribavirin appears to be beneficial for selected infants hospitalized with lower respiratory tract infection caused by RSV.

BACTERIAL PNEUMONIA

Bacterial pneumonia during childhood is not a common infection in the absence of an underlying chronic illness, such as cystic fibrosis or immunologic deficiency. An underlying disorder should be considered if a child experiences recurrent bacterial pneumonia.

Pneumococcal Pneumonia

Although the incidence of pneumococcal pneumonia has declined during the past several decades, *S. pneumoniae* is still the most common cause of bacterial infection of the lungs. One or more lobes or parts of lobes are usually involved. However, this pattern of lobar pneumonia is often not present in infants, who may have a more patchy and diffuse disease that follows a bronchial distribution and is characterized by many areas of consolidation around the smaller airways.

CLINICAL MANIFESTATIONS. The classic history of sudden onset with a shaking chill followed by a high fever, cough, and chest pain may be noted in older children, but it is rarely observed in infants and young children, in whom the clinical pattern is considerably more variable.

Infants. A mild upper respiratory tract infection characterized by stuffy nose, fretfulness, and diminished appetite usually precedes the onset of pneumococcal pneumonia in infants. This mild prodrome of several days' duration ends with abrupt onset of fever, restlessness, apprehension, and respiratory distress. Patients appear ill, with moderate to severe air hunger and often cyanosis. The respiratory distress is manifested by grunting; nasal flaring; retractions of the supraclavicular, intercostal, and subcostal areas; tachypnea; and tachycardia.

Physical examination of the chest is often unrevealing. Dullness to percussion overlying an area of consolidation associated with bronchial breath sounds and rales may be found. Abdominal distention may be prominent because of gastric dilation from swallowed air or ileus. The liver may seem enlarged because of downward displacement of the right diaphragm or superimposed congestive heart failure.

Children and Adolescents. The signs and symptoms are similar to those in adults. A brief, mild upper respiratory tract infection is often followed by onset of a shaking chill and then by high fever. This is accompanied by drowsiness with intermittent periods of restlessness; rapid respirations; a dry, hacking, unproductive cough; anxiety; and occasionally delirium. Circumoral cyanosis may be observed. Many children are noted to be splinting on the affected side to minimize pleuritic pain and improve ventilation; they may lie on their side with their knees drawn up to their chest. Abnormal chest findings include retractions, nasal flaring, dullness to percussion, diminished tactile and vocal fremitus, bronchial breath sounds, and rales. As resolution occurs, moist rales are heard, and the cough loosens and becomes productive of large amounts of blood-tinged mucus.

DIAGNOSIS. Pneumococcal pneumonia cannot be differentiated from other bacterial and viral pneumonias without appropriate microbiologic studies.

LABORATORY FINDINGS. The white blood cell count is usually elevated to 15,000–40,000 cells/mm^3, with a preponderance of polymorphonuclear cells.

RADIOGRAPHIC FINDINGS. Consolidation may be demonstrated by radiography before it can be detected by physical examination. Lobar consolidation is not as common in infants and young children as in older children.

TREATMENT. The drug of choice is penicillin G (100,000 units/kg/24 hr). A third-generation cephalosporin (cefotaxime, 150 mg/kg/24 hr, or ceftriaxone, 75 mg/kg/24 hr) should be used if the isolate of *S. pneumoniae* is resistant to penicillin (minimal inhibitory concentration > 2.0 μg/mL) but sensitive to the cephalosporin. Vancomycin (40 mg/kg/24 hr) should be used if the isolate is resistant to both penicillin and third-generation cephalosporins. The majority of older children with pneumococcal pneumonia can be treated at home; the decision to hospitalize depends on the severity of the illness. Pneumonia in young infants is best treated in the hospital.

Group A Streptococcal Pneumonia

Group A streptococci most commonly cause disease limited to the upper respiratory tract (pharyngitis), but the organisms may spread to other areas of the body, including the lower respiratory tract. The signs and symptoms of streptococcal pneumonia are similar to those of pneumococcal pneumonia. The drug of choice is penicillin G (100,000 units/kg/24 hr). Parenteral penicillin is used initially, and a 2–3-wk course may be completed orally after clinical improvement has begun in the hospital.

Staphylococcal Pneumonia

Pneumonia caused by *S. aureus* is a serious and rapidly progressive infection. It occurs less frequently than viral or pneumococcal pneumonia.

CLINICAL MANIFESTATIONS. Infants younger than 1 yr are most commonly affected and typically have a history of an upper respiratory tract infection for several days to 1 wk. An infant's condition changes abruptly, with the onset of high fever, cough, and evidence of respiratory distress. Signs and symptoms include tachypnea, grunting respirations, sternal and subcostal retractions, nasal flaring, cyanosis, and anxiety. If left undisturbed, infants are lethargic but on arousal are irritable and appear toxic. They may develop severe dyspnea and a shocklike state.

TREATMENT. Therapy consists of appropriate antibiotics and drainage of collections of pus. Infants should be given oxygen and placed in a semireclining position to relieve cyanosis and anxiety. During the acute phase, intravenous hydration and nutrition are indicated. Assisted ventilation may occasionally be needed. A semisynthetic, penicillinase-resistant penicillin should be administered intravenously immediately after cultures are obtained (e.g., nafcillin, 200 mg/kg/24 hr).

CHAPTER 128

Gastroenteritis

(Nelson Textbook, Chapter 176)

Infections of the gastrointestinal tract are caused by a wide variety of enteropathogens, including bacteria, viruses, and parasites. Clinical manifestations depend on the organism and host and include asymptomatic infection, watery diarrhea, bloody diarrhea, chronic diarrhea, and extraintestinal manifestations of infection. The two basic types of acute infectious diarrhea are inflammatory and noninflammatory. Enteropathogens elicit noninflammatory diarrhea through enterotoxin production by some bacteria, destruction of villus (surface) cells by viruses, adherence by parasites, and adherence and/or translocation by bacteria. Inflammatory diarrhea is usually caused by bacteria that invade the intestine directly or produce cytotoxins. Some enteropathogens possess more than one of these virulent properties.

EPIDEMIOLOGY. Diarrheal diseases are one of the leading causes of morbidity and mortality in children worldwide, causing 1 billion episodes of illness and 3–5 million deaths annually.

ETIOLOGY. The relative importance and epidemiologic characteristics of diarrheal pathogens vary by geographic location. Children in developing countries become infected with a diverse group of bacterial and parasitic pathogens, whereas all children in developed as well as developing countries acquire rotavirus and, in many cases, the other viral enteropathogens and *Giardia lamblia* during their first 5 yr of life.

Bacterial Enteropathogens. Antimicrobial therapy is administered to selected patients with diarrhea to shorten the clinical course, to decrease excretion of the causative organism, or to prevent complications. Indications for specific antimicrobial therapy of patients infected with bacterial enteropathogens are shown in Table 128–1.

Parasitic Enteropathogens. Patients with diarrhea normally do not need to have their stools examined for ova and parasites unless they have a history of recent travel to an endemic area, stool cultures are negative for other enteropathogens, and diarrhea persists for more than 1 wk; or unless they are part of an outbreak of diarrhea; or unless they are immunocompromised. Treatment of these organisms depends on the clinical condition and availability of effective therapy (Table 128–2).

Viral Enteropathogens. The four causes of viral gastroenteritis include rotavirus, enteric adenovirus, astrovirus, and calicivirus. Cytomegalovirus and herpes simplex virus have been associated with diarrhea and other gastrointestinal tract signs and symptoms, generally in immunocompromised hosts.

GENERAL APPROACH TO CHILDREN WITH ACUTE DIARRHEA. Enteric infections cause signs of gastrointestinal tract involvement as well as

TABLE 128-1 Antimicrobial Therapy for Bacterial Enteropathogens in Children

Organism	Antimicrobial Agent	Indication for Antimicrobial Therapy
Aeromonas	TMP/SMX	Dysentery-like illness, prolonged diarrhea
Campylobacter	Erythromycin*	Early in the course of illness
Clostridium difficile	Metronidazole or vancomycin	Moderate to severe disease
Escherichia coli		
Enterotoxigenic	TMP/SMX*	Severe or prolonged illness
Enteropathogenic	TMP/SMX	Nursery epidemics, life-threatening illness
Enteroinvasive	TMP/SMX*	All cases if organism susceptible
Salmonella	Ampicillin or chloramphenicol or TMP/SMX or cefotaxime*	Infants <3 mo, immunodeficient patients, typhoid fever *(Salmonella typhi)*, bacteremia, dissemination with localized suppuration
Shigella	TMP/SMX; cefixime or ceftriaxone for resistant strains*	All cases if organism susceptible
Vibrio cholerae	Tetracycline or doxycycline	All cases

*Quinolones (ciprofloxacin or ofloxacin) are recommended for persons ≥18 yr of age.
TMP-SMX = trimethoprim and sulfamethoxazole.

systemic manifestations and complications. Gastrointestinal tract involvement may include diarrhea, cramps, and emesis. Systemic manifestations may include fever, malaise, and seizures. Remote spread can result in endocarditis, osteomyelitis, meningitis, pneumonia, hepatitis, peritonitis, chorioamnionitis, soft tissue infection, and septic thrombophlebitis.

The main objectives in the approach to a child with acute

TABLE 128-2 Antimicrobial Therapy for Enteric Parasites in Children

Organism	Antimicrobial Agent
Giardia lamblia	Metronidazole or furazolidone or paromomycin
Entamoeba histolytica	Metronidazole followed by iodoquinol
Blastocystis hominis	Metronidazole or iodoquinol
Cryptosporidium parvum	None*
Cyclospora cayetanensis	Trimethoprim/sulfamethoxazole (TMP/SMX)
Isospora belli	TMP/SMX
Enterocytozoon bieneusi	Albendazole
Enterocytozoon intestinalis	Albendazole
Strongyloides stercoralis	Thiabendazole

*Paromomycin or azithromycin may be indicated in immunocompromised hosts.

diarrhea are to (1) assess the degree of dehydration and provide fluid and electrolyte replacement, (2) prevent spread of the enteropathogen, and (3) in select episodes determine the etiologic agent and provide specific therapy if indicated. Information about oral intake, frequency and volume of stool output, general appearance and activity of the child, and frequency of urination must be obtained. Information should be obtained about child care center attendance, recent travel to a diarrhea-endemic area, use of antimicrobial agents, exposure to contacts with similar symptoms, and intake of seafood, unwashed vegetables, unpasteurized milk, contaminated water, or uncooked meats. The duration and severity of diarrhea, stool consistency, presence of mucus and blood, and other associated symptomatology, such as fever, vomiting, and seizures, should be determined.

Examination of Stool. Stool specimens should be examined for mucus, blood, and leukocytes, the presence of which indicates colitis. Fecal leukocytes are produced in response to bacteria that invade the colonic mucosa diffusely. Stool cultures should be obtained as early in the course of the disease as possible from patients in whom the diagnosis of hemolytic-uremic syndrome is suspected, in patients with bloody diarrhea, if stools contain fecal leukocytes, during outbreaks of diarrhea, and in persons who have diarrhea and are immunosuppressed.

Management of Fluids and Electrolytes and Refeeding. Management of dehydration remains the cornerstone of therapy for diarrhea. Oral hydration usually is the treatment of choice for all but the most severely dehydrated patients whose caretakers cannot administer fluids. Once rehydration is complete, food should be reintroduced while the oral electrolyte solution is continued to replace ongoing losses from stools and for maintenance. Breast-feeding of infants should be resumed as soon as possible. Older children should be refed as soon as possible.

Antidiarrheal Compounds. Antidiarrheal compounds are generally not recommended for use in children with diarrhea because of their minimal benefit and potential for side effects.

PREVENTION. Patients who are hospitalized should be placed under contact precautions, including hand washing before and after patient contact, wearing gowns when soiling is likely, and wearing gloves when touching infected material. Patients and their families should be educated about the mode of acquisition of enteropathogens and methods to decrease transmission.

ACUTE FOODBORNE AND WATERBORNE DISEASE. Foodborne and waterborne diseases are major causes of morbidity and mortality in all developed countries, including the United States. The diagnosis of a foodborne or waterborne illness should be considered when two or more persons who have ingested common food or water develop a similar acute illness that usually is characterized by nausea, emesis, diarrhea, or neurologic symptoms.

Clinical Syndromes. Several clinical syndromes follow ingestion of contaminated food or water, including nausea and vomiting within 6 hr; paresthesia within 6 hr; neurologic and gastrointestinal tract symptoms within 2 hr; abdominal cramps and watery diarrhea within 16–48 hr; fever, abdominal cramps, and diarrhea within 8–72 hr; abdominal cramps and bloody diarrhea without fever within 72–120 hr; neurologic signs and symptoms within 6–24 hr; and nausea, vomiting, and paralysis within 18–48 hr.

Therapy for most persons with foodborne disease is supportive, because the majority of these illnesses are self-limited. The exceptions are botulism, paralytic shellfish poisoning, and long-acting mushroom poisoning, all of which may be fatal in previously healthy persons. If a foodborne or waterborne outbreak is suspected, public health officials should be notified.

Chapter 129

Viral Hepatitis

(Nelson Textbook, Chapter 177)

Six viruses are known to cause hepatitis as their primary disease manifestation (Table 129–1). The six hepatotropic viruses are a heterogeneous group of viruses that cause similar acute clinical illness, except for HGV, which appears to cause no or mild disease (Table 129–2).

HEPATITIS A

CLINICAL MANIFESTATIONS. The onset of HAV infection usually is abrupt and is accompanied by systemic complaints of fever, mal-

TABLE 129–1 Viral Hepatitis Nomenclature

Hepatotropic Viruses	Antigens	Identified Antibodies
Hepatitis A virus (HAV)	HAV	anti-HAV*
		IgM anti-HAV
Hepatitis B virus (HBV)	HBsAg*	anti-HBsAg*
		IgM anti-HBsAg*
	HBcAg	anti-HBcAg*
	HBeAg*	anti-HBeAg*
Hepatitis C virus (HCV)		anti-HCV*
Hepatitis D virus (HDV)	HDVAg	anti-HDV*
Hepatitis E virus (HEV)		anti-HEV
		IgM anti-HEV
Hepatitis G virus (HGV)		anti-HGV

*Assays are commercially available.

TABLE 129–2 Features of the Six Hepatotropic Viruses

	HAV	HBV	HCV	HDV	HEV	HGV
Nucleic acid	RNA	DNA	RNA	RNA	RNA	RNA
Incubation (mean)	30 days	100–120 days	7–9 wk	2–4 mo	40 days	Unknown
Transmission						
Percutaneous	Rare	Common	Common	Common	No	Common
Fecal-oral	Common	No	No	No	Common	No
Sexual	Rare	Common	Rare	Rare	Rare	Rare
Transplacental	No	Common	Rare	No	Probably no	Rare
Chronic infection	No	Yes	Yes	Yes	No	Yes
Fulminant disease	Rare	Yes	Rare	Yes	Rare	Probably no

aise, nausea, emesis, anorexia, and abdominal discomfort. This prodrome may be mild and often goes unnoticed in infants and preschool-aged children. Diarrhea often occurs in children. Jaundice may be so subtle in young children that it can be detected only by laboratory tests. When jaundice and dark urine occur, they usually develop after the systemic symptoms. Symptoms of HAV infection include right upper quadrant pain, dark-colored urine, and jaundice. The duration of symptoms usually is less than 1 mo, and appetite, exercise tolerance, and a feeling of well-being gradually return. Almost all patients with HAV infection recover completely, but a relapsing course can occur for several months. Fulminant hepatitis leading to death is rare. HAV is not associated with chronic liver disease, persistent viremia, or an intestinal carrier state.

DIAGNOSIS. The diagnosis of HAV infection should be considered when a history of jaundice exists in family contacts, friends, schoolmates, or child care playmates or personnel or if the child or family has traveled to an area endemic for HAV. The diagnosis is made by serologic criteria; liver biopsies rarely are performed. Anti-HAV is detected at the onset of symptoms of acute hepatitis A and persists for life (Fig. 129–1). The virus is excreted in stools from 2 wk before to 1 wk after the onset of illness. Rises are almost universally found in alanine aminotransferase, aspartate aminotransferase, bilirubin, alkaline phosphatase, 5'-nucleotidase, and γ-glutamyltransferase and do not help differentiate the etiology. The prothrombin time should always be measured in a child with hepatitis to help assess the extent of liver injury; prolongation is a serious sign mandating hospitalization.

COMPLICATIONS. Children almost universally recover from HAV infections. Rarely, fulminant hepatitis can occur.

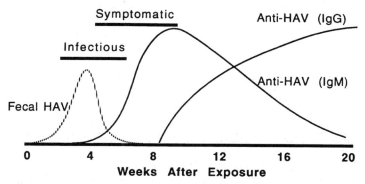

Figure 129–1 Pattern of response to hepatitis A virus (HAV) infection. IgM = immunoglobulin M; IgG = immunoglobulin G.

PREVENTION. Persons infected with HAV are contagious for about 7 days after the onset of jaundice and should be excluded from school, child care, or work during this period. Careful hand washing is necessary, particularly after changing diapers and before preparing or serving food. In hospital settings, contact as well as standard precautions, including strict hand washing, are recommended for diapered or incontinent patients for 1 wk after onset of symptoms.

Vaccine. The availability of two inactivated, highly immunogenic and safe HAV vaccines marks a major advance in the prevention of HAV infection.

Immunoglobulin. Indications for intramuscular administration of immunoglobulin include pre-exposure and postexposure prophylaxis (Table 129–3).

HEPATITIS B

CLINICAL MANIFESTATIONS. Many cases of HBV infection are asymptomatic, as evidenced by the high carriage rate of serum markers in persons who have no history of acute hepatitis. The usual acute symptomatic episode is similar to HAV and HCV infections but may be more severe and is more likely to include involvement of skin and joints. The first clinical evidence of HBV infection is elevation of the alanine aminotransferase level, which begins to rise just before development of lethargy, anorexia, and

TABLE 129–3 Hepatitis A Virus Prophylaxis

Age	Exposure	Dose
Pre-Exposure Prophylaxis (Travelers to Endemic Regions)		
<2 yr	Expected <3 mo	IG 0.02 mL/kg
	Expected 3–5 mo	IG 0.06 mL/kg
	Expected long term	IG 0.06 mL/kg at departure and every 5 mo thereafter
≥2 yr	Expected <3 mo	HAV vaccine* or IG 0.02 mL/kg
	Expected 3–5 mo	HAV vaccine* or IG 0.06 mL/kg
	Expected long term	HAV vaccine*
Postexposure Prophylaxis		
	Future exposure likely	
≥2 yr	≤2 wk since exposure	IG 0.02 mL/kg and HAV vaccine
	>2 wk since exposure	HAV vaccine*
	Future exposure unlikely	
All ages	≤2 wk since exposure	IG 0.02 mL/kg and HAV vaccine should be considered (if ≥2 years)
	>2 wk since exposure	No prophylaxis

*Two inactivated vaccines are approved for use in persons ≥2 yr of age.
IG = immunoglobulin.

malaise, which occur 6–7 wk after exposure. The illness may be preceded in a few children by a serum sickness–like prodrome marked by arthralgia or skin lesions, including urticarial, purpuric, macular, or maculopapular rashes. Jaundice, which may be present in about 25% of infected individuals, usually begins about 8 wk after exposure and lasts for about 4 wk. In the usual course of resolving HBV infection, symptoms are present for 6–8 wk. The percentage of children in whom clinical evidence of hepatitis develops is higher for HBV than for HAV, and the rate of fulminant hepatitis also is greater. Chronic hepatitis also occurs, and the chronic active form can result in cirrhosis and hepatocellular carcinoma, which occurs almost exclusively in patients with cirrhosis, typically 25–30 yr after HBV infection. On physical examination, symptomatic infection results in skin and mucous membranes that are icteric, especially the sclera and the mucosa under the tongue. The liver usually is enlarged and tender to palpation. When the liver is not palpable below the costal margin, tenderness can be demonstrated by gently striking the rib cage over the liver with a closed fist. Splenomegaly and lymphadenopathy are common.

DIAGNOSIS. The serologic pattern for HBV is more complex than for HAV and differs depending on whether the disease is acute, subclinical, or chronic (Fig. 129–2). Table 129–1 summarizes the several antigens and antibodies that can be used to confirm the diagnosis of acute HBV infection.

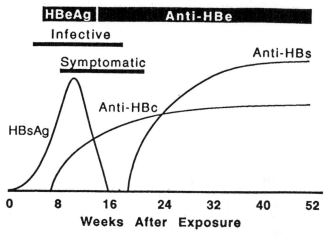

Figure 129–2 Pattern of response to hepatitis B virus infection. HBeAg = hepatitis B e antigen; HBsAg = hepatitis B surface antigen; HBc = hepatitis B core antigen.

TREATMENT. No available medical therapy is successful in the majority of persons infected with HBV. Interferon-α2b (IFN-α2b) is approved for treatment of chronic hepatitis B in patients age 18 yr or older with compensated liver disease and HBV replication. IFN-α2b also has been used in children, with long-term eradication rates similar to the 25% rate reported in adults.

COMPLICATIONS. Acute fulminant hepatitis with coagulopathy, encephalopathy, and cerebral edema occurs more frequently with HBV than with the other hepatotropic viruses, and the risk of fulminant hepatitis is further increased when there is co-infection or superinfection with HDV. Mortality due to fulminant hepatitis is greater than 30%.

PREVENTION. Hepatitis B vaccine and hepatitis B immunoglobulin (HBIG) are available for prevention of HBV infection. Universal immunization of all infants with hepatitis B vaccine is recommended in both pre-exposure and postexposure situations and provides long-term protection. In addition, all children who have not previously received the vaccine should be immunized by or before 11–12 yr of age, and catch-up programs should be implemented for unimmunized adolescents and high-risk adults. HBIG is indicated only for specific postexposure circumstances and provides temporary protection.

HEPATITIS C

ETIOLOGY. HCV is now recognized as the cause of almost all parenterally acquired cases of what was previously known as non-A, non-B hepatitis.

CLINICAL MANIFESTATIONS. The clinical pattern of the acute infection is similar to that of the other hepatitis viruses. Acute disease tends to be mild and insidious in onset. Fulminant liver failure rarely occurs. About 85% of HCV cases become chronic, with a fluctuating pattern of elevated hepatic transaminases. After 20–30 yr, about 25% ultimately progress to cirrhosis, liver failure, and occasionally primary hepatocellular carcinoma.

DIAGNOSIS. The clinically available assays for detection of HCV infection are based on detection of antibodies to HCV antigens or testing directly for the virus RNA.

TREATMENT. Treatment of HCV infection is provided to prevent progression to future complications. IFN-α2b is approved for treatment of chronic HCV in patients who are age 18 yr or older and who have compensated liver disease and a history of blood or blood product exposure or are anti-HCV positive. This treatment has also been used in children with a long-term response rate similar to the 25% rate reported in adults.

PREVENTION. No vaccine is available to prevent HCV. Immunoglobulin has not proved to be of benefit.

HEPATITIS D (HDV)

HDV cannot produce infection without a concurrent HBV infection.

CLINICAL MANIFESTATIONS. The symptoms of hepatitis D infection are similar to but usually more severe than those of the other hepatotropic viruses. In co-infection, acute hepatitis, which is much more severe than for HBV alone, is common, but the risk of developing chronic hepatitis is low.

PREVENTION. There is no vaccine for hepatitis D. However, because HDV replication cannot occur without hepatitis B co-infection, immunization against HBV also prevents HDV infection.

HEPATITIS IN NEONATES

Various infectious agents have been implicated in hepatic inflammation in neonates, including bacterial and viral pathogens. Hepatitis in neonates due to specific causes usually is distinguished from the term *neonatal hepatitis,* which has been used to designate hepatic inflammation of unknown cause. The six hepatotropic viruses that cause hepatitis as their primary disease manifestation rarely cause clinical hepatitis in neonates.

CLINICAL MANIFESTATIONS. Hepatitis in neonates may be characterized by jaundice, vomiting, poor feeding, and elevated hepatic enzyme levels. When infection is caused by an organism other than one of the six hepatotropic viruses, evidence of diffuse illness usually is present and may involve the skin, central nervous, cardiorespiratory, and musculoskeletal systems. A spectrum of illness, ranging from mild to fulminant disease, can occur with any of the infecting agents. Fulminant hepatitis is characterized by rapid progression to very high hepatic enzyme levels, decreased production of coagulation proteins, elevated serum ammonia level, shock, coma, or death.

HBV, the most common hepatotropic virus that infects neonates, usually results in an asymptomatic infection. Chronic infection can lead to cirrhosis usually in the 3rd and 4th decades of life, greatly increasing the risk of developing primary hepatocellular carcinoma.

TREATMENT. In addition to effective antimicrobial therapy for bacteria-associated hepatitis, acyclovir is effective against HSV and varicella virus, and ganciclovir and foscarnet can be used to treat cytomegalovirus infections.

PREVENTION. Women should be tested for HBsAg during routine prenatal care, and infants born to women who are HBsAg positive should receive hepatitis B vaccine and HBIG within 12 hr of birth.

CHAPTER 130

Osteomyelitis and Suppurative Arthritis

(Nelson Textbook, Chapter 178)

Suppurative infections of bones and joints in children are not common, but they are important because of their potential to cause permanent disability. The risk is greatest if the physis (the growth plate of bone) or the synovium is damaged.

ETIOLOGY. Bacteria are the usual pathogens in acute skeletal infections. Fungal infections usually occur as part of multisystem disseminated disease, and *Candida* arthritis or osteomyelitis sometimes complicates bloodstream infection in neonates with indwelling vascular catheters.

PATHOGENESIS. In newborns and young infants, blood vessels connect the metaphysis and epiphysis, so it is common for pus from the metaphysis to enter the joint space. In the latter part of the 1st yr of life, the physis forms, obliterating these transphyseal blood vessels. Bone is not distensible, and because pus under pressure is prevented from decompressing into the joint in these children, purulent material moves laterally through cortical vascular channels and accumulates under the loosely attached periosteum.

CLINICAL MANIFESTATIONS. The earliest signs and symptoms of skeletal infection are often subtle. This is particularly true of neonates, who characteristically do not appear ill and in half of cases do not have fever. Infants may have only pseudoparalysis of an extremity or apparent pain on movement of the affected extremity. Most older infants and children have fever and localizing signs.

Redness and swelling of the skin and soft tissue overlying the site of infection tend to be seen earlier in arthritis than in osteomyelitis. Local swelling and redness with osteomyelitis mean that the infection has spread out of the metaphysis into the subperiosteal space and denote a secondary soft tissue inflammatory response.

DIAGNOSIS. The diagnosis is most directly confirmed by needle aspiration of infected material for examination and culture when the history and physical findings indicate a strong likelihood of suppurative bone or joint disease.

Radiographic Findings. Radiologic studies are often helpful in evaluating suspected osteomyelitis and arthritis, but normal results of standard radiographs do not preclude those diagnoses. In osteomyelitis, destructive changes in bone do not appear radiographically for at least 10 days; however, effacement of normal deep soft tissue planes around bone is indicative of an inflammatory process. The findings in suppurative arthritis are a result of swelling of the capsule, joint space widening, and soft tissue swelling.

Differential Diagnosis. A great many noninfectious disorders affect the musculoskeletal system. It is common for children with acute leukemia to have bone or joint pain as an initial manifestation of disease.

TREATMENT

Antibiotic Therapy. In newborns, an antistaphylococcal penicillin, such as oxacillin (150–200 mg/kg/24 hr in 3–4 divided doses), and a broad-spectrum cephalosporin, such as cefotaxime (100–150 mg/kg/24 hr in 3–4 divided doses), provide coverage for the anticipated *S. aureus*, group B *Streptococcus*, and gram-negative bacilli. In infants and children up to 4–5 yr of age, the principal pathogens of infection are *S. aureus*, streptococci, and *Haemophilus influenzae* type b in children who have not received the *H. influenzae* vaccine. Most experience has been with cefuroxime (100–150 mg/kg/24 hr in 3 divided doses) or a third-generation cephalosporin (cefotaxime [150 mg/kg/24 hr in 3 divided doses] or ceftriaxone [50 mg/kg/24 hr given once daily]). Beyond 5 yr of age and in the absence of special circumstances, virtually all cases of osteomyelitis are caused by gram-positive cocci, so an antistaphylococcal antibiotic such as nafcillin (150 mg/kg/24 hr in 4 divided doses) or cephalothin (100–150 mg/ kg/24 hr in 4 divided doses) can be used; however, in children who have arthritis and who are older than 5 yr, the etiologic bacteria are more varied and broader-spectrum drugs (cefuroxime or a third-generation cephalosporin) are generally given unless gram-positive cocci are seen in the stain of synovial fluid. Special situations dictate deviations from the usual empirical antibiotic selection.

Surgical Therapy. Hip joint infection is considered a surgical emergency because of the vulnerability of the blood supply to the head of the femur. After a penetrating injury and when a foreign body is likely to be involved, surgical intervention is also indicated. In other situations, the need for surgery is individualized.

Physical Therapy. The major role of physical medicine is a preventive one.

CHAPTER 131

Infections in Immunocompromised Hosts

(Nelson Textbook, Chapter 179)

A compromised host is one who, at the time of microbial exposure, has a pre-existing condition that reduces one or more mechanisms for normal defense against infection.

CAUSES OF IMMUNOCOMPROMISE AND INFECTION. The major causes of increased risk for infection in immunocompromised hosts are listed in Table 131–1, and the most common causative organisms are listed in Table 131–2.

UNIQUE CLINICAL MANIFESTATIONS. Defects in the normal host response may be reflected in clinical manifestations. For example, extensive bacterial infection may occur in the lungs of severely neutropenic patients without an infiltrate discernible by chest radiography; the swelling and erythema of cellulitis may not be evident, and anemic and neutropenic patients may have acute otitis media without erythema and congestion of the tympanic membrane. Fever is a sensitive and specific sign of an infectious disease, even in an immunocompromised host. Almost all infec-

TABLE 131–1 Major Causes of Increased Risk for Infection in Immunocompromised Hosts

Primary	Secondary
Antibody deficiency (B-cell defects)	Human immunodeficiency virus
X-linked agammaglobulinemia	Malignancies
IgG subclass deficiencies	Transplantation
Common variable immunodeficiency	Bone marrow
Selective IgA deficiency	Solid organ
Cell-mediated deficiency (T-cell defects)	Burns
DiGeorge syndrome	Sickle cell disease
Hyper-IgM	Cystic fibrosis
CD8 lymphopenia	Diabetes mellitus
Cytokine deficiencies	Drugs: immunosuppressive
Defective T-cell receptor	Asplenia
T-cell activation defects	Implanted foreign body
Combined B- and T-cell defects	Malnutrition
Severe combined immunodeficiency	
Wiskott-Aldrich syndrome	
Ataxia telangiectasia	
Hyper-IgE syndrome	
Omenn syndrome	
Phagocyte defects	
Chronic granulomatous disease	
Congenital neutropenias	
Leukocyte adhesion disorder	
Other	
Complement deficiencies	

TABLE 131–2 Most Common Causes of Infections in Immunocompromised Children

Bacteria	**Viruses**
Escherichia coli	Varicella-zoster virus
Pseudomonas aeruginosa	Cytomegalovirus
Klebsiella species	Herpes simplex virus
Enterobacter species	Epstein-Barr virus
Haemophilus influenzae	Human herpesvirus 6
Staphylococcus aureus	Respiratory and enteric viruses
Staphylococcus, coagulase-negative	
Streptococcus pneumoniae	**Protozoa**
Bacillus species	*Pneumocystis carinii*
Corynebacterium species	*Toxoplasma gondii*
Viridans streptococcus group	*Cryptosporidium parvum*
Listeria monocytogenes	
Enterococcus faecalis	
Mycobacterium species	
Nocardia species	

Fungi

Candida albicans
Candida, not *albicans*
Aspergillus species
Cryptococcus neoformans
Zygomycetes

tions of significance are associated with a febrile response. Aside from fever, characteristic signs and symptoms of infection may be absent in a compromised host.

Extreme granulocytopenia with absolute neutrophil counts of less than 500 cells/mm^3 is predictive of impending infection. Multiple infections, either concomitant or sequential, are especially common in patients with prolonged immunocompromise.

CHAPTER 132

Infection Associated with Medical Devices

(Nelson Textbook, Chapter 180)

INTRAVASCULAR DEVICES. Intravascular access devices range from short stainless steel needles to multilumen implantable synthetic plastic catheters that are expected to remain in use for years. Infectious complications of intravascular devices include localized infections (exit site and tunnel tract infection and suppurative phlebitis) and synthetic infections (catheter-related bacteremia and fungemia).

The clinical manifestations of local infection include erythema, tenderness, and purulent discharge at the exit site or along the subcutaneous tunnel tract of the catheter. Catheter-related sepsis may also present as fever without an identifiable focus. The diagnosis of localized infection is made clinically.

If either localized or systemic catheter-related infection is diagnosed in a peripheral catheter or central venous catheter, the device should be removed. Antibiotics should be administered in cases of systemic infection, with the exception of uncomplicated coagulase-negative staphylococcal bacteremia in normal hosts. In patients with long-term vascular access devices in place (Hickman, Broviac, implanted ports), antibiotic treatment is successful in most systemic bacterial infections without removal of the device.

Prevention of Infection. Prevention of long-term vascular access device–related infection includes placement using meticulous surgical aseptic technique in an operating room–like environment, use of antibacterial ointment, avoidance of occlusive or semipermeable dressings, avoidance of bathing or swimming, and careful catheter care.

CEREBROSPINAL FLUID SHUNTS. Shunting is required for the treatment of many children with hydrocephalus. Four distinct clinical syndromes have been described: colonization of the shunt, wound infection, distal infection with peritonitis, and infection associated with meningitis.

Treatment of shunt colonization and distal infection with peritonitis includes the use of antibiotics against the specific organisms isolated and, in most situations, removal of the shunt. Intrashunt antibiotics are indicated because of the poor penetration of most antibiotics into the central nervous system across uninflamed meninges. If the isolate is susceptible, a parenteral antistaphylococcal penicillin plus intrashunt vancomycin is the treatment of choice. If the organism is resistant to the penicillins, systemic and intrashunt vancomycin is recommended.

CHAPTER 133

Animal and Human Bites

(Nelson Textbook, Chapter 181)

CLINICAL MANIFESTATIONS. Dog bite–related injuries can be divided almost equally into three categories: abrasions, puncture wounds, and lacerations with or without an associated avulsion of tissue. The most common type of injury from cat and rat bites is a puncture wound. Human bite injuries are of two types, an occlusion injury that is incurred when the upper and lower teeth come together on a body part and, in older children and young adults, a clenched-fist injury that occurs when the fist, usually of the dominant hand, comes in contact with the tooth of another individual.

EVALUATION. Careful attention should be paid to the circumstances surrounding the bite (type of animal [domestic or sylvatic, provoked or unprovoked] and location of the attack), a history of drug allergies, and the immunization status of the child and animal. During physical examination, meticulous attention should be paid to the type, size, and depth of the injury; the presence of foreign material in the wound; the status of underlying structures; and, in instances in which the bite is on an extremity, the range of motion of the affected area.

COMPLICATIONS. Infection is the most common complication of bite injuries, regardless of the species of biting animal. Unless they are deep and extensive, dog bite wounds that are less than 8 hr old do not need to be cultured unless contamination or early signs of infection are evident. It is prudent to obtain material for culture from all but the most trivial cat-inflicted wounds and from all other animal bite wounds, regardless of the species of the biting animal, that are not brought to medical attention within 8 hr. All human bite wounds, regardless of the mechanism of injury, should be regarded as at high risk for infection; culture is required. Because of the high incidence of anaerobic infection after bite wounds, it is important to obtain material for anaerobic as well as aerobic cultures.

TREATMENT. After the appropriate material has been obtained for bacterial culture, the wound should be anesthetized, cleaned, and vigorously irrigated with copious amounts of normal saline. Puncture wounds should be thoroughly cleaned and gently irrigated with a catheter or blunt-tipped needle; however, high-pressure irrigation should not be used. Avulsed or devitalized tissue should be débrided, and any fluctuant areas should be incised and drained.

All but the most trivial bite wounds of the hand should be immobilized in a position of function for 3–5 days, and patients with bite wounds of an extremity should be instructed to keep the affected extremity elevated for 24–36 hr or until the edema has resolved. All bite-wound victims should be re-evaluated within 24–36 hr after the injury.

Wound Closure. Much controversy and few data exist to determine whether bite wounds should undergo primary closure or delayed primary closure (after 3–5 days) or should be allowed to heal by secondary intention.

Antibiotic Therapy. Antibiotics should be administered after all human bites and after all but the most trivial of injuries from bites of dogs, cats, and rats, regardless of whether there is evidence of infection. Amoxicillin-clavulanate (40 mg/kg/24 hr) is an excellent choice for empirical oral prophylaxis or therapy for human and animal bite wounds because of its activity against the majority of strains of bacteria that have been isolated from infected bite injuries. Similarly, ticarcillin-clavulanate (200–300 mg/kg/24 hr) or ampicillin-sulbactam (100–200 mg/kg/24 hr) is preferred for patients who require empirical parenteral therapy. Procaine penicillin remains the drug of choice for prophylaxis and treatment of rat-inflicted injuries. No regimen is recognized to be effective for prophylaxis of cat-scratch disease *(B. henselae).*

Tetanus. Although the occurrence of tetanus after human or animal bite injuries is extremely rare, it is important to obtain a careful immunization history and to provide tetanus toxoid to all patients who are incompletely immunized or to adults who have not had tetanus immunization for more than 10 yr.

Rabies. The need for postexposure rabies vaccine in victims of dog and cat bites depends on whether the biting animal is known to have been vaccinated against rabies and, most importantly, on the local experience with rabid animals in the community. The local health department should be consulted for advice in all instances when the vaccination status of the biting animal is unknown and in instances when rabies is known to be endemic in the region.

SECTION 3

Gram-Positive Bacterial Infections
(Nelson Textbook, Chapters 182–190)

CHAPTER 134

Staphylococcal Infections
(Nelson Textbook, Chapter 182)

Staphylococcus aureus is the most common cause of pyogenic infection of the skin; it may also cause furuncles, carbuncles, osteomyelitis, septic arthritis, wound infection, abscesses, pneumonia, empyema, endocarditis, pericarditis, meningitis, and toxin-mediated diseases, including food poisoning, scalded skin syndrome, and toxic shock syndrome (TSS).

CLINICAL MANIFESTATIONS. The signs and symptoms vary with the location of the infection, which, although most commonly located on the skin, may involve any tissue. Disease states of various degrees of severity are generally a result of local suppuration, systemic dissemination with metastatic infection, or systemic effects of toxin production.

Skin. Pyogenic skin infections may be primary or secondary to wounds or may be a superinfection of other noninfectious skin disease (eczema) or of impetigo contagiosa.

Respiratory Tract. Infections of the upper respiratory tract and otitis media due to *S. aureus* are rare. Staphylococcal sinusitis is relatively common in children with cystic fibrosis or defects in white blood cell function. Bacterial tracheitis that complicates viral croup may be caused by *S. aureus* but also by other organisms.

Pneumonia due to *S. aureus* may be primary (hematogenous) or secondary after a viral infection such as influenza. High fever, abdominal pain, tachypnea, dyspnea, and localized or diffuse bronchopneumonia or lobar disease are common. Staphylococci cause a necrotizing pneumonitis; empyema, pneumatoceles, pyopneumothorax, and bronchopleural fistulas develop frequently.

Sepsis. Staphylococcal bacteremia and sepsis may be associated with any localized infection. The onset may be acute and marked by nausea, vomiting, myalgia, fever, and chills. Organisms may localize subsequently at any site but are found especially in the lungs, heart, joints, bones, kidneys, and brain.

Bones and Joints. *S. aureus* is the most common cause of osteomyelitis and suppurative arthritis in children.

Central Nervous System. Meningitis due to *S. aureus* is not common; it is associated with cranial trauma and neurosurgical procedures (e.g., craniotomy, cerebrospinal fluid shunt placement) and less frequently with endocarditis, parameningeal foci (e.g., epidural or brain abscess), diabetes mellitus, or malignancy.

DIAGNOSIS. The diagnosis of staphylococcal infection depends on isolation of the organisms from nonpermissive sites such as skin lesions, abscess cavities, blood, or other sites of infection.

TREATMENT. Antibiotic therapy alone is rarely effective in individuals with undrained abscesses or with infected foreign bodies. Loculated collections of purulent material should be relieved by incision and drainage. Foreign bodies should be removed, if possible. Therapy always should be initiated with a penicillinase-resistant antibiotic because more than 90% of all staphylococci isolated, regardless of source, are resistant to penicillin. For serious infections, parenteral treatment is indicated, at least at the outset, until symptoms are controlled. Serious staphylococcal infections, with or without abscesses, tend to persist and recur, necessitating prolonged therapy.

PREVENTION. Staphylococcal infection is transmitted primarily by direct contact. Strict attention to hand washing techniques is the most effective measure for preventing the spread of staphylococci from one individual to another.

TOXIC SHOCK SYNDROME

TSS is an acute multisystemic disease characterized by high fever, hypotension, vomiting, diarrhea, myalgias, nonfocal neurologic abnormalities, conjunctival hyperemia, strawberry tongue, and an erythematous rash with subsequent desquamation on the hands and feet.

PATHOGENESIS. A majority of *S. aureus* strains isolated from confirmed cases are phage group I and produce a number of extracellular toxins. The primary toxin associated with TSS is TSST-1.

CLINICAL MANIFESTATIONS. The onset is abrupt, with high fever, vomiting, and diarrhea, and is accompanied by sore throat, headache, and myalgias. A diffuse erythematous macular rash (sunburn-like or scarlatiniform) appears within 24 hr and may be associated with hyperemia of pharyngeal, conjunctival, and vaginal mucous membranes. A strawberry tongue is common. Symptoms often include alterations in the level of consciousness, oliguria, and hypotension, which in severe cases may progress to shock and disseminated intravascular coagulation.

TREATMENT. Parenteral administration of a β-lactamase–resistant antistaphylococcal antibiotic (e.g., nafcillin or a first-generation cephalosporin) is recommended after appropriate cultures have been obtained. Fluid replacement should be aggressive to prevent or treat hypotension, renal failure, and cardiovascular collapse. Isotropic agents may be needed to treat shock; corticosteroids and intravenous immunoglobulin are reserved for severe cases.

COAGULASE-NEGATIVE STAPHYLOCOCCI

S. epidermidis is one of many recognized species of coagulase-negative staphylococci (CONS) affecting or colonizing humans. Originally thought to be avirulent commensal bacteria, CONS, particularly *S. epidermidis*, is now known to produce nosocomial infections in patients with indwelling foreign devices.

CLINICAL MANIFESTATIONS. The low virulence of CONS usually requires the presence of another factor, such as immune compromise or a foreign body, for development of clinical disease.

TREATMENT. Most *S. epidermidis* is resistant to methicillin. Vancomycin is the drug of choice for methicillin-resistant *S. epidermidis*. The new quinolones and teicoplanin have some activity against CONS, and the addition of rifampin or gentamicin to vancomycin may increase antimicrobial efficacy.

CHAPTER 135

Streptococcus pneumoniae
(Pneumococcus) Infection
(Nelson Textbook, Chapter 183)

The pneumococcus *(Streptococcus pneumoniae),* a normal inhabitant of the upper respiratory tract, can cause local respiratory tract disease (otitis, sinusitis) and can also be an invasive pathogen (pneumonia, bacteremia, meningitis). *S. pneumoniae* is the most common cause of community-acquired bacterial pneumonia and otitis media and, with the widespread use of conjugated *Haemophilus influenzae* type b vaccines, has become the second most common cause of bacterial meningitis in children. The significance of this agent is accentuated by the emergence of penicillin-resistant and multidrug-resistant strains in many communities.

CLINICAL MANIFESTATION. The signs and symptoms are related to the site of infection. Local spread of infection may occur, causing empyema, pericarditis, mastoiditis, epidural abscess, or, rarely, meningitis.

DIAGNOSIS. The diagnosis is established by recovery of pneumococci from the site of infection or the blood. However, pneumococci found in the nose or throat of patients with otitis media, pneumonia, septicemia, or meningitis may not be related casually to their disease.

TREATMENT. Empirical treatment of pneumococcal disease should be based on knowledge of susceptibility patterns in specific communities. Penicillin G is the drug of choice for penicillin-susceptible strains. Oral penicillin V (50–100 mg/kg/24 hr every 6–8 hr) for minor infections, intravenous penicillin G (200,000–250,000 U/kg/24 hr every 4–6 hr) for bacteremia or pneumonia, and intravenous penicillin G (300,000 U/kg/24 hr every 4–6 hr) for meningitis are recommended. For serious infections (e.g., meningitis) with strains that are intermediately resistant to penicillin and for all infections with highly penicillin-resistant strains, vancomycin (60 mg/kg/24 hr every 6 hr) is the treatment of choice. Rifampin (20 mg/kg/24 hr every 12 hours) may be added in severe or unresponsive cases.

CHAPTER 136

Group A Streptococcus Infection

(Nelson Textbook, Chapter 184)

Streptococci are among the most common causes of bacterial infection in infancy and childhood. Group A *Streptococcus*, the most common bacterial cause of acute pharyngitis, also produces diverse other infections as well as nonsuppurative sequelae such as rheumatic fever and glomerulonephritis. Infection during the first 3 mo of life with group B β-hemolytic streptococci is common and may present as bacteremia, meningitis, osteomyelitis, or septic arthritis.

CLINICAL MANIFESTATIONS. The most common infections caused by group A β-hemolytic streptococci involve the respiratory tract, skin, soft tissues, and blood.

Skin Infections. The most common form of skin infection due to group A β-hemolytic streptococci is superficial pyoderma (impetigo). Colonization of unbroken skin precedes pyoderma by about 10 days. Skin lesions such as impetigo, ecthyma, and cellulitis develop after intradermal inoculation by insect bites, scabies, or minor trauma. Skin colonization or pyoderma may predispose patients to later pharyngeal colonization with the same strain.

Deeper soft tissue infections may occur. Erysipelas is an acute, well-demarcated infection of the skin with lymphangitis involving the face (associated with pharyngitis) and extremities (wounds). The skin is erythematous and indurated; the advancing margins of the lesions have raised, firm borders. The skin lesion usually is associated with fever, vomiting, and irritability. Streptococcal *cellulitis* is a painful, erythematous, indurated infection of the skin and subcutaneous tissues that commonly follows some injury to the skin. Certain streptococcal strains (i.e., those producing proteinase) may cause a more severe necrotizing fasciitis or myositis that results in a rapidly spreading tissue-destructive process that causes necrosis of involved soft tissues, including skin, fat, fasciae, and muscle. Lymphangitis and regional lymphadenitis are common.

Vaginitis. β-Hemolytic streptococci are a common cause of vaginitis in prepubertal girls. Patients usually have a serous discharge and marked erythema and irritation of the vulvar area, accompanied by discomfort in walking and in urination.

Bacteremia and Sepsis. Bacteremia and sepsis may follow a localized cutaneous (wounds, cellulitis, varicella lesions, hemangioma, abscess) or respiratory (pharyngitis, otitis media, sinusitis, pneumonia) infection in previously healthy or immunocompromised (malnutrition, malignancy) patients. Sepsis may be rapidly progressive, leading to a toxic shock–like illness with hypotension, fever, leukocytosis, disseminated intravascular coagulation, and peripheral gangrene. Metastatic foci may result in meningitis, brain abscess, osteomyelitis, septic arthritis, pneumonia, and peritonitis.

Scarlet Fever. This disease is a result of infection by streptococci that elaborate one of three pyrogenic (erythrogenic) exotoxins. The incubation period ranges from 1–7 days, with an average of 3 days. The onset is acute and is characterized by fever, vomiting, headache, toxicity, pharyngitis, and chills. Abdominal pain may be present; when this is associated with vomiting before the appearance of the rash, an abdominal surgical condition may be suggested. Within 12–48 hr, the typical rash appears. The tonsils are hyperemic and edematous and may be covered with a gray-white exudate. The pharynx is inflamed and covered by a membrane in severe cases. The tongue may be edematous and reddened.

The exanthem is red, is punctate or finely papular, and blanches on pressure. In some individuals, it may be palpated more readily than it is seen, having the texture of gooseflesh or coarse sandpaper. The rash appears initially in the axillae, groin, and neck but within 24 hr becomes generalized. Desquamation begins on the face in fine flakes toward the end of the 1st wk and proceeds over the trunk and finally to the hands and feet. The duration and extent of desquamation vary with the intensity of the rash; it may continue for as long as 6 wk.

Scarlet fever may follow infection of wounds (i.e., surgical scarlet fever), burns, or streptococcal skin infection. Clinical manifestations including the strawberry tongue are similar to those just described, but the tonsils and posterior pharynx generally are not involved.

TREATMENT. The goals of therapy are to decrease symptoms and prevent septic, suppurative, and nonsuppurative complications. Penicillin is the drug of choice for the treatment of streptococcal infections. All strains of group A β-hemolytic streptococci isolated to date have been sensitive to concentrations of penicillin (and many cephalosporins) achievable in vivo. Erythromycin (40 mg/kg/24 hr), clindamycin (30 mg/kg/24 hr), or the first-generation cephalosporins may be used for treating streptococcal pharyngitis in patients who are allergic to penicillin.

PREVENTION. Administration of penicillin prevents most cases of streptococcal disease if the drug is provided before the onset of symptoms. Except for rheumatic fever, indications for prophylaxis are not clear. Oral penicillin G or V (400,000 U/dose) may be provided four times each day for 10 days. Alternatively, 600,000 U of benzathine penicillin in combination with 600,000 U of aqueous procaine penicillin may be given as a single intramuscular injection. Treatment of carriers of group A β-hemolytic streptococci is controversial.

RHEUMATIC FEVER

ETIOLOGY. Group A β-hemolytic *Streptococcus* is the inciting agent leading to the development of acute rheumatic fever, although the exact pathogenetic mechanisms remain unexplained.

CLINICAL MANIFESTATIONS. No single specific clinical manifestation or specific laboratory test unequivocally establishes the diagnosis of rheumatic fever.

Carditis. This important finding in acute rheumatic fever is a pancarditis that involves the pericardium, epicardium, myocardium, and endocardium. Carditis is the only residual of acute rheumatic fever that results in chronic changes. Common manifestations include evidence of valvular insufficiency, most frequently affecting the mitral valve, but the mitral and aortic valves may be affected.

Polyarthritis. The arthritis of acute rheumatic fever is exquisitely tender. It is not uncommon for children with this form of arthritis to refuse to allow even bed sheets or clothing to cover an affected joint. The joints are red, warm, and swollen. The arthritis is migratory and affects several different joints: the elbows, knees, ankles, and wrists. It rarely occurs in the fingers, toes, or spine. The arthritis does *not* result in chronic joint disease.

Chorea. Sydenham chorea, a unique part of the rheumatic fever syndrome, occurs much later than other manifestations. These choreoathetoid movements may begin very subtly.

Erythema Marginatum. This unique rash seen in patients with rheumatic fever is another of the major manifestations that can be very difficult to diagnose. Although early in the disease it may be manifested as nonspecific pink macules that are usually seen over the trunk, later in its fully developed form, blanching occurs in the middle of the lesions, sometimes with fusing of the borders, resulting in a serpiginous-looking lesion. The rash does not itch.

Subcutaneous Nodules. These lesions occur infrequently and are most commonly observed in patients with severe carditis. These pea-sized nodules are firm and nontender, and there is no inflammation. They are characteristically seen on the extensor surfaces of the joints, such as the knees and elbows, and over the spine.

Minor Manifestations. The minor manifestations are much less specific but may be necessary to confirm a diagnosis of rheumatic fever. They include the clinical findings of fever and arthralgia. Arthralgia is present if a patient feels discomfort in a joint in the absence of objective findings (e.g., pain, redness, warmth) on physical examination.

DIAGNOSIS. A number of selective clinical findings, the Jones criteria, are used to determine the diagnosis of acute rheumatic fever (Table 136–1).

Evidence of Group A Streptococcal Infection. This is one of the most

TABLE 136–1 The Jones Criteria for Diagnosis of an Initial Attack of Rheumatic Fever

Major Criteria*	Minor Criteria
Carditis	Fever
Polyarthritis, migratory	Arthralgia
Erythema marginatum	Elevated acute-phase reactants (erythrocyte sedimentation rate, C-reactive protein)
Chorea	Prolonged PR interval on an electrocardiogram
Subcutaneous nodules	

plus

Evidence of a preceding group A streptococcal infection (culture, rapid antigen, antibody rise/elevation)

*Two major criteria or one major and two minor criteria plus evidence of a preceding streptococcal infection indicate a high probability of rheumatic fever. In the three special categories listed below, the diagnosis of rheumatic fever is acceptable without two major or one major and two minor criteria. However, only for 1 and 2 can the requirement for evidence of a preceding streptococcal infection be ignored.

    1. Chorea, if other causes have been precluded.
    2. Insidious or late-onset carditis with no other explanation.
    3. Rheumatic recurrence: In patients with documented rheumatic heart disease or prior rheumatic fever, the presence of one major criterion or of fever, arthralgia, or elevated acute-phase reactants suggests a presumptive diagnosis of recurrence. Evidence of previous streptococcal infection is needed here.

From Special Writing Group of the Committee on Rheumatic Fever, Endocarditis, and Kawasaki Disease of the Council on Cardiovascular Disease in the Young of the American Heart Association: Guidelines for the diagnosis of rheumatic fever. JAMA 268:2069, 1992. Copyright © 1992, American Medical Association.

important aspects of the Jones criteria. There must be evidence of a preceding group A streptococcal infection documented by a positive throat culture, a history of scarlet fever, or elevated streptococcal antibodies such as ASO, ADB, or AH.

TREATMENT. All patients presenting with acute rheumatic fever should be treated for a group A streptococcal infection at the time the diagnosis is made, whether or not the organism is initially isolated from the patient. Ten full days of an appropriate oral agent or a single intramuscular injection of 1.2 million units of benzathine penicillin G is recommended.

Therapy is given acutely for three systemic manifestations of acute rheumatic fever. These are arthritis, carditis, and Sydenham chorea. Salicylates provide prompt and dramatic relief for patients with the arthritis of acute rheumatic fever. For patients with mild carditis without evidence of congestive heart failure, salicylates alone are indicated. However, in patients with congestive heart failure or other significant manifestations of carditis, corticosteroids are required. Administration of corticosteroids should be limited both in amount and in duration to reduce their untoward side effects. Congestive heart failure should be treated by conventional techniques.

PREVENTION. Prevention and treatment of group A streptococcal infection can prevent rheumatic fever. Primary prophylaxis refers to antibiotic treatment of the streptococcal upper respiratory tract infection to prevent an initial attack of rheumatic fever. Secondary prophylaxis refers to the prevention of colonization or infection of the upper respiratory tract with group A β-hemolytic streptococci in individuals who have already had a previous attack of acute rheumatic fever. The recommended methods of secondary prevention include regular monthly (every 3–4 wk) injections of intramuscular benzathine penicillin G, daily administration of oral penicillin, daily administration of oral sulfadiazine, or daily oral administration of erythromycin (for individuals who cannot take any of the previously recommended antibiotics).

CHAPTER 137

Group B Streptococcus *Infection*
(Nelson Textbook, Chapter 185)

Group B *Streptococcus* (GBS) is a major cause of severe systemic and focal infections in newborns.

CLINICAL MANIFESTATIONS. The spectrum of early-onset infections ranges from asymptomatic bacteremia to septic shock. Early-onset disease may present at birth, and most infants become ill within 6 hr of birth. In utero infection may result in fetal asphyxia, coma, or shock. Respiratory symptoms are prominent and include cyanosis, apnea, tachypnea, grunting, flaring, retractions, and radiographic findings consisting of a reticulogranular pattern (50%), patchy pneumonic infiltrates (30%), and, less commonly, pleural effusions, pulmonary edema, cardiomegaly, and increased pulmonary vascular markings. Persistent fetal circulation or acute respiratory distress syndrome may develop. Bacteremia or sepsis without localization is noted in 30–40% of infants. Apnea or hypotension may be the initial presentation of sepsis. Meningitis occurs in about 10% of infants with early-onset infection. Patients with meningeal involvement may have seizures, lethargy, coma, and a bulging fontanel, but meningitis may be present without signs of meningeal involvement.

Late-onset GBS infection is manifested as bacteremia without a focus (55%), meningitis (35%), osteoarthritis, and soft tissue infection and is predominantly caused by the type III serotype. The presenting signs of late-onset GBS meningitis are usually fever and lethargy. Bulging fontanel and nuchal rigidity are more common in late-onset than early-onset meningitis.

DIAGNOSIS. The probability of infection increases with the presence of risk factors and colonization in the mother if untreated during labor. Diagnosis of GBS infection is confirmed by culture.

TREATMENT. GBS is uniformly sensitive to penicillin G, which is the treatment of choice of confirmed GBS infection. Empirical antimicrobial therapy is initiated with a penicillin (usually ampicillin) and an aminoglycoside until GBS has been identified by culture. GBS demonstrates a minimal inhibitory concentration (0.010.4 mg/mL) for penicillin G that is 4- to 10-fold greater than that of group A streptococci.

Penicillin should be used in high doses for the treatment of GBS meningitis (i.e., 300,000 units/kg/24 hr of penicillin G or 300 mg/kg/24 hr of ampicillin). Cerebrospinal fluid should be obtained within 48 hr of therapy for documented meningitis to determine whether persistent infection is present (>90% are sterile within 36 hr), owing to a high inoculum effect or tolerant GBS. If GBS continue to grow from the CSF, some authorities continue giving a combination of penicillin (or ampicillin) and gentamicin (for synergism) for the duration of treatment (2–3 wk).

Treatment of bacteremia with a soft tissue focus or pneumonia may be discontinued after 10 days. Arthritis may be treated in 2–3 wk and osteomyelitis and endocarditis in 3–4 wk.

Supportive care of infants with GBS infection is important, including the treatment of hypoxia and shock, disseminated intravascular coagulation, seizures, increased intracranial pressure, and inappropriate secretion of antidiuretic hormone.

PROGNOSIS. Mortality due to GBS disease is currently close to 10%. The principal predictor of mortality and morbidity is septic shock.

PREVENTION. Selective intrapartum chemoprophylaxis (SIC) has been repeatedly demonstrated to decrease the incidence of GBS early-onset disease but not late-onset disease. Intravenous penicillin G (5 million units initially and then 2.5 million units every 4 hr until delivery) or ampicillin (2 g initially and then 1 g every 4 hr until delivery) is given immediately to selected women at the onset of labor or when prolongation of membrane rupture is anticipated. Clindamycin (900 mg IV every 8 hr) is recommended for penicillin-allergic mothers. SIC should be implemented in communities and hospitals where GBS perinatal disease is prevalent. The selection of women for SIC remains controversial, and several strategies have been recommended. In all cases, maternal chorioamnionitis is an indication for treatment of the mother with broad-spectrum antibiotics.

Gram-Negative Bacterial Infections
(Nelson Textbook, Chapters 191– 207)

CHAPTER 138

Neisseria meningitidis (Meningococcus) Infection
(Nelson Textbook, Chapter 191)

EPIDEMIOLOGY. Meningococcal dissemination occurs as endemic disease punctuated by outbreaks of cases that are often clustered geographically. True epidemics have become rare in developed countries but remain a significant problem in much of the developing world.

PATHOGENESIS. *N. meningitidis* is thought to be acquired by a respiratory route. Colonization of the nasopharynx with meningococci usually leads to asymptomatic carriage, and only rarely does dissemination occur.

CLINICAL MANIFESTATIONS. The spectrum of meningococcal disease can vary widely, from fever and occult bacteremia to sepsis, shock, and death. Recognized patterns of disease are bacteremia without sepsis, meningococcemic sepsis without meningitis, meningitis with or without meningococcemia, meningoencephalitis, and infection of specific organs. A well-recognized entity is occult bacteremia in a febrile child. Upper respiratory or gastrointestinal symptoms or a maculopapular rash can be evident. The child often is sent home on no antibiotics or oral antibiotics for a minor infection. Spontaneous recovery without antibiotics has been reported, but some children have developed meningitis.

Acute meningococcemia initially can mimic a virus-like illness with pharyngitis, fever, myalgias, weakness, and headache. With widespread hematogenous dissemination, the disease rapidly progresses to septic shock characterized by hypotension, disseminated intravascular coagulation, acidosis, adrenal hemorrhage, renal failure, myocardial failure, and coma. Meningitis may or may not develop. Concomitant pneumonia, myocarditis, purulent pericarditis, and septic arthritis have been described. More often, meningococcal disease is manifested as acute meningitis that responds to appropriate antibiotics and supportive therapy.

DIAGNOSIS. Definitive diagnosis of meningococcal disease is made by isolation of the organism from a usually sterile body fluid such as blood, cerebrospinal fluid (CSF), or synovial fluid.

Isolation of meningococci from the nasopharynx is not diagnostic for disseminated disease. CSF cultures can be positive in patients with meningococcemia but without clinical evidence of meningitis or CSF pleocytosis.

Differential Diagnosis. This includes acute bacterial or viral meningitis, *Mycoplasma* infection, leptospirosis, syphilis, acute hemorrhagic encephalitis, encephalopathies, serum sickness, collagen vascular diseases, Henoch-Schönlein purpura, hemolytic-uremic syndrome, and ingestion of various poisons. The petechial or purpuric rash of meningococcemia is similar to that in any patient with a disease characterized by generalized vasculitis.

TREATMENT. Aqueous penicillin G is the drug of choice and should be given in doses of 250,000–300,000 U/kg/24 hr, administered intravenously in six divided doses. Cefotaxime (200 mg/kg/24 hr) and ceftriaxone (100 mg/kg/24 hr) are acceptable alternatives. Therapy is continued for 5–7 days.

COMPLICATIONS. Acute complications are related to the inflammatory changes, vasculitis, disseminated intravascular coagulation, and hypotension of invasive meningococcal disease. These can include adrenal hemorrhage, arthritis, myocarditis, pneumonia, lung abscess, peritonitis, and renal infarcts. The vasculitis can lead to skin loss with secondary infection, tissue necrosis, and gangrene.

PROGNOSIS. Despite the use of appropriate antibiotics, the mortality rate for disseminated meningococcal disease remains at 8–13% in the United States.

PREVENTION. Close contacts of patients with meningococcal disease are at increased risk of infection and should be carefully monitored and brought to medical attention if fever develops. Prophylaxis is indicated as soon as possible for household, daycare, and nursery school contacts. Prophylaxis is also recommended for persons who have had contact with patients' oral secretions. Prophylaxis is not routinely recommended for medical personnel, except those with intimate exposure, such as with mouth-to-mouth resuscitation, intubation, or suctioning before antibiotic therapy was begun. Rifampin is given (10 mg/kg; maximum dose, 600 mg) orally every 12 hr for 2 days (total of 4 doses). The dose is reduced to 5 mg/kg for infants younger than 1 mo.

Vaccine. A quadrivalent vaccine composed of capsular polysaccharide of meningococcal groups A, C, Y, and W135 is licensed in the United States. The vaccine is immunogenic in adults but is unreliable in children younger than 2 yr.

CHAPTER 139

Neisseria gonorrhoeae *(Gonococcus)* Infection

(Nelson Textbook, Chapter 192)

Neisseria gonorrhoeae produces various forms of gonorrhea, an infection of the genitourinary tract mucous membranes and rarely of the mucosa of the rectum, oropharynx, and conjunctiva. Gonorrhea transmitted by sexual contact or perinatally is the most frequently reported communicable disease in the United States and affects children of all ages.

CLINICAL MANIFESTATIONS. Gonorrhea is manifested by a spectrum of clinical presentations from asymptomatic carriage, to the characteristic localized urogenital infections, to disseminated systemic infection.

Asymptomatic Gonorrhea. The incidence of this form of gonorrhea in children has not been ascertained. Gonococci have been isolated from the oropharynx of young children who have been abused sexually by male contacts; oropharyngeal symptoms are usually absent. Most genital tract infections produce symptoms in children. However, as many as 80% of sexually mature females with urogenital gonorrhea infections are asymptomatic.

Uncomplicated Gonorrhea. Genital gonorrhea has an incubation period of 2–5 days in men and 5–10 days in women. Primary infection develops in the urethra of males, the vulva and vagina of prepubertal females, and the cervix of postpubertal females. Neonatal ophthalmitis occurs in both sexes.

Urethritis is usually characterized by a purulent discharge and by burning on urination without urgency or frequency. Untreated urethritis in males resolves spontaneously in several weeks or may be complicated by epididymitis, penile edema, lymphangitis, prostatitis, or seminal vesiculitis. Gram-negative intracellular diplococci are found in the discharge.

In prepubertal females, vulvovaginitis usually is characterized by a purulent vaginal discharge with a swollen, erythematous, tender, and excoriated vulva. Dysuria may occur. In postpubertal females, symptomatic gonococcal cervicitis and urethritis are characterized by purulent discharge, suprapubic pain, dysuria, intermenstrual bleeding, and dyspareunia. The cervix may be inflamed and tender.

Gonococcal ophthalmitis may be unilateral or bilateral. It may occur in any age group after inoculation of the eye with infected secretions. Ophthalmia neonatorum due to *N. gonorrhoea*e usually appears from 1–4 days after birth.

Disseminated Gonococcal Infection (DGI). Hematogenous dissemination occurs in 13% of all gonococcal infections. The most common manifestations are asymmetric arthralgia, petechial or pustular acral skin lesions, tenosynovitis, suppurative arthritis, and, rarely, carditis, meningitis, and osteomyelitis. The most common initial symptoms are acute onset of polyarthralgia with fever.

DIAGNOSIS. In males with symptomatic urethritis, a presumptive diagnosis of gonorrhea can be made by identification of gram-negative intracellular diplococci (within leukocytes) in the urethral discharge. A similar finding in females is not sufficient because *Mima polymorpha* and *Moraxella*, which are normal vaginal flora, have a similar appearance.

TREATMENT. General principles in the treatment of gonorrhea include the need to consider therapy for coexisting sexually transmitted diseases (syphilis, *Chlamydia* infection, human immunodeficiency virus infection) and infection due to resistant *N. gonorrhoeae*. It is recommended that *Chlamydia* infection be treated simultaneously with gonorrhea. Because of the increased prevalence of resistance of *N. gonorrhoeae* to penicillin, a third-generation cephalosporin, specifically ceftriaxone, is recommended as initial therapy for all ages. A single intramuscular injection of ceftriaxone (125 mg) for children and adults is the treatment of choice for uncomplicated urethritis, vulvovaginitis, proctitis, or pharyngitis. Ceftriaxone may also be effective against incubating syphilis but is ineffective against *Chlamydia* infections. The addition of doxycycline (100 mg PO bid for 7 days) or azithromycin 1 g PO in a single dose is recommended. Children younger than 9 yr and pregnant women should not be given tetracycline drugs, and erythromycin is recommended for them.

Ceftriaxone is recommended as the treatment of choice for DGI. Hospitalization is recommended. A 7-day course of parenteral ceftriaxone (50 mg/kg/24 hr; maximum 1 g/24 hr) given intravenously or intramuscularly is recommended. Neonates with gonococcal ophthalmitis must be hospitalized and evaluated for DGI. Nondisseminated infections including ophthalmia neonatorum should be treated with ceftriaxone (25–50 mg/kg IV or IM, not to exceed 125 mg) given once. Pelvic inflammatory disease (PID) requires hospitalization for evaluation and initiation of treatment. PID encompasses a spectrum of infectious diseases of the upper genital tract due to *N. gonorrhoeae, C. trachomatis,* and endogenous flora (streptococci, anaerobes, gram-negative bacilli). Therapy must cover a broad spectrum and must be given to adolescents as inpatients. A commonly recommended therapeutic regimen is 2 g of cefoxitin IV every 6 hr or 2 g of cefotetan IV every 12 hr, plus 100 mg of doxycycline PO or IV every 12 hr. Therapy is continued for at least 48 hr after a patient shows improvement. Thereafter, oral doxycycline is continued for a total of 10–14 days.

PREVENTION. Prevention of gonorrhea can be achieved through education, use of barrier contraceptives (especially condoms and spermicides), intensive epidemiologic and bacteriologic surveillance (screening and sexual contacts), and early identification and treatment of infected contacts. Gonococcal ophthalmia neonatorum can be prevented by instilling 2 drops of a 1% solution of silver nitrate into each conjunctival sac shortly after birth.

Chapter 140

Haemophilus influenzae *Infection*

(Nelson Textbook, Chapter 193)

CLINICAL MANIFESTATIONS AND TREATMENT. The clinical manifestations and treatment of all invasive *H. influenzae* disease are similar regardless of serotype. The initial antibiotic therapy of invasive infections possibly due to *H. influenzae* type b should be a parenterally administered antimicrobial agent effective in sterilizing all foci of infection and effective against ampicillin-resistant strains.

Meningitis. Antimicrobial therapy should be administered parenterally for 7–14 days for uncomplicated cases. Cefotaxime, ceftriaxone, ampicillin, and chloramphenicol all are thought to cross the blood-brain barrier during acute inflammation in concentrations adequate to render them effective for *H. influenzae* meningitis. Chloramphenicol has been administered orally to complete a therapeutic regimen for meningitis. Dexamethasone (0.6 mg/kg/ 24 hr divided every 6 hr for 2 days), particularly when given shortly before or concurrent with the initiation of antimicrobial therapy, decreases the incidence of hearing loss associated with *H. influenzae* type b meningitis.

Cellulitis. The head and neck, particularly the cheek and preseptal region, are the most common sites of involvement. The involved region generally has indistinct margins and is tender and indurated. Buccal cellulitis is classically erythematous with a violaceous hue. Parenteral antimicrobial therapy is indicated until patients become afebrile.

Preseptal Cellulitis. Infection involving the superficial tissue layers anterior to the orbital septum is termed preseptal cellulitis, which may be caused by *H. influenzae*. Patients with preseptal cellulitis without concurrent meningitis should receive parenteral therapy for about 5 days until fever and erythema have abated. In uncomplicated cases, antimicrobial therapy should be given for a total of 10 days.

Orbital Cellulitis. Orbital cellulitis may present as lid edema but is distinguished by the presence of proptosis, chemosis, impaired vision, limitation of the extraocular movements, decreased mobility of the globe, or pain on movement of the globe. Orbital infections are treated with parenteral therapy for at least 14 days. Underlying sinusitis may require surgical drainage. Abscesses in the orbit usually require prompt surgical drainage and more prolonged antimicrobial therapy.

Suppurative Arthritis. The signs and symptoms of septic arthritis due to *H. influenzae* are indistinguishable from those of arthritis caused by other bacteria.

Otitis Media. The most common bacterial pathogens are *Streptococcus pneumoniae, H. influenzae,* and *Moraxella catarrhalis.* Most *H. influenzae* isolates are nontypable. Amoxicillin (80–90 mg/kg/24 hr) is a suitable first-line oral antimicrobial agent.

Sinusitis. *H. influenzae* is an important cause of acute sinusitis in children, second in frequency only to *S. pneumoniae.* For uncomplicated sinusitis, amoxicillin is acceptable initial therapy.

PREVENTION OF SEROTYPE B INFECTIONS

Chemoprophylaxis. Unvaccinated close contacts younger than 48 mo of patients with invasive *H. influenzae* type b infections are at increased risk of invasive infection when exposed to an index case. Rifampin prophylaxis is indicated for all members of the close contact group, including the index patient, if one or more children younger than 48 mo are not fully immunized, defined as having received at least 1 dose of a *H. influenzae* type b conjugate vaccine at 15 mo of age or older, 2 doses at 12–14 mo of age, and 2 or more doses at 12 mo of age. For chemoprophylaxis, children should be given rifampin orally (0–1 mo of age, 10 mg/kg/dose; >1 mo, 20 mg/kg/dose, not to exceed 600 mg/dose), once each a day for 4 consecutive days. The adult dose is 600 mg once daily.

Vaccine. Currently available combinations are PRP-OMP combined with hepatitis B vaccine (Comvax) and HbOC combined with DTP (whole-cell pertussis vaccine) (Tetramune).

CHAPTER 141

Pertussis (Bordetella pertussis *and* B. parapertussis)

(Nelson Textbook, Chapter 195)

CLINICAL MANIFESTATIONS. Pertussis is a lengthy disease, divided into catarrhal, paroxysmal, and convalescent stages, each lasting 2 wk. Classically, after an incubation period ranging from 3–12 days, nondistinctive catarrhal symptoms of congestion and rhinorrhea occur, variably accompanied by low-grade fever, sneezing, lacrimation, and conjunctival suffusion. As symptoms wane, coughing begins first as a dry, intermittent, irritative hack and evolves into the inexorable paroxysms that are the hallmark of pertussis. After the most insignificant startle from a draft, light, sound, sucking, or stretching, a well-appearing young infant begins to choke, gasp, and flail extremities, with eyes watering and bulging and face reddened. Cough (expiratory grunt) may not be prominent at this stage. Whoop (forceful inspiratory gasp) infrequently occurs in infants younger than 3 mo who are exhausted or lack muscular strength to create sudden negative intrathoracic pressure. Post-tussive emesis is common in pertussis at all ages and is a major clue to the diagnosis in adolescents and adults. Post-tussive exhaustion is universal. The number and severity of paroxysms progress over days to a week (more rapidly in young infants) and remain at that plateau for days to weeks (longer in young infants). At the peak of the paroxysmal stage, patients may have more than one episode hourly. As paroxysmal stage fades into convalescence, the number, severity, and duration of episodes diminish. Paradoxically in infants, with growth and increased strength, cough and whoops may become louder and more classic in convalescence. Immunized children have foreshortening of all stages of pertussis.

DIAGNOSIS. Leukocytosis (15,000–100,000 cells/mm^3) due to absolute lymphocytosis is a characteristic in late catarrhal and paroxysmal stages. A severe course and death are correlated with extreme leukocytosis and thrombocytosis. Isolation of *B. pertussis* in culture remains the gold standard and is a more sensitive and specific method of diagnosis than direct fluorescent antibody (DFA) testing of nasopharyngeal secretions.

TREATMENT. Goals of therapy are to limit the number of paroxysms, to observe the severity of the cough to provide assistance when necessary, and to maximize nutrition, rest, and recovery without sequelae. Infants younger than 3 mo are admitted to the hospital almost without exception, at between 3 and 6 mo unless witnessed paroxysms are not severe, and at any age if significant complications occur. Prematurely born young infants and children with underlying cardiac, pulmonary, muscular, or neurologic disorders have a high risk for severe disease.

Antimicrobial Agents. An antimicrobial agent is always given when pertussis is suspected or confirmed for potential clinical benefit and to limit the spread of infection. Erythromycin, 40–50 mg/kg/24 hr PO in four divided doses (maximum 2 g/ 24 hr), for 14 days is standard treatment.

Isolation. Patients are placed in respiratory isolation for at least 5 days after initiation of erythromycin therapy.

Care of Household and Other Close Contacts. Erythromycin, 40–50 mg/kg/24 hr PO in four divided doses (maximum 2 g/24 hr) for 14 days should be given promptly to all household contacts and other close contacts, such as those in day care, regardless of age, history of immunization, or symptoms. Visitation and movement of coughing family members in the hospital must be assiduously controlled until erythromycin has been taken for 5 days. Close contacts younger than 7 yr who are underimmunized should be given a pertussis-containing vaccine, with further doses to complete recommended series.

COMPLICATIONS. Infants younger than 6 mo have excessive mortality and morbidity.

PREVENTION. Universal immunization of children with pertussis vaccine, beginning in infancy, is central to the control of pertussis.

CHAPTER 142

Salmonella
(Nelson Textbook, Chapter 196)

Acute gastroenteritis, the most frequent presentation, is usually self-limited, although bacteremia and focal extraintestinal infections may develop, especially in immunocompromised patients.

NONTYPHOIDAL SALMONELLOSIS

CLINICAL MANIFESTATIONS. Several distinct clinical syndromes can develop in children infected with nontyphoidal *Salmonella*, depending on host factors and the specific stereotype involved.

Acute Gastroenteritis. This is the most common clinical presentation. After an incubation period of 6–72 hr (mean, 24 hr), there is an abrupt onset of nausea, vomiting, and crampy abdominal pain primarily in the periumbilical area and right lower quadrant, followed by mild to severe watery diarrhea and sometimes by diarrhea containing blood and mucus. Moderate fever (temperature of 101–102°F [38.5–39°C]) affects about 70% of patients. Some children develop severe disease with high fever, headache, drowsiness, confusion, meningismus, seizures, and abdominal distention. Abdominal examination reveals some tenderness. The stool typically contains a moderate number of polymorphonuclear leukocytes and occult blood. Mild leukocytosis may be detected. Symptoms subside within 2–7 days in healthy children; fatalities are rare. In certain high-risk groups, the course of *Salmonella* gastroenteritis may be more complicated. Neonates, young infants, and children with primary or secondary immune deficiency may have symptoms persisting for several weeks. In patients with acquired immunodeficiency syndrome, the infection may become widespread and overwhelming, causing multisystem involvement, septic shock, and death.

Bacteremia. Transient bacteremia during nontyphoidal Salmonella gastroenteritis is thought to occur in 1–5% of patients. *Salmonella* bacteremia is associated with fever, chills, and often with a toxic appearance. Bacteremia has been documented, however, in afebrile, well-appearing children, especially neonates. Prolonged or intermittent bacteremia is associated with low-grade fever, anorexia, weight loss, diaphoresis, and myalgias.

Extraintestinal Focal Infections. After salmonellae have entered the bloodstream, they have a unique capability to metastasize and cause a focal suppurative infection of almost any organ.

DIAGNOSIS. Definitive diagnosis of the various clinical syndromes is based on culturing and subsequent identification of _Salmonella_ organisms.

TREATMENT. Assessment of the hydration status, correction of dehydration and electrolyte disturbances, and supportive care are the most important aspects of managing _Salmonella_ gastroenteritis in children. Antimotility agents prolong intestinal transit time and are thought to increase the risk of invasion; they should not be used when salmonellosis is suspected. In patients with gastroenteritis, antimicrobial agents do not shorten the clinical course, nor do they eliminate fecal excretion of _Salmonella_. By suppressing normal intestinal flora, antimicrobial agents may prolong the excretion of _Salmonella_ and increase the risk of creating the chronic carrier state.

Children with bacteremia or extraintestinal focal Salmonella infections should receive antimicrobial therapy. Ampicillin (200 mg/kg/24 hr in 4 divided doses) is efficacious and used to be the drug of choice; trimethoprim-sulfamethoxazole (TMP-SMX; 10–50 mg/kg/24 hr in 2 divided doses) and chloramphenicol (75 mg/kg/24 hr in 4 divided doses) are also effective. Because of the increasing worldwide antibiotic resistance of _Salmonella_ strains, it is necessary to perform susceptibility tests on all human isolates.

PROGNOSIS. Complete recovery is the rule in healthy children who develop _Salmonella_ gastroenteritis. The prognosis is poor for children with _Salmonella_ meningitis or endocarditis.

Chronic Carrier State. After clinical recovery from Salmonella gastroenteritis, asymptomatic fecal excretion of salmonellae occurs for several months, particularly in younger children or those treated with antibiotics. A prolonged carrier state after nontyphoidal salmonellosis is rare (<1%).

ENTERIC FEVER

Enteric fever is a systemic syndrome produced by certain _Salmonella_ organisms. It encompasses typhoid fever, caused by S. typhi, and paratyphoid fever, caused by _S. paratyphi_ A, _S. schottmuelleri_ (formerly _S. paratyphi_ B), _S. hirschfeldii_ (formerly _S. paratyphi_ C), and occasionally other _Salmonella_ serotypes. Typhoid fever, the most frequent enteric fever, tends to be more severe than the other forms.

CLINICAL MANIFESTATIONS. The incubation period is usually 7–14 days, but it may range from 3–30 days, depending mainly on the size of the ingested inoculum. The clinical manifestations of enteric fever depend on age.

School-Age Children and Adolescents. The onset of symptoms is insidious. Initial symptoms of fever, malaise, anorexia, myalgia, headache, and abdominal pain develop over 2–3 days. Although diarrhea having a pea soup consistency may be present during the early course of the disease, constipation later becomes a more prominent symptom. Severe lethargy may develop in some children. Temperature, which rises in a stepwise fashion, becomes an unremitting and high fever within 1 wk, often reaching 40°C (104°F). During the 2nd wk of illness, high fever is sustained, and fatigue, anorexia, cough, and abdominal symptoms increase in severity. Patients appear acutely ill, disoriented, and lethargic. Delirium and stupor may be observed. Physical findings include a relative bradycardia, which is disproportionate to the high fever. Hepatomegaly, splenomegaly, and distended abdomen with diffuse tenderness are very common. In about 50% of patients with enteric fever, a macular or maculopapular rash (i.e., rose spots) appears on about the 7th–10th day. If no complications occur, the symptoms and physical findings gradually resolve within 2–4 wk, but malaise and lethargy may persist for an additional 1–2 mo.

Infants and Young Children (<5 yr). Although clinical sepsis can occur, the disease is surprisingly mild at presentation, making the diagnosis difficult. Mild fever and malaise, misinterpreted as a viral syndrome, occur in infants with culture-proven typhoid fever. Diarrhea is more common in young children with typhoid fever than in adults, leading to a diagnosis of acute gastroenteritis.

Neonates. In addition to its ability to cause abortion and premature delivery, enteric fever during late pregnancy may be transmitted vertically. The neonatal disease usually begins within 3 days of delivery. Vomiting, diarrhea, and abdominal distention are common.

DIAGNOSIS. Results of blood cultures are positive in 40–60% of the patients seen early in the course of the disease, and stool and urine cultures become positive after the first week. A normochromic, normocytic anemia often develops after several weeks of illness and is related to intestinal blood loss or bone marrow suppression. Blood leukocyte counts are frequently low in relation to the fever and toxicity.

TREATMENT. Antimicrobial therapy is essential in treating enteric fever. Because of increasing antibiotic resistance, however, choosing the appropriate empirical therapy is problematic and controversial. Resistant strain are usually susceptible to third-generation cephalosporins. Chloramphenicol (50 mg/kg/24 hr PO or 75 mg/kg/24 hr IV in 4 equal doses), ampicillin (200 mg/kg/24 hr IV in 4 to 6 doses), amoxicillin (100 mg/kg/24 hr PO in 3 doses), and trimethoprim-sulfamethoxazole (10 mg of TMP and 50 mg of SMX/kg/24 hr PO in 2 doses) have demonstrated good clinical efficacy. Most children become afebrile within 7 days; treatment of uncomplicated cases should be continued for at least 14 days, or 5–7 days after defervescence.

In addition to antibiotic therapy, a short course of dexamethasone, using 3 mg/kg for the initial dose, followed by 1 mg/kg every 6 hr for 48 hr, improves the survival rate of patients with shock, obtundation, stupor, or coma.

COMPLICATIONS. Severe intestinal hemorrhage and intestinal perforation occur in 1–10% and 0.5–3% of the patients, respectively. These and most other complications usually occur after the 1st wk of the disease.

PREVENTION. In endemic areas, improved sanitation and clean running water are essential to control enteric fever. To minimize person-to-person transmission and food contamination, personal hygiene measures, hand washing, and attention to food preparation practices are necessary.

Vaccine. Three vaccines against *S. typhi* are commercially available. Typhoid vaccination is recommended to travelers to endemic areas, especially Latin America, Southeast Asia, and Africa.

CHAPTER 143

Shigella

(Nelson Textbook, Chapter 197)

Four species of *Shigella* are responsible for illness: *S. dysenteriae* (serogroup A), *S. flexneri* (serogroup B), *S. boydii* (serogroup C), and *S. sonnei* (serogroup D).

CLINICAL MANIFESTATIONS. Bacillary dysentery is clinically similar regardless of whether the disease is caused by an enteroinvasive *Escherichia coli* or any of the four species of *Shigella*; however, there are some clinical differences, particularly relating to the severity and risk of complications with *S. dysenteriae* serotype 1 infection.

Ingestion of shigellae is followed by an incubation period of 12 hr to several days before symptoms ensue. Severe abdominal pain, high fever, emesis, anorexia, generalized toxicity, urgency, and painful defecation characteristically occur. Physical examination at this point may show abdominal distention and tenderness, hyperactive bowel sounds, and a tender rectum on digital examination.

The diarrhea may be watery and of large volume initially, evolving into frequent small-volume, bloody mucoid stools; however, some children never progress to the stage of bloody diarrhea, whereas in others the first stools are bloody. Significant dehydration related to the fluid and electrolyte losses in both feces and emesis can occur. Untreated diarrhea may last 1–2 wk; only about 10% of patients have diarrhea persisting for more than 10 days.

Neurologic findings are among the most common extraintestinal manifestations of bacillary dysentery, occurring in as many as 40% of hospitalized infected children. Enteroinvasive *E. coli* can cause similar neurologic toxicity. Convulsions, headache, lethargy, confusion, nuchal rigidity, or hallucinations may be present before or after the onset of diarrhea.

The most common complication of shigellosis is dehydration, with its attendant risks of renal failure and death. Inappropriate secretion of antidiuretic hormone with profound hyponatremia may complicate dysentery, particularly when *S. dysenteriae* is the etiologic agent. Hypoglycemia and protein-loosing enteropathy are common. Other major complications, particularly in very young, malnourished children, include sepsis and disseminated intravascular coagulation.

TREATMENT. As with gastroenteritis of other causes, the first concern about a child with suspected shigellosis should be for fluid and electrolyte correction and maintenance. Drugs that retard intestinal motility should not be used because of the risk of prolonging the illness. Cefixime (8 mg/kg/24 hr PO in 2 divided doses for 5 days) or another oral third-generation cephalosporin, or ceftriaxone (50 mg/kg/24 hr as a single daily dose given parenterally for 2–5 days) can be used for empirical therapy. Treatment regimens are for a 5-day course.

PREVENTION. Two simple measures decrease the risk of shigellosis in children. The first is to encourage prolonged breast-feeding in regions in which shigellosis is common. The second measure is to educate families and child care center personnel in hand washing techniques, especially after defecation and before food preparation and consumption.

CHAPTER 144

Escherichia coli *Infection*

(Nelson Textbook, Chapter 198)

ETIOLOGY. Five classes of *E. coli* are recognized as agents associated with pediatric gastroenteritis.

Enterotoxigenic *E. coli* (ETEC) is a major cause of dehydrating infantile diarrhea in the developing world. The typical signs and symptoms include explosive watery diarrhea, abdominal pain, nausea, vomiting, and little or no fever. Resolution usually occurs in a matter of days. These infections have an untoward effect on infant nutritional status.

Enteroinvasive *E. coli* (EIEC) causes an illness that is indistinguishable from classic bacillary dysentery. Fever, systemic toxicity, crampy abdominal pain, tenesmus, and urgency with watery or bloody diarrhea are characteristic.

Enteropathogenic *E. coli* (EPEC) usually is isolated from infants and children who are in the first 2 yr of life and who have a nonbloody diarrhea with mucus; fever may occur. These organisms often cause a prolonged diarrheal disease.

Shigatoxin-producing *E. coli* (STEC) may cause a nondescript diarrheal illness or an illness characterized by abdominal pain with diarrhea that is initially watery but within a few days becomes blood streaked or grossly bloody (hemorrhagic colitis). Although this pattern resembles that of shigellosis or EIEC disease, it differs in that fever is an uncommon manifestation. The major risk with STEC is that 5–8% of symptomatic infections are complicated by development of hemolytic-uremic syndrome.

TREATMENT. The cornerstone of proper management is related to fluid and electrolyte therapy. In general, this therapy should include oral replacement and maintenance with rehydrating solutions. Early refeeding (within 8–12 hr of initiation of rehydration) with breast milk or dilute formula should be encouraged. Specific antimicrobial therapy of diarrheogenic *E. coli* is problematic because of the difficulty of making an accurate diagnosis of these pathogens and the unpredictability of antibiotic susceptibilities. Other than for a child recently returning from travel in the developing world, empirical treatment of severe watery diarrhea with antibiotics is seldom appropriate. Prophylactic antibiotic therapy is not recommended.

CHAPTER 145

Pseudomonas *Infection*

(Nelson Textbook, Chapter 203)

EPIDEMIOLOGY. *P. aeruginosa* and other pseudomonads frequently enter the hospital environment on the clothes, skin, or shoes of patients or hospital personnel, with plants or vegetables brought into the hospital, and in the gastrointestinal tracts of patients.

CLINICAL MANIFESTATIONS. Most clinical patterns (Table 145–1) are related to opportunistic infections or are associated with shunts and indwelling catheters. *P. aeruginosa* may be introduced into a minor wound of a healthy person as a secondary invader, and cellulitis and a localized abscess that exudes green or blue pus may follow. The characteristic skin lesions of *Pseudomonas*, ecthyma gangrenosum, whether caused by direct inoculation or secondary to septicemia, begin as pink macules and progress to

TABLE 145–1 *Pseudomonas aeruginosa* **Infections**

Infection	Common Clinical Characteristics
Endocarditis	Native right-sided (tricuspid) valve disease in intravenous drug addicts
Pneumonia	Compromised local (lung) or systemic host defense mechanisms. Nosocomial (respiratory), bacteremic (malignancy), or abnormal mucociliary clearance (cystic fibrosis) may be pathogenetic. Cystic fibrosis is associated with mucoid *P. aeruginosa* organisms producing capsular slime and *B. cepacia*
Central nervous system infection	Meningitis, brain abscess; contiguous spread (mastoiditis, dermal sinus tracts, sinusitis); bacteremia or direct inoculation (trauma, surgery)
External otitis	Swimmer's ear; humid warm climates, swimming pool contamination
Malignant otitis externa	Invasive, indolent, febrile toxic, destructive necrotizing lesion in young infants, immunosuppressed neutropenic patients, or diabetic patients; associated seventh nerve palsy and mastoiditis
Chronic mastoiditis	Ear drainage, swelling, erythema; perforated tympanic membrane
Keratitis	Corneal ulceration; contact lens keratitis
Endophthalmitis	Penetrating trauma, surgery, penetrating corneal ulceration; fulminant progression
Osteomyelitis/septic arthritis	Puncture wounds of foot and osteochondritis; intravenous drug abuse; fibrocartilaginous joints, sternum, vertebrae, pelvis; open fracture osteomyelitis; indolent; pyelonephritis and vertebral osteomyelitis
Urinary tract infection	Iatrogenic, nosocomial; recurrent urinary tract infections in children, instrumented patients, and those with obstruction or stones
Gastrointestinal tract infection	Immunocompromise, neutropenia, typhlitis, rectal abscess, ulceration, rarely diarrhea; peritonitis in peritoneal dialysis
Ecthyma gangrenosum	Metastatic dissemination; hemorrhage, necrosis, erythema, eschar, discrete lesions with bacterial invasion of blood vessels; also subcutaneous nodules, cellulitis, pustules, deep abscesses
Primary and secondary skin infections	Local infection; burns, trauma, decubitus ulcers, toe web infection, green nail (paronychia); whirlpool dermatitis: diffuse, pruritic, folliculitis, vesiculopustular or maculopapular, erythematous lesions

hemorrhagic nodules and eventually to ulcers with ecchymotic and gangrenous centers with eschar formation, surrounded by an intense red areola.

DIAGNOSIS. Diagnosis depends on recovery of the organism from the blood, cerebrospinal fluid, urine, or needle aspirate of the lung or from purulent material obtained by aspiration of subcutaneous abscesses or areas of cellulitis.

TREATMENT. Systemic infections with *Pseudomonas* should be treated promptly with an antibiotic to which the organism is susceptible in vitro. Response to treatment may be limited, and prolonged treatment may be necessary for systemic infection in compromised hosts.

SECTION 5

Anaerobic Bacterial Infections

(Nelson Textbook, Chapters 208–211)

CHAPTER 146

Botulism

(Nelson Textbook, Chapter 208)

Botulism is the acute, flaccid paralytic illness caused by the neurotoxin produced by *Clostridium botulinum* or, rarely, an equivalent neurotoxin produced by unique strains of *C. butyricum* and *C. baratii.* Three forms of human botulism are known: infant botulism (the most common in the United States), foodborne (classic) botulism, and wound botulism.

CLINICAL MANIFESTATIONS. Botulinum toxin is distributed hematogenously. All three forms of botulism manifest neurologically as a symmetric, descending flaccid paralysis of the cranial nerve musculature. Patients with evolving illness may already have generalized weakness and hypotonia in addition to bulbar palsies when first seen. In older children with foodborne or wound botulism, the onset of neurologic symptoms follows a characteristic pattern of diplopia, blurred vision, ptosis, dry mouth, dysphagia, dysphonia, and dysarthria, with decreased gag and corneal reflexes. Importantly, because the toxin acts only on motor nerves, paresthesias are not seen in botulism, except when a patient hyperventilates from anxiety. The sensorium remains clear, but this may be difficult to ascertain because of the slurred speech.

Foodborne botulism begins with gastrointestinal symptoms of nausea, vomiting, or diarrhea in about one third of cases. Constipation is common in foodborne botulism once flaccid paralysis becomes evident. Illness usually begins 18–36 hr after ingestion of the contaminated food but can range from as little as 2 hr to as long as 8 days. The incubation period in wound botulism is

4–14 days. All three forms of botulism display a wide spectrum in their clinical severity. *Fatigability with repetitive muscle activity is the clinical hallmark of botulism.*

Infant botulism differs in apparent initial symptoms of illness only because the infant cannot verbalize them. Usually, the first indication of illness is a decreased frequency or even absence of defecation. Parents typically notice inability to feed, lethargy, listlessness, weak cry, and diminished spontaneous movement. Dysphagia may be evident as secretions drooling from the mouth. Gag, suck, and corneal reflexes diminish as the paralysis advances. Loss of head control is typically a prominent sign. Respiratory arrest may occur suddenly from airway occlusion by unswallowed secretions or from obstructive flaccid pharyngeal musculature. In mild cases or in the early stages of illness, the physical signs of infant botulism may be subtle and easily missed.

DIAGNOSIS. The diagnosis of botulism is unequivocally established by demonstrating the presence of botulinum toxin in serum or of *C. botulinum* toxin or organisms in wound material or feces.

TREATMENT. Management of botulism rests on three principles: (1) fatigability with repetitive muscle activity is the clinical hallmark of the disease; (2) complications are best avoided by anticipating them; and (3) meticulous supportive care is a necessity. The first principle applies mainly to feeding and breathing. Correct positioning is imperative to protect the airway and improve respiratory mechanics. About one half of patients will require endotracheal intubation, which is best done prophylactically. Feeding should be done by a nasogastric or nasojejunal tube until sufficient oropharyngeal strength and coordination enables feeding by breast or bottle. Antibiotic therapy is not part of the treatment of uncomplicated infant or foodborne botulism because the toxin is primarily an intracellular molecule that is released into the intestinal lumen with vegetative bacterial cell death and lysis.

Botulism immune globulin (BIG) should be started as early in the illness as possible. In the United States, BIG may be obtained from the California Department of Health Services (24-hour telephone: 510-540-2646). Because sensation remains intact, providing auditory, tactile, and visual stimuli is beneficial. Maintaining strong central respiratory drive is essential, so sedatives or central nervous system depressants (e.g., metoclopramide [Reglan]) are contraindicated.

PREVENTION. Foodborne botulism is best prevented by adhering to safe methods of home canning (pressure cooker and acidification), by avoiding suspicious foods, and by heating all home-canned foods to 80°C for at least 5 min. Wound botulism is best prevented by thorough cleansing and surgical débridement of contaminated traumatic injuries with provision of appropriate antibiotics and by not using illicit drugs. Most infant botulism patients probably inhale and then swallow airborne clostridial spores; these cases are unpreventable. The one identified, avoidable source of botulinum spores for infants is honey.

CHAPTER 147

Tetanus

(Nelson Textbook, Chapter 209)

Tetanus (lockjaw) is an acute, spastic paralytic illness caused by tetanus toxin (tetanospasmin), the neurotoxin produced by *Clostridium tetani*.

CLINICAL MANIFESTATIONS. Tetanus may be either localized or generalized, the latter being more common. The incubation period typically is 2–14 days, but it may be as long as months after the injury. In generalized tetanus, trismus (masseter muscle spasm, or "lockjaw") is the presenting symptom in about half the cases. Headache, restlessness, and irritability are early symptoms, often followed by stiffness, difficulty chewing, dysphagia, and neck muscle spasm. The so-called sardonic smile of tetanus (risus sardonicus) results from intractable spasm of facial and buccal muscles. When the paralysis extends to abdominal, lumbar, hip, and thigh muscles, the patient may assume an arched posture, opisthotonos, in which only the back of the head and the heels touch ground. Laryngeal and respiratory muscle spasm can lead to airway obstruction and asphyxiation. Because tetanus toxin does not affect sensory nerves or cortical function, the patient unfortunately remains conscious, in extreme pain, and in fearful anticipation of the next tetanic seizure. These seizures are characterized by sudden, severe tonic contractions of the muscles, with fist clenching, flexion, and adduction of the arms and hyperextension of the legs. Without treatment, the seizures range from a few seconds to a few minutes in length with intervening respite periods, but as the illness progresses the spasms become sustained and exhausting. The smallest disturbance by sight, sound, or touch may trigger a tetanic spasm. Fever, occasionally with a temperature as high as 40°C (104°F), is common. Notable autonomic effects include tachycardia, arrhythmias, labile hypertension, diaphoresis, and cutaneous vasoconstriction.

Neonatal tetanus (tetanus neonatorum), the infantile form of generalized tetanus, typically manifests within 3–12 days of birth as progressive difficulty in feeding (i.e., sucking and swallowing), with associated hunger and crying. Paralysis or diminished movement, stiffness to the touch, and spasms, with or without opisthotonos, characterize the disease.

Localized tetanus results in painful spasms of the muscles adjacent to the wound site and may precede generalized tetanus.

TREATMENT. Management of tetanus requires eradication of *C. tetani* and the wound environment conducive to its anaerobic multiplication, neutralization of all accessible tetanus toxin, control of seizures and respiration, palliation and provision of meticulous supportive care, and, finally, prevention of recurrences. Surgical wound excision and débridement is often needed to remove the foreign body or devitalized tissue that created anaerobic growth conditions. Surgery should be done promptly, after the administration of human tetanus immune globulin (TIG) and antibiotics.

A single intramuscular injection of 500 U of TIG is sufficient to neutralize systemic tetanus toxin, but doses as high as 3,000–6,000 U are also recommended. If TIG is unavailable, use of human intravenous immune globulin (IVIG), which contains 4–90 U/mL of TIG, or of equine- or bovine-derived tetanus antitoxin (TAT), may be necessary. The usual dose of TAT is 50,000–100,000 U, with half given intramuscularly and half intravenously. When using TAT, it is essential to check for possible sensitivity to horse serum; desensitization may be needed.

Penicillin G remains the antibiotic of choice. The dose is 100,000 U/kg/24 hr divided and administered in every 4–6 hr for 10–14 days. Erythromycin and tetracycline (in patients older than 8 yr old) are alternatives for penicillin-allergic patients.

All patients with generalized tetanus need muscle relaxants. Diazepam provides both relaxation and seizure control; the initial dose of 0.1–0.2 mg/kg every 3–6 hr given intravenously is then titrated to control the tetanic spasms, after which it is sustained for 2–6 wk before its tapered withdrawal. Meticulous supportive care in a quiet, dark, secluded setting is most desirable. Because tetanic spasms may be triggered by minor stimuli, the patient should be sedated and protected from all unnecessary sounds, sights, and touch.

PREVENTION. Tetanus is an entirely preventable disease; a serum antibody titer of more than 0.01 U/mL is considered protective. Active immunization should begin in early infancy with combined diphtheria toxoid/tetanus toxoid/pertussis (DTaP is preferred over DTP) vaccine at 2, 4, and 6 mo of age, with a booster at 4–6 yr of age and at 10-yr intervals thereafter throughout adult life with tetanus/diphtheria (Td) toxoids.

Wound Management. Tetanus prevention measures after trauma consist of inducing active immunity to tetanus toxin and of passively providing antitoxic antibody. The wound should have immediate, thorough surgical cleansing and débridement to remove foreign bodies and any necrotic tissue in which anaerobic conditions might develop.

Mycobacterial Infections

(Nelson Textbook, Chapters 212–214)

CHAPTER 148

Tuberculosis

(Nelson Textbook, Chapter 212)

EPIDEMIOLOGY

Infection and Disease. Tuberculosis *infection* occurs after the inhalation of infective droplet nuclei containing *M. tuberculosis*. A reactive tuberculin skin test and the absence of clinical and radiographic manifestations are the hallmark of this stage. Tuberculosis *disease* occurs when signs and symptoms or radiographic changes become apparent. The word "tuberculosis" refers to disease. The World Health Organization estimates that one third of the world's population—2 billion people—are infected with *M. tuberculosis*.

Transmission. Transmission of *M. tuberculosis* is person to person, usually by airborne mucus droplet nuclei.

Tuberculin Skin Tests. The Mantoux tuberculin skin test is the intradermal injection of 0.1 mL, containing 5 tuberculin units (TU) of purified protein derivative (PPD) stabilized with Tween 80. The amount of induration in response to the test should be measured by a trained person 48–72 hr after administration. Tuberculin sensitivity develops 3 wk to 3 mo—most often 4–8 wk—after inhalation of organisms. Host-related factors, including very young age, malnutrition, immunosuppression by disease or drugs, viral infections (measles, mumps, varicella, influenza), live-virus vaccines, and overwhelming tuberculosis, can depress the skin test reaction in a child infected with *M. tuberculosis*. False-positive reactions to tuberculin can be caused by cross-sensitization to antigens of nontuberculous mycobacteria (NTM).

CLINICAL MANIFESTATIONS AND DIAGNOSIS

Primary Pulmonary Disease. The primary pulmonary complex includes the parenchymal focus and the regional lymph nodes. About 70% of lung foci are subpleural, and localized pleurisy is common. The hallmark of primary tuberculosis in the lung is the relatively large size of the regional lymphadenitis compared with the relatively small size of the initial lung focus. The common sequence is hilar adenopathy, focal hyperinflation, and then atelectasis. Most cases of tuberculous bronchial obstruction in children resolve fully with appropriate treatment. Children may have lobar pneumonia without impressive hilar adenopathy.

More than 50% of infants and children with radiographically moderate to severe pulmonary tuberculosis have no physical findings and are discovered only by contact tracing. Infants are more likely to experience signs and symptoms. Nonproductive cough and mild dyspnea are the most common symptoms. Systemic complaints such as fever, night sweats, anorexia, and decreased activity occur less often. The most specific confirmation of pulmonary tuberculosis is isolation of *M. tuberculosis*.

Lymphohematogenous (Disseminated) Disease. Tubercle bacilli are disseminated to distant sites, including liver, spleen, skin, and lung apices, in all cases of tuberculosis infection. Lymphohematogenous spread is usually asymptomatic. The most clinically significant form of disseminated tuberculosis is miliary disease, which occurs when massive numbers of tubercle bacilli are released into the bloodstream, causing disease in two or more organs. Miliary tuberculosis usually complicates the primary infection, occurring within 2–6 mo of the initial infection. Although this form of disease is most common in infants and young children, it is also found in adolescents and older adults. The clinical manifestations of miliary tuberculosis are protean, depending on the load of organisms that disseminate and where they lodge. This form of tuberculosis is most common in infants and malnourished or immunosuppressed patients. The onset of miliary tuberculosis is sometimes explosive, and the patient may become gravely ill in several days. More often, the onset is insidious with early systemic signs, including anorexia, weight loss, and low-grade fever. The resolution of miliary tuberculosis is slow, even with proper therapy.

Lymph Node Disease. Tuberculosis of the superficial lymph nodes, often referred to as scrofula, is the most common form of extrapulmonary tuberculosis in children. Most current cases occur within 6–9 mo of initial infection by *M. tuberculosis*, although some cases appear years later. The tonsillar, anterior cervical, submandibular, and supraclavicular nodes become involved secondary to extension of a primary lesion of the upper lung fields or abdomen. Lymph node tuberculosis may resolve if left untreated but more often progresses to caseation and necrosis. A definitive diagnosis of tuberculous adenitis usually requires histologic or bacteriologic confirmation, which is best accomplished by excisional biopsy of the involved node. The most frequent problem is distinguishing infection due to *M. tuberculosis* from lymphadenitis due to NTM in geographic areas where NTM are common.

Central Nervous System (CNS) Disease. Tuberculosis of the CNS is the most serious complication in children and is fatal without effective treatment. Tuberculous meningitis usually arises from the formation of a metastatic caseous lesion in the cerebral cortex or meninges that develops during the lymphohematogenous dissemination of the primary infection. The brain stem is often the site of greatest involvement, which accounts for the frequently associated dysfunction of cranial nerves III, VI, and VII. The combination of vasculitis, infarction, cerebral edema, and hydrocephalus results in the severe damage that can occur gradually or rapidly. Profound abnormalities in electrolyte metabolism, due to salt wasting or the syndrome of inappropriate antidiuretic hormone secretion, also contribute to the pathophysiology of tuberculous meningitis.

The clinical progression of tuberculous meningitis may be rapid or gradual. Rapid progression tends to occur more often in infants and young children, who may experience symptoms for only several days before the onset of acute hydrocephalus, seizures, and cerebral edema. More commonly, the signs and symptoms progress slowly over several weeks and can be divided into three stages. The prognosis of tuberculous meningitis correlates most closely with the clinical stage of illness at the time treatment is initiated. The prognosis for young infants is generally worse than for older children.

Perinatal Disease. Symptoms of congenital tuberculosis may be present at birth but more commonly begin by the 2nd or 3rd wk of life. The most common signs and symptoms are respiratory distress, fever, hepatic or splenic enlargement, poor feeding, lethargy or irritability, lymphadenopathy, abdominal distention, failure to thrive, ear drainage, and skin lesions. The clinical manifestations vary in relation to the site and size of the caseous lesions. Many infants have an abnormal chest radiograph, most often a miliary pattern. The clinical presentation of tuberculosis in newborns is similar to that caused by bacterial sepsis and other congenital infections, such as syphilis, toxoplasmosis, and cytomegalovirus. The most important clue for rapid diagnosis of congenital tuberculosis is a maternal or family history of tuberculosis.

TREATMENT. The major biologic determinant of the success of antituberculosis chemotherapy is the size of the bacillary population within the host. For patients with large bacterial populations, such as adults with cavities or extensive infiltrates, many naturally drug-resistant organisms are present and at least two antituberculosis drugs must be used to effect a cure. Conversely, for patients with infection (reactive skin test) but no disease, the bacterial population is small, drug-resistant organisms are rare or nonexistent, and a single drug can be used. Children with pulmonary tuberculosis and most patients with extrapulmonary tuberculosis have medium-sized populations in which significant numbers of naturally drug-resistant organisms may or may not be present. In general, these patients are treated with at least two drugs. The various antituberculosis drugs (Table 148–1) differ in their primary site of activity and their actions.

Treatment Regimens for Disease. The American Academy of Pediatrics and the Centers for Disease Control and Prevention have endorsed a regimen of 6 mo of isoniazid (INH) and rifampin (RIF)

TABLE 148–1 Most Commonly Used Antituberculosis Drugs

Drug	Daily Dose (mg/kg/24 hr)	Twice-Weekly Dose (mg/kg/dose)	Maximum Dose
Isoniazid (INH)*	10–15	20–30	Daily: 300 mg Twice weekly: 900 mg
Rifampin (RIF)*	10–20	10–20	600 mg
Pyrazinamide (PZA)*	20–40	40–60	2 g
Streptomycin (IM) (STM)	20–40	20–40	1 g
Ethambutol (EMB)	15–25	25–50	2.5 g
Ethionamide (ETH)	15–20 (1–3 divided doses)	—	1 g
Cycloserine	10–20 (1–2 divided doses)	—	1 g
Kanamycin or capreomycin (IM)	15–30	15–30	1 g
Amikacin (IV)	15–30	15–30	1 g

*Isoniazid (150 mg) and rifampin (300 mg) are combined in one preparation called Rifamate. Isoniazid, rifampin, and pyrazinamide are combined in one preparation called Rifater.

IM = Intramuscular; IV = intravenous.

supplemented during the first 2 mo by pyrazinamide (PZA) as standard therapy for intrathoracic tuberculosis in children. Most experts recommend that all drug administration be directly observed, meaning that a health care worker is physically present when the medications are administered to the patients. When directly observed therapy is used, intermittent (twice-weekly) administration of drugs after an initial period as short as 2 wk of daily therapy is as effective in children as daily therapy for the entire course. In locales where the community rate of INH resistance is greater than 5–10%, or when the adult source case is at increased risk for drug-resistant tuberculosis, most experts recommend adding a 4th drug—usually streptomycin (STM), ethambutol (EMB), or ethionamide (ETH)—to the initial regimen.

In general, the treatment for most forms of extrapulmonary tuberculosis in children is the same as for pulmonary tuberculosis. Exceptions are bone and joint, disseminated, and CNS tuberculosis for which there are inadequate data to recommend 6-mo therapy. These cases usually are treated for 9–12 mo.

Most experts believe that human immunodeficiency virus (HIV)–seropositive children with drug-susceptible tuberculosis should receive at least INH, RIF, and PZA for 2 mo followed by INH and RIF to complete a total treatment duration of 6–12 mo: It is recommended that all children with tuberculosis be evaluated for HIV infection because the presence of HIV may necessitate a longer duration of treatment.

Drug-Resistant Tuberculosis. When a child has possible drug-resistant tuberculosis, at least three and usually four or five drugs should be administered initially until the susceptibility pattern is determined and a more specific regimen can be designed.

Corticosteroids. There is convincing evidence that corticosteroids decrease mortality rates and long-term neurologic sequelae in some patients with tuberculosis meningitis. Short courses of corticosteroids also may be effective for children with endobronchial tuberculosis that causes respiratory distress, localized emphysema, or segmental pulmonary lesions. Corticosteroids can help relieve symptoms and constriction associated with acute tuberculous pericardial effusion. Corticosteroids may cause dramatic improvement in symptoms in some patients with tuberculous pleural effusion and shift of the mediastinum. Some children with severe miliary tuberculosis have dramatic improvement with corticosteroid therapy if the inflammatory reaction is so severe that alveolocapillary block is present. The most commonly prescribed regimen is prednisone, 1–2 mg/kg/24 hr in 1 to 2 divided doses for 4–6 wk with gradual tapering.

Treatment of Tuberculosis Infection Without Disease. INH therapy should be given to any child with a positive tuberculin skin test but no clinical or radiographic evidence of disease. The currently recommended regimen is 9 mo of daily INH therapy. INH can be given twice weekly under direct observation if adherence with daily treatment is likely to be poor. INH therapy also should be started for children younger than 6 yr of age with a negative tuberculin skin test who have had recent exposure to an adult with infectious tuberculosis, including infants born to mothers who have tuberculosis.

SECTION 7

Spirochetal Infections

(Nelson Textbook, Chapters 215–219)

CHAPTER 149

Syphilis (Treponema pallidum)

(Nelson Textbook, Chapter 215)

EPIDEMIOLOGY. Two forms of syphilis are encountered in children. *Acquired* syphilis is transmitted almost exclusively by sexual contact. *Congenital* syphilis results from transplacental transmission of spirochetes.

CLINICAL MANIFESTATIONS. Primary syphilis is characterized by syphilitic chancre and regional lymphadenitis. A painless papule appears at the site of inoculation 2–6 wk after *T. pallidum* has been introduced. The papule soon develops into a clean, painless ulcer with raised borders called a chancre. The chancre, usually on the genitals, contains viable *T. pallidum* and is highly contagious. Extragenital chancres can also be seen, depending on the site of primary inoculation. Adjacent lymph nodes are generally enlarged. The chancre heals spontaneously within 4–6 wk, leaving a thin scar. Untreated individuals develop manifestations of secondary syphilis 2–10 wk after the chancre heals. Manifestations of secondary syphilis are related to spirochetemia and include a nonpruritic maculopapular rash, which can cover the entire body involving palms and soles; pustular lesions may also develop. A flulike illness with low-grade fever, headache, malaise, anorexia, weight loss, sore throat, myalgias, and arthralgias, and generalized lymphadenopathy is often present. Meningitis occurs in 30% of patients with secondary syphilis, manifested by cerebrospinal fluid (CSF) pleocytosis and elevated protein levels, but the patient may not show neurologic symptoms. Secondary infection becomes latent within 1–2 mo after the onset of the rash.

After the 1st year, syphilis may be either asymptomatic (*late latent*) or symptomatic (*tertiary*).

Congenital Infection. Syphilis during pregnancy has a transmission rate approaching 100%. Fetal or perinatal death occurs in 40% of affected infants. Among survivors, manifestations have traditionally been divided into early and late stages. The former appear during the first 2 yr of life, whereas the latter appear gradually during the first 2 decades. Approximately two thirds of infants are asymptomatic at the time of birth and are identified only by routine prenatal screening; if they are untreated, symptoms develop within weeks or months.

The early manifestations of congenital infection are varied and involve multiple organ systems. Hepatosplenomegaly, jaundice, and elevated levels of liver enzymes are common. Lymphadenopathy tends to be diffuse and resolve spontaneously; shotty nodes may persist. Coombs-negative hemolytic anemia is characteristic. Thrombocytopenia is often associated with platelet trapping in an enlarged spleen. Characteristic osteochondritis and periostitis and mucocutaneous rash presenting with erythematous maculopapular or bullous lesions, followed by desquamation involving hands and feet, are common. Mucous patches, rhinitis (snuffles), and condylomatous lesions are highly characteristic features of mucous membrane involvement in congenital syphilis. Bone involvement occurs frequently. The osteochondritis is painful and often results in irritability and refusal to move the involved extremity (pseudoparalysis of Parrot). Central nervous system (CNS) abnormalities, failure to thrive, chorioretinitis, nephritis, and nephrotic syndrome may also be seen. Clinical manifestations of renal involvement include hypertension, hematuria, proteinuria, hypoproteinemia, hypercholesterolemia, and hypocomplementemia.

The late manifestations result primarily from chronic inflammation of bone, teeth, and the CNS. Skeletal changes due to persistent or recurrent periostitis and associated thickening of bone include frontal bossing, a bony prominence of the forehead ("olympian brow"); unilateral or bilateral thickening of the sternoclavicular portion of the clavicle; an anterior bowing of the middle portion of the tibia (saber shins); and scaphoid scapula, a convexity along its medial border. Dental abnormalities are common. A saddle nose, a depression of the nasal root, is a result of syphilitic rhinitis that destroys the adjacent bone and cartilage. A perforated nasal septum is an associated abnormality. Rhagades are linear scars that extend in a spokelike pattern from previous mucocutaneous fissures of the mouth, anus, and genitalia.

DIAGNOSIS. Diagnosis of primary syphilis is made with certainty when *T. pallidum* is demonstrated by darkfield microscopy or direct immunofluorescence on specimens from skin lesions, placenta, or umbilicus. However, serologic tests for syphilis are the principal means for diagnosis.

Nontreponemal tests, such as the Venereal Disease Research Laboratory (VDRL) and rapid plasma reagin (RPR) tests, detect antibodies against a cardiolipin-cholesterol-lecithin complex not specific for syphilis. Titers rise when disease is active (including treatment failure or reinfection) and fall when treatment is adequate. Treponemal tests, which measure antibody specific for *T. pallidum*, include the *T. pallidum* immobilization test (TPI), the fluorescent treponemal antibody absorption test (FTA-ABS), and the microhemagglutination assay for antibodies to *T. pallidum* (MHA-TP). Treponemal antibody titers become positive soon after initial infection and usually remain positive for life, even with adequate therapy. These antibody titers do not correlate with disease activity and are not quantified.

The Centers for Disease Control and Prevention (CDC) recommends that infants be treated if (1) they were born to mothers who had untreated syphilis at delivery; (2) there is evidence of maternal relapse or reinfection; (3) there is physical evidence of active disease; (4) there is radiologic evidence of syphilis; (5) there is a reactive CSF VDRL or, for infants born to seropositive

TABLE 149–1 Treatment of Syphilis

Stage	Treatment and Dosage	Alternatives
Primary, secondary, or early latent (<1 yr)	Penicillin G benzathine, 2.4 million U IM, in one dose	Tetracycline (500 mg PO qid for 2 wk) or doxycycline (100 mg PO bid for 2 wk) or erythromycin (500 mg PO qid for 2 wk)
Late latent (>1 yr), latent of unknown duration, or tertiary (gumma or cardiovascular syphilis)	Penicillin G benzathine, 2.4 million U IM, weekly for 3 doses	Tetracycline (500 mg PO qid for 4 wk) or doxycycline (100 mg PO bid for 4 wk)
Neurosyphilis	Aqueous crystalline penicillin G (12–24 million U/24 hr IV given as 2.4 million U every 4 hr) for 10–14 days	Penicillin G procaine (2.4 million U/day IM) *plus* probenicid (500 mg PO qid). Both for 10–14 days
Congenital syphilis	Aqueous crystalline penicillin G (100,000–150,000 U/kg/24 hr, given as 50,000 U/kg IV every 12 hr for the first 7 days and every 8 hr thereafter) for 10–14 days *or* Procaine penicillin G (50,000 U/kg IM daily in a single dose) for 10–14 days	

mothers, an abnormal CSF white blood cell count or protein, regardless of CSF serology; or (6) a serum quantitative nontreponemal serologic titer in the infant is at least fourfold greater than the mother's titer.

TREATMENT. Table 149–1 presents the recommended therapeutic regimens for syphilis.

PREVENTION. Testing is indicated at any time for persons with suspicious lesions, a history of recent sexual exposure to a person with syphilis, or diagnosis of another sexually transmitted infection, including human immunodeficiency virus infection. No newborn should leave the hospital without the maternal serologic status having been determined at least once during pregnancy.

Chapter 150

Lyme Disease (Borrelia burgdorferi)

(Nelson Textbook, Chapter 219)

Lyme disease is the most common vector-borne disease in the United States. It is a zoonosis caused by the transmission of *B. burgdorferi* to humans through the bite of an infected tick of the *Ixodes* species.

CLINICAL MANIFESTATIONS. The clinical manifestations of Lyme disease are divided into early and late stages. Early Lyme disease is further classified as early localized or early disseminated disease. Untreated patients may progressively develop clinical symptoms of each stage of the disease, or they may present with early disseminated or with late disease without apparently having had any symptoms of the earlier stages of Lyme disease.

Early Localized Disease. The first clinical manifestation of Lyme disease is the typical annular rash, named erythema migrans. Although it usually occurs 7–14 days after the bite, the onset of the rash has been reported from 3–32 days later. The initial lesion occurs at the site of the bite. The rash may be uniformly erythematous, or it may appear as a target lesion with central clearing or central vesicular or necrotic areas. Occasionally the rash may be itchy or painful. The lesion can occur anywhere on the body, although the most common locations are the axilla, the periumbilical area, the thigh, and the groin. Erythema migrans may be associated with systemic features including fever, myalgia, headache, or malaise. Without treatment, the rash gradually expands (hence the name migrans) to an average diameter of 15 cm and remains present for at least 1–2 wk.

Early Disseminated Disease. The secondary lesions, which may develop several days or even weeks after the first lesion, usually are smaller than the primary lesion and are often accompanied by fever, myalgia, headache, and malaise; conjunctivitis and lymph-adenopathy also may develop. Other manifestations may include aseptic meningitis, with signs of meningeal irritation such as nuchal rigidity; uveitis; focal neurologic findings, especially cranioneuropathies. Paralysis of the facial (7th) cranial nerve is relatively common in children and may be the initial or the only manifestation of Lyme disease. The paralysis usually lasts 2–8 wk and resolves completely in most cases.

Late Disease. Arthritis, beginning months after the initial infection, is the usual manifestation of late Lyme disease. Arthritis typically involves the large joints, especially the knee, which is affected in more than 90% of cases, but any joint may be affected. The joint is swollen and tender, but patients do not experience the exquisite pain that is typical of bacterial arthritis. The joint

---

TABLE 150–1 Antimicrobial Treatment of Lyme Borreliosis

Early Disease

Erythema Migrans and Disseminated Early Disease Without Focal Findings

Doxycycline, 100 mg twice daily for 14–21 days (do not use in children <8 yr)
or
Amoxicillin, 50 mg/kg/24 hr in 3 divided doses (maximum 500 mg/dose) for 14–21 days

Alternative agents for those who cannot take either amoxicillin or doxycycline are either erythromycin, 30–50 mg/kg/24 hr in 4 divided doses (maximum: 250 mg/dose) for 14–21 days, or cefuroxime, 30 mg/kg/24 hr in 2 divided doses (maximum: 500 mg/dose) for 14–21 days

Palsy of the Cranial Nerves (Including 7th Nerve Palsy)

Treat as for erythema migrans for 21–30 days. Do not use corticosteroids.

Carditis

Treat as for late neurologic disease.

Meningitis

Treat as for late neurologic disease.

Late Disease

Neurologic Disease*

Ceftriaxone, 50–80 mg/kg/24 hr in a single dose (maximum: 2 g) intravenously or intramuscularly for 14–21 days, or penicillin G, 200,000–400,000 U/kg/24 hr (maximum: 20 million units/24 hr) divided every 4 hr intravenously for 14–21 days.

Arthritis

Initial treatment is the same as for erythema migrans except treatment is continued for 30 days. If symptoms fail to resolve after 2 mo or there is a recurrence, then give either a second course or orally administered antimicrobial agents for 30 days or treat as for late neurologic disease.

---

*For isolated palsy of the facial nerve or of other cranial nerves, see Palsy of the Cranial Nerves.

swelling usually resolves within 1–2 wk before recurring, often in other joints. If the disease is not treated, the episodes of arthritis often increase in duration, sometimes lasting for months; but in most cases the disease eventually resolves.

TREATMENT. Recommendations for the treatment of children (Table 150–1) are extrapolated from studies of adults.

PREVENTION. Children in endemic areas are often bitten by deer ticks, but the overall risk of acquiring Lyme disease is low (1–2%). The most reasonable approach to preventing Lyme disease is to wear appropriate clothing when entering infested areas and to check for and remove ticks after spending time in such areas.

Section 8

Mycoplasmal Infections

(Nelson Textbook, Chapters 220 and 221)

Chapter 151

Mycoplasma pneumoniae *Infection*

(Nelson Textbook, Chapter 220)

Among the five *Mycoplasma* species isolated from the human respiratory tract, *Mycoplasma pneumoniae* is the only known human pathogen. It is a major cause of respiratory infections in school-aged children and young adults.

CLINICAL MANIFESTATIONS. Bronchopneumonia is the most commonly recognized clinical syndrome occurring after *M. pneumoniae* infections. Although the onset of illness may be abrupt, it is usually characterized by gradual onset of headache, malaise, fever, rhinorrhea, and sore throat, with progression of lower respiratory symptoms, including hoarseness and cough. Although the clinical course in untreated individuals is variable, coughing usually worsens during the first 2 wk of illness, and then all symptoms gradually resolve within 3–4 wk. The severity of symptoms is usually greater than the condition suggested by the physical signs, which appear later in the disease. Crackles or rales, which are often fine and crackling and resemble those heard in asthma and bronchiolitis, are the most prominent sign. With progression of the disease, the fever intensifies, the cough becomes more troublesome, and the patient may become dyspneic. Radiographic findings are not specific.

DIAGNOSIS. Cultures of the throat or sputum on special media may demonstrate *M. pneumoniae,* but growth is rarely detected earlier than within 1 wk. Serum cold hemagglutinins in a titer of 1:64 or greater or a positive IgM *M. pneumoniae* antibody supports the diagnosis. A rise or fall in convalescent-phase complement-fixing serum antibody to *M. pneumoniae* obtained after 10 days to 3 wk is diagnostic.

TREATMENT. In general, *M. pneumoniae* illness is mild and hospitalization is infrequently required. Erythromycin, clarithromycin, azithromycin, and the tetracyclines are effective in shortening the course of mycoplasmal illnesses.

SECTION 9

Chlamydial Infections

(Nelson Textbook, Chapters 222, 223, and 224)

CHAPTER 152

Chlamydia pneumoniae *Infection*

(Nelson Textbook, Chapter 222)

Chlamydia pneumoniae is increasingly recognized as a common cause of lower respiratory tract diseases, including pneumonia in children and bronchitis and pneumonia in adults.

CLINICAL MANIFESTATIONS. Infections caused by *C. pneumoniae* cannot be readily differentiated from those caused by other respiratory pathogens, especially *M. pneumoniae.* The pneumonia usually presents as a classic atypical (or nonbacterial) pneumonia characterized by mild to moderate constitutional symptoms, including fever, malaise, headache, cough, and frequently pharyngitis. *C. pneumoniae* may serve as an infectious trigger for asthma and can cause pulmonary exacerbations in patients with cystic fibrosis.

DIAGNOSIS. Specific diagnosis of *C. pneumoniae* infection is based on isolation of the organism in tissue culture and on serology.

TREATMENT. Erythromycin (40 mg/kg/24 hr divided into two doses orally for 10 days), clarithromycin (15 mg/kg/24 hr divided in two doses orally for 10 days), and azithromycin (10 mg/kg/24 on day 1, 5 mg/kg/24 hr on days 2–5) are effective for eradication of *C. pneumoniae* from the nasopharynx of children with pneumonia in approximately 80% of cases.

CONJUNCTIVITIS AND PNEUMONIA IN NEWBORNS

Newborns may acquire *C. trachomatis* at parturition from a mother with chlamydial infection.

CLINICAL MANIFESTATIONS. Approximately 70% of infected infants are infected in the nasopharynx. Clinically, the infant may develop conjunctivitis or pneumonia.

Inclusion Conjunctivitis. *C. trachomatis* is the most frequent identifiable infectious cause of neonatal conjunctivitis, the major clinical manifestation of neonatal chlamydial infection. Symptoms usually develop 5–14 days after delivery, or earlier if premature rupture of membranes has occurred. The presentation is extremely variable and ranges from mild conjunctival injection with scant mucoid discharge to severe conjunctivitis with copious purulent discharge, chemosis, and pseudomembrane formation.

Pneumonia. Pneumonia due to *C. trachomatis* develops in 10–20% of infants born to women with chlamydial infection. Onset usually appears between 1 and 3 mo of age and is often insidious, with persistent cough, tachypnea, and absence of fever. Auscultation reveals rales; wheezing is uncommon. The absence of fever and wheezing helps to distinguish *C. trachomatis* pneumonia from respiratory syncytial virus (RSV) pneumonia. A distinctive laboratory finding is the presence of peripheral eosinophilia (>400 cells/mm^3).

TREATMENT. The recommended treatment regimen for *C. trachomatis* conjunctivitis or pneumonia in infants is erythromycin (50 mg/kg/24 hr in two or four divided doses orally for 14 days). The failure rate with oral erythromycin remains 10–20%, and some infants require a second course of treatment.

SECTION 10

Rickettsial Infections

(Nelson Textbook, Chapters 225–229)

CHAPTER 153

Spotted Fever Group (Rickettsioses)

(Nelson Textbook, Chapter 225)

Many members of the spotted fever group of rickettsiae are pathogenic for humans (Table 153–1).

ROCKY MOUNTAIN SPOTTED FEVER *(RICKETTSIA RICKETTSII)*

Rocky Mountain spotted fever (RMSF) is the most frequently diagnosed rickettsial disease in the United States. While infre-

TABLE 153–1 Rickettsial Diseases of Humans: Summary of Pertinent Features

Group and Disease	Causative Agent	Arthropod Vector Transmission	Hosts	Confirmatory Tests*	Geographic Distribution
Spotted Fever					
Rocky Mountain spotted fever	*Rickettsia rickettsii*	Tick bite	Dogs, rodents	IFA, DFA, IH	Western hemisphere
Boutonneuse fever (Mediterranean spotted fever)	*Rickettsia conorii*	Tick bite	Dogs, rodents	IFA, DFA, IH	Africa, Mediterranean region, India, Middle East
Rickettsialpox	*Rickettsia akari*	Mite bite	Mice	IFA	North America, Russia, Ukraine, Adriatic region, Korea, South Africa
Scrub Typhus					
Scrub typhus	*Orientia tsutsugamushi*	Chigger bite	Rodents?	IFA	Southern Asia, Japan, Indonesia, Australia, Korea, Asiatic Russia, India, China
Typhus					
Murine typhus	*Rickettsia typhi/Rickettsia felis*	Rat flea or cat flea feces	Rats, opossums	IFA, DFA	Worldwide
Epidemic typhus	*Rickettsia prowazekii*	Louse feces	Humans	IFA	Africa, South America, Central America, Mexico, Asia
Brill-Zinsser disease (recrudescent typhus)	*Rickettsia prowazekii*	Reactivation of latent infection	Humans	IFA	Potentially worldwide; United States, Canada, Eastern Europe
Flying squirrel (sylvatic) typhus	*Rickettsia prowazekii*	Louse or flea of flying squirrel	Flying squirrels	IFA	Eastern United States
Ehrlichioses					
Human monocytic ehrlichiosis	*Ehrlichia chaffeensis*	Tick bite	Deer, dogs?	IFA, PCR	United States, Europe, Africa
Human granulocytic ehrlichiosis	*Ehrlichia phagocytophila* group	Tick bite	Rodents	IFA, PCR	United States, Europe
Sennetsu ehrlichiosis	*Ehrlichia sennetsu*	Unknown	Unknown	IFA	Japan, Malaysia
Q fever	*Coxiella burnetii*	Aerosols, ticks?	Cattle, sheep, goats, cats, rabbits	IFA	Worldwide

*DFA or IH test can be used to detect *Rickettsia* in tissue samples. PCR may be performed to detect *Ehrlichia* nucleic acids in acute phase blood using specific oligonucleotide primers. The preferred confirmatory serologic test is IFA. Cultivation may be attempted by specialized health laboratories.

IFA = indirect fluorescent antibody assay; DFA = direct fluorescent antibody; IH = immunohistology; PCR = polymerase chain reaction.

443

quently diagnosed, this potentially rapidly fatal infection is often considered in the differential diagnosis of patients with fever, headache, and rash in the summer months, especially after tick exposure.

CLINICAL MANIFESTATIONS. The incubation period in children varies from 2–14 days, with a median of 7 days. The illness is initially nonspecific with headache, fever, anorexia, myalgia, and restlessness. Gastrointestinal symptoms such as nausea, vomiting, diarrhea, or abdominal pain occur frequently (39–63%) early in the disease. Often considered the hallmark of rickettsial infection, rash is detected usually after the third day of illness, and the typical clinical triad of headache, fever, and rash is documented in only 3% of all patients at presentation. Discrete, pale, rose-red blanching macules or maculopapules appear initially, characteristically on the extremities including the ankles, wrists, or lower legs. The rash then spreads rapidly to involve the entire body, including the soles and palms. After several days, the rash becomes more petechial or hemorrhagic, with sometimes a palpable purpura. Fever and headache persist and are accompanied by severe myalgia and malaise. Splenomegaly and hepatomegaly are present in approximately 33% of patients. Central nervous system infection often produces changes in the sensorium, and delirium or coma may supervene.

Recommended treatment regimens for RMSF are doxycycline orally or intravenously (two loading doses of 2.2 mg/kg/dose at 12-hr intervals followed by 2.2 mg/kg/24 hr divided in two doses every 12 hr; maximum: 300 mg/dose); tetracycline orally (25–50 mg/kg/24 hr divided in four doses; maximum: 2 g/24 hr) or chloramphenicol (50–100 mg/kg/24 hr divided in four doses; maximum: 3 g/24 hr). Therapy should be continued for a minimum of 5 days and until the patient has been afebrile for at least 2–4 days to avoid relapse, especially in patients who were treated early.

Mycotic Infections

CHAPTER 154

Candida *Infection*

(Nelson Textbook, Chapter 230)

NEONATAL INFECTION

Candida species are a common cause of oral mucous membrane infections (thrush) and perineal skin infections (diaper dermatitis) in newborns. With the improved survival of very-low-birth-weight infants, disseminated *Candida* infections have become more frequent in special care nurseries.

CLINICAL MANIFESTATIONS. The manifestations of systemic infection vary in acuteness and severity. Fungemia may be asymptomatic or may be associated with sepsis and shock. The presentation of disseminated candidiasis mimics that of bacterial sepsis, with respiratory distress, apnea, bradycardia, temperature instability, glucose intolerance, and abdominal signs or symptoms. Cutaneous evidence of *Candida* infection may be seen in as many as half of these patients and manifests as a diffuse erythroderma or vesiculopustules from which the organism can be cultured. Renal involvement is found in more than 50% of patients and may be subclinical with persistent candiduria or may become manifest with a flank mass, hypertension, renal failure, renal abscesses, papillary necrosis, or fungal balls in the collecting system resulting in obstruction and hydronephrosis.

Central nervous system (CNS) involvement occurs in as many as one third of cases and may involve the meninges, ventricles, or cerebral cortex with abscess formation. Clinical manifestations of CNS disease may be inapparent, mandating evaluation of the cerebrospinal fluid in all patients with disseminated candidiasis regardless of CNS signs or symptoms. Because endophthalmitis is seen in 20–50% of cases, retinal examinations should be performed in neonates with systemic candidiasis; repeat examinations are necessary to monitor resolution of the retinal lesions.

TREATMENT. Amphotericin B (0.5–1.0 mg/kg/24 hr given intravenously) is the drug of choice for systemic candidiasis and is active against both yeast and mycelial forms. The duration of therapy varies widely according to the extent of infection, clinical response, and drug toxicity.

ORAL CANDIDIASIS. Oral thrush, or oral pseudomembranous candidiasis, is a superficial mucous membrane infection that affects

2–5% of normal newborns. Infants acquire *Candida* from their mothers at delivery and remain colonized. Thrush may develop as early as 7–10 days of age. The use of antibiotics, especially in the first year of fife, may lead to recurrent or persistent thrush. The plaques of thrush invade the mucosa superficially and may be found on the lips, buccal mucosa, tongue, and palate. Removal of plaques from these surfaces may cause mild punctate areas of bleeding, which helps to confirm the diagnosis. Thrush may be asymptomatic or may cause pain, fussiness, and decreased feeding. Treatment of mild cases may not be necessary. When treatment is warranted, the most commonly prescribed antifungal agent is nystatin.

DIAPER DERMATITIS. Diaper dermatitis is the most common infection caused by *Candida*. Primary infection generally occurs in the intertriginous areas of the perineum and presents as a confluent papular erythema with red satellite papules. *Candida* diaper dermatitis often complicates oral antibiotic treatment of otitis media as well as other noninfectious diaper dermatitides.

Treatment is usually performed with nystatin cream, powder, or ointment, clotrimazole 1% cream, miconazole 2% ointment, or amphotericin cream or ointment. If significant inflammation is present, the addition of hydrocortisone 1% may be useful for the first 1 or 2 days.

VULVOVAGINITIS. Vulvovaginitis is a common candidal infection of pubertal and postpubertal females that affects as many as 75% of females at one time or another. Candidal vulvovaginitis can be effectively treated with either vaginal creams or troches of nystatin, clotrimazole, or miconazole. Oral therapy with single-dose fluconazole has been found to be as effective as clotrimazole in women and may be useful in adolescent girls.

Viral Infections

(Nelson Textbook, Chapters 240–269)

CHAPTER 155

Measles

(Nelson Textbook, Chapter 240)

Measles (rubeola) is an important childhood disease that was historically widespread but is now very infrequent. It is an acute viral infection characterized by a final stage with a maculopapular rash erupting successively over the neck and face, body, arms, and legs and accompanied by a high fever.

CHAPTER 156

Rubella

(Nelson Textbook, Chapter 241)

Rubella (German or three-day measles) is an important childhood disease that was historically widespread but is now very infrequent. It is an acute viral infection ordinarily characterized by mild constitutional symptoms, a rash similar to that of mild rubeola or scarlet fever, and enlargement and tenderness of the postoccipital, retroauricular, and posterior cervical lymph nodes. Rubella in early pregnancy may cause the congenital rubella syndrome, a serious multisystemic disease with a wide spectrum of clinical expression and sequelae.

CHAPTER 157

Mumps

(Nelson Textbook, Chapter 242)

Mumps is an important childhood disease that was historically widespread but now occurs very infrequently. It is an acute viral infection characterized by painful enlargement of the salivary glands, chiefly the parotids, as the usual presenting sign.

CHAPTER 158

Enterovirus Infection

(Nelson Textbook, Chapter 243)

Enteroviruses are a large group of viral agents that inhabit the intestinal tract and are responsible for significant and frequent human illnesses that produce protean clinical manifestations.

POLIOVIRUSES

Poliovirus infections may follow one of several courses: inapparent infection, which occurs in 90–95% of cases and causes no disease and no sequelae; abortive poliomyelitis; nonparalytic poliomyelitis; or paralytic poliomyelitis.

NONPOLIO ENTEROVIRUSES

Coxsackieviral and echoviral infections are exceedingly common, and their spectrum of disease is protean. More than 90% of infections caused by nonpolio enteroviruses are asymptomatic or result in undifferentiated febrile illnesses. Some clinical syndromes are highly but not exclusively associated with certain serotypes.

CLINICAL MANIFESTATIONS

Nonspecific Febrile Illness. Nonspecific febrile illness is the most common manifestation of enteroviral infections. All viral types cause this clinical presentation. Onset of illness is usually abrupt and has no prodrome. In young children the initial finding is fever that may be associated with malaise. In older children headache and myalgia are usually also noted. Nonpolio enteroviruses are common causes of a large variety of skin manifestations.

Hand, Foot, and Mouth Disease. The clinical expression rate of this enanthem-exanthem complex is high, being close to 100% in young children, 38% in schoolchildren, and 11% in adults. The tongue and buccal mucosa are most frequently involved.

Herpangina. Herpangina is usually characterized by a sudden onset of fever. Older children frequently complain of headache and backache. The characteristic lesions are small, 1- to 2-mm vesicles and ulcers.

Acute Hemorrhagic Conjunctivitis. Enterovirus 70 has been the cause of a majority of epidemics of acute hemorrhagic conjunctivitis.

Respiratory Manifestations. Pharyngitis, tonsillitis, tonsillopharyngitis, and nasopharyngitis are common clinical manifestations of coxsackieviral and echoviral infections; probably all enteroviruses on occasion cause mild pharyngitis.

Gastrointestinal Manifestations. Gastrointestinal manifestations are common (7–30%) in patients with enteroviral infections. Vomiting and diarrhea are common manifestations of infections due to many coxsackieviral and echoviral types, along with other manifestations of the systemic illness.

Neurologic Manifestations. Aseptic meningitis resulting from enteroviruses occurs in epidemics and as isolated cases. Virtually all patients have fever, and many have mild pharyngitis; other respiratory manifestations are also common. Rash is common but varies with the specific viral agents; 30–50% of all patients with echovirus 9 meningitis have exanthem. Frequently, the rash is petechial, thus suggesting meningococcemia.

Pericarditis and Myocarditis. Cardiac manifestations have been noted in association with 27 different nonpolio enteroviruses.

Neonatal Infections. Nonpolio enteroviral infections in neonatal infants result in a wide variety of clinical manifestations, ranging from asymptomatic infection to sepsis-like illness, fatal encephalitis, and myocarditis.

PREVENTION. Vaccines for enteroviruses other than polioviruses are not available.

TREATMENT. There is no specific therapy for any enterovirus infection.

CHAPTER 159

Herpes Simplex Virus Infection

(Nelson Textbook, Chapter 245)

Herpes simplex virus (HSV) is common among humans and has a variety of clinical manifestations involving the skin, mucous membranes, eye, central nervous system (CNS), and genital tract. It also causes generalized systemic disease.

CLINICAL MANIFESTATIONS. HSV characteristically produces a vesicular lesion. Only rarely is there a viremic distribution that results in widespread systemic disease or neurogenic transmission that leads to meningoencephalitis.

Lesions of the Skin and Mucous Membranes. On the skin the lesion consists of aggregates of thin-walled vesicles on an erythematous base. These rupture, scab, and heal within 7–10 days without leaving a scar except after repeated attacks or secondary bacterial infections; temporary depigmentation may occur in darkly pigmented individuals. The lesions tend to recur at the same site, particularly at mucocutaneous junctions, but they may occur anywhere. Traumatic lesions of the skin or burns can be infected by HSV. Primary lesions can also occur on apparently unbroken skin, as, for example, on the chin of a drooling infant with herpetic stomatitis, in whom scattered isolated vesicles appear.

Acute Herpetic Gingivostomatitis. This primary infection, probably the most common cause of stomatitis in children 1–3 yr of age, can also occur in older children and adults. The symptoms may appear abruptly, with pain in the mouth, salivation, fetor oris, refusal to eat, and fever, often as high as 40–40.6°C (104–105°F).

Recurrent Stomatitis and Herpes Labialis. The typical oral recurrence of HSV is one or a few vesicles grouped at the mucocutaneous junction. Lesions are usually accompanied by local pain, tingling, or itching and last 3–7 days.

Eczema Herpeticum (Kaposi Varicelliform Eruption). This, the most serious manifestation of "traumatic herpes," results from a widespread infection of the eczematous skin with HSV.

Ocular Infections. *Conjunctivitis* and *keratoconjunctivitis* may occur as manifestations of either a primary or a recurrent infection. The conjunctiva appears congested and swollen, but there is little, if any, purulent discharge.

Genital Herpes. Genital infections with herpesvirus occur most commonly in adolescents and young adults, are usually due to HSV-2, and are usually spread by sexual activity.

Central Nervous System Infections. HSV has a predilection to infect the nervous system. Both types 1 and 2 may cause a meningoencephalitis as part of neonatal HSV. In patients with primary genital herpes, usually resulting from HSV-2, an aseptic meningitis syndrome may complicate the course. HSV-1 is an unusual cause of the aseptic meningitis syndrome, but it is the most common cause of fatal sporadic encephalitis. It has a striking predilection to involve the frontal and parietal areas. Typical signs and symptoms include fever, altered consciousness, headache, personality changes, seizures, dysphasia, and focal neurologic signs.

Immunocompromised Persons. Unusually severe HSV infection may occur in a variety of persons, including the newborn; the severely malnourished; and children with malignancies or other conditions necessitating immunosuppressive therapy, with the acquired immunodeficiency syndrome, with burns, or with primary immunodeficiency diseases that particularly impair cell-mediated immunity.

Perinatal Infections. Most cases of neonatal herpes occur due to infection during delivery, and 75–80% are HSV-2. Infection manifests in the first month of life, with 25% on the first day, and in two thirds by the first week. The hallmark of neonatal HSV infection—the vesicular, ulcerative skin lesions—are present in only 30–43% of children at presentation; one third will never manifest skin lesions. Symptoms of CNS involvement are found in 48–79% and include lethargy, poor feeding, irritability, poor tone, and seizures. Fever (7–14%) and respiratory distress (5–19%) may be present.

TREATMENT. Acyclovir (9-[-2-hydroxyethoxymethyl] guanine, a purine nucleoside analog) is the mainstay of therapy for HSV. Two recently licensed oral anti-herpes drugs simplify the therapy for genital herpes. Valacyclovir, a prodrug of acyclovir, and famciclovir, a prodrug of penciclovir, have excellent oral bioavailability (55–80%) and are converted in vivo to acyclovir and penciclovir, respectively. Topical acyclovir therapy for oral or genital herpes may decrease the period of viral shedding but has little effect on symptoms and is not recommended.

Lesions of the Skin and Mucous Membranes. Oral acyclovir (15 mg kg 5 times a day with a maximum dose of 1 g/24 hr for 7 days) started within 72 hr of onset of lesions has significant benefits in children with primary herpetic gingivostomatitis by decreasing drooling, gum swelling, pain, eating and drinking difficulties, and duration of lesions. Therapy for recurrent oral herpes with oral acyclovir has limited effects. Symptomatic and supportive therapy is of great importance. The recommended treatment regimen for initial genital herpes is valacyclovir (1000 mg/dose) or famciclovir (500 mg/dose) given twice daily for 10 days; these are equivalent to acyclovir 5 times a day. For HSV genital recurrence, valacyclovir (500 mg/dose) and famciclovir (125 mg/dose) given twice daily for 5 days are equivalent to acyclovir 5 times a day.

CNS and Systemic Infections. Intravenously administered acyclovir (10 mg/kg/dose given over 1 hr every 8 hr for 14–21 days) is the treatment of choice for herpes encephalitis. The drug is well tolerated. The best results are obtained when treatment is started early.

Perinatal Infections. As in other serious forms of HSV infection, intravenous acyclovir (60 mg/kg/24 hr in 3 divided doses for 14–21 days) is the drug of choice for neonatal HSV infection. For the neonate with HSV infection, intensive care is necessary initially to observe for signs of disseminated or CNS disease necessitating ventilatory control, seizure management, and intensive supportive care.

PREVENTION. Acyclovir administered during periods of high risk in immunocompromised hosts and administered chronically in individuals with frequently recurrent genital or oral disease markedly decreases the rate of recurrence. Acyclovir administered before a known trigger factor, such as intense sunlight, usually prevents recurrences.

Obstetric Management of the Woman with Genital HSV Infection. Recommendations are for a cesarean section if primary, first-episode, or recurrent HSV lesions are present at the onset of labor.

CHAPTER 160

Varicella-Zoster Virus Infection

(Nelson Textbook, Chapter 246)

The primary infection is manifested as varicella (chickenpox) and results in establishment of a lifelong latent infection of sensory ganglion neurons. Reactivation of the latent infection causes herpes zoster (shingles). Although often a mild illness of childhood, chickenpox can cause increased morbidity and mortality in adolescents and immunocompromised persons and predisposes to severe group A *Streptococcus* and *Staphylococcus aureus* infections.

CLINICAL MANIFESTATIONS. Varicella is an acute febrile illness, common in children who have not been immunized, that has variable severity and is usually self-limited. It may be associated with several complications, including congenital infection and perinatal transmission causing life-threatening infection in the fetus.

Varicella. The illness usually begins 14–16 days after exposure, although the incubation period can range from 10–21 days. Almost all exposed, susceptible children experience a rash, but illness may be limited to only a few lesions. Fever, malaise, anorexia, headache, and occasionally mild abdominal pain may occur 24–48 hr before the rash appears. Temperature elevation is usually moderate, usually from 100–102°F (37.8–38.9°C), but may be as high as 106°F (41.1°C); fever and other systemic symptoms persist during the first 2–4 days after the onset of the rash.

Varicella lesions often appear first on the scalp, face, or trunk. The initial exanthem consists of intensely pruritic erythematous macules that evolve to form clear, fluid-filled vesicles. Clouding and umbilication of the lesions begin in 24–48 hr. While the initial lesions are crusting, new crops form on the trunk and then the extremities; the simultaneous presence of lesions in various stages of evolution is characteristic of varicella. Ulcerative lesions involving the oropharynx and vagina are also common; many children have vesicular lesions on the eyelids and conjunctivae.

Neonatal Chickenpox. Delivery within 1 wk before or after the onset of maternal varicella frequently results in the newborn developing varicella, which may be severe. The initial infection is intrauterine, although the newborn often develops clinical chickenpox post partum.

TREATMENT. Antiviral treatment modifies the course of both varicella and herpes zoster.

Varicella. Acyclovir therapy is not recommended routinely for treatment of uncomplicated varicella in the otherwise healthy child because of the marginal benefit, the cost of the drug, and the low risk of complications. Oral therapy with acyclovir (20 mg/kg/dose; maximum of 800 mg/dose) given as 4 doses per day for 5 days should be used to treat uncomplicated varicella in nonpregnant individuals older than 13 yr of age and children older than 12 mo of age with chronic cutaneous or pulmonary disorders; receiving short-term, intermittent, or aerosolized corticosteroids; receiving long-term salicylate therapy; and possibly second cases in household contacts. Intravenous therapy is indicated for severe disease and for varicella in immunocompromised patients.

PREVENTION

Vaccine. Varicella is a vaccine-preventable disease. Live virus vaccine is recommended for routine administration in children at 12–18 mo of age.

Postexposure Prophylaxis. Varicella-zoster immune globulin (VZIG) postexposure prophylaxis is recommended for immunocompromised children, pregnant women, and newborns exposed to maternal varicella.

CHAPTER 161

Epstein-Barr Virus Infection

(Nelson Textbook, Chapter 247)

Infectious mononucleosis is the best-known clinical syndrome caused by Epstein-Barr virus (EBV). It is characterized by systemic somatic complaints consisting primarily of fatigue, malaise, fever, sore throat, and generalized lymphadenopathy.

CLINICAL MANIFESTATIONS. The incubation period of infectious mononucleosis in adolescents is 30–50 days. In children it may be shorter. The majority of cases of primary EBV infection in infants and young children are clinically silent. In older patients, the onset of illness is usually insidious and vague. Patients may complain of malaise, fatigue, fever, headache, sore throat, nausea, abdominal pain, and myalgia. This prodromal period may last 1–2 wk. Splenic enlargement may be rapid enough to cause left upper quadrant abdominal discomfort and tenderness.

The physical examination is characterized by generalized lymphadenopathy (90% of cases), splenomegaly (50% of cases), and hepatomegaly (10% of cases). Lymphadenopathy occurs most commonly in the anterior and posterior cervical nodes and the submandibular lymph nodes. Epitrochlear lymphadenopathy is particularly suggestive of infectious mononucleosis. The sore throat is often accompanied by moderate to severe pharyngitis with marked tonsillar enlargement, occasionally with exudates. The pharyngitis resembles that caused by streptococcal infection.

Routine Laboratory Tests. In more than 90% of cases there is leukocytosis of 10,000–20,000 cells/mm³, of which at least two thirds are lymphocytes; atypical lymphocytes usually account for 20–40% of the total number.

Heterophile Antibody Test. The heterophile antibodies of infectious mononucleosis agglutinate sheep or, for greater sensitivity, horse red cells but not guinea pig kidney cells.

Specific EBV Antibodies. EBV-specific antibody testing is useful to confirm acute EBV infection, especially in heterophile-negative cases, or to confirm past infection and determine susceptibility to future infection.

TREATMENT. There is no specific treatment for infectious mononucleosis. Rest and symptomatic therapy are the mainstays of management.

PROGNOSIS. The prognosis for complete recovery is excellent if no complications ensue during the acute illness. The major symptoms typically last 2–4 wk, followed by gradual recovery.

CHAPTER 162

Roseola
(Human Herpesvirus Types 6 and 7)
(Nelson Textbook, Chapter 249)

CLINICAL MANIFESTATIONS. Roseola is the prototypical HHV-6 infection, although nonspecific infections are common.

Roseola Infantum (Exanthem Subitum). Roseola is a mild febrile, exanthematous illness occurring almost exclusively during infancy. More than 95% of roseola cases occur in children younger than 3 yr, with a peak at 6–15 mo of age. Transplacental antibodies likely protect most infants until 6 mo of age.

The prodromal period of roseola is usually asymptomatic but may include mild upper respiratory tract signs, among them minimal rhinorrhea, slight pharyngeal inflammation, and mild conjunctival redness.

Clinical illness is generally heralded by high temperature, usually ranging from 37.9–40°C (100.2–104°F), with an average of 39°C (102.2°F). Some children may become irritable and anorexic during the febrile stage, but most behave normally despite high temperatures. Fever persists for 3–5 days, and then typically resolves rather abruptly ("crisis"). A rash appears within 12–24 hr of fever resolution. In many cases, the rash develops during defervescence or within a few hours of fever resolution. The rash of roseola is rose colored. The roseola rash begins as discrete, small (2–5 mm), slightly raised pink lesions on the trunk and usually spreads to the neck, face, and proximal extremities. The rash is not usually pruritic, and no vesicles or pustules develop.

Lesions typically remain discrete but occasionally may become almost confluent. After 1–3 days, the rash fades.

CHAPTER 163

Respiratory Syncytial Virus Infection
(Nelson Textbook, Chapter 253)

Respiratory syncytial virus (RSV) is the major cause of bronchiolitis and pneumonia in children younger than 1 yr. It is the most important respiratory tract pathogen of early childhood.

CLINICAL MANIFESTATIONS. The first signs of infection of the infant with RSV are rhinorrhea and pharyngitis. Cough may appear simultaneously but more often after an interval of 1–3 days, at which time there may also be sneezing and a low-grade fever. Soon after the cough develops, the child begins to wheeze audibly. If the disease is mild, the symptoms may not progress beyond this stage. Auscultation often reveals diffuse rhonchi, fine rales or crackles, and wheezes. Clear rhinorrhea usually persists throughout the illness, with intermittent fever. Radiographs of the chest at this stage are frequently normal.

If the illness progresses, cough and wheezing increase and air hunger ensues with increased respiratory rate, intercostal and subcostal retractions, hyperexpansion of the chest, restlessness, and peripheral cyanosis. Signs of severe, life-threatening illness are central cyanosis, tachypnea of more than 70 breaths/min, listlessness, and apneic spells. At this stage, the chest may be greatly hyperexpanded and almost silent to auscultation because of poor air exchange.

Chest radiographs of infants hospitalized with RSV bronchiolitis are normal in about 10% of cases; air trapping or hyperexpansion of the chest is evident in about 50%. Peribronchial thickening or interstitial pneumonia is seen in 50–80%. Segmental consolidation occurs in 10–25%. Pleural effusion is rarely, if ever, seen.

In some infants, the course of the illness may be more like that of pneumonia with the prodromal rhinorrhea and cough followed by dyspnea, poor feeding, and listlessness, with a minimum of wheezing and hyperexpansion. Fever is an inconstant sign in RSV infection.

TREATMENT. In uncomplicated cases of bronchiolitis, treatment is symptomatic. Humidified oxygen is usually indicated for hospitalized infants because most are hypoxic. Many infants are slightly to moderately dehydrated; therefore, fluids should be carefully administered in amounts somewhat greater than maintenance. Often intravenous or tube feeding is helpful when sucking is difficult due to tachypnea. Infants may breathe more easily when propped up at an angle of 10–30 degrees.

The antiviral drug ribavirin, delivered by small-particle aerosol and breathed, along with the required concentration of oxygen, for 20 of 24 hr/day for 3–5 days, has a modest beneficial effect on the course of RSV pneumonia. Its use is indicated only in very sick infants or in high-risk infants.

Passive Immunoprophylaxis. Administration of either palivizumab (15 mg/kg intramuscularly), a monoclonal antibody against RSV, or high-titered RSV intravenous immunoglobulin (RSVIVIG; 750 mg/kg) is recommended for protecting high-risk children against serious complications from RSV disease. There is not currently a vaccine against RSV.

CHAPTER 164

Adenovirus Infection

(Nelson Textbook, Chapter 254)

Adenoviruses cause 5–8% of acute respiratory disease in infants, plus a wide array of other syndromes, including pharyngoconjunctival fever, follicular conjunctivitis, epidemic keratoconjunctivitis, myocarditis, hemorrhagic cystitis, acute diarrhea, intussusception, and encephalomyelitis.

CLINICAL MANIFESTATIONS

Acute Respiratory Disease. This is the most common manifestation of adenovirus infection in children and adults. Acute adenovirus respiratory tract infections in infants and children are not clinically distinctive. Primary infections in infants are frequently associated with fever and respiratory symptoms and are complicated by otitis media in more than half of the patients. Adenovirus respiratory infections are associated with a significant incidence of diarrhea.

Conjunctivitis and Keratoconjunctivitis. Adenovirus is one of the most common causes of follicular conjunctivitis and keratoconjunctivitis.

TREATMENT. No agents are effective in treating adenovirus infections.

CHAPTER 165

Rotavirus and Other Agents of Viral Gastroenteritis

(Nelson Textbook, Chapter 256)

In early childhood, the single most important cause of severe dehydrating diarrhea is rotavirus infection. Rotavirus and other gastroenteritis viruses not only are major causes of pediatric mortality but also lead to significant morbidity as a result of malnutrition.

CLINICAL MANIFESTATIONS. Rotavirus infection typically begins after an incubation period of less than 48 hr, with mild to moderate fever and vomiting followed by the onset of frequent, watery stools. Vomiting and fever typically abate during the second day of illness, but diarrhea often continues for 5–7 days. The stool is without gross blood or white blood cells. Dehydration may develop and progress rapidly, particularly in infants.

The clinical course of astrovirus appears to be similar to that of rotavirus, with the notable exception that the disease tends to be milder, with less significant dehydration. Adenovirus enteritis tends to cause diarrhea of longer duration, often 10–14 days.

TREATMENT. Avoiding and treating dehydration are the main goals in treatment of viral enteritis. A secondary goal is maintenance of the nutritional status of the patient. There is no role for antiviral drug treatment of viral gastroenteritis. Antibiotics are similarly of no benefit.

CHAPTER 166

Acquired Immunodeficiency Syndrome (Human Immunodeficiency Virus Infection)

(Nelson Textbook, Chapter 268)

Most HIV-infected children are born in developing countries. HIV infection in children progresses more rapidly than in adults, and some children die within the first yr of life.

CLINICAL MANIFESTATIONS. The clinical manifestations of HIV infection vary widely among infants, children, and adolescents. In the majority of infants, physical examination at birth is normal. Initial symptoms may be subtle, such as lymphadenopathy and hepatosplenomegaly, or nonspecific, such as failure to thrive, chronic or recurrent diarrhea, interstitial pneumonia, or oral thrush; symptoms may be distinguishable only by their persistence. Whereas systemic and pulmonary findings are common in the United States and Europe, chronic diarrhea, wasting, and severe malnutrition predominate in Africa. Symptoms found more commonly in children than adults with HIV infection include recurrent bacterial infections, chronic parotid swelling, lymphocytic interstitial pneumonitis, and early onset of progressive neurologic deterioration.

Bacterial Infections. Approximately 20% of AIDS-defining illnesses in children are recurrent bacterial infections caused primarily by encapsulated organisms such as *Streptococcus pneumonia*e and *Salmonella* species. The most common serious infections are bacteremia, sepsis, and pneumonia, accounting for more than 50% of infections in HIV-infected children. Milder recurrent infections, such as otitis media, sinusitis, and skin and soft tissue infections are very common and may be chronic with atypical presentations.

Atypical Mycobacterial Infections. Atypical mycobacterial infections, particularly with *Mycobacterium avium complex* (MAC), may cause disseminated disease in HIV-infected children who are severely immunosuppressed.

Fungal Infections. Oral candidiasis is the most common fungal infection seen in HIV-infected children. Oral nystatin suspension (100,000 units/mL, 2–5 mL four times a day) is often effective. Oral thrush progresses to involve the esophagus in approximately 20% of children, who present with symptoms of anorexia, dysphagia, vomiting, and fever. Treatment with oral fluconazole (4–6 mg/kg/24 hr for 14 days) generally results in rapid improvement in symptoms.

***Pneumocystis carinii* Pneumonia.** The peak incidence of *P. carinii* pneumonia occurs at 3–6 mo of age, with the highest mortality rate in infants younger than 1 yr. However, newer, more aggressive approaches to treatment have improved the outcome substantially. The first-line therapy for *P. carinii* pneumonia is intravenous trimethoprim (TMP)/sulfamethoxazole (SMZ) (15–20 mg/kg/24 hr of TMP and 75–100 mg/kg/24 hr of SMZ divided every 6 hr) with adjunctive intravenous methylprednisolone (2 mg/kg/24 hr divided every 6 or 12 hr for 5–7 days).

Central Nervous System. The incidence of central nervous system involvement in perinatally infected children is 40–90%, with a median onset at 19 mo of age. The most common presentation is progressive encephalopathy with loss or plateau of developmental milestones, cognitive deterioration, impaired brain growth resulting in acquired microcephaly, and symmetric motor dysfunction. Encephalopathy may be the initial manifestation of the HIV infection, or it may present much later when severe immune suppression occurs.

Respiratory Tract. Recurrent upper respiratory tract infections such as otitis media and sinusitis are very common. Lymphocytic interstitial pneumonitis is the most common chronic lower respiratory tract abnormality, occurring in 30–50% of HIV-infected children. It is a chronic process with nodular lymphoid hyperplasia in the bronchial and bronchiolar epithelium that often leads to progressive alveolar capillary block developing over months to years. Clinically, there is an insidious onset of tachypnea, cough, and mild to moderate hypoxemia with normal auscultatory findings or minimal rales. Most symptomatic HIV-infected children experience at least one episode of pneumonia. *Streptococcus pneumoniae* is the most common bacterial pathogen.

Gastrointestinal and Hepatobiliary Tract. The most common symptoms of gastrointestinal disease are chronic or recurrent diarrhea with malabsorption, abdominal pain, dysphagia, and failure to thrive. Chronic liver inflammation, evidenced by fluctuating serum levels of hepatic transaminases with or without cholestasis, is relatively common, often without identification of an etiologic agent.

Hematologic Diseases. Anemia occurs in 20–70% of HIV-infected children, more commonly in children with AIDS. Leukopenia occurs in almost one third of untreated HIV-infected children, and neutropenia often occurs. In many cases, treatment with subcutaneous granulocyte colony-stimulating factor is successful. Thrombocytopenia occurs in 10–20% of patients. Treatment with IVIG or anti-D offers temporary improvement in many cases.

TREATMENT. HIV-infected children with symptoms or with evidence of immune dysfunction should be treated with antiretroviral therapy regardless of age or viral load. Infants younger than 1 yr are at high risk for disease progression, and immunologic and virologic tests to identify those likely to experience rapidly progressive disease are less predictive than in older children. Therefore, all such infants should be treated with antiretroviral agents as soon as the diagnosis of HIV infection has been confirmed, regardless of clinical or immunologic status or viral load.

Most clinicians advocate treating asymptomatic children older than 1 yr to prevent immunologic deterioration. However, when there are concerns regarding drug adherence, safety, and durability of antiretroviral response, some providers elect to delay treatment in the immunologically normal child older than 1 yr with a low viral load (<20,000 copies/mL), for whom the risk for clinical progression is low. Such children should be monitored regularly for evidence of virologic, immunologic, or clinical progression, at which point therapy should be initiated. Even before the new antiretroviral drugs were available, a significant impact on the quality of life and survival of HIV-infected children was achieved with intensive supportive treatment.

HIV-exposed and infected children can be given most standard pediatric immunizations, although live virus vaccines and live bacterial vaccines (e.g., bacille Calmette-Guérin) are generally contraindicated. Prophylactic regimens are an integral component for the care of HIV-infected children.

PREVENTION. Prevention of sexual transmission involves avoiding the exchange of body fluids. Interruption of perinatal transmission from mother to child can be achieved by administering zidovudine chemoprophylaxis to pregnant women and their offspring.

SECTION 13

Protozoan Diseases
(Nelson Textbook, Chapters 270–281)

CHAPTER 167

Giardiasis
(Nelson Textbook, Chapter 272)

Giardia lamblia is a flagellated protozoan that infects the duodenum and small intestine. Infection results in a wide variety of clinical manifestations ranging from asymptomatic colonization to acute or chronic diarrhea and malabsorption.

CLINICAL MANIFESTATION. Children who are exposed to *G. lamblia* may experience asymptomatic excretion of the organism, acute infectious diarrhea, or chronic diarrhea with persistent gastrointestinal tract signs and symptoms, including failure to thrive. Most infections, in both children and adults, are asymptomatic.

DIAGNOSIS. A definitive diagnosis of giardiasis is established by documentation of trophozoites, cysts, or *Giardia* antigens in stool specimens or duodenal fluid.

TREATMENT. There are several drugs available in the United States that are effective in the therapy of patients with giardiasis, including metronidazole, which is the drug of choice, and furazolidone and paromomycin.

CHAPTER 168

Trichomoniasis
(Nelson Textbook, Chapter 274)

Trichomonas vaginalis is a sexually transmitted protozoan parasite that primarily causes symptomatic vaginitis in women.

CLINICAL MANIFESTATIONS. Signs and symptoms most commonly associated with trichomoniasis include copious malodorous yellow vaginal discharge, vulvovaginal irritation, dysuria, and dyspareunia. On physical examination, a frothy discharge with vaginal erythema and cervical hemorrhages ("strawberry cervix") may be seen.

TREATMENT. The treatment of trichomoniasis is administration of a nitroimidazole. In the United States, metronidazole is used; in other countries tinidazole or ornidazole has been used with similar efficacy.

CHAPTER 169

Malaria (Plasmodium)

(Nelson Textbook, Chapter 278)

Malaria is an acute and chronic protozoan illness characterized by paroxysms of fever, chills, sweats, fatigue, anemia, and splenomegaly.

CLINICAL MANIFESTATIONS. The classic presentation of malaria includes febrile paroxysms alternating with periods of fatigue but otherwise relative wellness. Symptoms associated with febrile paroxysms include high fever, rigors, sweats, and headache, as well as myalgia, back pain, abdominal pain, nausea, vomiting, diarrhea, pallor, and jaundice. Paroxysms coincide with the rupture of schizonts that occurs every 48 hr with *P. vivax* and *P. ovale* and results in daily fever spikes; this rupture occurs every 72 hr with *P. malariae* and results in alternate-day or every-third-day fever spikes. Periodicity is less apparent with *P. falciparum* and mixed infections. Symptoms of malaria in children older than 2 mo of age who are nonimmune vary widely from low-grade fever and headache, to fever greater than 104°F (40°C) with headache, drowsiness, anorexia, nausea, vomiting, diarrhea, pallor, cyanosis, splenomegaly, hepatomegaly, anemia, thrombocytopenia, and a normal or low white blood cell count.

DIAGNOSIS. The diagnosis of malaria is established by identification of organisms on Giemsa-stained smears of peripheral blood.

TREATMENT. Physicians caring for patients with malaria or for those who are traveling to endemic areas need to be aware of current information regarding malaria. Resistance to antimalarial drugs is increasing and has greatly complicated therapy and prophylaxis. The best source for such information is the Centers for Disease Control and Prevention Malaria Hotline, which is available 24 hr a day (888-232-3228).

CHAPTER 170

Toxoplasmosis (Toxoplasma gondii)

(Nelson Textbook, Chapter 280)

In the immunologically normal child, the acute acquired infection may be asymptomatic, cause lymphadenopathy, or damage almost any organ. Once acquired, the latent encysted organism persists for the lifetime of the host. In the immunocompromised infant or child, either initial acquisition or recrudescence of latent organisms often causes signs or symptoms related to the central nervous system (CNS). Infection acquired congenitally, if untreated, almost always causes signs or symptoms in the perinatal period or later in life. The most frequent of these signs are due to chorioretinitis and CNS lesions. However, other manifestations, such as intrauterine growth retardation, fever, lymphadenopathy, rash, hearing loss, pneumonitis, hepatitis, and thrombocytopenia, also occur. Congenital toxoplasmosis in infants with human immunodeficiency virus (HIV) infection may be fulminant.

CLINICAL MANIFESTATIONS. The manifestations of primary infection with *T. gondii* are highly variable and influenced primarily by host immunocompetence. Reactivation of previously asymptomatic congenital toxoplasmosis is usually manifest as ocular toxoplasmosis.

TREATMENT. Pyrimethamine plus sulfadiazine or trisulfapyrimidines act synergistically against *Toxoplasma*. Combined therapy is indicated to treat many of the forms of toxoplasmosis. However, use of pyrimethamine is contraindicated during the first trimester of pregnancy. Spiramycin should be used to prevent transmission of infection to the fetus of acutely infected pregnant women and to treat congenital toxoplasmosis. Neutropenia is the most common side effect in treated infants. Seizures may occur with overdosage of pyrimethamine. Folinic acid (calcium leukovorin) should always be administered concomitantly with pyrimethamine to prevent suppression of the bone marrow.

SECTION 14

Helminthic Diseases

(Nelson Textbook, Chapters 282–300)

CHAPTER 171

Ascariasis (Ascaris lumbricoides)

(Nelson Textbook, Chapter 282)

Infection with *Ascaris lumbricoides* is the most prevalent human helminthiasis, causing an estimated 1 billion cases worldwide. Infection is most common in children of preschool or early school age.

CLINICAL MANIFESTATIONS. Although disease occurs in only a small proportion of infected individuals, this is a significant clinical problem because of the high incidence of ascariasis. Morbidity may be manifested during migration of the larvae through the lungs or may be associated with the presence of adult worms in the small intestine. Pulmonary ascariasis may occur after heavy exposure. The most characteristic features are cough, blood-stained sputum, and eosinophilia. This Löffler-like syndrome may be associated with transient pulmonary infiltrates. The presence of adult worms in the small intestine is associated with vague complaints such as abdominal pain and distention. Intestinal obstruction, although rare, may be due to a mass of worms in heavily infected children. The onset is usually sudden, with severe colicky abdominal pain and vomiting, which may be bile stained; these symptoms may progress rapidly and follow a course similar to acute intestinal obstruction due to any other cause.

TREATMENT. Several chemotherapeutic agents are effective against ascariasis; none, however, is useful during the pulmonary phase of the infection. The recommended treatment of uncomplicated gastrointestinal ascariasis is albendazole (400 mg as a single oral dose). Treatment of children with heavy infections should be approached with caution.

CHAPTER 172

Enterobiasis (Pinworm; Enterobius vermicularis)

(Nelson Textbook, Chapter 284)

This infection is essentially harmless and causes more social than medical problems in affected children and their families.

CLINICAL MANIFESTATIONS. Symptomatic individuals most commonly complain of nocturnal anal pruritus and sleeplessness.

DIAGNOSIS. Definitive diagnosis is established by either finding the parasite eggs or recovering worms.

TREATMENT. The recommended regimen for enterobiasis is albendazole (400 mg PO for children and adults, with a repeat dose in 2 wk).

SECTION 15

Preventive Measures

(Nelson Textbook, Chapters 301–304)

CHAPTER 173

Immunization Practices

(Nelson Textbook, Chapter 301)

VACCINES FOR ROUTINE USE IN CHILDREN AND ADOLESCENTS. All children should be vaccinated against diphtheria, tetanus, pertussis, poliomyelitis, measles, mumps, rubella, *Haemophilus influenzae* type b, hepatitis B, and varicella unless contraindicated. The first dose of hepatitis B vaccine is recommended to be given at birth. This is especially important for infants of hepatitis B surface antigen (HBsAg)-positive mothers. For poliomyelitis immunization, expanded use of inactivated poliovirus vaccine (IPV) is now recommended in the United States to reduce the risk of vaccine-associated paralytic poliomyelitis associated with oral poliovirus vaccine (OPV).

Acellular pertussis vaccine, combined with diphtheria and tetanus toxoids (DTaP), is now the preferred vaccine for pertussis immunization. After the 7th birthday, combined tetanus and diphtheria toxoids in the adult formulation (Td), containing a lesser amount of diphtheria toxoid, are recommended for both primary and booster vaccination. The first booster dose of Td is recommended at 11–12 yr of age and is followed by a booster at

10-yr intervals thereafter. The second dose of measles-containing vaccine (given as measles-mumps-rubella [MMR]) should be routinely given before school entry at 4–6 yr of age. Varicella vaccine is recommended beginning at 12 mo of age and for older children through 12 yr of age if they have not been previously immunized or if they lack a reliable history of chickenpox. Heptavalent pneumococcal conjugate vaccine (PCV7) is recommended for universal use in children 23 mo and younger.

VACCINES WITH SELECTED INDICATIONS. Vaccines with selected indications for children include influenza, hepatitis A, meningococcal polysaccharide, rabies, and those given primarily for international travel.

PART 16

The Digestive System

SECTION 1

Clinical Manifestations of Gastrointestinal Disease

CHAPTER 174

Normal Digestive Tract Phenomena
(Nelson Textbook, Chapter 305)

Gastrointestinal function varies with maturity; a symptom that might be abnormal at an older age, such as regurgitation, may be normal in an infant. A number of normal anatomic variations may be noted in the mouth. A short lingual frenulum ("tongue tie") may be worrisome to parents but only rarely interferes with eating or speech, generally requiring no treatment.

Regurgitation, the result of gastroesophageal reflux, occurs commonly in the first 12–18 mo of life. Effortless emesis may dribble out of an infant's mouth but also may be forceful. In an otherwise healthy infant with regurgitation, volumes of emesis are commonly 15–30 mL but may occasionally be much larger. Most often, the infant remains happy, although possibly hungry, after an episode of regurgitation. Episodes may occur from fewer than one to several times per day.

The *number, color,* and *consistency of stools* may vary greatly in the same infant and between infants of similar age without apparent explanation. A *protuberant abdomen* is often noted in infants and toddlers, especially after large feedings.

Blood loss from the gastrointestinal tract is never normal, but swallowed blood may be misinterpreted as gastrointestinal bleeding. *Jaundice* is common in neonates, especially among premature infants. An elevated direct bilirubin level is never normal and suggests liver disease.

CHAPTER 175

Major Symptoms and Signs of Digestive Tract Disorders

(Nelson Textbook, Chapter 306)

Disorders of organs outside the gastrointestinal tract can produce symptoms and signs that mimic digestive tract disorders and should be considered in the differential diagnosis.

DISORDERED INGESTION. Disordered ingestion may result from refusal to feed or from swallowing difficulty. Dysphagia, or difficulty swallowing, occurs at the level of the mouth, oropharynx, or esophagus and results from a motor disorder (e.g., cerebral palsy or achalasia) or mechanical obstruction (e.g., foreign body, webs, vascular rings, peptic stricture of the esophagus).

VOMITING. Vomiting is a highly coordinated reflex process that may be preceded by increased salivation and begins with involuntary retching. Many acute or chronic processes can cause vomiting (Table 175–1).

DIARRHEA. Diarrhea is best defined as excessive loss of fluid and electrolyte in the stool. The basis for all diarrhea is disturbed intestinal solute transport. The pathogenesis of most episodes of diarrhea can be explained by secretory, osmotic, or motility abnormalities or a combination of these.

Secretory diarrhea is often caused by a secretagogue, such as cholera toxin, binding to a receptor on the surface epithelium of the bowel and thereby stimulating intracellular accumulation of cyclic adenosine monophosphate or cyclic guanosine monophosphate. Osmotic diarrhea occurs after ingestion of a poorly absorbed solute. Motility disorders may be associated with rapid or delayed transit and generally are not associated with a large volume of diarrhea. Slowed motility may be associated with a large volume of diarrhea.

CONSTIPATION. Any definition of constipation is relative, dependent on stool consistency, stool frequency, and difficulty in passing the stool. Constipation tends to be self-perpetuating, whatever its cause.

ABDOMINAL PAIN. Individual children differ greatly in their perception of and tolerance for abdominal pain. A child with functional abdominal pain (i.e., no identifiable organic cause) may be as uncomfortable as one with an organic cause. In the gut, the usual stimulus provoking pain is tension or stretching.

GASTROINTESTINAL HEMORRHAGE. Bleeding may occur anywhere along the gastrointestinal tract, and identification of the site may be challenging. When bleeding originates in the esophagus, stomach, or duodenum, it may cause *hematemesis*. When exposed to gastric or intestinal juices, blood quickly darkens to resemble coffee grounds; massive bleeding is likely to be red. Red or ma-

TABLE 175–1 Differential Diagnosis of Emesis During Childhood

Infant	Child	Adolescent
Common		
Gastroenteritis	Gastroenteritis	Gastroenteritis
Gastroesophageal reflux	Systemic infection	Systemic infection
Overfeeding	Toxic ingestion	Toxic ingestion
Anatomic obstruction	Pertussis syndrome	Inflammatory bowel
Systemic infection	Medication	disease
Pertussis syndrome	Reflux	Appendicitis
		Migraine
		Pregnancy
		Medication
		Ipecac abuse/bulimia
Rare		
Adrenogenital syndrome	Reye syndrome	Reye syndrome
Inborn error of metabolism	Hepatitis	Hepatitis
Brain tumor (increased	Peptic ulcer	Peptic ulcer
intracranial pressure)	Pancreatitis	Pancreatitis
Subdural hemorrhage	Brain tumor	Brain tumor
Food poisoning	Increased	Increased
Rumination	intracranial	intracranial
Renal tubular acidosis	pressure	pressure
	Middle ear disease	Middle ear disease
	Chemotherapy	Chemotherapy
	Achalasia	Cyclic vomiting
	Cyclic vomiting	(migraine)
	(migraine)	Biliary colic
	Esophageal stricture	Renal colic
	Duodenal hematoma	
	Inborn error of	
	metabolism	

roon blood in stools, *hematochezia,* signifies either a distal bleeding site or massive hemorrhage above the distal ileum. Moderate to mild bleeding from sites above the distal ileum tends to cause blackened stools of tarry consistency, *melena,* and major hemorrhages in the duodenum or above may also be causative.

ABDOMINAL DISTENTION AND ABDOMINAL MASSES. Enlargement of the abdomen can result from diminished tone of the wall musculature or from increased content—fluid, gas, or solid.

The Oral Cavity

(Nelson Textbook, Chapters 307–317)

CHAPTER 176

Malocclusion

(Nelson Textbook, Chapter 309)

When teeth meet simultaneously, the force is distributed over a large area of the bone-to-tooth attachment. In malocclusion, when only a few teeth touch, the same force is exerted over a smaller area and may contribute to tooth loss in adulthood. Establishing a proper relationship between the mandibular and maxillary teeth is important for physiologic and cosmetic reasons.

In class I (normal) occlusion, the cusps of the posterior mandibular teeth interdigitate ahead and inside the corresponding cusps of the opposing maxillary teeth. This relationship provides a normal facial profile. In class II occlusion, the cusps of the posterior mandibular teeth are behind and inside the corresponding cusps of the maxillary teeth. This is the most common occlusal discrepancy, with approximately 45% of the population exhibiting some degree of this condition. The facial profile often gives the appearance of a "receding chin," also called retrognathia. In class III occlusion, the cusps of the posterior mandibular teeth interdigitate a tooth or more ahead of their opposing maxillary counterparts. The facial profile gives the appearance of a "protruding chin" (prognathia).

CHAPTER 177

Cleft Lip and Palate

(Nelson Textbook, Chapter 310)

CLINICAL MANIFESTATIONS. Cleft lip may vary from a small notch in the vermilion border to a complete separation extending into the floor of the nose. Clefts may be unilateral (more often on the left side) or bilateral and may involve the alveolar ridge. Deformed, supernumerary, or absent teeth are associated findings. Isolated cleft palate occurs in the midline and may involve only the uvula or may extend into or through the soft and hard palates to the incisive foramen. When associated with cleft lip, the defect may involve the midline of the soft palate and extend into the hard palate on one or both sides, exposing one or both of the nasal cavities as a unilateral or bilateral cleft palate.

TREATMENT. The most immediate problem in an infant born with a cleft lip or palate is feeding. Most feel that with the use of soft artificial nipples with large openings, a squeezable bottle, and proper instruction, feeding of infants with clefts can be achieved with relative ease and effectiveness. Surgical closure of a cleft lip is usually performed by 3 mo of age. The initial repair may be revised at 4 or 5 yr of age. Corrective surgery on the nose may be delayed until adolescence. Because clefts of the palate vary considerably in size, shape, and degree of deformity, the timing of surgical correction should be individualized.

PREOPERATIVE AND POSTOPERATIVE MANAGEMENT. Even the suspicion of infection is a contraindication to operation. During the immediate postoperative period, special nursing care is essential. Gentle aspiration of the nasopharynx minimizes the chances of the common complications of atelectasis or pneumonia. The primary considerations in postoperative care are maintenance of a clean suture line and avoidance of tension on the sutures.

Chapter 178

Dental Caries

(Nelson Textbook, Chapter 312)

CLINICAL MANIFESTATIONS. Dental caries of the primary dentition usually begin in the pits and fissures. Small lesions may be difficult to diagnose by visual inspection, but larger lesions present as cavitations of the occlusal surface. The second most frequent sites of caries occur on contact surfaces between the teeth, which in many cases can only be detected by intraoral radiographs. Rampant caries in infants and toddlers, referred to as early childhood caries (ECC), nursing bottle caries, or baby bottle tooth decay, has in the past been ascribed solely to inappropriate bottle-feeding. Early childhood caries is common, with a prevalence of 30% to 50% in children from low socioeconomic backgrounds. Children who develop caries at a young age are known to be at high risk for developing further caries as they get older.

TREATMENT. Dental treatment can restore many teeth affected with dental caries, using silver amalgam or plastic restorations and crowns. Clinical management of the pain and infection associated with untreated dental caries varies with the extent of involvement and the medical status of the patient.

PREVENTION. The most effective preventive measure against dental caries is optimizing the fluoride content of communal water supplies to 1 part per million. In fluoride-deficient water supplies, similar caries prevention benefits are obtained from dietary fluoride supplements. Thorough daily brushing and flossing of the teeth may help prevent dental caries and periodontal disease.

SECTION 3

The Esophagus
(Nelson Textbook, Chapters 318–327)

CHAPTER 179

Atresia and Tracheoesophageal Fistula
(Nelson Textbook, Chapter 319)

CLINICAL MANIFESTATIONS. Atresia of the esophagus should be suspected (1) in cases of maternal polyhydramnios; (2) if a catheter used at birth for resuscitation cannot be inserted into the stomach; (3) if a newborn has excessive oral secretions; or (4) if choking, cyanosis, or coughing occurs with an attempt at feeding. Suctioning of excess secretions from the mouth and pharynx frequently results in improvement, but symptoms quickly recur. The diagnosis may not be made until after an infant has aspirated feedings.

DIAGNOSIS. Inability to pass a catheter into the stomach confirms the suspicion. The presence of air in the abdomen indicates a fistula between the trachea and the distal esophagus.

TREATMENT. Esophageal atresia is a surgical emergency. Preoperatively, patients should be kept prone to decrease any tendency of gastric contents to reach the lungs. The esophageal pouch should be kept empty by constant suction to prevent aspiration of secretions. Structural malformations of the trachea are common in patients with esophageal atresia and fistula.

CHAPTER 180

Gastroesophageal Reflux (Chalasia)
(Nelson Textbook, Chapter 323)

When the lower esophageal sphincter (LES) is not competent, passive reflux of gastric contents may cause symptoms. The term *chalasia* describes free reflux across a dilated sphincter. Although many infants have minor degrees of reflux, about 1 in 300 has significant reflux and associated complications.

CLINICAL MANIFESTATIONS. The signs and symptoms relate directly to the exposure of the esophageal epithelium to refluxed gastric contents. In 85% of affected infants, excessive vomiting occurs during the 1st wk of life; an additional 10% have symptoms by 6 wk. Symptoms abate without treatment in 60% by the age of 2 yr as the child assumes a more upright posture and eats solid foods; the remainder continue to have symptoms until at least 4 yr of age. Iron-deficiency anemia is common in patients with severe esophagitis. Substernal pain is less common, but dysphagia may cause irritability and anorexia in advanced cases.

TREATMENT. Infants with significant symptoms should be kept prone, an exception to the usually recommended supine position. In older infants and children, raising the head of the bed and keeping a child upright are indicated. Thickening an infant's formula with cereal decreases crying and the volume of vomitus. If symptoms do not improve with a prolonged trial of intensive medical therapy, surgery may be indicated. A shortened trial of medical therapy may be indicated in cases of recurrent aspiration or apnea.

SECTION 4

Stomach and Intestines
(Nelson Textbook, Chapters 328–346)

CHAPTER 181

Pyloric Stenosis and Other Congenital Anomalies of the Stomach
(Nelson Textbook, Chapter 329)

CLINICAL MANIFESTATIONS. Nonbilious vomiting is the initial symptom of pyloric stenosis. The vomiting may or may not be projectile initially but is usually progressive, occurring immediately after a feeding. Emesis may follow each feeding, or it may be intermittent. The vomiting usually starts after 3 wk of age, but symptoms may develop as early as the 1st wk of life and as late as the 5th mo. After vomiting, the infant is hungry and wants to feed again. As vomiting continues, a progressive loss of fluid, hydrogen ion, and chloride leads to a hypochloremic metabolic alkalosis.

The diagnosis has traditionally been established by palpating the pyloric mass. The mass is firm, movable, approximately 2 cm in length, olive shaped, hard, best palpated from the left side, and located above and to the right of the umbilicus in the mid epigastrium beneath the liver edge. Ultrasound examination confirms the diagnosis in the majority of cases.

TREATMENT. The preoperative treatment is directed toward correcting the fluid, acid-base, and electrolyte losses. Fluid therapy should be continued until the infant is rehydrated and the serum bicarbonate concentration is less than 30 mEq/dL, which implies that the alkalosis has been corrected. The surgical procedure of choice is the Ramstedt pyloromyotomy. The underlying pyloric mass is split without cutting the mucosa, and the incision is closed. In most infants, feedings can be initiated within 12–24 hr after surgery and advanced to maintenance oral feedings within 36–48 hr of the surgery.

CHAPTER 182

Intestinal Atresia, Stenosis, and Malrotation

(Nelson Textbook, Chapter 330)

GENERAL CONSIDERATIONS. Intestinal obstruction occurs in approximately 1 in 1500 live births. Obstruction may be partial or complete and may arise from intrinsic abnormalities of the gut. Simple obstruction is associated with the failure of progression of aboral flow of luminal contents. Strangulating obstruction is associated with impaired blood flow to the intestine in addition to obstruction of the flow of luminal contents. If strangulating obstruction is not promptly relieved, it may lead to bowel infarction and perforation. Obstruction is typically associated with an accumulation of ingested food, gas, and intestinal secretions proximal to the point of obstruction, leading to distention of the bowel. As the bowel dilates, intestinal absorption decreases and secretion of fluid and electrolytes increases. The shift in fluid and electrolytes results in isotonic intravascular depletion usually associated with hypokalemia.

When the obstruction is *complete*, there should be little difficulty in clinical recognition, but when it is incomplete, diagnosis may pose considerable difficulty. When obstruction is *incomplete* (e.g., as with intestinal stenosis, constricting bands, duplications, and incomplete volvulus), signs (vomiting, abdominal distention, obstipation) may appear shortly after birth or may be delayed an indeterminate time. Atresia refers to complete obstruction of the bowel lumen, and stenosis refers to a partial block of luminal contents. Intestinal atresia is common in the duodenum, jejunum, and ileum and rare in the colon.

Blood flow to the obstructed bowel decreases as the bowel dilates. Blood flow is shifted away from the mucosa, with loss of mucosal integrity. Bacteria proliferate in the stagnant bowel, with a predominance of coliforms and anaerobes. The rapid proliferation of bacteria coupled with the loss of mucosal integrity allows bacterial translocation across the bowel wall, resulting in endotoxemia, bacteremia, and sepsis.

The clinical presentation of intestinal obstruction varies with the cause, level of obstruction, and time between the obstructing event and the patient's evaluation. The classic symptoms of obstruction include nausea and vomiting, abdominal distention, and obstipation. Obstruction high in the intestinal tract involving the duodenum or proximal jejunum results in large-volume, frequent, bilious emesis. Pain is intermittent and is usually relieved by vomiting. The pain is localized to the epigastrium or periumbilical area, and there is little abdominal distention. Obstruction in the distal small bowel leads to moderate or marked abdominal distention with emesis that is progressively feculent. Pain is usually diffuse over the entire abdomen.

No laboratory studies are diagnostic of obstruction or differentiate simple obstruction from obstruction associated with bowel infarction. Bowel obstruction is almost always suggested on the basis of history and physical examination. Imaging is used to confirm the diagnosis and localize the area of obstruction. Plain supine and erect or decubitus radiographs are the initial studies.

MANAGEMENT. Initial treatment must be directed at fluid resuscitation and stabilizing the patient. Nasogastric decompression usually provides relief from pain and vomiting. After appropriate cultures, broad-spectrum antibiotics are usually started in neonates with bowel obstruction and those with suspected strangulating infarction. Patients with strangulation must have immediate surgical relief before the bowel infarcts, resulting in gangrene and intestinal perforation. Nonoperative conservative management is usually limited to children with suspected adhesions or inflammatory strictures that may resolve with nasogastric decompression or anti-inflammatory medications. If clinical signs of improvement are not evident within 12–24 hr, then operative intervention is usually indicated.

DUODENAL OBSTRUCTION

CLINICAL MANIFESTATIONS. The hallmark of duodenal obstruction is bilious vomiting without abdominal distention, which is usually noted on the 1st day of life. Peristaltic waves may be visualized early in the disease process. A history of polyhydramnios is present in half the pregnancies. Jaundice is present in one third of the infants. The diagnosis is suggested by the presence of a "double-bubble sign" on plain abdominal radiographs.

TREATMENT. The usual surgical repair for duodenal atresia is duodenoduodenostomy. A gastrostomy tube may be placed to drain the stomach and protect the airway.

JEJUNAL AND ILEAL ATRESIA AND OBSTRUCTION

Jejunoileal atresias have been attributed to intrauterine vascular obstructive accidents of the bowel.

CLINICAL MANIFESTATIONS. In contrast to duodenal atresia, extragastrointestinal anomalies are less common in atresia of the remaining intestine. Most infants become symptomatic during the 1st day of life with abdominal distention and bile-stained emesis or gastric aspirate. Sixty to 75 percent of the infants fail to pass meconium. Jaundice has been found in one fifth to one third of the patients. Plain radiographs demonstrate many air-fluid levels or peritoneal calcification associated with meconium peritonitis. It is impossible to consistently distinguish small bowel from large bowel by studying plain radiographs of the abdomen in newborns and infants.

TREATMENT. Ileal or jejunal atresia requires resection of the dilated proximal portion of the bowel followed by end-to-end anastomosis. If a simple mucosal diaphragm is present, jejunoplasty or ileoplasty with partial excision of the web is an acceptable alternative to resection. With meconium ileus, an attempt to reduce obstruction with a Gastrografin enema containing polysorbate and a detergent (Tween 80) is usually indicated.

MALROTATION

Malrotation is incomplete rotation of the intestine during fetal development.

CLINICAL MANIFESTATIONS. The majority of patients present within the 1st yr of life with symptoms of acute or chronic obstruction. Infants often present within the 1st wk of life with bilious emesis and acute bowel obstruction. Older infants present with episodes of recurrent abdominal pain that may mimic colic. An acute presentation of small bowel obstruction is usually a result of volvulus associated with malrotation. This is a life-threatening complication of malrotation and the main reason symptoms suggestive of malrotation must always be investigated. Surgical intervention is recommended for any patient with a significant rotational abnormality, regardless of age.

CHAPTER 183

Motility Disorders and Hirschsprung Disease
(Nelson Textbook, Chapter 332)

Chronic intestinal pseudo-obstruction comprises a group of disorders characterized by signs and symptoms of intestinal obstruction in the absence of an anatomic lesion.

SUPERIOR MESENTERIC ARTERY SYNDROME. The classic example is an adolescent who starts vomiting after application of a body cast for orthopedic surgery.

CONGENITAL AGANGLIONIC MEGACOLON (HIRSCHSPRUNG DISEASE)

This is caused by abnormal innervation of the bowel, beginning in the internal anal sphincter and extending proximally to involve a variable length of gut.

CLINICAL MANIFESTATIONS. The clinical symptoms of Hirschsprung disease usually begin at birth with the delayed passage of meconium. Ninety-nine percent of full-term infants pass meconium within 48 hr of birth. Hirschsprung disease should be suspected in any full-term infant (the disease is unusual in preterm infants) with delayed passage of stool. Some infants pass meconium normally but subsequently present with a history of chronic constipation. Hirschsprung disease in older patients must be distinguished from other causes of abdominal distention and chronic constipation.

DIAGNOSIS. Rectal manometry and rectal suction biopsy are the easiest and most reliable indicators of Hirschsprung disease.

TREATMENT. Once the diagnosis is established, the definitive treatment is operative intervention.

CHAPTER 184

Ileus, Adhesions, Intussusception, and Closed-Loop Obstructions

(Nelson Textbook, Chapter 333)

ILEUS. Ileus is the failure of intestinal peristalsis without evidence of mechanical obstruction. Lack of normal gut motility interferes with aboral movement of intestinal contents and in children is most often associated with abdominal surgery or infection (pneumonia, gastroenteritis, peritonitis). Ileus presents as increasing abdominal distention and initially minimal pain. Pain increases with increasing distention. Bowel sounds are minimal or absent, in contrast to early mechanical obstruction, when they are hyperactive. Treatment of ileus involves correction of the underlying abnormality.

ADHESIONS. Adhesions are fibrous bands of tissue that are a common cause of postoperative small bowel obstruction after abdominal surgery.

INTUSSUSCEPTION

Intussusception occurs when a portion of the alimentary tract is telescoped into a segment just caudad to it.

CLINICAL MANIFESTATIONS. In typical cases there is sudden onset, in a previously well child, of severe paroxysmal colicky pain that recurs at frequent intervals and is accompanied by straining efforts with legs and knees flexed and loud cries. The infant may initially be comfortable and play normally between the paroxysms of pain, but if the intussusception is not reduced, the infant becomes progressively weaker and more lethargic. Palpation of the abdomen usually reveals a slightly tender sausage-shaped mass, sometimes ill defined, which may increase in size and firmness during a paroxysm of pain and is most often in the right upper abdomen, with its long axis cephalocaudal.

TREATMENT. Reduction of an acute intussusception is an emergency procedure and performed immediately after diagnosis in preparation for possible surgery.

CHAPTER 185

Anorectal Malformations

(Nelson Textbook, Chapter 335)

Anorectal malformations refers to a spectrum of defects. Some are complex, difficult to manage, and associated with important anatomic deficiencies and therefore have poor functional prognosis.

DIAGNOSIS AND EARLY MANAGEMENT. The most important decision regarding a newborn with an anorectal malformation is whether the patient needs a diverting-decompression colostomy and emergency urinary diversion for an associated obstructive uropathy. About 50% of children with anorectal anomalies have a urologic problem.

TREATMENT. Perineal fistulas are treated by a simple anoplasty without a protective colostomy; the operation is performed during the newborn period. All other defects are best managed during the newborn period with a protective colostomy. Later in life (1–12 mo), corrective surgical repair is performed.

CHAPTER 186

Ulcer Disease

(Nelson Textbook, Chapter 336)

Ulcers and gastritis are classified as primary (peptic) or secondary, caused by factors known to affect the integrity of the gastric or duodenal mucosa. Ulcers and gastritis are closely related. Primary peptic ulcers are usually chronic, duodenal, and related to *Helicobacter pylori* gastritis, whereas secondary ulcers are usually acute and gastric. Infection with *H. pylori* usually leads to clinically silent gastritis. The eradication of *H. pylori* is strongly recommended if patients have peptic ulcer disease, active or inactive, bleeding or not, on the basis of unequivocal evidence. Effective treatment prevents recurrence of ulcer disease.

PRIMARY (PEPTIC) ULCERS

CLINICAL MANIFESTATIONS. The manifestations of peptic ulcer disease include pain, vomiting, acute and chronic gastrointestinal blood loss, and a strong familial incidence. In the 1st mo of life, the two main manifestations are gastrointestinal hemorrhage and perforation.

TREATMENT. The goal is to hasten healing of the ulcer, to relieve pain, and to prevent complications. If present, hemorrhagic shock and anemia must be treated as a first priority. Although antacids, sucralfate, and misoprostol are capable of healing an ulcer, primary ulcers have a high likelihood of recurring unless the associated *H. pylori* gastritis is effectively treated.

SECONDARY OR STRESS (PEPTIC) ULCER DISEASE

CLINICAL MANIFESTATIONS. In infants, stress ulcers are usually due to sepsis, respiratory or cardiac insufficiency, trauma, or dehydration. In older children, they are related to trauma or other life-threatening conditions. Most stress ulcers are asymptomatic, are often multiple, and may be terminal events. They can be associated with severe hemorrhage or perforation.

TREATMENT. Treatment of secondary ulcers is similar to that of primary ulcers. The inciting cause should be removed if possible. Bleeding and less often perforation are common presentations and must be addressed immediately.

CHAPTER 187

Inflammatory Bowel Disease
(Nelson Textbook, Chapter 337)

Inflammatory bowel disease (IBD), a group of idiopathic, chronic disorders, includes Crohn disease and ulcerative colitis. The most common time of onset of IBD is during adolescence and young adulthood. Nonetheless, IBD may begin in the 1st yr of life.

CHRONIC ULCERATIVE COLITIS

CLINICAL MANIFESTATIONS. Symptoms of mild dysentery (bloody diarrhea with mucus) are the typical presentations of ulcerative colitis. Symptoms such as tenesmus, urgency, crampy abdominal pain (especially with bowel movements), and nocturnal bowel movements suggest a more severe colitis. The onset may be insidious with gradual progression of symptoms, but can be fulminant. Chronicity is an important part of the diagnosis. Extraintestinal manifestations that tend to occur more commonly with ulcerative colitis than with Crohn disease include pyoderma gangrenosum, sclerosing cholangitis, chronic active hepatitis, and ankylosing spondylitis. Any of the extraintestinal disorders described for IBD may occur with ulcerative colitis. The clinical course of ulcerative colitis is marked by exacerbations, often without apparent explanation. Typically, the disease may be quieted with medication but eventually recurs.

TREATMENT. A medical cure for ulcerative colitis is not available; treatment is aimed at controlling symptoms and reducing the risk of recurrence. The first drug to be used with mild colitis is an aminosalicylate. Sulfasalazine has been used extensively over many years, and its effects are well characterized. Children with moderate to severe pancolitis or colitis that is responsive to 5-aminosalicylate therapy should be treated with oral corticosteroids, most commonly prednisone. Surgical treatment for intractable or fulminant colitis is total colectomy.

CROHN DISEASE (REGIONAL ENTERITIS, REGIONAL ILEITIS, GRANULOMATOUS COLITIS)

Crohn disease, an idiopathic, chronic inflammatory disorder of the bowel, involves any region of the alimentary tract from the mouth to the anus. The inflammatory process tends to be eccentric and segmental, often with skip areas (normal regions of bowel between inflamed areas). Although inflammation in ulcerative colitis is limited to the mucosa (except in toxic megacolon), gastrointestinal involvement in Crohn disease is transmural.

CLINICAL MANIFESTATIONS. Crohn disease presents in many forms; the manifestations tend to be dictated by the region of bowel involved, the degree of inflammation, and the presence of complications such as stricture or fistula. Children with ileocolitis typically have crampy abdominal pain and diarrhea, sometimes with blood. Ileitis may present as right lower quadrant abdominal pain alone. Crohn colitis may be associated with bloody diarrhea, tenesmus, and urgency. Systemic signs and symptoms are more common in Crohn disease than in ulcerative colitis. Fever, malaise, and easy fatigability are common. Extraintestinal manifestations occur more commonly with Crohn disease than with ulcerative colitis; those that are especially associated with Crohn disease include oral aphthous ulcers, peripheral arthritis, erythema nodosum, digital clubbing, episcleritis, renal stones (uric acid, oxalate), and gallstones.

DIAGNOSIS. The diagnosis of Crohn disease is dependent on finding typical clinical features of the disorder (history, physical examination, laboratory studies, and endoscopic or radiologic findings) and ruling out specific entities that mimic chronicity.

TREATMENT. The aim of treatment is largely to alleviate symptoms; treatment is dictated by the symptoms present. If disease is largely limited to small bowel, oral prednisone, 1–2 mg/kg/24 hr, is often the first treatment (maximum dose of 60 mg). Aminosalicylates have been used in the treatment of colon disease and are sometimes more effective than corticosteroids in this region. Nutritional therapy is an effective primary treatment. Total parenteral nutrition is effective not only in nutritional repletion but also in quieting active disease. Surgical therapy should be reserved for very specific indications.

PROGNOSIS. Crohn disease is a chronic disorder that is associated with a high morbidity but low mortality.

CHAPTER 188

Malabsorptive Disorders
(Nelson Textbook, Chapter 340)

Malabsorptive disorders (syndromes) are conditions that cause insufficient assimilation of ingested nutrients as a result of either maldigestion or malabsorption (Table 188–1). Previously known as celiac syndromes, this term is best avoided because of potential confusion with the specific entity celiac disease (gluten-sensitive enteropathy). Disorders that cause generalized defects in assimilation of nutrients tend to present with similar signs and symptoms: abdominal distention; pale, foul-smelling, bulky stools; muscle wasting; poor weight gain or weight loss; and growth retardation. Stools may appear greasy and may be associated with an oil slick in the toilet; with mild steatorrhea, the stools may appear normal.

Congenital disorders affecting individual intestinal digestive enzymes or transport processes have also been identified. The clinical features of these disorders typically differ from those of the generalized malabsorption syndromes; some present without gastrointestinal symptoms. The disaccharidase deficiencies are the most common of these entities.

TABLE 188–1   Generalized Malabsorptive States in Childhood

Site	More Common	Less Common
Exocrine pancreas	Cystic fibrosis	Shwachman-Diamond syndrome
	Chronic protein-calorie malnutrition	Chronic pancreatitis
Liver, biliary tree	Biliary atresia	Other cholestatic states (including Alagille syndrome, familial neonatal hepatitis)
Intestine		
Anatomic defects	Massive resection	Congenitally short gut
	Stagnant loop syndrome	
Chronic infection	Giardiasis	Immune deficiency
Others	Celiac disease	Tropical sprue
	Dietary protein intolerance (milk, soy)	Idiopathic diffuse mucosal lesions

CHAPTER 189

Acute Appendicitis

(Nelson Textbook, Chapter 343)

Acute appendicitis is the most common condition requiring emergency abdominal operation in childhood.

CLINICAL MANIFESTATIONS. The clinical signs and symptoms depend on the pathologic phase of appendicitis at examination. The classic triad consists of pain, vomiting, and fever. In the initial stage of appendiceal obstruction, the pain is periumbilical. Emesis usually follows the onset of pain and is infrequent. Anorexia is more common. Fever is low grade unless perforation with peritonitis has occurred. As the inflammation progresses to involve the serosa and overlying peritoneum, the pain migrates to the area of peritoneal irritation, usually the right lower quadrant. If the appendix is retrocecal, the pain will be lateral or posterior. With perforation, the pain becomes generalized unless the contamination is well localized to produce a discrete abscess, usually of the right lower quadrant.

The child with appendicitis frequently moves tentatively and slowly, hunched forward, and often with a slight limp. The child may protect the right lower quadrant with a hand and may be reluctant to climb onto the examining table. Early in appendicitis, the abdomen is flat. Abdominal distention indicates a complication such as perforation or obstruction. Auscultation may reveal normal or hyperactive bowel sounds in early appendicitis to be replaced with hypoactive bowel sounds as it progresses to perforation. The most important physical finding in appendicitis is persistent, direct tenderness to palpation and rigidity of the overlying rectus muscle.

Laboratory Findings. The primary role of laboratory studies is to exclude alternative diagnoses such as urinary tract infection, hemolytic-uremic syndrome, Henoch-Schönlein purpura, and so on.

Imaging Studies. The imaging studies that may be helpful in evaluating children with suspected appendicitis include plain radiographs of the abdomen or chest, ultrasonography, computed tomography, and, rarely, barium enema.

TREATMENT. Children with nonperforated appendicitis require minimal preoperative preparation with intravenous fluids and antibiotics. If the appendix has perforated, especially with generalized peritonitis, significant fluid resuscitation and broad-spectrum antibiotics may be required a few hours before appendectomy.

CHAPTER 190

Inguinal Hernias
(Nelson Textbook, Chapter 346)

An inguinal hernia is the most common condition requiring operation in the pediatric age group.

CLINICAL MANIFESTATIONS. An inguinal hernia usually appears as a bulge in the inguinal region and extends toward or into the scrotum. Occasionally, an infant presents with a swelling of the scrotum without a prior bulge in the inguinal region. Physical examination reveals an inguinal bulge at the level of the internal or external ring or a scrotal swelling that is reducible or fluctuates in size.

TREATMENT. The treatment of choice is operative repair; an inguinal hernia does not resolve spontaneously. The operation should be carried out electively shortly after diagnosis because of the high risk of later incarceration, especially during the 1st yr of life.

PREMATURE INFANT. The premature infant has a higher incidence of inguinal hernia and incarceration. Because the incidence of incarceration approaches 30% in this patient population, elective hernia repair should be considered before discharge from the neonatal intensive care nursery.

SECTION 5

Exocrine Pancreas
(Nelson Textbook, Chapters 347–353)

CHAPTER 191

Pancreatitis
(Nelson Textbook, Chapter 351)

After cystic fibrosis, acute pancreatitis is probably the most common pancreatic disorder in children. Blunt abdominal injuries, mumps and other viral illnesses, multisystem disease, congenital anomalies, and biliary microlithiasis (sludging) account for most known causes.

CLINICAL MANIFESTATIONS. The patient with acute pancreatitis has abdominal pain, persistent vomiting, and fever. The pain is epigastric and steady, often resulting in the child's assuming an antalgic position with hips and knees flexed, sitting upright, or lying on the side. The child is very uncomfortable and irritable and appears acutely ill. The abdomen may be distended and tender. A mass may be palpable.

DIAGNOSIS. Acute pancreatitis is usually diagnosed by measurement of serum amylase and lipase activities. The serum amylase level is typically elevated for up to 4 days. A variety of other conditions may also cause hyperamylasemia without pancreatitis. Ultrasonography and computed tomography have major roles in the diagnosis and follow-up of children with pancreatitis.

TREATMENT. Meperidine is the drug of choice for pain relief and should be given in adequate doses. Fluid, electrolyte, and mineral balance should be restored and maintained. The patient should be maintained with nothing by mouth. The response to treatment is usually complete over 2–4 days. Refeeding may commence when the serum amylase value has normalized and clinical symptoms have resolved.

SECTION 6

The Liver and Biliary System
(Nelson Textbook, Chapters 354–368)

CHAPTER 192

Cholestasis
(Nelson Textbook, Chapter 356)

NEONATAL CHOLESTASIS

Neonatal cholestasis is defined as prolonged elevation of serum levels of conjugated bilirubin beyond the first 14 days of life. Cholestasis in a newborn may be due to infectious, genetic, metabolic, or undefined abnormalities giving rise either to mechanical obstruction of bile flow or to functional impairment of hepatic excretory function and bile secretion.

EVALUATION. The clinical features of infants with neonatal cholestasis provide very few clues about etiology. Affected infants have icterus, dark urine, light or acholic stools, and hepatomegaly, all reflecting decreased bile flow resulting from either liver cell injury or bile duct obstruction. Hepatic synthetic dysfunction may lead to hypoprothrombinemia and a bleeding disorder; administration of vitamin K should be considered in the initial treatment of cholestatic infants to prevent hemorrhage.

Most infants with neonatal cholestasis come to medical attention in the 1st mo of life. Prompt differentiation of conjugated from unconjugated hyperbilirubinemia is imperative because the findings of cholestasis are more ominous. The initial step in identification of cholestasis is finding a significantly elevated level of total bilirubin, more than 20% of which is conjugated bilirubin. The next step is prompt recognition of any specific or treatable primary causes of cholestasis, such as *sepsis*, an *endocrinopathy* (hypothyroidism or panhypopituitarism), *nutritional hepatotoxicity* caused by a specific metabolic illness (galactosemia), or other *metabolic diseases* (tyrosinemia). The final step is to differentiate extrahepatic biliary atresia from neonatal hepatitis.

NEONATAL HEPATITIS SYNDROME (INTRAHEPATIC CHOLESTASIS). The term *neonatal hepatitis* implies intrahepatic cholestasis, which has various forms:

1. *Idiopathic neonatal hepatitis.* These patients presumably are afflicted with a specific yet undefined metabolic or viral disease.

2. *Infectious hepatitis in a neonate.* This may be shown to be due to a specific virus, such as herpes simplex, enteroviruses, cytomegalovirus, or, rarely, hepatitis B.

3. *Intrahepatic bile duct paucity.* Some syndromes characterized morphologically by intrahepatic cholestasis may be clinically manifested either as neonatal hepatitis or as cholestasis in an older child. As patients mature, clinical and histologic features may suggest a specific syndrome. *Alagille syndrome* (arteriohepatic dysplasia) is the most common syndrome incorporating intrahepatic bile duct paucity.

BILIARY ATRESIA

A more appropriate terminology would reflect the pathophysiology, namely, *progressive obliterative cholangiopathy.*

DIFFERENTIATION OF IDIOPATHIC NEONATAL HEPATITIS FROM BILIARY ATRESIA. No single biochemical test or imaging procedure is entirely satisfactory. Idiopathic neonatal hepatitis has a familial incidence of approximately 20%, whereas extrahepatic biliary atresia is unlikely to recur within the same family. Some infants with biliary atresia have an increased incidence of other abnormalities. Neonatal hepatitis appears to be more common in premature or small-for-gestational-age infants. Persistently acholic stools suggest biliary obstruction (biliary atresia), but patients with severe idiopathic neonatal hepatitis may have a transient, severe impairment of bile excretion. On the other hand, consistently pigmented stools rule against biliary atresia. The finding of bile-stained fluid on duodenal intubation also excludes biliary atresia. Palpation of the liver may find an abnormal size or consistency in patients with extrahepatic biliary atresia; this is less common with neonatal hepatitis. Ultrasonography may detect a choledochal cyst or another unsuspected cause of cholestasis associated with dilatation of the biliary tract. Hepatobiliary scintigraphy using imidodiacetic acid analogs has been used by some clinicians to differentiate biliary atresia from neonatal hepatitis. Liver biopsy provides the most reliable discriminatory evidence.

MANAGEMENT OF PATIENTS WITH SUSPECTED BILIARY ATRESIA. In infants in whom clinical features and liver biopsy suggest biliary obstruction, exploratory laparotomy and direct cholangiography should be performed to determine the presence and site of obstruction. For patients with correctable lesions, direct drainage can be accomplished. For patients in whom no correctable lesion is found, the hepatoportoenterostomy procedure of Kasai can be carried out. If flow is not rapidly established within the first months of life, progressive obliteration and cirrhosis ensue.

MANAGEMENT OF CHRONIC CHOLESTASIS

Treatment of chronic cholestasis is empirical, and the best guide is careful monitoring. At present, no therapy is known to be effective in halting the progression of cholestasis or in preventing further hepatocellular damage and cirrhosis. A major concern is growth failure, which is related in part to malabsorption and malnutrition resulting from ineffective digestion and absorption of dietary fat.

CHAPTER **193**

Metabolic Diseases of the Liver
(Nelson Textbook, Chapter 357)

Because the liver has a central role in synthetic, degradative, and regulatory pathways involving carbohydrate, protein, lipid, trace element, and vitamin metabolism, many metabolic abnormalities or specific enzyme deficiencies affect the liver primarily or secondarily (Table 193–1).

TABLE 193–1 Inborn Errors of Metabolism Manifested as Hepatobiliary Dysfunction

Disorders of Carbohydrate Metabolism

Disorders of galactose metabolism
  Galactosemia
Disorders of fructose metabolism
  Hereditary fructose intolerance (aldolase deficiency)
  Fructose-1,6 diphosphatase deficiency

TABLE 193–1   Inborn Errors of Metabolism Manifested as Hepatobiliary Dysfunction *Continued*

Glycogen storage diseases
    Type I
        Von Gierke (1a)
        Type 1b
    Type III (Cori/Forbes)
    Type IV (Andersen)
    Type VI (Hers)

Disorders of Amino Acid and Protein Metabolism

Disorders of tyrosine metabolism
    Transient
        Neonatal
        Associated with severe liver disease (e.g., cirrhosis)
    Nontransient
        Hereditary tyrosinemia (type I)
        Tyrosinemia, type II
Inherited urea cycle enzyme defects
    CPS deficiency
    OTC deficiency (X-linked dominant)
    Citrullinemia
    Argininosuccinic aciduria
    Argininemia
    N-AGS deficiency

Disorders of Lipid Metabolism

Wolman disease
Cholesteryl ester storage disease
Gaucher disease
Niemann-Pick type C

Disorders of Bile Acid Metabolism

Isomerase deficiency
Reductase deficiency
Zellweger syndrome (cerebrohepatorenal)

Disorders of Metal Metabolism

Wilson disease
Hepatic copper overload
Indian childhood cirrhosis
Neonatal iron storage disease (perinatal hemochromatosis)

Disorders of Bilirubin Metabolism

Crigler-Najjar
    Type I
    Type II—Arias
    Gilbert disease
    Dubin-Johnson
    Rotor

Miscellaneous

α_1-Antitrypsin deficiency
Cystic fibrosis
Erythropoietic protoporphyria

CPS = Carbamoyl phosphate synthetase; OTC = ornithine transcarbamoylase; N-AGS = N-acetylglutamate synthetase.

CHAPTER 194

Autoimmune (Chronic) Hepatitis

(Nelson Textbook, Chapter 361)

Autoimmune hepatitis is a continuing hepatic inflammatory process manifested by elevated serum aminotransaminase concentrations and liver-associated serum autoantibodies. Chronic hepatitis can also be caused by persistent viral infection, metabolic diseases, or unknown factors.

CLINICAL MANIFESTATIONS. The clinical features and course of autoimmune hepatitis are extremely variable. Signs and symptoms at the time of presentation include a wide spectrum of disease including a substantial number of asymptomatic patients and some who have an acute, even fulminant, onset. In 25–30% of patients with autoimmune hepatitis, the illness may mimic acute viral hepatitis. In most, the onset is insidious. Patients may be asymptomatic or have fatigue, malaise, behavioral changes, anorexia, and amenorrhea, sometimes for many months before jaundice or stigmata of chronic liver disease are recognized. There is usually mild to moderate jaundice. Spider telangiectasia and palmar erythema may be present. The liver is often tender and slightly enlarged but may not be felt in patients with cirrhosis. The spleen is commonly enlarged. Extrahepatic manifestations may include arthritis, vasculitis, nephritis, thyroiditis, Coombs-positive anemia, and rash. Some patients' initial clinical features may reflect cirrhosis (ascites, bleeding esophageal varices, or hepatic encephalopathy).

LABORATORY FINDINGS. There is a moderate elevation (usually less than 1000 IU/L) of serum aminotransferase activities. Serum bilirubin concentrations (predominantly the direct reacting fraction) are commonly 2–10 mg/dL. Hypoalbuminemia is common. The prothrombin time is prolonged. A normochromic normocytic anemia, leukopenia, and thrombocytopenia are present and become more severe with the development of portal hypertension and hypersplenism. Most patients with autoimmune hepatitis have hypergammaglobulinemia.

TREATMENT. Corticosteroid therapy, with or without low doses of azathioprine, improves the clinical, biochemical, and histologic features in most patients with autoimmune hepatitis and prolongs survival in most patients with severe disease.

CHAPTER 195

Drug- and Toxin-Induced Liver Injury

(Nelson Textbook, Chapter 362)

Clinical manifestations may be mild and nonspecific, such as fever and malaise. Fever, rash, and arthralgia may be prominent in cases of hypersensitivity. In ill, hospitalized patients, the signs and symptoms of hepatic drug toxicity may be difficult to separate from the underlying illness.

The laboratory features of drug- or toxin-related liver disease are extremely variable. Hepatocyte damage may lead to elevations of serum aminotransferase activities and serum bilirubin levels and to impaired synthetic function, as evidenced by decreased serum coagulation factors and albumin. Hyperammonemia may occur with liver failure or with selective inhibition of the urea cycle (sodium valproate). Toxicologic screening of blood and urine specimens may aid in the detection of drug or toxin exposure.

Treatment of drug- or toxin-related liver injury is mainly supportive. Contact with the offending agent should be avoided. Corticosteroids may have a role in immune-mediated disease. N-acetylcysteine therapy, by stimulating glutathione synthesis, is effective in preventing hepatotoxicity when administered within 16 hr after an acute overdose of acetaminophen and appears to improve survival in patients with severe liver injury even up to 36 hr after ingestion. Orthotopic liver transplantation may be required for treatment of drug- or toxin-induced hepatic failure.

CHAPTER 196

Fulminant Hepatic Failure

(Nelson Textbook, Chapter 363)

Fulminant hepatic failure is a clinical syndrome resulting from massive necrosis of hepatocytes or from severe functional impairment of hepatocytes in a patient who does not have a pre-existing liver disease. The disorder usually evolves over a period of less than 8 wk.

CLINICAL MANIFESTATIONS. Fulminant hepatic failure may complicate previously known acute liver disease or be the presenting feature of liver disease. A child with fulminant hepatic failure has usually been previously healthy and most often has no risk factors for liver disease such as hepatitis or blood product exposure. Progressive jaundice, fetor hepaticus, fever, anorexia, vomiting, and abdominal pain are common. A rapid decrease in liver size without clinical improvement is an ominous sign. A hemorrhagic diathesis and ascites may develop. Patients should be closely observed for hepatic encephalopathy, which is initially character-ized by minor disturbances of consciousness or motor function. Irritability, poor feeding, and a change in sleep rhythm may be the only findings in infants; asterixis may be demonstrable in older children. Patients are often somnolent or confused or com-bative on arousal and eventually may become responsive only to painful stimuli.

LABORATORY FINDINGS. Serum direct and indirect bilirubin levels and serum aminotransferase activities may be markedly elevated. The blood ammonia concentration is usually increased. Prothrom-bin time is always prolonged and often does not improve after parenteral administration of vitamin K.

TREATMENT. Management of fulminant hepatic failure is suppor-tive. No therapy is known to reverse hepatocyte injury or to promote hepatic regeneration. An infant or child with advanced hepatic coma should be treated in an intensive care unit, where continuous monitoring of vital functions is possible. Controlled trials have shown a worsened outcome of fulminant hepatic fail-ure in patients treated with corticosteroids.

CHAPTER 197

Portal Hypertension and Varices

(Nelson Textbook, Chapter 366)

Portal hypertension—defined as an elevation of portal pressure above 10–12 mm Hg—is a major cause of morbidity and mortality in children with liver disease. The clinical features of the various forms of portal hypertension may be similar, but the associated complications, management, and prognosis can vary significantly and depend on whether the process is complicated by hepatic insufficiency.

CLINICAL MANIFESTATIONS. Bleeding from esophageal varices is the most common presentation. In patients with underlying hepatic disease, physical examination may show jaundice and stigmas of cirrhosis such as palmar erythema and vascular telangiectasia. Ascites may be present in patients with intrahepatic causes of portal hypertension but is uncommon with portal vein obstruc-tion. Dilated cutaneous collateral vessels carrying blood from the portal to systemic circulation may be apparent in the periumbilical region. In the absence of clinical or biochemical features of liver disease and a liver of normal size, portal vein obstruction is most likely. The bleeding may become apparent with hematemesis or with melena. Splenomegaly, sometimes with hypersplenism, is the next most common presenting feature in portal vein obstruc-tion and may be discovered first on routine physical examination.

Children with portal hypertension, regardless of the underlying cause, may have recurrent bouts of life-threatening hemorrhage.

TREATMENT. Treatment of patients with variceal hemorrhage must focus on fluid resuscitation initially in the form of crystalloid infusion followed by the replacement of red blood cells. Correction of coagulopathy by administration of vitamin K, the infusion of platelets or fresh frozen plasma, or both therapies may be required. An H_2 receptor blocker such as ranitidine should be given intravenously to reduce the risk of bleeding from gastric erosions. Pharmacologic therapy to decrease portal pressure may be considered in patients with continued bleeding. Vasopressin or one of its analogs has been commonly used.

After an episode of variceal hemorrhage or in patients in whom bleeding cannot be controlled, endoscopic sclerosis of esophageal varices is an important option. In patients who continue to bleed despite pharmacologic and endoscopic methods to control hemorrhage, a Sengstaken-Blakemore tube may be placed to stop hemorrhage by mechanically compressing esophageal and gastric varices. Various surgical procedures have been devised to divert portal blood flow and to decrease portal pressure. A portacaval shunt diverts nearly all of the portal blood flow into the subhepatic inferior right vena cava.

SECTION 7

Peritoneum

(Nelson Textbook, Chapters 368–372)

CHAPTER 198

Peritonitis

(Nelson Textbook, Chapter 370)

Inflammation of the peritoneal lining of the abdominal cavity may result from infectious, autoimmune, and chemical processes. Infectious peritonitis is usually defined as primary (spontaneous) or secondary. In primary peritonitis, the source of infection originates outside the abdomen and seeds the peritoneal cavity via hematogenous or lymphatic spread. Secondary peritonitis arises from the abdominal cavity itself through either extension from or rupture of an intra-abdominal viscus or an abscess within an organ.

ACUTE PRIMARY PERITONITIS

CLINICAL MANIFESTATIONS. Onset may be insidious or rapid and is characterized by fever, abdominal pain, vomiting, diarrhea, and a "toxic appearance." Hypotension and tachycardia are common, along with shallow, rapid respirations because of discomfort associated with breathing. Abdominal palpation may demonstrate rebound tenderness and rigidity. Bowel sounds are hypoactive or absent.

DIAGNOSIS AND TREATMENT. In a child with known renal or hepatic disease and ascites, the presence of peritoneal signs should prompt a diagnostic paracentesis. Infected fluid usually reveals a white blood cell count of 250 cells/mm or greater, with more than 50% polymorphonuclear cells. Gram stain of the ascitic fluid characteristically reveals a single species of gram-positive or, less often, gram-negative bacteria. The presence of mixed bacterial flora on ascitic fluid examination or free air on abdominal radiograph in children with presumed primary peritonitis mandates laparotomy to localize an intestinal perforation as a likely intraabdominal source of the infection. Parenteral antibiotic therapy with cefotaxime and an aminoglycoside should be started promptly, with subsequent changes depending on sensitivity testing.

ACUTE SECONDARY PERITONITIS

This is most often due to the entry of enteric bacteria into the peritoneal cavity through a necrotic defect in the wall of the intestines or other viscus as a result of obstruction or infarction or after rupture of an intra-abdominal visceral abscess.

CLINICAL MANIFESTATIONS. Similar to primary peritonitis, characteristic symptoms include fever (39.5°C or more), diffuse abdominal pain, nausea, and vomiting. Physical findings of peritoneal inflammation include rebound tenderness, abdominal wall rigidity, a paucity of body motion (lying still), and decreased or absent bowel sounds from a paralytic ileus. A "toxic appearance," irritability, and restlessness are common.

TREATMENT. Aggressive fluid resuscitation and support of cardiovascular function should begin immediately. Stabilization of the patient before surgical intervention is mandatory. Antibiotic therapy must provide coverage for those organisms that predominate at the site or presumed origin of the infection. Surgery to repair a perforated viscus should proceed after the patient is stabilized and the antibiotic therapy is initiated.

CHAPTER 199

Diaphragmatic Hernia

(Nelson Textbook, Chapter 371)

Herniation of abdominal contents into the thoracic cavity may occur as a result of a congenital or traumatic defect in the diaphragm.

CLINICAL MANIFESTATIONS. Although many cases are identified by prenatal ultrasonography, the majority of infants with congenital diaphragmatic hernia experience severe respiratory distress within the first hours of life. A small group will present beyond the neonatal period. Occasionally, incarceration of the intestine will proceed to ischemia with sepsis and cardiorespiratory collapse. The absence of breath sounds and shift of heart sounds common to congenital diaphragmatic hernia and pneumothorax will be accompanied by a scaphoid abdomen in the infants with congenital diaphragmatic hernia. Chest radiograph is usually diagnostic.

TREATMENT. The availability of extracorporeal membrane oxygenation (ECMO) and the utility of preoperative stabilization have been the major stimuli to aggressive therapy. Initial resuscitation has traditionally consisted of attempted stabilization with sedation and paralysis and modest hyperventilation. If the infant stabilizes and demonstrates stable pulmonary vascular resistance without significant right-to-left shunting, repair of the diaphragm is performed at 24–72 hr of age. The abdominal surgical approach is favored because the accompanying malrotation may be addressed if necessary.

PART 17

The Respiratory System

SECTION 1

Development and Function
(Nelson Textbook, Chapters 373–377)

CHAPTER 200

Respiratory Pathophysiology
(Nelson Textbook, Chapter 375)

RESPIRATORY FAILURE

CLINICAL MANIFESTATION AND DIAGNOSIS. The limited ability of the developing respiratory system to compensate for disease-induced mechanical abnormalities makes the early recognition of respiratory failure critical. Respiratory failure should be anticipated rather than recognized so that alterations in gas exchange can be prevented.

In a child suspected of respiratory failure, this evaluation should always start with a rapid assessment of the adequacy of ventilation, including the presence and vigor of the respiratory movements, breathing rate, extent of the respiratory movements, the presence of cyanosis, and the presence of signs of upper airway obstruction. A child with grossly inadequate respiratory efforts or complete airway obstruction will not survive long unless ventilation of the lungs is restored immediately. In addition, special attention must be paid to the patient's state of consciousness. Hypoxemia and hypercarbia frequently cause lethargy and confusion alternating with agitation.

TREATMENT. The goal of treatment of respiratory failure is the restoration of adequate gas exchange with a minimum of complications. Specific therapy for the initiating or underlying disease is essential. Administration of supplemental oxygen is a safe and wise precaution in all patients at risk for respiratory failure, even if there is no initial evidence of hypoxemia. The indication for ventilatory support in a child with respiratory failure is usually based on the persistence or worsening of gas exchange abnormalities. On occasion, ventilatory support must be instituted in the absence of alterations in the $Paco_2$, when the dysfunction of other systems places gas exchange in jeopardy by severely limiting the compensatory ability of the respiratory system. Cardiovascular

494

shock is a typical example. Ventilatory support usually (but not always) requires intubation of the trachea with an endotracheal tube or less often a tracheostomy cannula.

SECTION 2

Upper Respiratory Tract
(Nelson Textbook, Chapters 378–383)

CHAPTER 201

Congenital Disorder of the Nose
(Nelson Textbook, Chapter 378)

CHOANAL ATRESIA

CLINICAL MANIFESTATIONS. This is the most common congenital anomaly of the nose. Because newborns have a variable ability to breathe through their mouths, nasal obstruction does not produce the same symptoms in every infant. When only one side is affected, the infant usually does not have severe symptoms at birth and may be asymptomatic for a prolonged period, often until the first respiratory infection, when the diagnosis may be suggested by unilateral nasal discharge or disproportionately severe nasal obstruction. Infants with bilateral choanal atresia who have difficulty with mouth breathing make vigorous attempts to inspire, often suck in their lips, and develop cyanosis. Distressed children then cry (which relieves the cyanosis) and become more calm, only to repeat the cycle after closing their mouths. Those who are able to breathe through their mouths at once experience difficulty when sucking and swallowing, becoming cyanotic when they attempt to feed.

DIAGNOSIS. This is established by the inability to pass a firm catheter through each nostril 3–4 cm into the nasopharynx.

TREATMENT. Initially, this consists of promptly providing an oral airway, maintaining the mouth in an open position, or intubation. Passage of an orogastric tube is often sufficient to prevent the complete opposition of tongue and soft palate and to ensure an open airway. In bilateral cases, intubation or tracheotomy may be indicated. If the child is free of other serious medical problems, operative intervention can be considered in the neonate. Operative correction of unilateral obstruction may be deferred for several years. In both unilateral and bilateral cases, restenosis necessitating dilation or reoperation, or both, is common.

CHAPTER 202

Acquired Disorders of the Nose

(Nelson Textbook, Chapter 379)

FOREIGN BODY

Food, crayons, small toys, erasers, paper wads, beads, beans, stones, pieces of sponge, and other foreign bodies are frequently introduced into the nose by children. Initial symptoms are local obstruction, sneezing, relatively mild discomfort, and, rarely, pain. Unilateral nasal discharge and obstruction should suggest the presence of a foreign body, which can often be seen on examination with a nasal speculum or otoscope placed in the nose. Removal should be carried out promptly to minimize the danger of aspiration and prevent local tissue necrosis.

EPISTAXIS

Nosebleeds are rare in infancy and common in childhood; their incidence decreases after puberty.

CLINICAL MANIFESTATIONS. Epistaxis usually occurs without warning, with blood flowing slowly but freely from one nostril or occasionally from both. When bleeding occurs at night, the blood may be swallowed and may become apparent only when the child vomits or passes blood in the stools.

TREATMENT. Most nosebleeds stop spontaneously in a few minutes. The nares should be compressed and the child kept as quiet as possible, in an upright position with the head tilted forward to avoid blood trickling posteriorly into the pharynx. Cold compresses applied to the nose may also help. If these measures do not stop the bleeding, local application of a solution of oxymetazoline (Afrin) or Neo-Synephrine (0.25–1%) may be useful. If bleeding persists, an anterior nasal pack may need to be inserted; if bleeding originates in the posterior nasal cavity, combined anterior and posterior packing is necessary. After bleeding has been controlled and if a bleeding site is identified, its obliteration by cautery with silver nitrate may prevent further difficulties.

CHAPTER 203

Infections of the Upper Respiratory Tract

(Nelson Textbook, Chapter 381)

Upper respiratory infections (URIs) are the most frequently occurring illnesses in childhood.

CLINICAL MANIFESTATIONS. In older children and adults, the initial symptoms are usually nasal irritation and a scratchy throat. Most individuals can usually sense a cold that is about to start. Within hours, a thin nasal discharge and sneezing are present. A sore throat is common, partly due to postnasal drip and mouth breathing. Myalgia, a feeling of "being cold," headache, malaise, and decreased appetite are often present. Children may complain of headache and eye irritation and may have a low-grade fever. By the 2nd to 3rd days, the nasal discharge becomes thicker and is often purulent. Although the child usually feels better, sneezing, sore throat, and night-time cough (the latter two symptoms due to postnasal drip) are common. The nose may become tender and excoriated. The nasal secretions become progressively more purulent. Most systemic symptoms subside within 5 days. Infants have a more variable presentation, frequently with a fever. Infants with URIs are often irritable and restless. Nasal congestion may make feeding and sleeping difficult, and cough may lead to vomiting.

TREATMENT. For most URIs the best treatment is no pharmacologic treatment. Therapy should be directed toward a specific symptom that is causing discomfort. Acetaminophen (10–15 mg/kg/dose) or ibuprofen (10 mg/kg/dose) is often helpful in relieving the constitutional symptoms and the fever that may be present during the 1st day or two.

SINUSITIS

CLINICAL MANIFESTATIONS. Headaches, facial pain, tenderness, and facial edema occur in adolescents and adults but are not common in preadolescents. Cough and nasal discharge are the most common clinical manifestations of acute sinusitis in children. Sore throat secondary to postnasal drip may be present, and the child may sniff or snort to clear the drainage. Most URIs improve by 7 to 10 days. If symptoms persist without improvement for more than 10 days, a diagnosis of acute sinusitis should be considered. A less common but more severe form of acute sinusitis can occur with symptoms for less than 10 days in the child with fever higher than 39°C (102.2°F), purulent nasal discharge, headache, and eye swelling.

On physical examination, the nasal mucosa is usually erythematous and swollen. If allergic rhinitis is a contributing factor, the turbinates may be pale and boggy. Mucopurulent material sometimes can be seen draining into the posterior nasopharynx. Palpation of the bones overlying the sinuses may elicit pain, particularly in older children.

TREATMENT. This consists primarily of effective antimicrobial therapy. Amoxicillin is a reasonable initial choice.

ACUTE PHARYNGITIS

Pharyngitis is part of most URIs; however, in the strict sense, *acute pharyngitis* refers to conditions in which the principal involvement is in the throat.

CLINICAL MANIFESTATIONS. Viral and streptococcal pharyngitis have many overlapping signs and symptoms. *Viral pharyngitis* is generally considered a disease of relatively gradual onset, with early signs of fever, malaise, and anorexia with moderate throat pain. Frequently, a close contact has a common cold. Conjunctivitis, rhinitis, cough, hoarseness, coryza, anterior stomatitis, discrete ulcerative lesions, viral exanthems, and diarrhea strongly suggest that a viral agent rather than *Streptococcus* is the cause. Small ulcers may form on the soft palate and the posterior pharyngeal wall. Exudates may appear on lymphoid follicles of the palate and tonsils and may be indistinguishable from exudates encountered with streptococcal disease. The cervical lymph nodes are often moderately enlarged and firm and may or may not be tender.

Streptococcal pharyngitis in a child older than 2 yr may begin with nonspecific complaints of headache, abdominal pain, and vomiting. These symptoms may be associated with a fever as high as 40°C (104°F). Hours after the initial complaints, the throat may become sore; however, only one third of patients demonstrate the classic tonsillar enlargement, exudates, and pharyngeal erythema. Anterior cervical lymphadenopathy usually occurs early, and the nodes are often tender.

TREATMENT. Because even exudative tonsillitis is usually of viral origin, for which there is no specific therapy, the use of antibiotics should be guided by the results of antigen detection tests or cultures, unless there are strong clinical and epidemiologic grounds to suspect a streptococcal infection. Treatment within the first 9 days after onset of symptoms is effective in preventing the long-term sequelae of rheumatic fever. Streptococcal pharyngitis is best treated orally with penicillin (125 mg for children weighing < 60 lb; 250 mg for older children and adults; 3 times daily for 10 days).

CHAPTER 204

Tonsils and Adenoids

(Nelson Textbook, Chapter 382)

The term *tonsils* is used in its commonly accepted sense of indicating the two faucial tonsils; the term *adenoids* refers to the nasopharyngeal tonsil.

CHRONIC TONSILLITIS (CHRONICALLY HYPERTROPHIC AND INFECTED TONSILS)

CLINICAL MANIFESTATIONS. These vary considerably; the significant features are recurrent or persistent sore throat, pain with swallowing, and obstruction to swallowing or breathing. There may be a sense of dryness and irritation in the throat, and the breath may be offensive; these symptoms may be more common with chronic mouth breathing. Children with chronic tonsillitis may also have adenotonsillar hypertrophy causing symptoms of airway obstruction. Symptoms of adenotonsillar hypertrophy include snoring, mouth breathing, gasping and pausing during sleep, and apnea.

INDICATIONS FOR TONSILLECTOMY

CHRONIC TONSILLITIS. For children with recurrent throat infections (7 in the past year, 5 in each of the past 2 yr, 3 in each of the past 3 yr, or more than any of these), tonsillectomy decreases the number of throat infections in the subsequent 2 yr, compared with no tonsillectomy. However, many children meeting these criteria who have not had tonsillectomy also have a decline in the number of throat infections.

HYPERTROPHIC TONSILS AND ADENOIDS. Large size alone, without symptoms of obstruction or infection, is not an indication to remove the tonsils. Hypertrophy sufficient to obstruct swallowing or breathing is often detectable; such tonsils practically meet in the midline when the throat is examined. However, before tonsillectomy is recommended, it should be ascertained that the hypertrophy is chronic and not the result of a recent acute infection.

TONSILLECTOMY IN RELATION TO THE AGE OF THE CHILD. Tonsillectomy in children younger than 2–3 yr is generally performed for obstructive sleep symptoms rather than tonsillitis, which is more common in older children.

TONSILLECTOMY IN RELATION TO ACTIVE INFECTION. Tonsillectomy should be postponed until 2–3 wk after subsidence of an infection, except in rare cases of acute respiratory obstruction with pulmonary artery hypertension and cor pulmonale.

ADENOIDAL HYPERTROPHY (HYPERTROPHY OF PHARYNGEAL TONSILS; "ADENOIDS")

CLINICAL MANIFESTATIONS. Mouth breathing and persistent rhinitis and nasal drainage are the most characteristic symptoms. Mouth breathing may be present only during sleep, especially when the child lies supine, when snoring is also likely to occur. Chronic nasopharyngitis may be constantly present or recur frequently. The voice is altered, with a nasal, muffled quality. The breath is offensive, and taste and smell are impaired. Chronic otitis media may be associated with infected, hypertrophied adenoids and blockage of the eustachian tube orifices; hearing loss is often present secondary to middle ear fluid.

TREATMENT. Adenoidectomy may be indicated for symptoms such as persistent mouth breathing, hyponasal speech, adenoid facies, repeated or chronic otitis media with effusion, and persistent or recurring nasopharyngitis when these seem to be related to infected hypertrophied adenoid tissue.

CHAPTER 205

Obstructive Sleep Apnea and Hypoventilation in Children

(Nelson Textbook, Chapter 383)

Obstructive sleep apnea/hypoventilation is a common problem in children that is characterized by a combination of prolonged partial upper airway obstruction and intermittent complete obstruction (obstructive apnea) that disrupts sleep and breathing patterns. It can lead to impaired daytime performance as well as more serious complications such as heart failure, developmental delay, poor growth, and death. Habitual snoring, the most common symptom, occurs in 8–10% of young schoolchildren.

CLINICAL MANIFESTATIONS. The majority of children with obstructive sleep apnea/hypoventilation do not present with dramatic, repetitive obstructive apnea. Instead, obstruction is partial and tonic. Common clinical manifestations of obstructive sleep apnea/hyperventilation include chronic mouth breathing, snoring, and restlessness during sleep with or without frequent awakening.

TREATMENT. Because adenotonsillar hyperplasia is the most common condition associated with pediatric obstructive sleep apnea/hypoventilation, adenotonsillectomy provides definitive relief of obstruction in the majority of patients. Medical management with nasal continuous positive airway pressure is an option in children in whom adenotonsillectomy fails, thus avoiding the need for a tracheostomy.

Lower Respiratory Tract

(Nelson Textbook, Chapters 384–417)

CHAPTER 206

Acute Inflammatory Upper Airway Obstruction

(Nelson Textbook, Chapter 385)

Inflammation involving the vocal cords and structures inferior to the cords is called laryngitis, laryngotracheitis, or laryngotracheobronchitis, and inflammation of the structures superior to the cords (i.e., arytenoids, aryepiglottic folds ["false cords"], epiglottis) is called supraglottitis. *Croup* is a generic term encompassing a heterogeneous group of relatively acute conditions (mostly infectious) characterized by a peculiarly brassy or "croupy" cough, which may or may not be accompanied by inspiratory stridor, hoarseness, and signs of respiratory distress due to various degrees of laryngeal obstruction. Such infection in infants and small children is rarely limited to a single area of the respiratory tract; it usually affects, to some degree, the larynx, trachea, and bronchi.

INFECTIOUS UPPER AIRWAY OBSTRUCTION

ETIOLOGY AND EPIDEMIOLOGY. Viral agents account for most acute infectious upper airway obstructions except those associated with diphtheria, bacterial tracheitis, and acute epiglottitis. Most patients who have viral croup are between the ages of 3 mo and 5 yr, but disease due to *Haemophilus influenzae* and *Corynebacterium diphtheriae* is more common from 3–7 yr of age.

CLINICAL MANIFESTATIONS

Croup (Laryngotracheobronchitis). Croup, the most common form of acute upper airway obstruction, is caused primarily by viruses. Most patients have an upper respiratory tract infection for several days before cough becomes apparent. At first, there is only a mild, brassy cough with intermittent inspiratory stridor. As obstruction increases, stridor becomes continuous and is associated with worsening cough, nasal flaring, and suprasternal, infrasternal, and intercostal retractions. As inflammation extends to the bronchi and bronchioles, respiratory difficulty increases, and the expiratory phase of respiration also becomes labored and prolonged. The temperature may be only slightly elevated; it rarely reaches 39–40°C (102.2–104°F). Symptoms are characteristically worse at night and often recur with decreasing intensity for several days.

The duration of illness ranges from several days to, rarely, several weeks; recurrences are frequent from 3–6 yr of age, decreasing with growth of the airway.

There may be diminished breath sounds, rhonchi, and scattered crackles. With further compromise of the airway, air hunger and restlessness occur and are then superseded by severe hypoxemia, hypercapnia, and weakness, accompanied by decreased air exchange and stridor, tachycardia, and eventual death from hypoventilation. In the hypoxemic child who may be cyanotic, pale, or obtunded, any manipulation of the pharynx, including use of a tongue depressor, may result in sudden cardiorespiratory arrest. This examination therefore should be deferred, and oxygen should be administered until the patient is transferred to a place in the hospital where optimal management of the airway and shock is possible.

Acute Epiglottitis (Supraglottitis). This dramatic, potentially lethal condition usually occurs in children aged 2–7 yr. It is seen much less commonly since the widespread use of immunization against *H. influenzae* type b. Epiglottitis is characterized by a fulminating course of high fever, sore throat, dyspnea, rapidly progressive respiratory obstruction, and prostration, although respiratory distress is frequently the first manifestation. Within a matter of hours it may progress to complete obstruction of the airway and death unless adequate treatment is provided. With adequate treatment the illness rarely lasts for more than 2–3 days. Often the child, particularly the younger patient, is apparently well at bedtime but awakens later in the evening with high fever, aphonia, drooling, and moderate or severe respiratory distress with stridor. Severe respiratory distress may ensue within minutes or hours of the onset, with inspiratory stridor, hoarseness, brassy cough (less commonly), irritability, and restlessness.

The physical examination may disclose moderate or severe respiratory distress with inspiratory and sometimes expiratory stridor, flaring of the alae nasi, and inspiratory retractions of the suprasternal notch, supraclavicular and intercostal spaces, and subcostal area. The diagnosis requires visualization of a large, swollen, cherry-red epiglottis by direct examination or laryngoscopy.

Acute Infectious Laryngitis. Laryngitis is a common illness. The onset is usually characterized by an upper respiratory tract infection during which sore throat, cough, and hoarseness appear. Hoarseness and loss of voice may be out of proportion to systemic signs and symptoms.

Acute Spasmodic Laryngitis (Spasmodic Croup). Spasmodic croup occurs most often in children 1–3 yr of age and is clinically similar to acute laryngotracheobronchitis, except that findings of infection in the patient and family are frequently absent. Occurring most frequently in the evening or night time, spasmodic croup begins with a sudden onset that may be preceded by mild to moderate coryza and hoarseness. The child awakens with a characteristic barking, metallic cough, noisy inspiration, and respiratory distress and appears anxious and frightened. The patient is usually afebrile.

TREATMENT. Therapy for *infectious croup* consists primarily of maintaining or providing for adequate respiratory exchange and depends, in part, on the primary location of the disease and its cause. In the bacterial forms, antibiotic therapy is also important. Most afebrile children with acute spasmodic croup or febrile patients with mild *laryngotracheobronchitis* can usually be managed safely and effectively at home. The use of steam from a shower or bath in a closed bathroom, steam from a vaporizer, or "cold steam" from a nebulizer (which has a safety and perhaps efficacy advantage) often terminates acute laryngeal spasm and respiratory distress within minutes. Children with croup should be hospitalized for any of the following: actual or suspected epiglottitis, progressive stridor, severe stridor at rest, respiratory distress, hypoxemia, restlessness, cyanosis, pallor, depressed sensorium, or high fever in a toxic-appearing child.

At home or in the hospital, the patient with croup should be watched carefully for intensification of symptoms of respiratory obstruction. The hospitalized child is usually placed in an atmosphere of cool humidity to lessen irritation and drying of secretions and perhaps to lessen edema. The patient should be disturbed as little as possible. Oxygen should be used to alleviate hypoxemia and apprehension, but because the oxygen reduces cyanosis, which is an indication for tracheotomy or nasotracheal intubation, these patients must be observed particularly closely. Racemic epinephrine by aerosol (2.25% solution diluted 1:8 with water in doses of 2–4 mL for 15 min) often results in transient relief of symptoms; close observation and repeated treatments usually are necessary. The use of corticosteroids is probably indicated for the hospitalized child with croup.

Epiglottitis is a medical emergency. It should be treated immediately with an artificial airway inserted under controlled conditions, usually in an operating room. All patients should receive oxygen en route to the operating room unless it is contraindicated by the increased agitation caused by the mask. Racemic epinephrine and corticosteroids are ineffective.

CHAPTER 207

Foreign Bodies in the Larynx, Trachea, and Bronchi

(Nelson Textbook, Chapter 386)

LARYNGEAL FOREIGN BODIES

CLINICAL MANIFESTATIONS. A laryngeal foreign body causes a cough that soon becomes croupy and hoarse; with profound obstruction, aphonia is seen. Hemoptysis, dyspnea with wheezing, and cyanosis may occur.

DIAGNOSIS. Radiographic and direct laryngoscopic examinations usually reveal or suggest the presence of a foreign body in the larynx. Direct laryngoscopy with a rigid open-tube endoscope, usually performed by an otolaryngologist, confirms the diagnosis and provides access for removal of the foreign body.

BRONCHIAL FOREIGN BODIES

CLINICAL MANIFESTATIONS. The initial symptoms of a bronchial foreign body are usually similar to those of foreign bodies in the larynx or trachea. Cough, wheeze, blood-streaked sputum, and metallic taste with metallic foreign bodies also may be produced by bronchial foreign bodies. A nonobstructing, nonirritating foreign body may produce few symptoms, even after a prolonged time. An obstructing foreign body quickly produces symptoms and signs and pathologic changes. If the obstruction allows air entry but not exit (i.e., check valve or ball valve obstruction), obstructive overinflation ensues. In the case of complete obstruction, which allows neither air entry nor exit, obstructive atelectasis is produced as the air distal to the obstruction is absorbed.

There is usually an immediate episode of choking, gagging, and paroxysmal coughing, which may lead to medical consultation. If this acute episode does not occur or is missed or if its importance is underestimated by the parents, a latent period of minutes to months may pass with only occasional cough or slight wheezing; the patient may acquire recurrent lobar pneumonia or intractable "asthma," often with bilateral wheezing and many episodes of status asthmaticus.

TREATMENT. Endoscopy and removal of the foreign body with a rigid open-tube bronchoscope under direct visualization should be performed as soon as possible. Emergency treatment of local upper airway obstruction is part of the basic rescuer course in cardiopulmonary resuscitation.

CHAPTER 208

Bronchitis

(Nelson Textbook, Chapter 390)

CLINICAL MANIFESTATIONS. Acute bronchitis is usually preceded by a viral upper respiratory infection. Typically, the child presents a frequent, dry, hacking, unproductive cough of relatively gradual onset, beginning 3–4 days after the appearance of rhinitis. Low substernal discomfort or burning anterior chest pain is often present and may be aggravated by coughing. As the illness progresses, the patient may be bothered by whistling sounds during respiration (probably rhonchi), soreness of the chest, and occasionally shortness of breath. Initially, the child is usually afebrile or has low-grade fever, and there are signs of nasopharyngitis, conjunctival infection, and rhinitis. Later, auscultation reveals roughening of breath sounds, coarse and fine moist rales, and rhonchi that may be high-pitched, resembling the wheezing of asthma.

TREATMENT. There is no specific therapy; most patients recover uneventfully without any treatment. In small infants, pulmonary drainage is facilitated by frequent shifts in position. Older children are more comfortable in high humidity, but there is no evidence that this shortens the duration of illness.

CHAPTER 209

Bronchiolitis

(Nelson Textbook, Chapter 391)

Acute bronchiolitis, a common disease of the lower respiratory tract in infants, results from inflammatory obstruction of the small airways. It occurs during the first 2 yr of life, with a peak incidence at approximately 6 mo of age. Acute bronchiolitis is predominantly a viral illness. The respiratory syncytial virus is the causative agent in more than 50% of cases.

CLINICAL MANIFESTATIONS. Most affected infants have a history of exposure to older children or adults with minor respiratory diseases within the week preceding the onset of illness. The infant first has a mild upper respiratory tract infection with serous nasal discharge and sneezing. These symptoms usually last several days and may be accompanied by diminished appetite and fever of 38.5–39°C (101.3–102.2°F), although the temperature may range from subnormal to markedly elevated. The gradual development of respiratory distress is characterized by paroxysmal wheezy cough, dyspnea, and irritability. In mild cases, symptoms disappear in 1–3 days. In more severely affected patients, symptoms may develop within several hours and the course is protracted.

An examination reveals a tachypneic infant, with a hyperexpanded chest and often in extreme distress. Respirations range from 60–80 breaths/min; severe air hunger and cyanosis may occur. The alae nasi flare, and use of the accessory muscles of respiration results in intercostal and subcostal retractions, which are shallow because of the persistent distention of the lungs by the trapped air. The depression of the liver and spleen by the overinflated lungs may result in their being palpable below the costal margin. Widespread fine crackles may be heard at the end of inspiration and in early expiration. The expiratory phase of breathing is prolonged, and wheezes are usually audible.

COURSE AND PROGNOSIS. The most critical phase of illness occurs during the first 48–72 hr after the onset of cough and dyspnea. During this period, the infant appears desperately ill, apneic spells occur in the very young infant, and respiratory acidosis is likely to be noticed. After the critical period, improvement occurs rapidly and often dramatically.

TREATMENT. Infants with respiratory distress should be hospitalized, but only supportive treatment is indicated. The child is commonly placed in an atmosphere of cool, humidified oxygen to relieve hypoxemia and reduce insensible water loss from tachypnea; this treatment usually relieves the dyspnea and cyanosis and allays anxiety and restlessness. The infant is usually more comfortable sitting at a 30- to 40-degree angle or with the head and chest slightly elevated so that the neck is somewhat extended.

Ribavirin (Vibrazole), an antiviral agent administered by aerosol, may be considered for infants with congenital heart disease or bronchopulmonary dysplasia. Antibiotics have no therapeutic value unless there is secondary bacterial pneumonia. Corticosteroids are not beneficial and may be harmful under certain conditions. Bronchodilating aerosolized drugs (e.g., albuterol) are frequently used empirically.

Chapter 210

Aspiration Pneumonias and Gastroesophageal Reflux–Related Respiratory Disease

(Nelson Textbook, Chapter 393)

ASPIRATION PNEUMONIA

ASPIRATION OF FOOD AND VOMITUS. Infants with obstructive lesions such as esophageal atresia or duodenal obstruction; hypotonic, weak, and debilitated infants and children with no obstructive lesions; patients with familial dysautonomia; and patients with impaired consciousness may aspirate or regurgitate and then aspirate food and vomitus, causing a chemical pneumonia. After aspiration of gastric contents, there frequently is a relatively brief latent period before the onset of signs and symptoms of pneumonia. More than 90% of patients have symptoms within 1 hr, and almost all patients have symptoms within 2 hr. Fever, tachypnea, and cough are common. Apnea and shock may also occur. Physical examination reveals diffuse crackles, wheezing, and possibly cyanosis. Chest radiographs reveal alveolar and, occasionally, reticular infiltrates that may be localized but often are more extensive and are frequently bilateral.

Treatment by immediate suctioning of the airway and administering oxygen is indicated for aspiration. Endotracheal intubation with suctioning and mechanical ventilation is often required for severe cases.

HYDROCARBON PNEUMONIA

ETIOLOGY. Hydrocarbons, such as furniture polish, kerosene, charcoal lighter fluid, and gasoline, occasionally are accidentally ingested by young children, causing a secondary pneumonitis.

CLINICAL MANIFESTATIONS. Coughing and vomiting follow ingestion almost immediately. Within hours, there may be temperature elevation (38–40°C [100.4–104°F]). However, with less extensive aspiration, the onset of pulmonary symptoms and inflammation may be delayed 12–24 hr. The pulmonary findings may include dyspnea, diminished resonance on percussion, suppressed or tubular breath sounds, and crackles. Radiographs may occasionally show minimal changes a few hours after ingestion, only to progress rapidly after that time with extensive infiltrates. Despite what may be a stormy clinical course, which averages 2–5 days, recovery occurs in most cases. Systemic symptoms of hydrocarbon ingestion, including somnolence, convulsions, and coma, may occur and sometimes dominate the course.

TREATMENT. Symptoms and radiologic infiltrates may be delayed, and no patient should be sent home in less than 6 hr, even if there are no symptoms. Patients who are symptomatic when they are first examined, patients who become symptomatic during 6 hr of observation, and all patients who ingested a particularly toxic agent (e.g., furniture polish) should be admitted to the hospital. No pulmonary therapy is indicated before symptoms develop.

After ingestion of small to moderate amounts of hydrocarbons, induction of vomiting or gastric lavage is contraindicated because of the risk of aspiration, especially if several hours have elapsed. If a large volume of hydrocarbon is thought to be in the stomach, nasogastric suction performed with great care to avoid aspiration rarely may be necessary to reduce the other dangers of hydrocarbon poisoning, including central nervous system toxicity.

CHAPTER 211

Hypersensitivity to Inhaled Materials

(Nelson Textbook, Chapter 396)

CLINICAL MANIFESTATIONS. The signs and symptoms are similar in all of these diseases. Within several hours after exposure, cough, dyspnea, chest pain, and sometimes fever occur with few physical findings, although occasional wheezes and moist rales may be audible. If no further exposure occurs, the symptoms abate over a period of several days; if contact with the responsible antigen continues, symptoms progress to severe dyspnea and cyanosis associated with diffuse, fine, interstitial or nodular densities and peripheral alveolar infiltrates on chest radiograph and occasionally irreversible loss of pulmonary function.

TREATMENT. Optimal therapy requires complete elimination of exposure to the suspected or proven antigen. Administration of adrenal corticosteroids (e.g., prednisone in initial dosage of 1–1.5 mg/kg/24 hr) usually results in prompt remission of symptoms; continued use for 1–6 mo may prevent subsequent development of pulmonary fibrosis in cases of chronic exposure.

CHAPTER 212

Pulmonary Hemosiderosis (Pulmonary Hemorrhage)

(Nelson Textbook, Chapter 402)

Bleeding in the lower respiratory tract in children is unusual but can be life threatening. During infancy and prepubertal childhood, infections, trauma, and foreign bodies are probably the most common causes of pulmonary hemorrhage. More extensive hemorrhage in this range can arise from any of the remaining secondary and primary causes listed in Table 212–1.

TABLE 212–1 Causes of Pulmonary Hemorrhage

Infection (extensive)
  Bacterial, fungal, parasitic
  Chronic with bronchiectasis*
Trauma
  Crush injury, suffocation, foreign body
Cardiovascular
  Increased pulmonary venous pressure
  Arteriovenous malformations
  Pulmonary emboli, infarcts
Vasculitis
  Autoimmune disorders*
  Immune complex disorders*
  Anti–glomerular basement membrane antibodies*
Toxic (penicillamine, cocaine)
Neoplasia (carcinoid)
Associated with antibodies to cow's milk proteins
Idiopathic

*Limited to school-aged children and older.

CHAPTER 213

Atelectasis

(Nelson Textbook, Chapter 406)

ACQUIRED ATELECTASIS

CLINICAL MANIFESTATIONS. Symptoms vary with the cause and extent of the atelectasis. A small area is likely to be asymptomatic. When a large area of previously normal lung becomes atelectatic, especially when it does so suddenly, dyspnea accompanied by rapid shallow respirations, tachycardia, and often cyanosis occurs. If the obstruction is removed, the symptoms disappear rapidly.

TREATMENT. Bronchoscopic examination is immediately indicated if atelectasis is the result of a foreign body or any other bronchial obstruction that may be relieved. It is also indicated when an isolated area of atelectasis persists for several weeks. It is usually advisable to suction the orifice of the involved bronchus; a *mucous plug* can occasionally be removed, with prompt re-expansion. Frequent changes in the child's position and deep breathing may be beneficial. Oxygen therapy is indicated when there is dyspnea or substantial hemoglobin desaturation.

MASSIVE PULMONARY ATELECTASIS

Massive collapse of one or both lungs is most often a postoperative complication but occasionally results from other causes, such as trauma, asthma, pneumonia, tension pneumothorax, aspiration of foreign material, following extubation, or paralysis.

CLINICAL MANIFESTATIONS. The onset in postoperative cases usually occurs within 24 hr after operation but may not occur for several days, with dyspnea, cyanosis, and tachycardia. An affected child is extremely anxious and, if old enough, complains of chest pain. Prostration is likely. The temperature may be as high as 39.5–40°C (103.1–104°F). The chest appears flat on the affected side, where decreased respiratory excursion, dullness to percussion, and feeble or absent breath and voice sounds are also noted.

TREATMENT. For bilateral atelectasis, bronchoscopic aspiration should be performed immediately. For unilateral atelectasis, the child should be placed on the unaffected side; forced coughing or crying while the child is lying on the unaffected side may also be helpful, as is positive-pressure ventilation; but when these measures are unsuccessful, bronchoscopic aspiration should be performed.

CHAPTER 214

Chronic or Recurrent Respiratory Symptoms

(Nelson Textbook, Chapter 415)

Respiratory tract symptoms such as cough, wheeze, and stridor may occur frequently or persist for long periods in a substantial number of children; others may have persistent or recurring lung infiltrates with or without symptoms. Determining the cause of these chronic findings can be difficult because symptoms may be caused by a rapid succession of unrelated acute respiratory tract infections or by a single pathophysiologic process, and there is a paucity of easily performed, specific diagnostic tests for many acute and chronic respiratory conditions.

A systemic approach to the diagnosis and treatment of these children consists of assessing whether the symptoms are the manifestation of a minor problem or a life-threatening process; determining the most likely underlying pathogenic mechanism; selecting the simplest effective therapy for the underlying process, which may often be only symptomatic therapy; and carefully evaluating the effect of the therapy. Failure of this approach to identify the process responsible or to effect improvement signals the need for more extensive and perhaps invasive diagnostic efforts, including bronchoscopy.

CHAPTER 215

Cystic Fibrosis
(Nelson Textbook, Chapter 416)

Cystic fibrosis (CF) is an inherited multisystem disorder of children and adults, characterized chiefly by obstruction and infection of airways and by maldigestion and its consequences. CF is inherited as an autosomal recessive trait. All of the more than 700 gene mutations that contribute to the CF syndrome occur at a single locus on the long arm of chromosome 7.

CLINICAL MANIFESTATIONS. Mutational heterogeneity and environmental factors appear responsible for highly variable involvement of the lung, pancreas, and other organs.

Respiratory Tract. Cough is the most constant symptom of pulmonary involvement. At first, the cough may be dry and hacking, but eventually it becomes loose and productive. Some patients remain asymptomatic for long periods or seem to have only prolonged, acute respiratory tract infections. Others acquire a chronic cough within the first weeks of life or they repeatedly have pneumonia. Extensive bronchiolitis is attended by wheezing, which is a frequent symptom during the first years of life. As lung disease progresses, exercise intolerance, shortness of breath, and failure to gain weight or grow are noted. Finally, cor pulmonale, respiratory failure, and death supervene. The rate of progression of lung disease is the chief determinant of morbidity and mortality.

Intestinal Tract. In 15–20% of newborns with CF, the ileum is completely obstructed by meconium (meconium ileus). More than 85% of affected children show evidence of maldigestion due to exocrine pancreatic insufficiency. Symptoms include frequent, bulky, greasy stools and failure to gain weight even when food intake appears to be large. Characteristically, stools contain readily visible droplets of fat. A protuberant abdomen, decreased muscle mass, poor growth, and delayed maturation are typical physical signs.

Pancreas. In addition to exocrine pancreatic insufficiency, evidence for hyperglycemia and glycosuria including polyuria and weight loss may appear, especially after 10 yr of age, when 8% of individuals acquire diabetes.

Genitourinary Tract. More than 95% of males are azoospermic because of failure of development of wolffian duct structures, but sexual function is generally unimpaired. The female fertility rate is diminished.

Sweat Glands. Excessive loss of salt in the sweat predisposes young children to salt depletion episodes, especially during gastroenteritis and during warm weather.

DIAGNOSIS AND ASSESSMENT. New diagnostic criteria have been recommended to include additional testing procedures (Table 215–1).

TREATMENT. The treatment plan should be comprehensive and linked to close monitoring and early, aggressive intervention.

General Approach to Care. A period of hospitalization for accurate diagnosis, baseline assessment, initiation of treatment, clearing of pulmonary involvement, and education of the patient and parents is recommended. Follow-up outpatient visits are scheduled every 2–3 mo because many aspects of the condition require careful monitoring.

Pulmonary Therapy. The object is to clear secretions from airways and to control infection. Aerosol therapy is used to deliver medications and water to the lower respiratory tract, usually before or after segmental postural drainage. Chest physical therapy usually consists of chest percussion combined with postural drainage, but chest vibrations are required to move secretions from small airways, where expiratory flow rates are low. Antibiotics are the mainstay of therapy designed to control progression of lung infection. Treatment may include use of β-adrenergic agonists by aerosol. Treatment of obstructed airways sometimes includes tracheobronchial suctioning or lavage, especially if atelectasis or mucoid impaction is present.

TABLE 215–1 Diagnostic Criteria for Cystic Fibrosis (CF)

Presence of typical clinical features (respiratory, gastrointestinal, or genitourinary)

or

A history of CF in a sibling

or

A positive newborn screening test

plus

Laboratory evidence for CFTR dysfunction:
  Two elevated sweat chloride concentrations obtained on separate days

  or

  Identification of two CF mutations

  or

  An abnormal nasal potential difference measurement

Disease of the Pleura

(Nelson Textbook, Chapters 418–423)

CHAPTER 216

Pneumothorax

(Nelson Textbook, Chapter 419)

Pneumothorax is the accumulation of extrapulmonary air within the chest.

CLINICAL MANIFESTATIONS AND DIAGNOSIS. The onset is usually abrupt, and the severity of symptoms depends on the extent of the lung collapse and on the amount of pre-existing lung disease. Extensive pneumothorax may involve pain, dyspnea, and cyanosis. Usually, there is respiratory distress, retractions, and markedly decreased breath sounds over the involved lung. The percussion note over the involved area is tympanitic. The larynx, trachea, and heart may be shifted toward the unaffected side. The diagnosis can usually be established by radiographic examination.

TREATMENT. A small or even moderate-sized pneumothorax in an otherwise normal child may resolve without specific treatment, usually within about 1 wk. A small (<5%) pneumothorax complicating asthma may also resolve spontaneously. Administering 100% oxygen may hasten resolution by increasing the nitrogen pressure gradient between the pleural air and the blood. Closed thoracotomy (i.e., simple insertion of a chest tube) and drainage of the trapped air through a catheter, the external opening of which is kept in a dependent position under water, are adequate to re-expand the lung in most patients.

PART 18

The Cardiovascular System

SECTION 1

Developmental Biology of the Cardiovascular System

CHAPTER 217

Cardiac Development and the Transition from Fetal to Neonatal Circulations

(Nelson Textbook, Chapters 427 and 428)

Knowledge of the cellular and molecular mechanisms of cardiac development is necessary to understand congenital heart defects and develop strategies for prevention. Developmental cardiologists traditionally grouped defects based on common morphologic patterns, for example, abnormalities of the outflow tracts (the conotruncal lesions such as tetralogy of Fallot and truncus arteriosus) or abnormalities of atrioventricular septation (primum atrial septal defect, complete atrioventricular canal defect). These morphologic categories do not provide an understanding of the mechanisms of heart malformations and their linkage to genetic alterations.

Much of the information concerning the fetal circulation has been derived from studies in fetal sheep. The human fetal circulation and its adjustments after birth are probably similar to those of other large mammals. At birth, the fetal circulation must immediately adapt to extrauterine life as gas exchange is transferred from the placenta to the lung. Some of these changes are virtually instantaneous with the first breath, and others are affected over hours or days.

Evaluation of the Cardiovascular System

CHAPTER 218

History and Physical Examination and Laboratory Evaluation

(Nelson Textbook, Chapters 429 and 430)

The importance of the history and physical examination cannot be overemphasized in the evaluation of infants and children with suspected cardiovascular disorders. After this assessment, patients may require further laboratory evaluation and eventual treatment or the family may be reassured that no significant problem exists.

RADIOLOGIC ASSESSMENT. The chest radiograph may provide information about cardiac size and shape, pulmonary blood flow (vascularity), pulmonary edema, and associated lung and thoracic anomalies that may be associated with congenital syndromes (skeletal dysplasias, extra or deficient numbers of ribs, previous cardiac surgery).

ELECTROCARDIOGRAPHY. The marked changes that occur in cardiac physiology and chamber dominance during the perinatal transition are reflected in the evolution of the electrocardiogram during the neonatal time period.

ECHOCARDIOGRAPHY. This has dramatically reduced the requirement for invasive studies such as cardiac catheterization. The echocardiographic examination can be used to evaluate cardiac structure in congenital heart lesions, estimate intracardiac pressures and gradients across stenotic valves and vessels, quantitate cardiac contractile function (both systolic and diastolic), determine the direction of flow across a defect, examine the integrity of the coronary arteries, evaluate the presence of vegetations due to endocarditis, and evaluate the presence of pericardial fluid, cardiac tumors, or chamber thrombi. Echocardiography may also be used to assist in the performance of pericardiocentesis, balloon atrial septostomy, and endocardial biopsy and in the placement of flow-directed pulmonary arterial (Swan-Ganz) monitoring catheters.

CARDIAC CATHETERIZATION. During catheterization, blood samples are obtained for measuring oxygen saturation and calculating shunt volumes, pressures are measured for calculating gradients and valve areas, and contrast medium is injected to delineate structures.

515

Congenital Heart Disease

CHAPTER 219

Evaluation of the Infant or Child with Congenital Heart Disease

(Nelson Textbook, Chapter 432)

The initial evaluation of the infant or child suspected of having congenital heart disease involves a systematic approach with three major components. First, congenital cardiac defects can be divided into two major groups based on the presence or absence of cyanosis, which can be determined by physical examination aided by pulse oximetry. Second, these two groups can be further subdivided based on whether the chest radiograph shows evidence of increased, normal, or decreased pulmonary vascular markings. Finally, the electrocardiogram can be used to determine whether right, left, or biventricular hypertrophy exists. The character of the heart sounds and the presence and character of any murmurs further narrow the differential diagnosis. The final diagnosis is then confirmed by echocardiography or cardiac catheterization or both.

ACYANOTIC CONGENITAL HEART LESIONS

Acyanotic congenital heart lesions can be classified according to the predominant physiologic load they place on the heart. The most common lesions are those that produce a *volume load*. The second major class of lesions causes an increase in *pressure load.*

LESIONS RESULTING IN INCREASED VOLUME LOAD. The most common lesions in this group are those that cause left-to-right shunting: atrial septal defect, ventricular septal defect, atrioventricular septal defects (atrioventricular canal), and patent ductus arteriosus. The pathophysiologic common denominator in this group is a communication between the systemic and pulmonary sides of the circulation, resulting in the shunting of fully oxygenated blood back into the lungs. This shunt can be quantitated by calculating the ratio of pulmonary to systemic blood flow, or $Q_P:Q_s$. Thus, a 2:1 shunt implies that there is twice the normal pulmonary blood flow.

The direction and magnitude of the shunt across such a communication depend on the size of the defect and the relative pulmonary and systemic pressures and vascular resistances. These factors are dynamic and may change dramatically with age: intracardiac defects may grow smaller with time; pulmonary vascular resistance, which is high in the immediate newborn period, decreases to normal adult levels by several weeks of life; and chronic exposure of the pulmonary circulation to high pressure and blood flow results in a gradual increase in pulmonary vascular resistance. Thus, in a lesion such as a large ventricular septal defect, there may be little shunting and few symptoms during the first weeks of life. When the pulmonary vascular resistance declines over the next several weeks, the volume of the left-to-right shunt increases, and symptoms begin to appear.

The increased volume of blood in the lungs decreases pulmonary compliance and increases the work of breathing. Fluid leaks into the interstitial space and alveoli, causing pulmonary edema. The infant acquires the symptoms we refer to as *heart failure*, such as tachypnea, chest retractions, nasal flaring, and wheezing.

Additional lesions that impose a volume load on the heart include the regurgitant lesions and the cardiomyopathies. Regurgitation of the atrioventricular valves is most commonly encountered in patients with partial or complete atrioventricular septal defects (atrioseptal defects, atrioventricular canal). Cardiomyopathies may affect systolic contractility or diastolic relaxation or both. The major causes of cardiomyopathy in infants and children include viral myocarditis, metabolic disorders, and genetic defects.

LESIONS RESULTING IN INCREASED PRESSURE LOAD. The pathophysiologic common denominator of these lesions is an obstruction to normal blood flow. The most common are obstructions to ventricular outflow: valvar pulmonic stenosis, valvar aortic stenosis, and coarctation of the aorta. Less common are obstructions to ventricular inflow: tricuspid or mitral stenosis and cor triatriatum. Unless the obstruction is severe, cardiac output will be maintained and clinical symptoms of heart failure will be either subtle or absent. The clinical picture is different when obstruction to outflow is severe, usually encountered in the immediate newborn period. The infant may become critically ill within several hours of birth.

CYANOTIC CONGENITAL HEART LESIONS

This group of congenital heart lesions can also be further divided based on pathophysiology, whether pulmonary blood flow is decreased (tetralogy of Fallot, pulmonary atresia with intact septum, tricuspid atresia, total anomalous pulmonary venous return with obstruction) or increased (transposition of the great vessels, single ventricle, truncus arteriosus, total anomalous pulmonary venous return without obstruction). The chest radiograph is a valuable tool for initial differentiation between these two categories.

CYANOTIC LESIONS WITH DECREASED PULMONARY BLOOD FLOW. These lesions must include both an obstruction to pulmonary blood flow (at the tricuspid valve or right ventricular or pulmonary valve level) and a pathway by which systemic venous blood can shunt from right to left and enter the systemic circulation (via a patent foramen ovale, atrial septal defect, or ventricular septal defect). In these lesions, the degree of cyanosis depends on the degree of obstruction to pulmonary blood flow. If the obstruction is mild, cyanosis may be absent at rest. These patients may acquire hypercyanotic ("tet") spells during conditions of stress. In contrast, if the obstruction is severe, pulmonary blood flow may be dependent on the patency of the ductus arteriosus. When the ductus closes during the first few days of life, the neonate presents with profound hypoxemia and shock.

CYANOTIC LESIONS WITH INCREASED PULMONARY BLOOD FLOW. In this group of lesions, there is no obstruction to pulmonary blood flow. Cyanosis is caused by either abnormal ventriculoarterial connections or by total mixing of systemic venous and pulmonary venous blood within the heart. Transposition of the great vessels is the most common of the former group of lesions. The total mixing lesions include those cardiac defects with a common atrium or ventricle, total anomalous pulmonary venous return, and truncus arteriosus. In this group, deoxygenated systemic venous blood and oxygenated pulmonary venous blood mix completely in the heart, resulting in equal oxygen saturations in the pulmonary artery and aorta. If there is no obstruction to pulmonary blood flow, these infants present with a combination of cyanosis and heart failure. In contrast, if pulmonary stenosis is present, these infants present with cyanosis alone, similar to patients with tetralogy of Fallot.

CHAPTER 220

General Principles of Treatment of Congenital Heart Disease

(Nelson Textbook, Chapter 441)

Most patients who have mild congenital heart disease require no treatment. Even patients with moderate to severe heart disease need not be markedly restricted in physical activities. Physical education should be modified appropriately to the child's capacity to participate. This can usually be accomplished best by exercise testing. Competitive sports for most of these patients should be discouraged. Patients with severe heart disease and decreased exercise tolerance usually tend to limit their own activities. Dyspnea, headache, and fatigability in cyanotic patients may be a sign of increasing hypoxemia and may require some limitation of activities among those for whom specific medical or surgical treatment is not available.

Bacterial infections should be treated vigorously, but the presence of congenital heart disease is not an appropriate reason to use antibiotics indiscriminately. Prophylaxis against infective endocarditis should be carried out during dental procedures, during instrumentation of the urinary tract, and before lower gastrointestinal tract manipulation.

Cyanotic patients need to be monitored for a multitude of noncardiac manifestations of oxygen deficiency. Treatment of iron deficiency anemia is important in cyanotic patients who show improved exercise tolerance and general well-being with adequate hemoglobin levels. These patients should also be carefully observed for excessive polycythemia. Cyanotic patients should avoid situations in which dehydration may occur, which leads to increased viscosity and increases the risk of stroke. Diuretics may need to be decreased or temporarily discontinued during episodes of acute gastroenteritis. High altitudes and sudden changes in thermal environment should also be avoided. Patients with severe congenital heart disease or a history of rhythm disturbance should be carefully monitored during anesthesia for even routine surgical procedures. Pregnancy may be extremely dangerous for patients with chronic cyanosis or pulmonary artery hypertension, or both.

POSTOPERATIVE MANAGEMENT. Immediate postoperative care should be provided in an intensive care unit staffed by a team of physicians, nurses, and technicians experienced with the unique problems encountered after open heart surgery. *Respiratory failure* is a major postoperative complication encountered after open heart surgery.

The electrocardiogram should be monitored continuously during the postoperative period. A change in the heart rate may be the first indication of a serious complication, such as hemorrhage, hypothermia, hypoventilation, or heart failure. *Cardiac rhythm disorders* must be diagnosed quickly because a prolonged untreated arrhythmia may add a severe hemodynamic burden to the heart in the critical early postoperative period. Injury to the heart's conduction system during surgery can cause postoperative *complete heart block.*

Heart failure with poor cardiac output following cardiac surgery may be secondary to respiratory failure, serious arrhythmias, myocardial injury, blood loss, hypervolemia or hypovolemia, or a significant residual hemodynamic abnormality. Treatment specific to the cause should be instituted. *Acidosis* secondary to low cardiac output, renal failure, or hypovolemia must be prevented or promptly corrected. *Kidney function* may be compromised by congestive heart failure and further impaired by prolonged cardiopulmonary bypass. Blood and fluid replacement, cardiac inotropic agents, and sometimes vasodilators will usually reestablish normal urine flow in patients with hypovolemia or cardiac failure.

The *postpericardiotomy syndrome* may occur toward the end of the first postoperative week or sometimes be delayed until weeks or months after operation. This febrile illness is characterized by pericarditis and pleurisy, decreased appetite, nausea, and vomiting. In most instances it is self-limiting and associated with a benign course. *Infection* is another potential postoperative problem. Patients usually receive a broad-spectrum antibiotic for the initial postoperative period.

SECTION 4

Cardiac Arrhythmias

CHAPTER 221

Disturbances of Rate and Rhythm of the Heart

(Nelson Textbook, Chapter 442)

Pediatric arrhythmias may be transient or permanent; congenital (in a structurally normal or abnormal heart) or acquired (rheumatic fever, myocarditis); or caused by a toxin (diphtheria), cocaine, or theophylline or by proarrhythmic or antiarrhythmic drugs; or they may be a sequela of surgical correction of congenital heart disease. The major risk of any arrhythmia is either severe tachycardia or bradycardia leading to decreased cardiac output or degeneration into a more severe arrhythmia, for example, ventricular fibrillation. These complications may lead to syncope, which itself can be dangerous under certain circumstances (e.g., swimming, driving), or to sudden death. When a patient has an arrhythmia, one of the major management issues is to determine whether the particular rhythm is prone to deteriorate into a life-threatening tachyarrhythmia or bradyarrhythmia. Some rhythm abnormalities, such as single premature atrial and ventricular beats, are common among children without heart disease and in the great majority of instances do not pose a risk to the patient.

The majority of rhythm disturbances in children can be reliably controlled with a single pharmacologic agent. For patients with tachyarrhythmias that are resistant to medical therapy, transcatheter radiofrequency ablation or surgical intervention is available. For patients with bradyarrhythmias, implantable pacemakers are small enough for use in premature infants. Automatic implantable cardioverter-defibrillators (AICDs) are available for use in high-risk patients with malignant ventricular arrhythmias.

Section 5

Acquired Heart Disease

Chapter 222

Infective Endocarditis
(Nelson Textbook, Chapter 443)

Infective endocarditis includes acute and subacute bacterial endocarditis as well as nonbacterial endocarditis caused by viruses, fungi, and other microbiologic agents. It is a significant cause of morbidity and mortality among children and adolescents despite advances in the management and prophylaxis of the disease with antimicrobial agents.

CLINICAL MANIFESTATIONS (Table 222–1). The early symptoms and signs are usually mild, especially when *Streptococcus viridans* is the infecting organism. Prolonged fever, without other manifestations (except occasionally weight loss) and persisting for as long as several months, may often be the only medical history. Alternatively, the onset may be acute and severe, with high, intermittent fever and prostration. Usually the onset and course vary between these two extremes. The symptoms are often nonspecific. New or changing heart murmurs are common. Splenomegaly and petechiae are relatively common. Many of the classic skin manifestations develop late in the course of the disease.

LABORATORY DIAGNOSIS. The critical information for appropriate treatment of infective endocarditis is obtained from blood cultures.

TREATMENT. Antibiotic therapy should be instituted immediately on diagnosis. Treatment for 4–6 wk is recommended.

PREVENTION. Antimicrobial prophylaxis before various procedures, including dental cleaning and other forms of dental manipulation, reduces the incidence of infective endocarditis in susceptible patients.

TABLE 222–1 Manifestations of Infective Endocarditis

History

Prior congenital or rheumatic heart disease
Preceding dental, urinary tract, or intestinal procedure
Intravenous drug use
Central venous catheter
Prosthetic heart valve

Symptoms

Fever
Chills
Chest and abdominal pain
Arthralgia, myalgia
Dyspnea
Malaise
Night sweats
Weight loss
CNS manifestations (stroke, seizures, headache)

Signs

Elevated temperature
Tachycardia
Embolic phenomena (Roth spots, petechiae, splinter nailbed hemorrhages, Osler
  nodes, CNS or ocular lesions)
Janeway lesions
New or changing murmur
Splenomegaly
Arthritis
Heart failure
Arrhythmias
Metastatic infection (arthritis, meningitis, mycotic arterial aneurysm, pericarditis,
  abscesses, septic pulmonary emboli)
Clubbing

Laboratory

Positive blood culture result
Elevated erythrocyte sedimentation rate; may be low with heart or renal failure
Elevated C-reactive protein
Anemia
Leukocytosis
Immune complexes
Hypergammaglobulinemia
Hypocomplementemia
Cryoglobulinemia
Rheumatoid factor
Hematuria
Renal failure: azotemia, high creatinine (glomerulonephritis)
Echocardiographic evidence of valve vegetations, prosthetic valve dysfunction or
  leak, or myocardial abscess

CNS = central nervous system.

CHAPTER 223

Rheumatic Heart Disease

(Nelson Textbook, Chapter 444)

Rheumatic involvement of the valves and endocardium is the most important manifestation of rheumatic fever. The mitral valve is affected most often, followed in frequency by the aortic valve.

MITRAL INSUFFICIENCY

CLINICAL MANIFESTATIONS. The physical signs of mitral insufficiency depend on its severity. With mild disease, signs of heart failure are not present, the precordium is quiet, and auscultation reveals a high-pitched holosystolic murmur at the apex, radiating to the axilla. With severe mitral insufficiency, signs of chronic heart failure may be noted. The heart is enlarged, with a heaving apical left ventricular impulse and often an apical systolic thrill. The second heart sound may be accentuated if pulmonary hypertension is present. A third heart sound is usually prominent. A holosystolic murmur is heard at the apex radiating to the axilla. A short mid-diastolic rumbling murmur is caused by increased blood flow across the mitral valve as a result of the insufficiency.

The electrocardiogram and radiographs are normal if the lesion is mild. With more severe insufficiency, the electrocardiogram shows prominent bifid P waves, signs of left ventricular hypertrophy, and associated right ventricular hypertrophy if pulmonary hypertension is present. Radiographically, there is prominence of the left atrium and ventricle.

TREATMENT. In patients with mild mitral insufficiency, prophylaxis against recurrences of rheumatic fever is all that is required. Surgical treatment is indicated in patients who, despite adequate medical therapy, have recurrent episodes of heart failure, dyspnea with moderate activity, and progressive cardiomegaly, often with pulmonary hypertension.

MITRAL STENOSIS

CLINICAL MANIFESTATIONS. Generally, there is a good correlation between symptoms and the severity of obstruction. Patients with mild lesions are asymptomatic. More severe degrees of obstruction are associated with exercise intolerance and dyspnea. Critical lesions can result in orthopnea, paroxysmal nocturnal dyspnea, and overt pulmonary edema as well as atrial arrhythmias. In mild disease, the heart size is normal; however, moderate cardiomegaly is usual with severe mitral stenosis. Cardiac enlargement can be massive when atrial fibrillation and heart failure supervene. The principal auscultatory findings are a loud first heart sound, an opening snap of the mitral valve, and a long, low-pitched, rumbling mitral diastolic murmur with presystolic accentuation at the apex. In the presence of pulmonary hypertension, the pulmonic component of the second heart sound is accentuated. Electrocardiograms and radiographs are normal if the lesion is mild; as the severity increases, there are prominent and notched P waves and varying degrees of right ventricular hypertrophy.

TREATMENT. Surgical or balloon catheter mitral valvotomy generally yields good results; valve replacement is avoided unless absolutely necessary.

AORTIC INSUFFICIENCY

Combined mitral and aortic insufficiency are more common than aortic involvement alone.

CLINICAL MANIFESTATIONS. Symptoms are unusual except in severe aortic insufficiency. The pulse pressure is wide, with bounding peripheral pulses. The systolic blood pressure is elevated, and the diastolic pressure is lowered. In severe aortic insufficiency, the heart is enlarged and there is a left ventricular apical heave. The typical murmur begins immediately with the second heart sound and continues until late in diastole. The murmur is heard over the upper and middle left sternal border, with radiation to the apex and to the aortic area. Characteristically, it has a high-pitched blowing quality and is easily audible in full expiration, with the diaphragm of the stethoscope placed firmly on the chest and the patient leaning forward. A systolic ejection murmur is frequent because of the increased stroke volume.

Radiographs show enlargement of the left ventricle and aorta. The electrocardiogram may be normal but in advanced cases reveals signs of left ventricular hypertrophy and strain with prominent P waves. The echocardiogram shows a large left ventricle and diastolic mitral valve flutter or oscillation caused by regurgitant flow hitting the valve leaflets.

SECTION 6

Disease of the Myocardium and Pericardium

(Nelson Textbook, Chapters 445–447)

CHAPTER 224

Disease of the Myocardium

(Nelson Textbook, Chapter 445)

DILATED CARDIOMYOPATHY

ETIOLOGY. The cause in the vast majority of pediatric cases is unknown *(idiopathic dilated cardiomyopathy).*

CLINICAL MANIFESTATIONS. All age groups may be affected. Usually the onset is insidious, but sometimes symptoms of heart failure occur suddenly. Irritability, anorexia, abdominal pain, cough due to pulmonary congestion, and dyspnea with exertion are common. When the disease is fully established, the skin is cool and pale, the arterial pulse is decreased, the pulse pressure is narrow, and tachycardia is present. The heart is enlarged, and holosystolic murmurs of mitral and tricuspid insufficiency may be present. A summation gallop rhythm is usually audible.

LABORATORY DIAGNOSIS. The electrocardiogram shows a combination of atrial enlargement, varying degrees of left ventricular hypertrophy, and nonspecific T-wave abnormalities. The radiograph confirms the cardiomegaly.

PROGNOSIS AND MANAGEMENT. The course of the disease is usually progressively downhill, although some patients may remain stable for years. Vigorous treatment of heart failure may result in a temporary remission, but relapses are common, and in time patients tend to become resistant to therapy. When medical therapy fails, heart transplantation has been used in infants and children with dilated cardiomyopathy.

HYPERTROPHIC CARDIOMYOPATHY

EPIDEMIOLOGY. Hypertrophic cardiomyopathy is most often inherited in an autosomal dominant pattern with a wide variability in penetrance.

CLINICAL MANIFESTATIONS. Many children are asymptomatic, and about 50% of cases are first evaluated because of either a heart murmur or an affected family member. In others, the clinical pattern is dominated by weakness, fatigue, dyspnea on effort, palpitations, angina pectoris, dizziness, and syncope. There is risk of sudden death even in asymptomatic children. The pulse is brisk because of the early systolic ejection of blood from the ventricle. There is a prominent left ventricular lift and double apical impulse. The systolic murmur is ejection in type and of medium intensity; it is heard maximally at the left sternal edge and apex.

TREATMENT. There is no standardized therapy. Competitive sports and strenuous physical activity should be discouraged because most sudden deaths occur after physical exertion. Patients with arrhythmias should be treated aggressively.

MYOCARDITIS

Myocarditis refers to inflammation, necrosis, or myocytolysis that may be caused by many infectious, connective tissue, granulomatous, toxic, or idiopathic processes affecting the myocardium with or without associated systemic manifestations of the disease process or involvement of the endocardium or pericardium.

CLINICAL MANIFESTATIONS. The presentation depends on the patient's age and the acute or chronic nature of the infection. The neonate may present with fever, severe heart failure, respiratory distress, cyanosis, distant heart sounds, weak pulses, tachycardia out of proportion to the fever, mitral insufficiency caused by dilatation of the valve annulus, a gallop rhythm, acidosis, and shock. In the most fulminant form, death may occur within 1–7 days of the onset of symptoms. The chest radiograph demonstrates an enormously enlarged heart and pulmonary edema; the electrocardiogram reveals sinus tachycardia, reduced QRS complex voltage, and ST segment and T-wave abnormalities. Arrhythmias may be the first clinical manifestation and in the presence of fever and a large heart strongly suggest acute myocarditis. The older patient with acute myocarditis may also present with acute congestive heart failure; however, more commonly patients present with the gradual onset of congestive heart failure or the sudden onset of ventricular arrhythmias. In these patients, the acute infectious phase has usually passed and an idiopathic dilated cardiomyopathy is present.

TREATMENT. The approach to treating acute myocarditis involves supportive measures for severe congestive heart failure. Arrhythmias should be treated aggressively. For infants and children having cardiogenic shock, extracorporeal membrane oxygenation may be indicated. In larger children and adolescents, implantation of a left ventricular assist device has been performed, usually as a bridge to the heart transplantation, which is the treatment of choice in patients with refractory heart failure.

Cardiac Therapeutics
(Nelson Textbook, Chapters 448 and 449)

CHAPTER 225

Heart Failure
(Nelson Textbook, Chapter 448)

CLINICAL MANIFESTATIONS. A critically ill infant or child who has exhausted the compensatory mechanisms to the point that cardiac output is no longer sufficient to meet the basal metabolic needs of the body is symptomatic at rest. Other patients may be comfortable when quiet but are incapable of increasing cardiac output in response to even mild activity without experiencing significant symptoms. The infant with heart failure often takes less volume per feeding, becomes dyspneic while sucking, and may perspire profusely. Eliciting a history of fatigue in an older child requires specific questions about activity.

In children, the signs and symptoms of heart failure are similar to those in adults and include fatigue, effort intolerance, anorexia, abdominal pain, and cough. Dyspnea is a reflection of pulmonary congestion. Elevation of systemic venous pressure may be gauged by clinical assessment of the jugular venous pressure and liver enlargement. Orthopnea and basilar rales may be present; edema is usually discernible in dependent portions of the body, or anasarca may be present. A gallop rhythm is common.

In infants, heart failure may be more difficult to identify. Prominent manifestations include tachypnea, feeding difficulties, poor weight gain, excessive perspiration, irritability, weak cry, and noisy, labored respirations with intercostal and subcostal retractions as well as flaring of the alae nasi. The signs of cardiac pulmonary congestion may be indistinguishable from those of bronchiolitis; wheezing is the most prominent finding. Pneumonitis with or without atelectasis is common, especially of the right middle and lower lobes; it is due to bronchial compression by the enlarged heart. Hepatomegaly usually occurs, and cardiomegaly is invariably present. In spite of pronounced tachycardia, a gallop rhythm can frequently be recognized. Edema may be generalized, usually involving the eyelids as well as the sacrum and less often the legs and feet.

LABORATORY DIAGNOSIS. Radiographs of the chest show cardiac enlargement. Echocardiographic techniques are useful in assessing ventricular function. The most commonly used parameter is the fractional shortening, determined as the difference between end-systolic and end-diastolic diameters divided by the end-diastolic diameter.

TREATMENT. The underlying cause of cardiac failure must be removed or alleviated if possible.

General Measures. Strict bed rest is rarely necessary except in extreme cases, but it is important that the child rest often and sleep adequately.

Diet. Increasing daily calories is an important aspect of management. Severely ill infants may lack sufficient strength for effective sucking because of extreme fatigue, rapid respirations, and generalized weakness. In these circumstances, nasogastric feeding may be helpful.

Digitalis. Digoxin is the digitalis glycoside used most often in the pediatric patient. *Rapid digitalization* of infants and children in heart failure may be carried out intravenously. The dose depends on the patient's age. The recommended schedule is to give one half of the total digitalizing dose immediately and the succeeding 2 one-quarter doses at 12-hr intervals later. *Maintenance digitalis* therapy is started approximately 12 hr after full digitalization. The daily dosage is divided in two and given at 12-hr intervals for more consistent blood levels and more flexibility in case of toxicity. The dosage is one quarter of the total digitalizing dose. *Patients who are not critically ill* may be given digitalis initially by the oral route, and in most instances digitalization is completed within 24 hr.

Diuretics. Diuretics are most often used in conjunction with digitalis therapy in patients with severe congestive heart failure. Furosemide is the most commonly used diuretic in patients with heart failure.

Afterload-Reducing Agents. This group of drugs reduces ventricular afterload by decreasing peripheral vascular resistance, thereby improving myocardial performance. Afterload reducers are especially useful in children with heart failure secondary to cardiomyopathy and in patients with severe mitral or aortic insufficiency.

SECTION 8

Disease of the Peripheral Vascular System

(Nelson Textbook, Chapters 450 and 451)

CHAPTER 226

Systemic Hypertension

(Nelson Textbook, Chapter 451)

In infants and younger children, systemic hypertension is uncommon, and when present it is usually indicative of an underlying disease process *(secondary hypertension)*. Older children and particularly adolescents may acquire *primary* or *essential hypertension* (with no underlying cause); hypertension may track into adulthood.

CLINICAL MANIFESTATIONS. Children and adolescents with essential hypertension are usually asymptomatic; the blood pressure elevation is usually mild and is detected during a routine examination or evaluation before athletic participation. These children may have mild to moderate obesity. Children with secondary hypertension can have blood pressure elevations ranging from mild to severe. Unless the pressure has been sustained or is rising rapidly, hypertension does not usually produce symptoms. Therefore, clinical manifestations of the underlying disease, such as growth failure in children with chronic renal disease, are the most frequent reasons for detecting the hypertension. With substantial hypertension, however, headache, dizziness, epistaxis, anorexia, visual changes, and seizures may occur. Hypertensive encephalopathy is suggested by the presence of vomiting, temperature elevation, ataxia, stupor, and seizures. Young children and infants with unexplained heart failure or seizures should have their blood pressure measured.

TREATMENT. Adolescents with essential hypertension are usually best managed initially with *nonpharmacologic* therapy. Intervention should focus on the risk factors that were cited as important in prevention. Because many patients with mild elevation of pressure are obese, weight reduction may result in a 5–10 mm Hg reduction in systolic pressure. A reduction in sodium intake often lowers pressure by a similar amount. A consistent program of aerobic exercise also has been noted to reduce blood pressure in patients with mild essential hypertension.

A number of antihypertensive drugs are available for both hypertensive emergencies and chronic therapy. In most *hypertensive emergencies*, the drugs of choice are intravenous labetalol or nitroprusside or sublingual nifedipine. In selecting a drug regimen for long-term use, an understanding of the underlying pathophysiology is helpful. Young patients with essential hypertension who require drug therapy may be treated initially with a diuretic or a β-blocking agent. Patients with volume-dependent hypertension usually have an adequate response to diuretics; those with high-renin, high cardiac output physiology respond best to β-blockers. If the pressure is not lowered adequately, a calcium channel blocker may be added to the diuretic and an angiotensin-converting enzyme inhibitor may replace the β-blocker.

PART 19

Disease of the Blood

CHAPTER 227

The Anemias

(Nelson Textbook, Chapter 453)

Anemia is defined as a reduction of the red blood cell (RBC) volume of hemoglobin concentration below the range of values occurring in healthy persons. Although a reduction in the amount of circulating hemoglobin decreases the oxygen-carrying capacity of the blood, few clinical disturbances occur until the hemoglobin level falls below 7–8 g/dL. Below this level, pallor becomes evident in the skin and in the mucous membranes. A useful classification of the anemias of childhood divides them into three groups by the RBC mean corpuscular volume: microcytic, macrocytic, or normocytic. Table 227–1 classifies the important anemias of childhood by the mean corpuscular volume.

TABLE 227–1 Classification of Anemia

Microcytic

Iron deficiency
Thalassemias
Lead poisoning
Chronic disease
  Infection
  Cancer
  Inflammation
  Renal disease
Vitamin B_6 responsive
Copper deficiency
Sideroblastic (some)

Normocytic

Decreased production
  Aplastic anemia
    Congenital
    Acquired

Table continued on following page

TABLE 227–1 Classification of Anemia *Continued*

Normocytic (Continued)

Pure RBC aplasia
  Congenital (Diamond-Blackfan)
  Acquired (transient erythroblastopenia)
Bone marrow replacement
  Leukemia
  Tumors
  Storage diseases
  Osteopetrosis
  Myelofibrosis
Blood loss
  Internal or external
Sequestration
Hemolysis: Intrinsic RBC abnormalities
  Hemoglobinopathies
  Enzymopathies
  Membrane disorders
    Hereditary spherocytosis
    Acquired: paroxysmal nocturnal hemoglobinuria
Hemolysis: Extrinsic RBC abnormalities
  Immunologic
    Passive (hemolytic disease of the newborn)
    Active: Autoimmune
  Toxins
  Infections
  Microangiopathic
    Disseminated intravascular coagulation (DIC)
    Hemolytic uremic syndrome
    Hypertension
    Cardiac disease

Macrocytic

Normal newborn (spurious)
Reticulocytosis (spurious)
Vitamin B_{12} deficiency
Folate deficiency
Oroticaciduria
Myelodysplasia
Liver disease
Hypothyroidism (some)
Vitamin B_6 deficiency (some)
Thiamine deficiency

Anemias of Inadequate Production

(Nelson Textbook, Chapters 454–462)

CHAPTER 228

Physiologic Anemia of Infancy

(Nelson Textbook, Chapter 459)

Normal newborns have higher hemoglobin and hematocrit levels with larger red blood cells (RBCs) than older children and adults. Within the first week of life, a progressive decline in hemoglobin level begins and persists for 6–8 wk. The result of this decline is generally referred to as *physiologic anemia of infancy*. When the hemoglobin level has fallen to 9–11 g/dL at 2–3 mo of age in full-term infants, erythropoiesis resumes. This "anemia" should be viewed as a physiologic adaptation to extrauterine life.

Premature infants also develop a physiologic anemia. The same factors are operative as in term infants, but they are exaggerated. The decline in hemoglobin level is both more extreme and more rapid. Minimal hemoglobin levels of 7–9 g/dL commonly occur by 3–6 wk of age, and in very small premature infants levels may be even lower.

The marginal erythropoietic equilibrium responsible for physiologic anemia can add to anemia-accompanying processes with increased hemolysis, such as congenital hemolytic states, which may be associated with severe anemia in the early weeks of life. Dietary factors may also aggravate physiologic anemia. Deficiency of folic acid superimposed on the physiologic process may result in more severe anemia.

TREATMENT. Physiologic anemia usually requires no therapy other than ensuring that the diet of the infant contains essential nutrients for normal hematopoiesis, especially folic acid and iron. Premature infants who are feeding well and growing normally rarely need transfusion unless iatrogenic blood loss has been significant. In otherwise healthy premature infants, hemoglobin levels as low as 6.5 g/dL are usually well tolerated. When transfusions are necessary, a volume of RBCs of 10–15 mL/kg is recommended.

Chapter 229

Megaloblastic Anemias

(Nelson Textbook, Chapter 460)

The megaloblastic anemias have in common certain abnormalities of red blood cell (RBC) morphology and maturation. The RBCs at every stage of development are larger than normal and have an open, finely dispersed nuclear chromatin and an asynchrony between maturation of nucleus and cytoplasm, with the delay in nuclear progression being more evident with further cell divisions.

MEGALOBLASTIC ANEMIA OF INFANCY

This disease is caused by a deficient intake or absorption of folic acid.

CLINICAL MANIFESTATIONS. Mild megaloblastic anemia has been reported in very-low-birth-weight infants, and routine folic acid supplementation is advised. Megaloblastic anemia has its peak incidence at 4–7 mo of age, somewhat earlier than iron deficiency anemia, although the two may be present concomitantly in infants with poor nutrition. Besides having the usual clinical features of anemia, affected infants with folate deficiency are irritable, fail to gain weight adequately, and have chronic diarrhea.

LABORATORY FINDINGS. The anemia is macrocytic (mean corpuscular volume > 100 fL). Variations in RBC shape and size are common. The reticulocyte count is low, and nucleated RBCs demonstrating megaloblastic morphology are often seen in the blood. Neutropenia and thrombocytopenia may be present, particularly in infants with long-standing deficiencies.

TREATMENT. When the diagnosis is established or in severely ill children, folic acid may be administered orally or parenterally in a dose of 1–5 mg/24 hr.

Chapter 230

Iron Deficiency Anemia

(Nelson Textbook, Chapter 461)

Anemia resulting from lack of sufficient iron for synthesis of hemoglobin is the most common hematologic disease of infancy and childhood.

CLINICAL MANIFESTATIONS. Pallor is the most important clue to iron deficiency. Blue scleras are also common, although they are also found in normal infants. In mild to moderate iron deficiency (hemoglobin levels of 6–10 g/dL), compensatory mechanisms may be so effective that few symptoms of anemia are noted, although affected children may be irritable. Pagophagia, the desire to ingest unusual substances such as ice or dirt, may be present. In some children, ingestion of lead-containing substances may lead to concomitant plumbism. When the hemoglobin level falls below 5 g/dL, irritability and anorexia are prominent. Tachycardia and cardiac dilation occur, and systolic murmurs are often present.

LABORATORY FINDINGS. In progressive iron deficiency, a sequence of biochemical and hematologic events occurs. First, the tissue iron stores represented by bone marrow hemosiderin disappear. The level of serum ferritin, an iron-storage protein, provides a relatively accurate estimate of body iron stores in the absence of inflammatory disease. Normal ranges are age dependent, and decreased levels accompany iron deficiency. Next, serum iron level decreases (also age dependent), the iron-binding capacity of the serum increases, and the percent saturation falls below normal (also varies with age). When the availability of iron becomes rate limiting for hemoglobin synthesis, a moderate accumulation of heme precursors, free erythrocyte protoporphyrins, results. As the deficiency progresses, the RBCs become smaller than normal and their hemoglobin content decreases. With increasing deficiency, the RBCs become deformed and misshapen and present characteristic microcytosis, hypochromia, poikilocytosis, and increased RBC distribution width.

TREATMENT. The regular response of iron deficiency anemia to adequate amounts of iron is an important diagnostic and therapeutic feature. Oral administration of simple ferrous salts (sulfate, gluconate, fumarate) provides inexpensive and satisfactory therapy. A daily total of 6 mg/kg of elemental iron in 3 divided doses provides an optimal amount of iron for the stimulated bone marrow to use. While adequate iron medication is given, the family must be educated about the patient's diet, and the consumption of milk should be limited to a reasonable quantity, preferably 500 mL (1 pint)/24 hr or less. Within 72–96 hr after administration of iron to an anemic child, peripheral reticulocytosis is noted. Reticulocytosis is followed by a rise in the hemoglobin level. Because a rapid hematologic response can be confidently predicted in typical iron deficiency, blood transfusion is indicated only when the anemia is very severe or when superimposed infection may interfere with the response.

Hemolytic Anemias

(Nelson Textbook, Chapters 463–471)

CHAPTER 231

Definitions and Classifications of Hemolytic Anemias

(Nelson Textbook, Chapter 463)

Hemolysis is defined as the premature destruction of red blood cells (RBCs). If the rate of destruction exceeds the capacity of the marrow to produce RBCs, anemia results. During hemolysis, RBC survival is shortened, and increased marrow activity results in a heightened reticulocyte percentage and number. Hemolysis should be suspected as a cause of anemia if an elevated reticulocyte count is present in the absence of bleeding or administration of hematinic therapy. The hematocrit during hemolysis is dependent on the severity of the hemolysis and on the marrow response in producing RBCs.

The hemolytic anemias may be classified as either (1) cellular, resulting from intrinsic abnormalities of the membrane, enzymes, or hemoglobin, or (2) extracellular, resulting from antibodies, mechanical factors, or plasma factors. Most of the cellular defects are inherited (paroxysmal nocturnal hemoglobinuria is acquired), and most of the extracellular defects are acquired (abetalipoproteinemia with acanthocytosis is inherited).

CHAPTER 232

Hereditary Spherocytosis

(Nelson Textbook, Chapter 464)

Hereditary spherocytosis is a common cause of hemolysis and hemolytic anemia.

CLINICAL MANIFESTATIONS. Hereditary spherocytosis may be a cause of hemolytic disease in the newborn and may present as anemia and hyperbilirubinemia sufficiently severe to require phototherapy or exchange transfusions. Some children remain asymptomatic into adulthood, but others may have severe anemia with pallor, jaundice, fatigue, and exercise intolerance. After infancy, the spleen is usually enlarged, and pigmentary (bilirubin) gallstones may form as early as age 4–5 yr. Because of the high red blood cell (RBC) turnover and heightened erythroid marrow activity, children with hereditary spherocytosis are susceptible to aplastic crisis, primarily as a result of parvovirus, and to hypoplastic crises associated with various other infections.

LABORATORY FINDINGS. Evidence for hemolysis includes reticulocytosis and hyperbilirubinemia. The hemoglobin level usually is 6–10 g/dL, but it can be in the normal range. The reticulocyte count often is heightened to 6–20%, with a mean of approximately 10%. The mean corpuscular volume is normal, whereas the mean corpuscular hemoglobin concentration often is increased (36–38 g/dL RBCs). The RBCs on the blood film vary in size and include polychromatophilic reticulocytes and spherocytes. The spherocytes are smaller in diameter and on the blood film are hyperchromic as a result of the high hemoglobin concentration.

TREATMENT. Because the spherocytes in hereditary spherocytosis are destroyed almost exclusively in the spleen, splenectomy eliminates most of the hemolysis associated with this disorder. For patients with more severe anemia and reticulocytosis or those with hypoplastic or aplastic crises, poor growth, or cardiomegaly, splenectomy is recommended after age 5–6 yr to avoid the heightened risk of postsplenectomy sepsis in younger children.

Chapter 233

Hemoglobin Disorders

(Nelson Textbook, Chapter 468)

The hemoglobin disorders are subdivided into three major groups. The *structural abnormalities*, including the hemoglobinopathies, result from changes in the amino acid sequences of the globin chains. Most have a single amino acid substitution; in others, however, amino acids may be deleted or inserted, or other, more complex structural changes may be present. The *thalassemias* are expressed as quantitative defects, in which the synthesis of one or more of the globin chains is decreased or, in the most severe forms, is totally suppressed. The *hereditary persistence of fetal hemoglobin (HPFH) syndromes* is characterized by elevated levels of Hb F continuing throughout adult life. Almost all these abnormalities result from the same types of molecular defect: nucleotides may be substituted, deleted, or inserted into globin-gene DNA.

SICKLE CELL ANEMIA

This disorder (homozygous Hb S) is characterized by severe, chronic hemolytic disease resulting from premature destruction of the brittle, poorly deformable red blood cells (RBCs).

CLINICAL MANIFESTATIONS. Affected newborns seldom exhibit clinical features of sickle cell disease; hemolytic anemia gradually develops over the first 2–4 mo, paralleling the replacement of much of the fetal hemoglobin by Hb S. Clinical manifestations are uncommon before 5–6 mo of age. Acute sickle dactylitis, presenting as the *hand-foot syndrome*, is frequently the first overt evidence that sickle cell disease is present in an infant. Its associated findings include painful, usually symmetric swelling of the hands and feet.

Acute, painful episodes represent the most frequent and prominent manifestation of sickle cell disease. Most patients experience some pain on a nearly daily basis. Episodes of severe pain that require hospitalization and parenteral analgesic administration average about 1/yr in children with Hb SS, but this interval varies considerably. More extensive vaso-occlusive events in these patients can produce gross ischemic damage. Splenic infarcts are common in children, causing pain and contributing to the process of "autosplenectomy." Pulmonary infarction, often occurring in association with pneumonitis or microscopic fat emboli (from bone marrow infarction), may produce the severe clinical picture of acute chest syndrome. Strokes caused by cerebrovascular occlusion are among the most catastrophic acute events and are a frequent cause of hemiplegia.

Young children with Hb SS may have splenic enlargement associated with their hemolytic disease, with progression to the syndrome of *hypersplenism* accompanied by worsening anemia and sometimes thrombocytopenia. Acute splenic sequestration is a distinct and episodic event that occurs in infants and young children with sickle cell anemia, often following an acute febrile illness. Altered splenic function in young children with sickle cell disease is a significant factor leading to their increased susceptibility to meningitis, sepsis, and other serious infections. In common with patients having other forms of chronic hemolytic anemia, children with Hb SS are at risk of developing a rapid, potentially life-threatening decrease in their hemoglobin level (aplastic episodes) in association with parvovirus B19 infection.

LABORATORY FINDINGS. Hemoglobin concentrations usually range from 5–9 g/dL. The peripheral blood smear typically contains target cells, poikilocytes, and irreversibly sickled cells.

DIAGNOSIS. The diagnosis is normally established by hemoglobin electrophoresis.

TREATMENT. Maintaining full immunization status is particularly important. Prophylactic penicillin is highly effective in preventing serious pneumococcal infections and should be administered to all young children with sickle cell disease. They should also receive conjugate pneumococcal vaccine. Parents of children with Hb SS need to be aware of the need to bring the child promptly to medical attention for acute illness, especially for a temperature exceeding 38.5°C (101.3°F) regardless of the use of prophylaxis. Parents and caretakers of these children should also be informed about the manifestations of acute splenic sequestration and the need for immediate medical attention for a child with rapid splenic enlargement and pallor.

Painful episodes can frequently be managed with oral acetaminophen, alone or with codeine. More severe episodes may require hospitalization and parenteral administration of narcotics. Dehydration or acidosis should be rapidly corrected by the intravenous route, but overhydration should be avoided. For patients with disabling chronic pain, for those with ischemic organ damage (acute chest, priapism) or stroke, or in preparation for major surgery, however, transfusions of normal RBCs can provide symptomatic relief and prevent further ischemic complications. A first stroke may be prevented by transfusion of children with sickle cell disease and abnormal results of transcranial Doppler ultrasonography.

Bone marrow transplantation from a normal donor can be curative in patients with sickle cell disease, but the risks and morbidity associated with this procedure limit its application to highly selected patients.

THALASSEMIA SYNDROMES

The thalassemias are a heterogeneous group of heritable hypochromic anemias of various degrees of severity.

Homozygous β-Thalassemia (Cooley Anemia, Thalassemia Major)

CLINICAL MANIFESTATIONS. Homozygous β-thalassemia usually becomes symptomatic as a severe, progressive hemolytic anemia during the second 6 mo of life. Regular blood transfusions are necessary in these patients to prevent the profound weakness and cardiac decompensation caused by the anemia. Without transfusion, life expectancy is no more than a few years. In untreated cases or in those receiving infrequent transfusions at times of severe anemia, hypertrophy of erythropoietic tissue occurs in medullary and extramedullary locations. The bones become thin, and pathologic fractures may occur. Massive expansion of the marrow of the face and skull produces characteristic facies. Pallor, hemosiderosis, and jaundice combine to produce a greenish brown complexion. The spleen and liver are enlarged by extramedullary hematopoiesis and hemosiderosis. Growth is impaired in older children; puberty is delayed or absent because of secondary endocrine abnormalities. Diabetes mellitus resulting from pancreatic siderosis may also occur. Cardiac complications, including intractable arrhythmias and chronic congestive failure caused by myocardial siderosis, have been common terminal events.

LABORATORY FINDINGS. In addition to severe hypochromia and microcytosis, many bizarre, fragmented poikilocytes and target cells are present. Large numbers of nucleated RBCs circulate, especially after splenectomy. The hemoglobin level falls progressively to lower than 5 g/dL unless transfusions are given. The unconjugated serum bilirubin level is elevated. The serum iron level is high, with saturation of the transferrin. A striking feature is the presence of very high levels of Hb F in the RBCs.

TREATMENT. Transfusions are given on a regular basis to maintain the hemoglobin level above 10 g/dL. *Hemosiderosis* is an inevitable consequence of prolonged transfusion therapy. Bone marrow transplantation is curative in these patients and has been performed with increasing success, even in patients who have been transfused extensively.

Section 4

Polycythemia (Erythrocytosis)

(Nelson Textbook, Chapters 472 and 473)

Chapter 234

Secondary Polycythemia

(Nelson Textbook, Chapter 473)

The differential diagnosis of secondary polycythemia is shown in Table 234–1. Clinical findings usually include cyanosis, hyperemia of the scleras and mucous membranes, and clubbing of the fingers. As the hematocrit rises above 65%, clinical manifestations of hyperviscosity, such as headache and hypertension, may require phlebotomy. On the other hand, the increased demand for red blood cell production may cause iron deficiency. Periodic phlebotomies may prevent or decrease symptoms. Apheresed blood should be replace with plasma or saline to prevent hypovolemia in patients accustomed to a chronically elevated total blood volume.

TABLE 234–1 Differential Diagnosis of Polycythemia

Primary (Polycythemia Vera)

Secondary

Neonatal
  Normal intrauterine environment
  Twin-twin or maternal-fetal hemorrhage
  Infants of diabetic mothers
  Intrauterine growth retardation
  Trisomies 13, 18, or 21
  Adrenal hyperplasia
  Thyrotoxicosis
Hypoxia
  Altitude
  Cardiac disease
  Lung disease
  Central hypoventilation
Hemoglobinopathy
  High oxygen affinity variants
  Methemoglobin reductase deficiency
  Chronic carbon monoxide exposure
Hormonal
  Malignant tumors
    Renal, hepatic, adrenal, cerebellar, other
  Renal disease
    Cysts, hydronephrosis
  Adrenal disease
    Virilizing hyperplasia, Cushing syndrome
  Anabolic steroid therapy
Familial

Spurious (Plasma Volume Decrease)

The Pancytopenias
(Nelson Textbook, Chapters 474–480)

CHAPTER 235

The Constitutional Pancytopenias
(Nelson Textbook, Chapter 474)

ETIOLOGY. Although Fanconi anemia is the best recognized constitutional pancytopenia, a number of other infrequent genetic disorders have also been implicated.

CLINICAL MANIFESTATIONS. Various physical abnormalities accompany most of the congenital pancytopenias, particularly Fanconi anemia and dyskeratosis congenita. Patients having Fanconi anemia are characterized by hyperpigmentation and café-au-lait spots, skeletal abnormalities (especially absent or hypoplastic thumbs), short stature, and a wide array of integumentary and organ abnormalities. Dyskeratosis congenita is also very commonly associated with hyperpigmentation as well as nail dystrophy of both the hands and feet, leukoplakia, and a number of ocular abnormalities, including epiphora, blepharitis, and cataracts.

LABORATORY FINDINGS. Depending on the specific disorder, thrombocytopenia, leukopenia, lymphopenia, or anemia generally precedes the onset of pancytopenia. Children with Fanconi anemia and dyskeratosis congenita generally have macrocytosis as well as mild poikilocytosis and anisocytosis, and their red blood cells contain higher levels of i antigen and hemoglobin F than are found in acquired aplasia.

TREATMENT. The traditional backbone of therapy for patients with congenital anemias has been corticosteroids and androgens (especially oxymetholone or nandrolone), alone or in combination. These therapies have been shown to prolong life by approximately 2 yr and hence can be considered palliative only. The only "curative" therapy to date has been bone marrow transplantation. However, patients with congenital pancytopenias also have an increased predisposition to malignancy, and the preparative regimens generally used during bone marrow transplantation can adversely affect this susceptibility. Encouraging results have been reported when granulocyte-macrophage colony-stimulating factor was administered subcutaneously to children with Fanconi anemia and pancytopenia.

CHAPTER 236

The Acquired Pancytopenias

(Nelson Textbook, Chapter 475)

ETIOLOGY AND EPIDEMIOLOGY. Various drugs, chemicals, toxins, infectious agents, radiation, or immune disorders can result in pancytopenia, either by direct destruction of hematopoietic progenitors, by disruption or destruction of the supporting marrow microenvironment and its necessary growth factors, or by direct or indirect (e.g., virus-related) immune-mediated destruction of marrow elements.

CLINICAL MANIFESTATIONS, LABORATORY FINDINGS, AND DIFFERENTIAL DIAGNOSIS. Acquired pancytopenia is usually characterized by anemia, leukopenia, and thrombocytopenia in the setting of elevated serum cytosine levels. The pancytopenia results in increased risks of fatigue, cardiac failure, infection, and bleeding. Other treatable disorders, such as cancer, collagen vascular disorders, paroxysmal nocturnal hemoglobinuria, or infections that may respond to specific therapies, should be considered in the differential diagnosis. In children, the possibility of a congenital pancytopenia must always be considered and chromosomal breakage should be evaluated. The presence of fetal hemoglobin suggests a congenital pancytopenia but is not diagnostic.

TREATMENT. As with congenital pancytopenias, the treatment of the children with acquired pancytopenia requires comprehensive supportive care coupled with an attempt to treat the underlying marrow failure. For patients with a matched sibling donor, allogeneic bone marrow transplantation offers a 45–70% chance of long-term survival.

Hemorrhagic and Thrombotic Diseases

(Nelson Textbook, Chapters 481–490)

CHAPTER 237

Hemostasis

(Nelson Textbook, Chapter 481)

THE CLINICAL AND LABORATORY EVALUATION

HISTORY. For most hemostatic disorders, whether they be hemorrhagic or thrombotic, the clinical history provides the most useful information.

PHYSICAL EXAMINATION. The physical examination should focus on whether symptoms are primarily associated with the mucous membranes or skin (mucocutaneous bleeding) or the muscles and joints (deep bleeding). The examination should determine the presence of petechiae, ecchymoses, hematomas, hemarthroses, or mucous membrane bleeding. Patients with defects in platelet/blood vessel wall interaction (von Willebrand disease or platelet function defects) usually have mucous membrane bleeding (epistaxis, menorrhagia, hematuria, gastrointestinal bleeding); petechiae on the skin and mucous membranes; and small, ecchymotic lesions of the skin sometimes associated with hematomas. Individuals with a clotting factor deficiency such as factor VIII or factor IX deficiency have symptoms of deep bleeding into muscles and joints with much more extensive ecchymoses and hematoma formation. Patients with mild von Willebrand disease or other mild bleeding disorders may have no abnormal findings on physical examination.

LABORATORY TESTS. Patients who have a positive bleeding history or are actively hemorrhaging should have a platelet count, bleeding time, partial thromboplastin time, and prothrombin time (PT). If these are normal, a thrombin time and von Willebrand factor testing should be considered. In individuals with abnormal screening tests, further specific factor workup should be undertaken. In a patient with an abnormal bleeding history and a positive family history, normal screening tests should not preclude further laboratory evaluation.

There are no effective routine screening tests for hereditary thrombotic disorders. If the family history is positive or the clinical thrombosis is unexplained, specific anticoagulant assays should be undertaken. Thrombosis is rare in children, and, when present, the possibility of a hereditary predisposition must be considered and evaluated in the laboratory.

Bleeding Time. The bleeding time assesses the function of platelets and their interaction with the vascular wall.

Platelet Count. The platelet count is essential in the evaluation of the child with a positive bleeding history because thrombocytopenia is the most common acquired cause of a bleeding diathesis in children. Patients with a platelet count above 50,000/mm³ rarely have significant clinical bleeding.

"Activated" Partial Thromboplastin Time (PTT). This test measures the initiation of clotting at the level of factor XII through sequential steps to the final clot endpoint. It does not measure factor VII, factor XIII, or anticoagulants.

Prothrombin Time. The PT measures the extrinsic clotting system after the activation of clotting by tissue factor (thromboplastin) in the presence of calcium. It is not prolonged with deficiencies of factors VIII, IX, XI, or XII. In most laboratories the normal PT ranges between 10 and 13 sec.

Thrombin Time. The thrombin time measures the final step of the clotting cascade, in which fibrinogen is converted to fibrin. The normal thrombin time varies between laboratories but is usually between 11 and 15 sec. Prolongation of the thrombin time occurs with reduced fibrinogen levels (hypofibrinogenemia or afibrinogenemia), with dysfunctional fibrinogen (dysfibrinogenemia), or by substances that interfere with fibrin polymerization such as heparin or fibrin split products.

HEMOSTASIS IN THE NEWBORN. The normal newborn has a reduced level of most procoagulants and anticoagulants. This renders the newborn at simultaneous increased risk for both hemorrhage and thrombosis.

CHAPTER 238

Hereditary Clotting Factor Deficiencies (Bleeding Disorders)

(Nelson Textbook, Chapter 482)

FACTOR VIII OR FACTOR IX DEFICIENCY (HEMOPHILIA A OR B)

Factor VIII and factor IX deficiencies are the most common severe, inherited bleeding disorders.

CLINICAL MANIFESTATIONS. Neither factor VIII nor factor IX crosses the placenta; thus, bleeding symptoms may be present from birth or occur in the fetus. Occasionally, neonates with hemophilia may sustain intracranial hemorrhage. Surprisingly, only about

30% of affected male infants with hemophilia bleed with circumcision. Thus, if the family history does not alert the physician to be suspicious of its presence, hemophilia may go undiagnosed in the newborn. It is only when a child begins to crawl and walk that mobility causes the initiation of easy bruising, intramuscular hematomas, and hemarthroses. Bleeding from minor traumatic lacerations of the mouth may persist for hours or days and may cause the parents to seek medical evaluation. Even in patients with severe hemophilia, only 90% have evidence of increased bleeding by 1 yr of age. Although bleeding may occur in any area of the body, the hallmark of hemophilia is the hemarthrosis. Whereas most muscular hemorrhages are visible, iliopsoas bleeding requires specific mention. Patients may lose large volumes of blood into the iliopsoas muscle and verge on hypovolemic shock, with only a vague area of referred pain in the groin.

Life-threatening bleeding in the hemophilic patient is caused by bleeding into vital structures (central nervous system, upper airway) or by exsanguination (external, gastrointestinal, or iliopsoas hemorrhage). Prompt treatment with clotting factor concentrate for these life-threatening hemorrhages is imperative. Patients with mild hemophilia who have factor VIII activities greater than 5% usually do not have spontaneous hemorrhaging.

LABORATORY FINDINGS. In severe hemophilia, the activated partial thromboplastin time is usually 2 to 3 times the upper limits of normal. The other screening tests of the hemostatic mechanism (platelet count, bleeding time, prothrombin time, and thrombin time) are normal. The specific assay for factor VIII and factor IX will confirm the diagnosis of hemophilia.

TREATMENT. The prevention of trauma is important to the care of the child with hemophilia, but bleeding may occur in the absence of trauma. Early psychosocial intervention helps the family achieve a balance between overprotection and permissiveness. Aspirin and other nonsteroidal anti-inflammatory drugs that affect platelet function should be avoided by patients with hemophilia.

REPLACEMENT THERAPY. When bleeding occurs, the factor VIII level must be raised to hemostatic levels (35–40%) or for life-threatening or major hemorrhages to 100% (100 U/dL). With mild factor VIII hemophilia, the patient's endogenously produced factor VIII can be released by the administration of desmopressin acetate (DDAVP). DDAVP is not effective in the treatment of factor IX–deficient hemophilia B.

CHRONIC COMPLICATIONS. The long-term complications of hemophilia A and B include chronic joint destruction, the risk of transfusion-transmitted infectious diseases, and the development of an inhibitor to either factor VIII or factor IX.

von Willebrand Disease

(Nelson Textbook, Chapter 483)

Von Willebrand disease is the most common hereditary bleeding disorder.

CLINICAL MANIFESTATIONS. Patients with von Willebrand disease usually have symptoms of mucocutaneous hemorrhage, including excessive bruising, epistaxis, menorrhagia, and postoperative hemorrhage, particularly after mucosal surgery such as tonsillectomy or wisdom tooth extraction. In patients with type 3 or homozygous von Willebrand disease, bleeding symptoms are much more profound.

LABORATORY FINDINGS. Patients with von Willebrand disease are said to have a long bleeding time and a long partial thromboplastin time. These tests are not universally prolonged except in patients with type 3 von Willebrand disease. Therefore, normal screening tests do not preclude the diagnosis of von Willebrand disease. If the history is suggestive of a bleeding disorder, von Willebrand testing must be undertaken, including a quantitative assay for von Willebrand factor (vWf) antigen, vWf activity (ristocetin cofactor activity, or vWf R:Co), and plasma factor VIII activity, determination of vWf structure (vWf multimers), and a platelet count.

TREATMENT. Treatment of von Willebrand disease is directed toward increasing the plasma level of vWf and factor VIII. Because the gene for factor VIII is normal in patients with von Willebrand disease, elevating the plasma concentration of vWf will permit the normal recovery and survival of the endogenously produced factor VIII. The most common form of von Willebrand disease is type 1. In these patients the synthetic drug desmopressin (DDAVP) induces the release of vWf from the endothelial cells.

CHAPTER 240

Hereditary Predisposition to Thrombosis

(Nelson Textbook, Chapter 484)

PATHOPHYSIOLOGY AND CLINICAL MANIFESTATIONS. The major causes of hereditary predisposition to thrombosis include deficiencies of protein C, protein S, plasminogen, and antithrombin III and, more commonly, mutations of the genes for factor V and prothrombin. The hereditary mutation of factor V, termed *factor V Leiden,* results in a factor V molecule that, when activated, is not

547

subsequently inactivated by activated protein C. This leaves the patient with unregulated "active" factor V. Children with these hereditary mutations have an increased frequency of venous thrombosis. Adolescents may have recurrent abortions. Whereas patients with heterozygous deficiencies may be predisposed to thrombosis, those with *homozygous protein C deficiency* have fatal purpura fulminans in the neonatal period if untreated. The physiologic deficiency of protein C in the newborn coupled with true sepsis may also lead to nearly undetectable levels of protein C.

LABORATORY FINDINGS. There are no screening tests for hereditary deficiencies of anticoagulants such as protein C, protein S, antithrombin III, or factor V Leiden and prothrombin 20210; thus, specific testing is required. A careful family history is perhaps the most productive investigation and often reveals thromboembolic diseases in family members at a young age. If hereditary deficiency of anticoagulant or regulatory proteins is suspected, specific assays should be undertaken.

TREATMENT. Homozygous deficiency of protein C presents as purpura fulminans in the first few hours of life. Because no licensed protein C concentrate is currently available, fresh frozen plasma (FFP) is the only immediately available source of protein C. Amelioration of symptoms usually requires 10–15 mL/kg of FFP every 8–12 hr. When the infant is beyond the neonatal period, high-dose warfarin (to achieve an INR of 4–5) may prevent most of the thrombotic problems, but acute intermittent thromboses require additional FFP or protein C concentrate.

CHAPTER 241

Disseminated Intravascular Coagulation (Consumptive Coagulopathy)

(Nelson Textbook, Chapter 489)

Consumption coagulopathy refers to a large group of conditions, including disseminated intravascular coagulation (DIC). Consequences of this process include widespread intravascular deposition of fibrin, which may lead to tissue ischemia and necrosis, a generalized hemorrhagic state, and hemolytic anemia.

CLINICAL MANIFESTATIONS. Most frequently, DIC accompanies a severe systemic disease process. Bleeding frequently first occurs from sites of venipuncture or surgical incision. The skin may show petechiae and ecchymoses. Tissue necrosis may involve many organs and can be most spectacularly seen as infarction of large areas of skin, subcutaneous tissue, or kidneys. Anemia caused by hemolysis may develop rapidly owing to a microangio-pathic hemolytic process.

LABORATORY FINDINGS. There is no well-defined sequence of events. The consumption coagulation factors (II, V, VIII, and fibrinogen) and platelets may be consumed by the ongoing intravascular clotting process, with prolongation of the prothrombin, partial thromboplastin, and thrombin times. Platelet counts may be profoundly depressed. The blood smear may contain fragmented, burr, and helmet-shaped red blood cells (schizocytes). In addition, because the fibrinolytic mechanism is activated, fibrinogen degradation products (FDPs) appear in the blood. The D-dimer assay is equally sensitive and more specific for DIC than the FDP test. The D-dimer is formed by fibrinolysis of a cross-linked fibrin clot.

TREATMENT. The most important component of therapy is control or reversal of the process that initiated the DIC. Infection, shock, acidosis, and hypoxia must be treated promptly and vigorously. Blood components are used for replacement therapy in patients who have hemorrhage. In some patients the treatment of the primary disease may be inadequate or incomplete, or the replacement therapy may not be effective in controlling the hemorrhage. When this occurs the DIC may be treated with heparin to prevent ongoing consumption of factors. Because administering heparin to patients with a deficiency of both clotting factors and platelets may result in profound hemorrhage, the heparin is usually started together with clotting factor and platelet replacement.

CHAPTER 242

Disorder of the Platelets and the Blood Vessels

(Nelson Textbook, Chapter 490)

IDIOPATHIC THROMBOCYTOPENIC PURPURA

The most common cause of acute onset of thrombocytopenia in an otherwise well child is (autoimmune) idiopathic thrombocytopenic purpura (ITP).

CLINICAL MANIFESTATIONS. The classic presentation of ITP is that of a perfectly healthy 1- to 4-yr-old child who has the sudden onset of generalized petechiae and purpura. Often there is bleeding from the gums and mucous membrane, particularly with profound thrombocytopenia (platelet count $< 10 \times 10^9/L$). There is a history of a preceding viral infection 1–4 wk before onset of the thrombocytopenia. Results of the physical examination are normal other than the finding of petechiae and purpura. Seventy to 80 percent of children who present with acute ITP will have spontaneous resolution of their ITP within 6 mo. Therapy does not appear to affect the natural history of the illness. Nevertheless, the objective of early therapy is to raise the platelet count to more than $20 \times 10^9/L$ and prevent the rare development of intracranial hemorrhage. Ten to 20 percent of children who present with acute thrombotic thrombocytopenic purpura go on to develop chronic ITP.

LABORATORY FINDINGS. Severe thrombocytopenia (platelet count $< 20 \times 10^9/L$) is common, and platelet size is normal or increased, reflective of increased platelet turnover. In acute ITP, the hemoglobin, white blood cell count, and differential should be normal.

TREATMENT. There are no data that treatment affects either short- or long-term clinical outcome of ITP. Initial treatment options include the following:

1. *Intravenous immunoglobulin* (IVIG) in a dose of 0.8 to 1 g/kg/day × 1–2 days induces a rapid rise in platelet count (usually $> 20 \times 10^9/L$) in 95% of patients within 48 hr.

2. *Prednisone* in doses of 1–4 mg/kg/24 hr appears to induce a more rapid rise in platelet counts than in untreated patients with ITP.

SECTION 7

The Spleen and Lymphatic System

(Nelson Textbook, Chapters 491–496)

CHAPTER 243

Splenomegaly

(Nelson Textbook, Chapter 492)

CLINICAL MANIFESTATION. A soft, thin spleen may be palpable in 15% of neonates, 10% of normal children, and 5% of adolescents. However, in most individuals, the spleen must be two to three times its normal size before it is palpable. Superficial abdominal venous distention may be present when splenomegaly is a result of portal hypertension.

TABLE 243–1 Common Causes of Splenomegaly

Infections

Bacterial: typhoid fever, endocarditis, septicemia, abscess
Viral: Epstein-Barr, cytomegalovirus, and others
Protozoal: malaria, toxoplasmosis

Hematologic Processes

Hemolytic anemia: congenital, acquired
Extramedullary hematopoiesis: thalassemia, osteopetrosis, myelofibrosis

Neoplasms

Malignant: leukemia, lymphoma, metastatic disease
Benign: hemangioma, hamartoma

Infiltration and Storage Diseases

Lipidoses: Niemann-Pick, Gaucher diseases
Mucopolysaccharidosis infiltration: histiocytosis

Congestion

Cirrhosis or hepatic fibrosis
Hepatic portal or splenic vein obstruction
Congestive heart failure

Cysts

Congenital (true cysts)
Acquired (pseudocysts)

Miscellaneous

Lupus erythematosus, sarcoidosis, rheumatoid arthritis

DIFFERENTIAL DIAGNOSIS. Specific causes of splenomegaly are listed in Table 243–1.

CHAPTER 244

Lymphadenopathy

(Nelson Textbook, Chapter 239)

Generalized adenopathy (enlargement of more than two non-contiguous node regions) is due to systemic disease (Table 244–1) and is often accompanied by abnormal physical findings in other systems. In contrast, localized adenopathy is most frequently due to infection in the involved node or its drainage area.

TABLE 244-1 Common Causes of Generalized Lymphadenopathy

Infections

Typhoid fever, tuberculosis, acquired immunodeficiency syndrome, mononucleosis, cytomegalovirus, rubella, varicella, rubeola, histoplasmosis, toxoplasmosis, other

Autoimmune Diseases

Rheumatoid arthritis, lupus erythematosus, dermatomyositis

Malignancies

Primary: Hodgkin disease, non-Hodgkin lymphoma, histiocytic disorders
Metastatic: leukemia, neuroblastoma, rhabdomyosarcoma, other

Lipid Storage Diseases

Gaucher disease, Niemann-Pick disease

Drug Reactions

Other

Sarcoidosis, serum sickness

PART 20

Neoplastic Disease and Tumors

(Nelson Textbook, Chapters 497–515)

CHAPTER 245

Principles of Diagnosis

(Nelson Textbook, Chapter 500)

The majority of childhood cancers are curable. The prognosis relates most strongly to tumor type, extent of disease at diagnosis, and effectiveness of the treatment. Rapid diagnosis helps to ensure that the appropriate therapy is given in a timely fashion and hence optimizes the chances of cure. Because most physicians in general practice rarely encounter children with cancer, they should be alert for an atypical course of a common childhood condition (Table 245–1). When a malignant neoplasm is suspected, the immediate goal is to determine its nature and extent. A thorough search for metastatic disease usually precedes biopsy of a suspicious lesion. Central to diagnosis of any tumor is histologic examination.

TABLE 245–1 Common Manifestations of Childhood Malignancy

Sign/Symptom	Nonmalignant Condition Mimicked
Hematologic	
Pallor, anemia	Iron-deficiency anemia, blood loss
Petechiae, thrombocytopenia	Idiopathic thrombocytopenic purpura
Fever, pharyngitis, neutropenia	Streptococcal/viral pharyngitis
Systemic	
Bone pain, limp, arthralgia	Osteomyelitis, rheumatologic disease, trauma
Fever of unknown origin, weight loss, night sweats	Collagen vascular disease, chronic infection
Painless lymphadenopathy	Epstein-Barr virus, cytomegalovirus
Cutaneous lesion	Abscess, trauma
Abdominal mass	Organomegaly, hydronephrosis, constipation
Hypertension	Renovascular disease, nephritis
Diarrhea	Inflammatory bowel disease
Soft tissue mass	Abscess
Vaginal bleeding	Foreign body, coagulopathy
Emesis, visual disturbances, ataxia, headache, papilledema	Migraine
Chronic ear discharge	Otitis media

Table continued on following page

TABLE 245–1 Common Manifestations of Childhood Malignancy
Continued

Sign/Symptom	Nonmalignant Condition Mimicked
Ophthalmologic Signs	
Leukocoria	Cataract, glaucoma
Periorbital ecchymosis	Trauma
Miosis, ptosis, heterochromia	Third nerve paresis
Opsoclonus/ataxia	Drug reaction
Exophthalmos, proptosis	Graves disease
Thoracic Mass	
Anterior mediastinal	Infection (tuberculosis), lymphadenopathy, sarcoidosis
Posterior mediastinal	Esophageal disease

Modified from Behrman R, Kliegman R (eds): Nelson Essentials of Pediatrics, 2nd ed. Philadelphia, WB Saunders, 1994.

CHAPTER 246

Principles of Treatment

(Nelson Textbook, Chapter 501)

Treatment of children with cancer is complex, requiring the expertise of teams of specialized health care providers. The best chance for cure exists during the initial course of treatment; patients should be referred to an appropriate specialized center as soon as possible when the diagnosis of cancer is suspected.

Whenever possible, treatment is given on an outpatient basis. Children should remain at home and in school as much as possible throughout treatment. The intensity of many treatment regimens is such that some patients miss a considerable amount of school in the first year after diagnosis. Tutoring should be encouraged so children do not fall behind; counseling should be provided as appropriate.

Local therapy with surgery or irradiation or both is an important component of treatment for most solid tumors, but systemic multiagent chemotherapy is usually necessary because tumor dissemination is generally present, even if undetectable.

CHEMOTHERAPY

Traditional drugs for treatment of cancer are selected from several classes of agents, including hormones, antimetabolites, antibiotics, plant alkaloids, and alkylating agents. Most of these agents can produce cytotoxicity to both malignant and normal cells. The increased metabolic and cell cycle activity of malignant cells makes them more susceptible to the cytotoxic effects of chemotherapy.

ACUTE COMPLICATIONS AND SUPPORTIVE CARE

Early complications of therapy include metabolic disorders, bone marrow suppression, and immunosuppression. Patients with a large tumor burden may have had substantial breakdown of tumor cells; renal function can be impaired by tubular precipitates of uric acid crystals. Symptomatic hyperkalemia and hyperphosphatemia with subsequent hypocalcemia develop in the setting of inadequate renal function.

Tumors that invade and replace bone marrow can cause pancytopenia; all chemotherapy regimens can produce *myelosuppression*. Anemia can be corrected by transfusions of packed red blood cells, and thrombocytopenia can be corrected by platelet infusions. Patients receiving immunosuppressive therapy should receive irradiated blood products to prevent graft versus host disease. Febrile granulocytopenic patients should be hospitalized and treated with empirical broad-spectrum intravenous antimicrobial therapy pending the results of appropriate cultures of blood, urine, or any obvious sites of infection. Patients should not be given live virus vaccines.

It is common for patients undergoing cancer therapy to lose 10% or more of their body weight. If oral supplementation proves inadequate, patients may require enteral tube feedings or parenteral hyperalimentation.

LATE SEQUELAE

Late consequences of therapy (Table 246–1) can cause significant morbidity. Successful surgical resection may require the sacrifice of important functional structures. Irradiation can produce irreversible organ damage. Chemotherapy also carries the risk of long-lasting organ damage. Perhaps the most serious late effect is the occurrence of second cancers in patients successfully cured of a first malignancy.

BONE MARROW TRANSPLANT

In some malignancies and certain other disease states, use of bone marrow or peripheral blood stem cells (PBSCs) together with chemotherapy given at very high doses, with or without irradiation, may provide lifesaving treatment. If the source of stem cells used is the patient, the transplant is termed *autologous*. Syngeneic stem cells are obtained from an identical twin. If the stem cells are from a nonidentical individual, the transplant is termed *allogeneic*. For neoplastic diseases that can be effectively

TABLE 246–1 Long-Term Sequelae of Cancer Therapy

Problem	Etiology
Infertility	Alkylating agents; radiation
Second cancers	Genetic predisposition; radiation, alkylating agents
Sepsis	Splenectomy
Hepatotoxicity	Methotrexate, 6-mercaptopurine, radiation
Amputation	Surgery for osteogenic sarcoma
Scoliosis	Radiation, surgery
Pulmonary (pneumonia, fibrosis)	Radiation, bleomycin, busulfan, nitrosoureas
Cardiomyopathy	Doxorubicin, daunomycin; radiation
Leukoencephalopathy	Cranial irradiation ± methotrexate
Impaired cognition/intelligence	Cranial irradiation ± methotrexate
Pituitary dysfunction (isolated growth hormone deficiency, panhypopituitary)	Cranial irradiation
Hypothyroidism	Neck irradiation

treated with high-dose chemotherapy followed by autologous transplantation, autologous PBSCs have become the most widely used source of hematopoietic stem cells. *Autologous stem cell transplantation* is used for various high-risk chemotherapy-responsive neoplastic diseases, including many of the common childhood cancers that are known to be at high risk of treatment failure with standard therapy because of previous relapse or initial extent of disease. *Allogeneic transplantation* remains a high morbidity and mortality procedure.

PALLIATIVE CARE

For a minority of children with cancer, the disease is lethal. At all stages of caring for children with cancer, particularly dying patients, principles of palliative care should be applied to relieve pain and suffering and to provide comfort.

CHAPTER 247

The Leukemias
(Nelson Textbook, Chapter 502)

Leukemias, the most common childhood cancers, account for about one third of pediatric malignancies. Acute lymphoblastic leukemia (ALL) represents about 75% of all cases in children and has a peak incidence at age 4 yr. Acute myeloid leukemia (AML) accounts for about 20% of leukemias, with an incidence that is stable from birth through age 10 and increases slightly during the teenage years. Most of the remaining leukemias are of the chronic myeloid form; chronic lymphoid leukemia rarely affects children.

ACUTE LYMPHOBLASTIC LEUKEMIA

Childhood ALL was the first form of disseminated cancer shown to be curable with chemotherapy and irradiation.

CLINICAL MANIFESTATIONS. About two thirds of children with ALL have had signs and symptoms of their disease for less than 4 wk at the time of diagnosis. The first symptoms are usually nonspecific and may include anorexia, irritability, and lethargy. Patients may have a history of viral respiratory infection or exanthem from which they have not appeared to recover fully. Progressive bone marrow failure leads to pallor, bleeding, petechiae, and fever—the features that usually prompt diagnostic studies. Lymphadenopathy is occasionally prominent; splenomegaly is found in about 60% of patients, whereas hepatomegaly is less common.

DIAGNOSIS. On initial examination, most patients have anemia, although only about 25% have hemoglobin levels below 6 g/dL. Most patients also have thrombocytopenia, but as many as 25% have platelet counts greater than 100,000/mm³. About half of the patients have white blood cell (WBC) counts less than 10,000/mm³, and about 20% have counts greater than 50,000/mm³. The diagnosis of leukemia is suggested by the presence of blast cells on a peripheral blood smear but is confirmed by examination of bone marrow, which is usually completely replaced by leukemic lymphoblasts.

TREATMENT. Contemporary treatment of ALL is based on clinical risk. In general, patients with a standard or average risk of relapse are between the ages of 1 and 10 yr, have a WBC count under 100,000/mm³, lack evidence of a mediastinal mass or central nervous system leukemia, and have a B-progenitor cell immunophenotype. The treatment program for standard-risk patients includes administration of induction chemotherapy until the bone marrow no longer shows morphologically identifiable leukemic cells, "prophylactic" treatment of the central nervous system, and continuation of chemotherapy. A combination of prednisone, vincristine, and asparaginase produces remission in about 98% of children with standard-risk ALL within 4 wk. Consolidation and intensification phases of therapy using several chemotherapeutic agents are often given after the induction of remission to produce further rapid reduction in leukemic cell number and improve ultimate outcome. Systemic continuation therapy includes the antimetabolites methotrexate and 6-mercaptopurine plus vincristine and prednisone, which should be given for 2 to 3 yr.

RELAPSE. The bone marrow is the most common site of relapse, although any site can be affected. In most centers, bone marrow is examined at infrequent intervals to confirm continued remission. If bone marrow relapse is detected, intensive retrieval therapy that includes drugs not used previously may achieve cures in 15–20% of patients, especially those who have had a long first remission (>18 mo).

PROGNOSIS. The overall cure rate for childhood ALL is estimated at about 80%.

ACUTE MYELOID LEUKEMIA

CLINICAL MANIFESTATIONS. AML may present with signs and symptoms related to anemia, thrombocytopenia, or neutropenia. Children may present with fatigue and pallor or heart failure secondary to anemia. Bruising, petechiae, epistaxis, or gum bleeding secondary to thrombocytopenia may be presenting manifestations, as may fever secondary to infection associated with neutropenia. Patients sometimes have hepatic or splenic enlargement, lymphadenopathy, or gum hypertrophy. A localized mass of leukemic cells, known as a chloroma, may herald the onset of AML.

DIAGNOSIS. The diagnosis of AML requires demonstration of greater than 25% myeloblasts in the bone marrow.

TREATMENT. With aggressive initial induction regimens containing an anthracycline and cytarabine with or without other agents, remission can be achieved in 80% or more of patients. About 10% of patients die early (i.e., during induction therapy) as a result of induction failure, overwhelming infection, or hemorrhage.

CHAPTER 248

Lymphoma

(Nelson Textbook, Chapter 503)

Lymphoma is the third most common cancer in children in the United States.

HODGKIN'S DISEASE

Hodgkin's disease accounts for about 5% of cancers in children and adolescents younger than 15 yr in the United States.

CLINICAL MANIFESTATIONS. Painless, firm, cervical or supraclavicular adenopathy is the most common presenting sign. Depending on the extent and location of nodal and extranodal disease, patients might present with symptoms and signs of airway obstruction, pleural or pericardial effusion, hepatocellular dysfunction, or bone marrow infiltration (anemia, neutropenia, or thrombocytopenia). Systemic symptoms considered important in staging are unexplained fever, weight loss, or drenching night sweats.

DIAGNOSIS. Any patient with persistent, unexplained adenopathy unassociated with an obvious underlying inflammatory or infectious process should have a chest radiograph to identify the presence of a mediastinal mass before undergoing node biopsy. Unless signs or symptoms dictate otherwise, additional laboratory studies can be delayed until the biopsy results are available.

TREATMENT. Multiagent chemotherapy is the cornerstone of treatment, supplemented in selected cases by relatively low-dose involved-field irradiation (2000–2500 cGy). Treatment is largely determined by the disease stage, the patient's age at diagnosis, the presence or absence of B "symptoms," and the presence of bulky nodal disease.

Early Stage Disease (Stages I, II, and IIIA). Cure rates with radiation alone (3500–4500 cGy) in *surgically staged* early-stage disease range from 40–80%, and the overwhelming majority of those who suffer relapse can be salvaged with a combination of multiagent chemotherapy or additional irradiation or both, resulting in cure rates of 90% or more. Unfortunately, this approach produces growth retardation in skeletally immature children and in some fully grown individuals and is associated with significant long-term morbidity, including thyroid failure, cardiac and pulmonary dysfunction, and an increased risk of breast cancer. For these reasons, many centers treating children and adolescents use combined modality therapy or even chemotherapy alone.

Advanced Disease (Stages IIIB and IV). Chemotherapy, based on the same regimens as used in early-stage disease, is considered the primary treatment for patients with advanced disease.

NON-HODGKIN'S LYMPHOMA

Non-Hodgkin's lymphoma (NHL) results from malignant clonal proliferation of lymphocytes of T-, B-, or indeterminate cell origin.

PATHOLOGY AND PATHOGENESIS. Most cases of NHL in children are high-grade, diffuse neoplasms. Three histologic subtypes are recognized: lymphoblastic (usually of T-cell origin); large cell (of T-, B-, or indeterminate cell origin); and small, noncleaved cell lymphoma (SNCCL, Burkitt's and non-Burkitt's subtypes, B-cell origin).

CLINICAL MANIFESTATIONS. Presenting signs and symptoms vary with disease site and extent, and these in turn correlate with histologic subtype. Lymphoblastic lymphoma often presents as an intrathoracic tumor (usually a mediastinal mass) with associated dyspnea, chest pain, dysphagia, pleural effusion, or superior vena cava syndrome. Cervical or axillary adenopathy is present in up to 80% of patients at diagnosis. SNCCL presents as an abdominal tumor in 80% of U.S. cases with abdominal pain or distention, bowel obstruction, change in bowel habits, intestinal bleeding, or, rarely, intestinal perforation. Large cell lymphomas occur in many sites, including the abdomen and mediastinum.

DIAGNOSIS AND STAGING. Prompt tissue diagnosis and staging is important because of the rapid growth rate of lymphomas, especially SNCCL.

TREATMENT AND PROGNOSIS. Surgical excision of localized intra-abdominal tumors often precedes the diagnosis of NHL. In this and other situations, multiagent chemotherapy is the primary treatment. Tumor lysis syndrome (i.e., high serum potassium, uric acid, and high phosphorus with low calcium levels) frequently complicates initial treatment of disseminated disease. NHL, unlike Hodgkin's disease, is considered a disseminated disease from the time of diagnosis. Even patients with limited-stage disease require chemotherapy.

CHAPTER 249

Neuroblastoma
(Nelson Textbook, Chapter 504)

Neuroblastoma, a common tumor of neural crest origin, demonstrates an extremely variable clinical presentation and biologic behavior.

CLINICAL PRESENTATION. Neuroblastoma may develop at any site of sympathetic nervous system tissue. Most tumors arise in the abdomen, either in the adrenal gland or in retroperitoneal sympathetic ganglia. About 30% of tumors arise in the cervical, thoracic, or pelvic ganglia. The signs and symptoms of neuroblastoma reflect the tumor site and extent of disease. Metastatic disease can be associated with myriad signs and symptoms, including fever, irritability, failure to thrive, bone pain, bluish subcutaneous nodules, orbital proptosis, and periorbital ecchymoses.

DIAGNOSIS AND STAGING. Neuroblastoma is generally discovered as a mass or multiple masses on plain radiographs, computed tomography, or magnetic resonance imaging. A pathologic diagnosis is made from tumor tissue obtained by biopsy. The International Neuroblastoma Staging System (INSS) is universally used. In the INSS, stage 1 includes tumors confined to the organ or structure of origin. Stage 2 tumors extend beyond the structure of origin but not across the midline, with (stage 2B) or without (stage 2A) ipsilateral lymph node involvement. Stage 3 tumors extend beyond the midline, with or without bilateral lymph node involvement. Stage 4 tumors are disseminated to distant sites (e.g., bone, bone marrow, liver, distant lymph nodes, other organs). The most important clinical and biologic prognostic factors

TABLE 249–1 Prognostic Factors in Neuroblastoma

	Three-Yr Survival		
	95%	*25–50%*	*<5%*
Age	<1 yr	>1 yr	1–5 yr
International Neuroblastoma Staging System	1, 2, 4S	3, 4	3, 4
MYCN	Normal	Normal	Amplified
Chromosome 1p depletion	<5%	25–50%	80–90%

Adapted from Brodeur GM, Maris JM, Yamashiro DJ, et al: Biology and genetics of human neuroblastomas. J Pediatr Hematol Oncol 19:93, 1997.

are the age of the patient at diagnosis, extent of tumor, *MYCN* status, and presence of 1p deletions in the tumor (Table 249–1).

TREATMENT. The respective roles of surgery, irradiation, and chemotherapy depend on the stage of the disease. In general, infants and children with early stage disease without *MYCN* amplification or 1p deletion can often be cured by surgery alone. Infants with more advanced disease require addition of chemotherapy (i.e., cisplatin, etoposide, vincristine, cyclophosphamide), as do older children.

CHAPTER **250**

Neoplasms of the Kidney

(Nelson Textbook, Chapter 505)

WILMS TUMOR

Wilms tumor accounts for most renal neoplasms in childhood. An important feature of Wilms tumor is its association with congenital anomalies, the most common being genitourinary anomalies (4.4%), hemihypertrophy (2.9%), and sporadic aniridia (1.1%).

CLINICAL MANIFESTATIONS. The median age at diagnosis of unilateral Wilms tumor is about 3 yr. The most frequent sign is an abdominal or flank mass, which is often asymptomatic. The mass is generally smooth and firm and rarely crosses the midline.

DIAGNOSIS. The major differential diagnostic consideration is neuroblastoma. The typical Wilms tumor arises from the kidney as an inhomogeneous mass with areas of low density indicating necrosis on computed tomography without contrast medium enhancement.

TREATMENT. The immediate treatment for unilateral tumors is surgical removal of the affected kidney through a flank incision even if pulmonary metastases are present. Combination chemotherapy with vincristine and dactinomycin is superior to single-agent therapy in localized disease, and doxorubicin is a significant addition to the treatment of advanced disease. For patients with advanced-stage disease who require irradiation in addition to surgery and chemotherapy, the dosage and fields have been modified to reduce the incidence of scoliosis.

PART 21

Nephrology

SECTION 1

Glomerular Disease

CHAPTER 251

Introduction to Glomerular Diseases
(Nelson Textbook, Chapter 516)

PATHOGENESIS. Glomerular injury may be a result of immunologic, inherited (presumably biochemical), or coagulation disorders. Immunologic injury is the most common cause and results in glomerulonephritis, which is both a generic term for several diseases and a histopathologic term signifying inflammation of the glomerular capillaries. There appear to be two major mechanisms of immunologic injury: (1) localization of circulating antigen-antibody immune complexes and (2) interaction of antibody with local antigen in situ.

In immune complex–mediated diseases, antibody is produced against and combines with a circulating antigen that is usually unrelated to the kidney. The immune complexes accumulate in glomeruli and activate the complement system, leading to immune injury. Experimental studies suggest that the complexes are formed in the circulation and deposited in the kidney.

An example of in situ antigen-antibody interaction is anti–glomerular membrane antibody disease, in which antibody reacts with antigen(s) of the glomerular basement membrane (GBM). Immunopathologic studies reveal linear deposition of immunoglobulin and complement on the GBM, similar to that in Goodpasture disease and certain types of rapidly progressive glomerulonephritis. The inflammatory reaction that follows immunologic injury results from activation of one or more mediator pathways. The most important of these is the complement system.

PATHOLOGY. The glomerulus may be injured by several mechanisms but has only a limited number of histopathologic responses; accordingly, different disease states may produce similar microscopic changes. Proliferation of glomerular cells occurs in most forms of glomerulonephritis and may be generalized, involving all glomeruli, or focal, involving only some glomeruli while sparing others. Crescent formation in the Bowman space (capsule) is a result of proliferation of parietal epithelial cells. In addition to proliferation, certain forms of acute glomerulonephritis show glomerular exudation of blood cells, most commonly neutrophils; eosinophils, basophils, and mononuclear cells may be seen in lesser numbers. The thickened appearance of the GBM may result from a true increase in the width of the membrane (as seen in membranous glomerulopathy). Sclerosis refers to the presence of scar tissue within the glomerulus.

Section 2

Conditions Particularly Associated with Hematuria

(Nelson Textbook, Chapters 517–530)

Chapter 252

Clinical Evaluation of the Child with Hematuria

(Nelson Textbook, Chapter 517)

Hematuria may be gross (visible to the naked eye) or microscopic (detected only by dipstick and confirmed by microscopic examination of the urine sediment). Gross hematuria may originate from the kidney, in which case it is generally brown or cola colored and may contain red blood cell (RBC) casts, or from the lower urinary tract (bladder and urethra), in which case the urine is red to pink and may contain clots. Gross hematuria may be associated with edema, hypertension, and renal insufficiency. The urine may be colored by pigments other than blood.

In children, microscopic hematuria is most commonly discovered at periodic health examinations, by dipstick or by microscopic examination of the urine sediment. A positive result of a dipstick test for blood indicates the need for a urinalysis. Microscopic hematuria is defined as more than 5 RBCs per high power field in the sediment from 10 mL of centrifuged freshly voided urine.

Causes of hematuria are listed in Table 252–1. Children with gross hematuria should be evaluated carefully because of the increased likelihood of finding hypertension and renal failure. Children having persistent microscopic hematuria (more than 5 RBCs per high power field on three urinalyses at monthly intervals) should undergo outpatient evaluation. In the evaluation of

TABLE 252–1 Causes of Hematuria in Children

Glomerular Diseases

Recurrent gross hematuria syndrome
  IgA nephropathy
  Idiopathic (benign familial)
  hematuria
  Alport syndrome
Acute poststreptococcal
  glomerulonephritis
Membranous glomerulopathy
Systemic lupus erythematosus
Membranoproliferative
  glomerulonephritis
Nephritis of chronic infection
Rapidly progressive
  glomerulonephritis
Goodpasture disease
Anaphylactoid purpura
Hemolytic-uremic syndrome

Infection

Bacterial
Tuberculosis
Viral

Hematologic

Coagulopathies
Thrombocytopenia
Sickle cell disease
Renal vein thrombosis

Stones and Hypercalciuria

Anatomic Abnormalities

Congenital anomalies
Trauma
Polycystic kidneys
Vascular abnormalities
Tumors

Exercise

Drugs

a child with hematuria, a thorough history and physical examination and screening laboratory tests may give clues to the cause of hematuria. Laboratory evaluation of a child with hematuria is done in steps, beginning with the studies most likely to reveal the etiology (Table 252–2).

TABLE 252–2 Evaluation of the Child with Hematuria

Step 1: Studies Performed on All Patients

Complete blood cell count
Urine culture
Serum creatinine level
24-hr urine collection for
  Creatinine
  Protein
  Calcium
Serum C3 level
Ultrasonography or intravenous pyelography

Step 2: Studies Performed on Selected Patients

DNase B titer or Streptozyme test if hematuria is of <6 mo duration
Skin or throat cultures when appropriate
Antinuclear antibody titer
Urine erythrocyte morphology
Coagulation studies/platelet count when suggested by history

Table continued on following page

TABLE 252–2 Evaluation of the Child with Hematuria *Continued*

Step 2: Studies Performed on Selected Patients (Continued)

Sickle cell screen in all black patients
Voiding cystourethrography with infection, or when a lower tract lesion is
    suspected

Step 3: Invasive Procedures

Renal biopsy indicated for
1. Persistent high-grade microscopic hematuria
2. Microscopic hematuria plus any of the following
    a. Diminished renal function
    b. Proteinuria exceeding 150 mg/24 hr (0.15 g/24 hr)
    c. Hypertension
3. Second episode of gross hematuria
Cystoscopy indicated for pink to red hematuria, dysuria, and sterile urine culture

CHAPTER 253

Recurrent Gross Hematuria

(Nelson Textbook, Chapter 518)

In patients having a syndrome of recurrent gross hematuria, recurrent episodes of generally painless hematuria occur (mild flank pain may be felt). The gross hematuria usually develops 1–2 days after the onset of a presumably viral upper respiratory tract infection. Patients with recurrent gross hematuria do not have manifestations of the acute nephritic syndrome (edema, hypertension, or renal insufficiency). Diseases causing recurrent gross hematuria may also present as persistent microscopic hematuria without episodes of gross hematuria.

In patients with recurrent gross hematuria, routine radiographic and laboratory studies may fail to reveal a cause of hematuria. The gross hematuria resolves over 1–2 wk, but microscopic hematuria usually persists. Later, with another respiratory infection, gross hematuria recurs. Renal biopsy is indicated after the second episode to determine the nature of any underlying disease, which most frequently is IgA nephropathy, idiopathic hematuria, or familial nephritis (Alport syndrome).

IgA NEPHROPATHY (BERGER NEPHROPATHY). Patients with this disorder have glomerulonephritis with IgA as the predominant immunoglobulin in mesangial deposits, in the absence of any systemic disease such as systemic lupus erythematosus or Henoch-Schönlein purpura.

Prognosis and Treatment. IgA nephropathy does not lead to significant kidney damage in most patients. Treatment is supportive, and activity need not be restricted. Progressive disease develops in 30% of patients.

CHAPTER 254

Gross or Microscopic Hematuria
(Nelson Textbook, Chapter 519)

ETIOLOGY AND EPIDEMIOLOGY. Acute poststreptococcal glomerulonephritis follows infection of the throat or skin with certain "nephritogenic" strains of group A β-hemolytic streptococci.

CLINICAL MANIFESTATIONS. The typical patient develops an acute nephritic syndrome 1–2 wk after an antecedent streptococcal infection. The severity of renal involvement may vary from asymptomatic microscopic hematuria with normal renal function to acute renal failure. Depending on the severity of renal involvement, patients may develop various degrees of edema, hypertension, and oliguria. Encephalopathy or heart failure due to hypertension or both may also develop. Nonspecific symptoms such as malaise, lethargy, abdominal or flank pain, and fever are common. The acute phase generally resolves within 2 mo after onset, but urinary abnormalities may persist for more than 1 yr.

DIAGNOSIS. Urinalysis demonstrates red blood cells (RBCs), frequently in association with RBC casts and proteinuria; polymorphonuclear leukocytes are common. A mild normochromic anemia may be present, owing to hemodilution and low-grade hemolysis. The serum C3 level is usually reduced.

Confirmation of the diagnosis requires clear evidence of invasive streptococcal skin infections. The best single antibody titer to measure is that to the deoxyribonuclease (DNase) B antigen.

TREATMENT. Because there is no specific therapy for acute poststreptococcal glomerulonephritis, the management is that of acute renal failure. Although a 10-day course of systemic antibiotic therapy, generally with penicillin, is recommended to limit the spread of the nephritogenic organisms, no evidence shows that antibiotic therapy affects the natural history of glomerulonephritis. Antihypertensive medications (diuretics, angiotensin-converting enzyme inhibitors) are indicated to treat hypertension and to avoid hypertensive complications.

CHAPTER 255

Hemolytic-Uremic Syndrome
(Nelson Textbook, Chapter 526)

The hemolytic-uremic syndrome is the most common cause of acute renal failure in young children; the incidence is increasing. The primary event in pathogenesis of the syndrome appears to be endothelial cell injury.

CLINICAL MANIFESTATIONS. The syndrome is most common in children younger than 4 yr. The onset is usually preceded by gastro-enteritis (fever, vomiting, abdominal pain, and diarrhea, which is often bloody) or, less commonly, by an upper respiratory tract infection. This is followed in 5–10 days by the sudden onset of pallor, irritability, weakness, lethargy, and oliguria. Physical examination may reveal dehydration, edema, petechiae, hepato-splenomegaly, and marked irritability.

DIAGNOSIS. The diagnosis is supported by the findings of mi-croangiopathic hemolytic anemia, thrombocytopenia, and acute renal failure. The hemoglobin level is commonly in the range of 5–9 g/dL. The blood film reveals helmet cells, burr cells, and fragmented red blood cells. Plasma hemoglobin levels are ele-vated, and plasma haptoglobin levels are diminished. The reticu-locyte count is moderately elevated.

PROGNOSIS AND TREATMENT. With aggressive management of the acute renal failure, more than 90% of patients survive the acute phase, and the majority of these recover normal renal function. Careful medical management of the hematologic and renal mani-festations, in conjunction with early and frequent peritoneal dial-ysis, offers the best chance of recovery from the acute phase.

SECTION 3

Conditions Particularly Associated with Proteinuria

(Nelson Textbook, Chapters 531–535)

CHAPTER 256

Nonpathologic Proteinuria

(Nelson Textbook, Chapter 532)

Protein may be found in the urine of healthy children. A reasonable upper limit of normal protein excretion in healthy children is 150 mg/24 hr (0.15 g/24 hr). Proteinuria in excess of 150 mg/24 hr (0.15 g/24 hr) may be divided into two categories (Table 256–1). In the first category, nonpathologic proteinuria, the excessive protein excretion is apparently not a result of a disease state. The level of proteinuria in this category is never associated with edema.

TABLE 256–1 Classification of Proteinuria

Nonpathologic Proteinuria

Postural (orthostatic)
Febrile
Exercise

Pathologic Proteinuria

Tubular
  Hereditary
  Cystinosis
  Wilson disease
  Lowe syndrome
  Proximal renal tubular acidosis
  Galactosemia
  Acquired
  Antibiotics
  Interstitial nephritis
  Acute tubular necrosis
  Cystic diseases
  Heavy metal poisoning (mercury, gold, lead, bismuth,
    cadmium, chromium, copper)
Glomerular
  Persistent asymptomatic
  Nephrotic syndrome
    Idiopathic nephrotic syndrome
      Minimal change
      Mesangial proliferation
      Focal sclerosis
    Glomerulonephritis
    Tumors
    Drugs
    Congenital

CHAPTER 257

Pathologic Proteinuria

(Nelson Textbook, Chapter 533)

The second category of proteinuria may result from glomerular or tubular disorders.

TUBULAR PROTEINURIA. Healthy individuals filter large amounts of proteins of lower molecular weight than albumin (lysozyme, light chains of immunoglobulin, β_2-microglobulin, insulin, growth hormone); these are normally reabsorbed in the proximal tubule. Injury to the proximal tubules results in diminished reabsorptive capacity and the loss of these low molecular weight proteins in the urine; such proteinuria rarely exceeds 1 g/24 hr; it is not associated with edema. Tubular proteinuria may be associated with other defects of proximal tubular function, such as glucosuria, phosphaturia, bicarbonate wasting, and aminoaciduria. Tubular proteinuria rarely presents a diagnostic dilemma because the underlying disease is usually detected before the proteinuria. In tubular proteinuria, the low-molecular-weight proteins migrate primarily in the α and β regions and little or no albumin is detected, whereas in glomerular proteinuria the major protein is albumin.

GLOMERULAR PROTEINURIA. The most common cause of proteinuria is increased permeability of the glomerular capillary wall. The amount of glomerular proteinuria may range from less than 1 to more than 30 g/24 hr. Glomerular proteinuria may be termed selective (loss of plasma proteins of molecular weight up to and including albumin) or nonselective (loss of albumin and of larger molecular weight proteins such as IgG). Most forms of glomerulonephritis are accompanied by nonselective proteinuria.

CHAPTER 258

Nephrotic Syndrome
(Nelson Textbook, Chapter 535)

The nephrotic syndrome is characterized by proteinuria, hypoproteinemia, edema, and hyperlipidemia.

ETIOLOGY. Most (90%) children with nephrosis have some form of the idiopathic nephrotic syndrome; minimal-change disease is found in approximately 85%, mesangial proliferation in 5%, and focal sclerosis in 10%. In the remaining 10% of children with nephrosis, the nephrotic syndrome is largely mediated by some form of glomerulonephritis, with membranous and membranoproliferative being most common.

PATHOPHYSIOLOGY. The underlying pathogenetic abnormality in nephrosis is proteinuria, which results from an increase in glomerular capillary wall permeability.

CLINICAL MANIFEESTATIONS. The idiopathic nephrotic syndrome is more common in boys than in girls (2:1) and most commonly appears between the ages of 2 and 6 yr. The initial episode and subsequent relapses may follow an apparent viral upper respiratory tract infection. The disease usually presents as edema, which is initially noted around the eyes and in the lower extremities, where it is "pitting" in nature. With time, the edema becomes generalized and may be associated with weight gain, the development of ascites or pleural effusions, and declining urine output. Anorexia, abdominal pain, and diarrhea are common; hypertension is uncommon.

DIAGNOSIS. Urinalysis reveals 3 + or 4 + proteinuria; microscopic hematuria may be present, but gross hematuria is rare. Renal function may be normal or reduced. Protein excretion exceeds 2 g/24 hr. The serum cholesterol and triglyceride levels are elevated, the serum albumin level is generally less than 2 g/dL, and the total serum calcium level is diminished, owing to a reduction in the albumin-bound fraction.

TREATMENT. Children with the first episode of nephrosis may be hospitalized or managed as outpatients for diagnostic, educational, and therapeutic purposes. When edema develops, sodium intake is reduced by the initiation of a "no added salt diet." Salt restriction is terminated when the edema resolves. If the edema becomes severe, resulting in respiratory distress from massive pleural effusions and ascites or in severe scrotal edema, the child should be hospitalized. Diuresis may be initiated by oral administration of furosemide (1–2 mg/kg every 4 hr) in conjunction with metolazone (0.2–0.4 mg/kg/24 hr in two divided doses.

Remission is induced by administration of prednisone at a dosage of 60 mg/m^2/24 hr (maximum daily dose 60 mg). The time needed for response to prednisone averages about 2 wk, the response being defined as the point at which urine becomes free of protein. If a child continues to have proteinuria (2 + or greater) after 1 mo of continuous daily divided-dose prednisone, the nephrosis is termed *steroid resistant* and renal biopsy is indicated to determine the precise cause of the disease. Five days after the urine becomes protein free (negative, trace, or 1 + on the dipstick) the scheduling of prednisone is changed to 60 mg/m^2 (maximum dose of 60 mg) taken every other day as a single dose with breakfast. This alternate-day regimen is continued for 3–6 mo.

SECTION 4

Tubular Disorders

(Nelson Textbook, Chapters 536–540)

CHAPTER 259

Renal Tubular Acidosis

(Nelson Textbook, Chapter 537)

Renal tubular acidosis (RTA) is a clinical state of systemic hyperchloremic acidosis resulting from impaired urinary acidification. Three types exist: distal RTA (type I), proximal RTA (type II), and mineralocorticoid deficiency (type IV). A proposed type

III has been found to be a variant of type I. All types are associated with a normal anion gap (Table 259–1).

PATHOGENESIS

PROXIMAL RENAL TUBULAR ACIDOSIS. Proximal RTA results from reduced proximal tubular reabsorption of bicarbonate, presumably owing to deficient carbonic anhydrase production or hydrogen ion secretion. Proximal RTA may occur as an isolated disorder not associated with other diseases or with other abnormalities of proximal tubular function.

DISTAL RENAL TUBULAR ACIDOSIS. The genesis of distal RTA is best explained as a deficiency of hydrogen ion secretion by the distal tubule and collecting duct, although other mechanisms may also be involved.

MINERALOCORTICOID DEFICIENCY. This form of RTA results from inadequate production of or reduced distal tubular responsiveness to aldosterone.

MANAGEMENT

CLINICAL MANIFESTATIONS. Children having isolated forms of proximal or distal RTA commonly present with growth failure toward the end of the 1st yr of life. Symptoms may include polyuria, dehydration, anorexia, vomiting, constipation, and hypotonia. Children having secondary forms of proximal or distal RTA may present in a similar fashion or with complaints unique to their fundamental disease. Mineralocorticoid deficiency is usually found as an underlying feature of a primary kidney disease. Distal RTA is complicated by hypercalciuria, which may lead to nephrocalcinosis, nephrolithiasis, and renal parenchymal destruction. Proximal RTA may be complicated by rickets, which may be due to phosphate wasting or insufficient production of 1,25-dihydroxyvitamin D.

DIAGNOSIS. In patients who have substantial systemic acidosis (serum bicarbonate level < 18 mEq/L), a urine pH of less than 5.6 supports the diagnosis of proximal RTA, whereas patients with distal RTA have a urine pH of 5.8 or greater.

TREATMENT. The goals of therapy are correction of the acidosis and maintenance of normal serum bicarbonate and potassium levels. The least expensive and easiest alkalizing solution for oral use is Shohl solution containing 1 mEq/mL of "bicarbonate equivalent" as sodium citrate. For patients requiring potassium supplementation, potassium citrate can be added. Patients with Fanconi syndrome may require phosphate and vitamin D supplements. Patients having mineralocorticoid-deficiency RTA may require diuretics or polystyrene sulfonate resin.

TABLE 259–1 Classification of Renal Tubular Acidosis

Proximal	Distal	Mineralocorticoid Deficiency
Isolated	Isolated	Adrenal disorders ($\downarrow$ A, $\uparrow$ R)*
Sporadic	Sporadic	Addison disease
Hereditary	Hereditary	Congenital hyperplasia
Fanconi syndrome	Secondary	Primary hypoaldosteronism
Primary	Interstitial nephritis	Hyporeninemic hypoaldosteronism ($\downarrow$ A, $\downarrow$ R)
Secondary	Obstructive	Obstruction
Inherited	Reflux	Pyelonephritis
Cystinosis	Pyelonephritis	Interstitial nephritis
Lowe syndrome	Transplant rejection	Diabetes mellitus
Galactosemia	Sickle cell nephropathy	Nephrosclerosis
Hereditary fructose intolerance	Lupus nephritis	Pseudohypoaldosteronism ($\uparrow$ A, $\uparrow$ R)
Tyrosinemia	Ehlers-Danlos syndrome	
Wilson disease	Nephrocalcinosis	
Medullary cystic disease	Hepatic cirrhosis	
Mitochondrial cytopathies	Elliptocytosis	
Acquired	Medullary sponge kidney	
Heavy metals	Toxins	
Outdated tetracycline	Amphotericin B	
Proteinuria	Lithium	
Interstitial nephritis	Toluene	
Hyperparathyroidism		
Vitamin D-deficiency rickets		
Gentamicin		
Cyclosporine		

*A = aldosterone; R = renin.

Toxic Nephropathies— Renal Failure
(Nelson Textbook, Chapters 541–544)

CHAPTER 260

Renal Failure
(Nelson Textbook, Chapter 543)

ACUTE RENAL FAILURE

Acute renal failure develops when renal function is diminished to the point where body fluid homeostasis can no longer be maintained. Although oliguria (daily urine volume < 400 mL/m²) is common in renal failure, the urine volume may approximate normal (nonoliguric renal failure) in certain types of acute renal failure (aminoglycoside nephrotoxicity).

CLINICAL MANIFESTATIONS. The presenting signs and symptoms may be dominated or modified by the precipitating disease. Clinical findings related to the renal failure include pallor (anemia), diminished urine output, edema (salt and water overload), hypertension, vomiting, and lethargy (uremic encephalopathy). Complications of acute renal failure include volume overload with heart failure and pulmonary edema, arrhythmias, gastrointestinal bleeding due to stress ulcers or gastritis, seizures, coma, and behavioral changes.

TREATMENT. In children with *hypovolemia*, the need for volume replacement may be critical. In patients with hypovolemia, the urine is concentrated (urine osmolality > 500 mOsm/kg), its sodium content is usually less than 20 mEq/L, and the fractional excretion of sodium (urine/plasma sodium concentration divided by the urine/plasma creatinine concentration × 100) is usually less than 1%. By contrast, in patients with acute tubular necrosis, the urine is dilute (osmolality < 350 mOsm/kg), the sodium concentration usually exceeds 40 mEq/L (mmol/L), and the fractional excretion of sodium usually exceeds 1%. If hypovolemia is detected, intravascular volume should be expanded by intravenous administration of isotonic saline, 20 mL/kg, over 30 min.

Fluid restriction is essential for patients who fail to produce adequate urine output after volume expansion or the administration of diuretics. For patients with oliguria or anuria having a relatively normal intravascular volume, fluid administration should initially be limited to 400 mL/m²/24 hr (insensible losses) plus an amount of fluid equal to the urine output for that day.

Markedly hypervolemic patients may require almost total fluid restriction.

In acute renal failure, rapid development of hyperkalemia (serum level > 6 mEq/L) may lead to cardiac arrhythmia and death. Patients should receive no potassium-containing fluid, foods, or medications until adequate renal function is re-established. In children with acute renal failure, procedures to deplete body potassium are initiated when the serum potassium value rises to 5.5 mEq/L (mmol/L). Sodium polystyrene sulfonate resin (Kayexalate), 1 g/kg, should be given orally or by retention enema. If the serum potassium rises above 7 mEq/L (mmol/L), emergency measures in addition to Kayexalate must be initiated:

1. Calcium gluconate 10% solution, 0.5 mL/kg IV, over 10 min
2. Sodium bicarbonate 7.5% solution, 3 mEq/kg IV
3. Glucose 50% solution, 1 mL/kg, with regular insulin, 1 unit/ 5 g of glucose, given IV over 1 hr

Acidosis should be corrected only partially by the intravenous route, generally giving enough bicarbonate to raise the arterial pH to 7.20. *Hypocalcemia* is treated by lowering the serum phosphorus level. *Hyponatremia* may be corrected by fluid restriction. When the serum sodium falls below 120 mEq/L (mmol/L), it may be elevated to 125 mEq/L (mmol/L) by intravenous infusion of hypertonic (3%) sodium chloride.

In patients with renal failure and hypertension, salt and water restriction is critical. In children with severe acute symptomatic hypertension, diazoxide is a useful drug. Diazepam is the most effective agent in controlling seizures.

Continuous hemofiltration is useful in patients with acute renal failure. In certain patients with acute renal failure, careful medical management may minimize complications and delay the need for dialysis; other patients eventually require dialysis for the uremic state itself. The life-threatening complications of uremia are hemorrhage, pericarditis, and central nervous system dysfunction. The risk of developing these complications correlates more closely with the level of blood urea nitrogen than with that of creatinine.

CHRONIC RENAL FAILURE

CLINICAL MANIFESTATIONS. In patients developing chronic renal failure from glomerular or hereditary diseases, the renal disease is usually detected because of clinical manifestations apparent before the onset of renal insufficiency. The development of renal failure may be insidious, however, in patients having anatomic abnormalities; their presenting complaints may be nonspecific (headache, fatigue, lethargy, anorexia, vomiting, polydipsia, polyuria, growth failure). Most patients with chronic renal failure appear pale and weak and have hypertension. Patients having anatomic abnormalities, in whom the renal failure has developed slowly over several years, may also have growth retardation and rickets.

TREATMENT. The management of chronic renal failure requires close monitoring of a patient's clinical (physical examination, growth, and blood pressure) and laboratory status.

Diet in Chronic Renal Failure. The optimal caloric intake in renal insufficiency is unknown, but an attempt should be made to equal or exceed (in patients with growth failure) the recommended daily caloric allowance for age. Recombinant human growth hormone therapy combined with optimal dialysis improves linear growth.

Water and Electrolyte Management in Chronic Renal Failure. Until the development of end-stage renal failure requires the initiation of dialysis, water restriction is rarely necessary in children with renal insufficiency, because water needs are regulated by the thirst center in the brain.

Acidosis in Chronic Renal Failure. Acidosis develops in almost all children with renal insufficiency and need not be treated unless the serum bicarbonate falls below 20 mEq/L (mmol/L).

Renal Osteodystrophy. The term *renal osteodystrophy* is used to indicate a spectrum of bone diseases resulting from defective mineralization due to renal failure. The goals of treatment include normalization of the serum calcium and phosphorus levels and maintenance of the intact parathyroid hormone level in the range of 200–400 pg/mL. Hyperphosphatemia may be controlled with a low-phosphate formula (Similac PM 60/40) and by enhancing fecal phosphate excretion by using oral calcium carbonate, an antacid that also binds phosphate in the intestinal tract. If the serum calcium level remains low after correction of the serum phosphorus level, oral calcium supplements at a dose of 500–2000 mg/24 hr can be administered. Vitamin D therapy is indicated (1) in patients having persistent hypocalcemia despite reduction of the serum phosphorus level below 6 mg/dL and the addition of oral calcium supplements and (2) in patients with osteodystrophy.

Anemia in Chronic Renal Failure. If the hemoglobin falls below 6 g/dL, 10 mL/kg of packed red blood cells should be administered cautiously. Erythropoietin can be administered subcutaneously to predialysis and peritoneal dialysis patients and intravenously to patients on hemodialysis.

Hypertension in Chronic Renal Failure. Hypertensive emergencies should be treated with oral nifedipine (0.25–0.5 mg/kg) or intravenous administration of diazoxide. Treatment of sustained hypertension may include a combination of salt restriction (2–3 g/24 hr), furosemide (1–4 mg/kg/24 hr), propranolol (1–6 mg/kg/24 hr), hydralazine (1–6 mg/kg/24 hr), and nifedipine (0.2–2.0 mg/kg/24 hr).

PART 22

Urologic Disorders in Infants and Children

(Nelson Textbook, Chapters 545–555)

CHAPTER 261

Urinary Tract Infections

(Nelson Textbook, Chapter 546)

CLASSIFICATION OF URINARY TRACT INFECTION (UTI). There are three basic forms of UTI: pyelonephritis, cystitis, and asymptomatic bacteriuria. *Clinical pyelonephritis* is characterized by any or all of the following: abdominal or flank pain, fever, malaise, nausea, vomiting, jaundice in neonates, and occasionally diarrhea. Some newborns and infants may show nonspecific symptoms such as poor feeding, irritability, and weight loss. These symptoms are an indication that there is bacterial involvement of the upper urinary tract. Involvement of the renal parenchyma is termed *acute pyelonephritis*, whereas if there is no parenchymal involvement, the condition may be termed *pyelitis*. Acute pyelonephritis may result in renal injury, which is termed *pyelonephritic scarring*.

Cystitis indicates that there is bladder involvement and includes dysuria, urgency, frequency, suprapubic pain, incontinence, and malodorous urine. Cystitis does not cause fever and does not result in renal injury.

Asymptomatic bacteriuria refers to children who have a positive urine culture without any manifestations of infection and occurs almost exclusively in girls. This condition is benign and does not cause renal injury, except in pregnant women. Some girls are mistakenly identified as having asymptomatic bacteriuria when they actually are symptomatic, experiencing day or night incontinence or perineal discomfort.

DIAGNOSIS. To make the diagnosis of UTI, the urine must be cultured.

TREATMENT. Acute cystitis should be treated promptly to prevent its possible progression to pyelonephritis. If the symptoms are severe, a specimen of bladder urine is obtained for culture and treatment is started immediately. If the symptoms are mild or the diagnosis doubtful, treatment can be delayed until the results of culture are known. If treatment is initiated before the results of culture and sensitivity testing are available, a 3- to 5-day course of therapy with trimethoprim-sulfamethoxazole is effective against most strains of *Escherichia coli*. Nitrofurantoin (5–7 mg/kg/24 hr in 3 to 4 divided doses) is also effective and has the advantage of being active against *Klebsiella* and *Enterobacter* organisms.

In acute febrile infections suggestive of pyelonephritis, a 14-day course of broad-spectrum antibiotics capable of reaching significant tissue levels is preferable. If the child is acutely ill, parenteral treatment with ceftriaxone (50–75 mg/kg/24 hr, not to exceed 2 g) or ampicillin (100 mg/kg/24 hr) with an aminoglycoside such as gentamicin (3 to 5 mg/kg/24 hr in 3 divided doses) is preferable.

Children with a renal or perirenal abscess or with infection in obstructed urinary tracts require surgical or percutaneous drainage in addition to antibiotic therapy and other supportive measures.

A urine culture should be performed 1 wk after the termination of treatment of any UTI to ensure that the urine remains sterile.

IMAGING STUDIES. The goal of imaging studies in children with a UTI is to identify anatomic abnormalities that predispose to infection. A renal ultrasonogram should be obtained to rule out hydronephrosis and renal or perirenal abscesses; ultrasonography also may show acute pyelonephritis (in 30% of cases) by demonstrating an enlarged kidney. A voiding cystourethrogram is also indicated in all children younger than 5 yr with a UTI, any child with a febrile UTI, school-aged girls who have had two or more UTIs, and any male with a UTI. When the diagnosis of acute pyelonephritis is uncertain, renal scanning with technetium-labeled DMSA or glucoheptonate is useful. If vesicoureteral reflux is present, a DMSA scan often is performed to assess whether renal scarring is present.

Chapter 262

Vesicoureteral Reflux

(Nelson Textbook, Chapter 547)

Vesicoureteral reflux is the retrograde flow of urine from the bladder to the ureter and renal pelvis. Reflux predisposes to renal infection (pyelonephritis) by facilitating the transport of bacteria from the bladder to the upper urinary tract. The inflammatory reaction caused by a pyelonephritic infection may result in renal injury or scarring. Extensive renal scarring impairs renal function and may result in renin-mediated hypertension, reflux nephropathy, renal insufficiency, end-stage renal disease, reduced somatic growth, and morbidity during pregnancy.

CLASSIFICATION. Reflux severity is graded using the International Study of Classification of I to V and is based on the appearance of the urinary tract on a contrast medium–enhanced voiding cystourethrogram. The more severe the reflux, the higher the rates of renal injury. Reflux may be primary or secondary (Table 262–1).

CLINICAL MANIFESTATIONS. Usually reflux is discovered during an evaluation for a urinary tract infection.

TREATMENT. The goals of treatment are to prevent pyelonephritis, renal injury, and other complications of reflux. Continuous antibiotic prophylaxis is the cornerstone in the initial management of children with reflux. Drugs commonly used for prophylaxis include sulfamethoxazole-trimethoprim, trimethoprim alone, and nitrofurantoin, generally administered once daily at a dose of one fourth to one third of the dose necessary to treat an acute infection. Prophylaxis is usually continued until reflux resolves or until the risk of reflux to the individual is considered to be low. In children with ongoing reflux, follow-up evaluation should be performed at least annually, at which time the child's height, weight, and blood pressure should be recorded. Open surgical management involves modifying the abnormal ureterovesical attachment to create a 4:1 to 5:1 ratio of intramural ureter length: ureteral diameter. The technique of endoscopic repair of reflux involves injection of a bulking agent via a cystoscope under the ureteral orifice, creating an artificial flap-valve.

TABLE 262–1 Classification of Vesicoureteral Reflux

Type	Cause
Primary	Congenital incompetence of the valvular mechanism of the vesicoureteral junction
Primary associated with other malformations of the ureterovesical junction	Ureteral duplication Ureterocele with duplication Ureteral ectopia Paraureteral diverticula
Secondary to increased intravesical pressure	Neuropathic bladder Non-neuropathic bladder dysfunction Bladder outlet obstruction
Secondary to inflammatory processes	Severe bacterial cystitis Foreign bodies Vesical calculi Clinical cystitis
Secondary to surgical procedures involving the ureterovesical junction	

CHAPTER 263

Voiding Dysfunction

(Nelson Textbook, Chapter 551)

NORMAL VOIDING AND TOILET TRAINING

Girls typically acquire bladder control before boys, and bowel control is typically achieved before urinary control. By 5 yr of age, 90–95% are nearly completely continent during the day and 80–85% are continent at night.

NOCTURNAL ENURESIS

Nocturnal enuresis is the occurrence of involuntary voiding at night at 5 yr, the age when volitional control of micturition is expected. Nocturnal enuresis without overt daytime voiding symptoms affects up to 20% of children at the age of 5 yr; it ceases spontaneously in approximately 15% of involved children every year thereafter. A careful history should be obtained, especially with respect to fluid intake at night and pattern of nocturnal enuresis. A complete physical examination should include palpation of the abdomen and rectal examination after voiding to assess the possibility of a chronically distended bladder. The child with nocturnal enuresis should be examined carefully for neurologic and spinal abnormalities.

The best approach to treatment is to reassure parents that the condition is self-limited and to avoid punitive measures that may affect the child's psychologic development adversely. Fluid intake in the evening should be restricted. In addition, the parents should be certain that the child voids at bedtime. If the child snores and the adenoids are enlarged, referral to an otolaryngologist should be considered, because adenoidectomy may result in cure of the enuresis.

Active treatment should be avoided in children younger than 6 yr because enuresis is extremely common in younger children. The simplest initial measure is motivational and includes a star chart for dry nights. Waking the child a few hours after the child goes to sleep for voiding often allows the child to awaken dry, although this measure is not curative. Conditioning therapy involves use of an auditory alarm attached to electrodes in the underwear. The primary role of psychologic therapy is to help the child deal with enuresis psychologically and help motivate the child to get up to void at night if awakening with a full bladder. Pharmacologic therapy is intended to treat the symptom of enuresis and is not curative. One form of treatment is desmopressin acetate, which is a synthetic analog of antidiuretic hormone and reduces urine production overnight. It is available as a tablet, with a dosage of 0.2–0.6 mg at bedtime. Another pharmacologic agent is imipramine, which is a tricyclic antidepressant. The dose

TABLE 263–1 Causes of Urinary Incontinence in Childhood

Pediatric unstable bladder (uninhibited bladder)
Infrequent voiding
Detrusor-sphincter dyssynergia
Non-neurogenic neurogenic bladder (Hinman syndrome)
Vaginal voiding
Giggle incontinence
Cystitis
Bladder outlet obstruction (posterior urethral valves)
Ectopic ureter and fistula
Sphincter abnormality (epispadias, exstrophy; urogenital sinus abnormality)
Neurogenic
Overflow incontinence
Traumatic
Iatrogenic
Behavioral
Combination

of imipramine is 25 mg in children 6–8 yr, 50 mg in children 9–12 yr, and 75 mg in teenagers.

DIURNAL INCONTINENCE

Daytime incontinence not secondary to neurologic abnormalities is common in children. The most common cause of daytime incontinence is a pediatric unstable bladder (also termed *uninhibited bladder, bladder spasms*). Table 263–1 lists this and other causes of diurnal incontinence in children. A pediatric unstable bladder is smaller than normal and exhibits strong uninhibited contractions. These children typically exhibit urinary frequency, urgency, and urge incontinence. Initial therapy is timed voiding every 1.5–2 hr and anticholinergic therapy with oxybutynin chloride or hyoscyamine. Constipation and urinary tract infections also should be addressed.

CHAPTER 264

Anomalies of the Penis and Urethra

(Nelson Textbook, Chapter 552)

HYPOSPADIAS. Hypospadias refers to a urethral opening that is on the ventral surface of the penile shaft and affects 1 in 250 male newborns. There is incomplete development of the prepuce, termed a *dorsal hood,* in which the foreskin is on the sides and dorsal aspect of the penile shaft and absent ventrally. Some boys, particularly those with proximal hypospadias, have chordee, in which there is ventral penile curvature during erection. Hypospadias usually is an isolated anomaly.

The treatment begins in the newborn period. Circumcision should be avoided, becauses the foreskin is often essential for the repair. The ideal age for repair in a healthy infant is 6–12 mo. Most cases are repaired in a single operation on an outpatient basis.

PHIMOSIS AND PARAPHIMOSIS. Phimosis refers to the inability to retract the prepuce. At birth phimosis is physiologic. Over time the adhesions between the prepuce and glans lyse and the distal phimotic ring loosens so that in 90% of uncircumcised males the prepuce becomes retractable by the age of 3 yr. In boys with persistent phimosis, application of a steroid cream to the foreskin three times daily for 1 mo can loosen the phimotic ring.

Paraphimosis occurs when the foreskin is retracted behind the coronal sulcus and the prepuce cannot be pulled back over the glans. Painful venous stasis in the foreskin distal to the corona results, with edema leading to severe pain and inability to reduce the foreskin. Treatment includes lubrication of the foreskin and glans and then compressing the glans and simultaneously placing distal traction on the foreskin to try to push the phimotic ring beyond the coronal sulcus.

CHAPTER 265

Disorders and Anomalies of the Scrotal Contents

(Nelson Textbook, Chapter 553)

UNDESCENDED AND RETRACTILE TESTES. Failure to find one or both testes in the scrotum may indicate that the testis is undescended, absent, or retractile. An undescended testis is the most common disorder of sexual differentiation in boys. The majority of undescended testes descend spontaneously during the first 3 mo of life. If the testis has not descended by 6 mo, it will remain undescended. Undescended testes are usually in the inguinal canal.

The consequences of cryptorchidism include infertility, malignancy, associated hernias, torsion of the cryptorchid testis, and the possible psychologic effects of an empty scrotum. *Indirect inguinal hernias* usually accompany undescended testes but are rarely symptomatic. *Retractile testes* often are misdiagnosed as undescended testes.

Treatment of the undescended testis is recommended at 9–15 mo. Most testes can be brought down to the scrotum with an operation (orchiopexy). If the testis is nonpalpable, diagnostic laparoscopy is performed to determine its location.

TESTICULAR (SPERMATIC CORD) TORSION. Testicular torsion requires prompt diagnosis and treatment to save the testis. Torsion is the most common cause of testicular pain in boys 12 yr and older and is uncommon in those younger than 10 yr. It is caused by inadequate fixation of the testis within the scrotum. Testicular torsion produces acute pain and swelling of the scrotum. On examination, the scrotum is swollen, tender, and often difficult to examine. If the pain has lasted less than 4–6 hr, manual detorsion may be attempted. Treatment is prompt surgical exploration and detorsion.

TORSION OF THE APPENDIX TESTIS. Torsion of the appendix testis is the most common cause of testicular pain in boys between 2 and 11 yr but is rare in adolescents. The onset of pain is usually gradual. Palpation of the testis usually reveals a 3- to 5-mm tender indurated mass on the upper pole. The natural history of torsion of the appendix testis is for the inflammation to resolve in 3–10 days. Nonoperative treatment is recommended, including bed rest and analgesia with nonsteroidal anti-inflammatory medication for 5 days.

PART 23

Gynecologic Problems of Childhood

(Nelson Textbook, Chapters 556–565)

CHAPTER 266

Vulvovaginitis

(Nelson Textbook, Chapter 557)

Vulvovaginitis is the most common childhood or adolescent gynecologic problem. The main clinical manifestations, in order of frequency, include vaginal discharge, erythema, and pruritus. Vaginal culture, cytology, and vaginoscopy may be indicated for evaluation of pediatric patients with vulvovaginitis. Infections are primarily located in the vulva and vagina (57%) in the majority of patients. *Candida* species are very commonly identified, followed by β-hemolytic streptococci group B and enterococci species.

PATHOLOGIC VAGINAL DISCHARGE. In pediatric patients, vaginal discharge is a common presenting complaint. It is often the primary symptom of vulvitis, vaginitis, or vulvovaginitis. Pruritus, frequent urination, dysuria, or enuresis may be associated signs and symptoms. Vulvitis is manifested primarily by dysuria and pruritus, associated with erythema of the vulva. It commonly has a more protracted course than vaginitis; the latter is characterized by discharge without associated dysuria, pruritus, or erythema. Vulvovaginitis involves a combination of these manifestations. The color, odor, and duration of the discharge should be noted. Although there are a number of causes of vulvovaginitis in pediatric patients, the more common ones include poor perineal hygiene, *Candida* infection, and a foreign body.

NONSPECIFIC VULVOVAGINITIS. Patients with poor perineal hygiene often develop a condition known as nonspecific vulvovaginitis. Overall, nonspecific vulvovaginitis accounts for 70% of all pediatric vulvovaginitis cases. The discharge is characteristically brown or green, has a fetid odor, and is associated with a vaginal pH of 4.7–6.5. Successful treatment of nonspecific vulvovaginitis should include instruction in perineal hygiene, switching from tight-fitting underwear, the use of sitz baths with mild soap, and air drying the vulva. Patients should be instructed in appropriate bowel and bladder habits, emphasizing the need to wipe fecal material away from the vulvovaginal area. Recurrent vulvovaginitis should be treated with systemic antibiotics such as amoxicillin or cephalosporins. Topical estrogen cream or polysporin ointment is often helpful.

SPECIFIC VULVOVAGINITIS. Treatment depends on the offending organism.

PART 24

The Endocrine System

SECTION 1

Disorders of the Hypothalamus and Pituitary Gland

(Nelson Textbook, Chapters 566–572)

CHAPTER 267

Hypopituitarism

(Nelson Textbook, Chapter 567)

Hypopituitary states associated with a deficiency of growth hormone (GH), with or without a deficiency of other pituitary hormones, are summarized in Table 267–1. Affected children have in common a phenotype of growth impairment that is specifically corrected by a replacement of GH.

CLINICAL MANIFESTATIONS

Patients without Demonstrable Lesions of the Pituitary. The child with hypopituitarism is usually of normal size and weight at birth. Children with severe defects in GH production or action fall more than 4 SD below the mean by 1 yr of age. Others with less severe deficiencies may have regular but slow growth in height, with the increments always below the normal percentiles, or periods of lack of growth may alternate with short spurts of growth. Without treatment, adult heights are 4 to 12 SD below the mean.

Infants with congenital defects of the pituitary or hypothalamus usually present neonatal emergencies such as apnea, cyanosis, or severe hypoglycemia. Microphallus in the male provides an additional diagnostic clue. Prolonged neonatal jaundice is common.

The head is round, and the face is short and broad. The frontal bone is prominent, and the bridge of the nose is depressed and saddle-shaped. The nose is small, and the nasolabial folds are well developed. The eyes are somewhat bulging. The mandible and the chin are underdeveloped and infantile, and the teeth, which erupt late, are frequently crowded. The voice is high pitched and remains high after puberty. The genitalia is usually underdeveloped for the child's age, and sexual maturation may be delayed

586

TABLE 267–1   Etiologic Classification of Hypopituitarism

Development Defects

Anencephaly
Holoprosencephaly (i.e., cyclopia, cebocephaly, orbital hypotelorism)
Midfacial anomalies (e.g., hypertelorism)
Septo-optic dysplasia (de Morsier syndrome)
Cleft lip and palate
Solitary maxillary central incisor
Hall-Pallister syndrome (i.e., hypothalamic hamartoblastoma, imperforate anus, polydactyly)
Rieger syndrome with mutations in the Ptx-2 or Rieg1 gene

Genetic Defects of GH or GHRH

Isolated GH deficiency
Autosomal recessive type I
  Type IA with deletions of the *GH1* gene
  Type IB with mutations in *GH1* or other genes
  Type IB with mutations in the GHRH-receptor gene
Autosomal dominant type II with mutations in *GH1* or other genes
X-linked type III with or without hypogammaglobulinemia
Multiple pituitary deficiencies
  Autosomal recessive type I
    GH, TSH, ACTH, LH, and FSH ± ACTH deficiency with mutations in the *PROP1* gene
    GH, TSH, and PRL deficiencies with mutations in the *POU1F1* gene
  Autosomal dominant type II
    GH, TSH, and PRL deficiencies with mutations in the *POU1F1* gene
  X-linked type III
    GH, TSH, ACTH, LH, and FSH deficiency

Destructive Lesions

Trauma
  Perinatal trauma (e.g., trauma, anoxia, hemorrhagic infarction)
  Basal skull fractures
  Child abuse

Infiltrative Lesions

Tumors
Histiocytosis X

GH = growth hormone; GHRH = growth hormone-releasing hormone; TSH = thyroid-stimulating hormone; ACTH = adrenocorticotropic hormone (corticotropin); LH = luteinizing hormone; FSH = follicle-stimulating hormone; PRL = prolactin.

or absent. Facial, axillary, and pubic hair usually is lacking, and the scalp hair is fine. Intelligence is usually normal.

Patients with Demonstrable Lesions of the Pituitary. The child is normal initially, and manifestations similar to those seen in idiopathic pituitary growth failure gradually appear and progress. When complete or almost complete destruction of the pituitary gland occurs, signs of pituitary insufficiency are present. Atrophy of the adrenal cortex, thyroid, and gonads results in loss of weight, asthenia, sensitivity to cold, mental torpor, and absence of sweating. Sexual maturation fails to take place or regresses if already present. There is a tendency to hypoglycemia and coma. Growth ceases.

If the lesion is an expanding tumor, symptoms such as headache, vomiting, visual disturbances, pathologic sleep patterns, decreased school performance, seizures, polyuria, and growth failure may occur. In children with craniopharyngiomas, visual field defects, optic atrophy, papilledema, and cranial nerve palsy are common.

LABORATORY FINDINGS. The diagnosis of classic GH deficiency is suspected in cases of profound postnatal growth failure, with heights more than 3 SD below the mean for age and gender. Acquired GH deficiency can occur at any age. Definitive diagnosis rests on demonstration of absent or low levels of GH in response to stimulation. Radiographs of the skull are most helpful when there is a destructive or space-occupying lesion causing hypopituitarism. Enlargement of the sella, especially ballooning with erosion and calcifications within or above the sella, may be detected. Magnetic resonance imaging is indicated in all patients with hypopituitarism.

TREATMENT. In children with classic GH deficiency, treatment should be started as soon as possible to narrow the gap in height between patients and their classmates during childhood and to have the greatest effect on mature height. The recommended dose of hGH is 0.18–0.3 mg/kg/wk. Maximum response to GH occurs in the first year of treatment. With each successive year of treatment, the response tends to decrease.

CHAPTER 268

Diabetes Insipidus
(Nelson Textbook, Chapter 568)

Diabetes insipidus (DI) is a disease characterized by polyuria and excessive thirst. DI may result from either a lack of arginine vasopressin (AVP; antidiuretic hormone) or failure of AVP-sensitive epithelial cells of the kidney collecting duct to respond normally to the hormone (NDI).

CLINICAL MANIFESTATIONS. Although polyuria and polydipsia are the hallmarks of DI, these symptoms may not be recognized immediately by either family members or caregivers. Often, the clinical features of NDI are dominated by signs and symptoms of chronic dehydration. In infants with NDI, such symptoms include irritability, poor feeding, growth failure, and intermittent high fevers. If unrecognized, intervals of dehydration and hypernatremia may result in brain damage. In children who have acquired bladder control, enuresis may be the first symptom. Patients with hypothalamic tumors may have disturbances in growth, progressive cachexia or obesity, hyperpyrexia, sleep disturbance, sexual precocity, or emotional disorders. Long-standing states of polyuria may cause the development of megacystis.

DIAGNOSIS AND TREATMENT. Often the diagnosis of either central DI or NDI requires either a water deprivation test or administration of desmopressin acetate (DDAVP) to test whether the patient is capable of responding to AVP. In central DI, administration of desmopressin acetate either intranasally or by intravenous infusion raises urine osmolality. Although individuals with NDI may also exhibit increases in serum osmolality after 3–8 hr of water deprivation, their corresponding urine osmolality does not increase. Moreover, administration of either intranasal or intravenous desmopressin acetate produces no increase in urine osmolality.

The cornerstone of therapy for central DI is administration of desmopressin acetate, usually via an intranasal route. The usual intranasal dose used for treatment of central DI ranges from 5–10 μg, given in single or divided doses. Therapy for NDI should ensure a sufficient intake of water to replace the large urinary water losses. Because renal water requirements are directly proportional to renal osmolar solute loads, restriction of sodium intake reduces obligatory water losses by the kidney. Thus, a diet containing low sodium (less than 1 mmol/kg/24 hr), adequate protein (2 g/kg/24 hr), and 300–400 mL/kg of water is recommended. Thiazide diuretics (hydrochlorothiazide, 2–4 mg/kg/24 hr) may reduce urine output by 50% but may produce hypokalemia.

CHAPTER 269

Disorders of Pubertal Development
(Nelson Textbook, Chapter 572)

Precocious puberty is generally defined as the onset of secondary sexual characteristics before 8 yr of age in girls and 9 yr in boys. Precocious pubertal development may be classified as gonadotropin dependent, also called true or central precocious puberty, or gonadotropin independent, also called peripheral precocious puberty or precocious pseudopuberty (Table 269–1). True precocious puberty is always isosexual and stems from hypothalamic-pituitary-gonadal activation. The gonadotropin-mediated increase in the size and activity of the gonads leads to increasing sex hormone secretion and progressive sexual maturation. In precocious pseudopuberty, some of the secondary sex characteristics appear, but there is no activation of the normal hypothalamic-pituitary-gonadal interplay. In this latter group, the sex characteristics may be isosexual or heterosexual.

Precocious pseudopuberty may induce maturation of the hypothalamic-pituitary-gonadal axis and eventually trigger the onset

TABLE 269–1 Conditions Causing Precocious Puberty

Gonadotropin-Dependent Puberty (True Precocious Puberty)

Idiopathic (constitutional, functional)
Organic brain lesions
  Hypothalamic hamartoma
  Brain tumors, hydrocephalus, severe head trauma
Hypothyroidism, prolonged and untreated

Combined Gonadotropin-Dependent and Gonadotropin-Independent Puberty

Treated congenital adrenal hyperplasia
McCune-Albright syndrome, late
Familial male precocious puberty, late

Gonadotropin-Independent Puberty (Precocious Pseudopuberty)

Females
  Isosexual (feminizing) conditions
    McCune-Albright syndrome
    Autonomous ovarian cysts
    Ovarian tumors
      Granulosa-theca cell tumor associated with Ollier disease
      Teratoma, chorionepithelioma
      Sex cord tumor with annular tubules (SCTAT) associated with Peutz-Jeghers
        syndrome
      Feminizing adrenocortical tumor
      Exogenous estrogens
  Heterosexual (masculinizing) conditions
    Congenital adrenal hyperplasia
    Adrenal tumors
    Ovarian tumors
    Glucocorticoid receptor defect
    Exogenous androgens
Males
  Isosexual (masculinizing) conditions
    Congenital adrenal hyperplasia
    Adrenocortical tumor
    Leydig cell tumor
    Familial male precocious puberty
    Isolated
    Associated with pseudohypoparathyroidism
    hCG-secreting tumors
      Central nervous system
      Hepatoblastoma
      Mediastinal tumor associated with Klinefelter syndrome
    Teratoma
    Glucocorticoid receptor defect
    Exogenous androgen
  Heterosexual (feminizing) conditions
    Feminizing adrenocortical tumor
    Sex-cord tumor with annular tubules (SCTAT) associated with Peutz-Jeghers
      syndrome
    Exogenous estrogens

Incomplete (Partial) Precocious Puberty

Premature thelarche
Premature adrenarche
Premature menarche

hCG = human chorionic gonadotropin.

of true sexual precocity. This mixed type of precocious puberty occurs commonly in conditions such as congenital adrenal hyperplasia and McCune-Albright syndrome, when the bone age reaches the pubertal range (10.5–12.5 yr).

CLINICAL MANIFESTATIONS. Sexual development may begin at any age and generally follows the sequence observed in normal puberty. In girls, the first sign is development of the breast; pubic hair may appear simultaneously but more often appears later. Maturation of the external genitalia, the appearance of axillary hair, and the onset of menstruation follow. In boys, enlargement of the testes is followed by enlargement of the penis, appearance of pubic hair, and acne. Erections are common, and nocturnal emissions may occur. The voice deepens, and linear growth is accelerated. In affected girls and boys, height, weight, and osseous maturation are advanced.

LABORATORY FINDINGS. Sensitive immunometric (including immunoradiometric, immunofluorimetric, and chemiluminescent) assays for luteinizing hormone (LH) have largely replaced the traditional LH radioimmunoassays and offer greater diagnostic sensitivity using random blood samples.

TREATMENT. The observation that the pituitary gonadotropic cells require pulsatile, rather than continuous, stimulation by GnRH to maintain the ongoing release of gonadotropins provides the rationale for using GnRH agonists for treatment of central precocious puberty. Depot preparations of long-acting GnRH analogs, which maintain fairly constant serum concentration of the drug for weeks, constitute the preparations of choice for treatment of central precocious puberty.

SECTION 2

Disorders of the Thyroid Gland

(Nelson Textbook, Chapters 573–579)

CHAPTER 270

Hypothyroidism

(Nelson Textbook, Chapter 575)

Hypothyroidism results from deficient production of thyroid hormone or a defect in thyroid hormonal β-receptor activity (Table 270–1). The term *cretinism* is often used synonymously with congenital hypothyroidism but should be avoided.

TABLE 270–1 Etiologic Classification of Hypothyroidism

Pit-1 (homeobox protein) mutations
   Deficiency of thyrotropin, growth hormone, and prolactin
Thyrotropin-releasing hormone (TRH) deficiency
   Isolated?
   Multiple hypothalamic deficiencies (e.g., craniopharyngioma)
TRH unresponsiveness
   Mutations in TRH receptor
Thyrotropin (TSH) deficiency
   Mutations in β-chain
   Multiple pituitary deficiencies
Thyrotropin unresponsiveness
   $G_s\alpha$ mutation (e.g., type IA pseudohypoparathyroidism)
   Mutation in TSH receptor
Defect of fetal thyroid development
   Aplasia, ectopia (dysgenesis)
Defect in thyroid hormone synthesis (e.g., goitrous hypothyroidism)
   Iodide transport defect
   Thyroid peroxidase defect
   Thyroglobulin synthesis defect
   Deiodination defect
Iodine deficiency (endemic goiter)
   Neurologic type
   Myxedematous type
Maternal antibodies
   Thyrotropin receptor-blocking antibody (TRBAb)
   (Also termed thyrotropin binding inhibitor immunoglobulin)
Maternal medications
   Radioiodine, iodides
   Propylthiouracil, methimazole
   Amiodarone
Autoimmune (acquired hypothyroidism)
   Hashimoto's thyroiditis
   Polyglandular autoimmune syndrome, types I, II, and III
Iatrogenic
Propylthiouracil, methimazole, iodides, lithium, amiodarone
Irradiation
   Radioiodine
   Radiographs (neck or whole body)
Thyroidectomy
Systemic disease
   Cystinosis
   Histocytic infiltration
Resistance to thyroid hormone (only occasional clinical manifestations of
   hypothyroidism)

CONGENITAL HYPOTHYROIDISM

Congenital causes of hypothyroidism may be sporadic or familial, goitrous or nongoitrous. In many cases, the deficiency of thyroid hormone is severe and symptoms develop in the early weeks of life. In others, lesser degrees of deficiency occur and manifestations may be delayed for months.

CLINICAL MANIFESTATIONS. Before neonatal screening programs, congenital hypothyroidism was rarely recognized in the newborn because the signs and symptoms are usually not sufficiently developed. Birth weight and length are normal, but head size may be slightly increased because of myxedema of the brain. Prolongation of physiologic icterus, caused by delayed maturation of glucuronide conjugation, may be the earliest sign. Feeding difficulties, especially sluggishness, lack of interest, somnolence, and choking spells during nursing, are often present during the first mo of life. Respiratory difficulties, due in part to the large tongue, include apneic episodes, noisy respirations, and nasal obstruction. Typical respiratory distress syndrome may also occur. Affected infants cry little, sleep much, have poor appetites, and are generally sluggish. There may be constipation. The abdomen is large, and an umbilical hernia is usually present. The temperature is subnormal, often less than 35°C (95°F), and the skin, particularly that of the extremities, may be cold and mottled.

These manifestations progress; retardation of physical and mental development becomes greater during the following months, and by 36 mo of age the clinical picture is fully developed. When there is only a partial deficiency of thyroid hormone, the symptoms may be milder, the syndrome incomplete, and the onset delayed. The child's growth is stunted, the extremities are short, and the head size is normal or even increased. The anterior and posterior fontanels are open widely. Development is usually retarded. Hypothyroid infants appear lethargic and are late in learning to sit and stand. The voice is hoarse, and they do not learn to talk.

LABORATORY FINDINGS. Most newborn screening programs in North America measure levels of thyroxine, supplemented by measurement of thyroid-stimulating hormone when thyroxine is low.

TREATMENT. Sodium-L-thyroxine given orally is the treatment of choice. In neonates, the initial starting dose is 10–15 μg/kg (37.5 or 50 μg/24 hr). Children with hypothyroidism require about 4 μg/kg/24 hr.

ACQUIRED HYPOTHYROIDISM

ETIOLOGY. The most common cause of acquired hypothyroidism is lymphocytic thyroiditis.

CLINICAL MANIFESTATIONS. Deceleration of growth is usually the first clinical manifestation. Myxedematous changes of the skin, constipation, cold intolerance, decreased energy, and an increased need for sleep develop insidiously. Osseous maturation is delayed, often strikingly.

Diagnostic studies and treatment are the same as those described for congenital hypothyroidism.

CHAPTER 271

Thyroiditis

(Nelson Textbook, Chapter 576)

LYMPHOCYTIC THYROIDITIS (HASHIMOTO'S THYROIDITIS; AUTOIMMUNE THYROIDITIS)

Lymphocytic thyroiditis is the most common cause of thyroid disease in children and adolescents and accounts for many of the enlarged thyroids formerly designated "adolescent" or "simple" goiter. It is also the most common cause of acquired hypothyroidism, with or without goiter.

CLINICAL MANIFESTATIONS. The most common clinical manifestations are growth retardation and goiter. In most patients, the thyroid is diffusely enlarged, firm, and nontender. Most of the affected children are clinically euthyroid and asymptomatic. Some children have clinical signs of hypothyroidism, but others who appear clinically euthyroid have laboratory evidence of hypothyroidism. A few children have manifestations suggestive of hyperthyroidism, such as nervousness, irritability, increased sweating, or hyperactivity. The clinical course is variable. The goiter may become smaller or may disappear spontaneously, or it may persist unchanged for years while the patient remains euthyroid.

TREATMENT. If there is evidence of hypothyroidism, replacement treatment with sodium-L-thyroxine (50–150 μg daily) is indicated. Because the disease may be self-limited in some instances, the need for continued therapy requires periodic reevaluation.

CHAPTER 272

Goiter

(Nelson Textbook, Chapter 577)

A goiter is an enlargement of the thyroid gland. Persons with enlarged thyroids may have normal function of the gland *(euthyroidism)*, thyroid deficiency *(hypothyroidism)*, or overproduction of the hormones *(hyperthyroidism)*. Goiter may be congenital or acquired, endemic or sporadic.

CONGENITAL GOITER

Congenital goiter is usually sporadic and may result from a fetal thyroxine (T_4) synthetic defect or the administration of antithyroid drugs or iodides during pregnancy for the treatment of thyrotoxicosis. Goiter is almost always present in the congenitally hyperthyroid infant. Iodine deficiency as a cause of congenital goiters has become rare but persists in isolated endemic areas.

ENDEMIC GOITER AND CRETINISM

The association between dietary deficiency of iodine and the prevalence of goiter or cretinism has been recognized for more than half a century.

CLINICAL MANIFESTATIONS. If the deficiency of iodine is mild, thyroid enlargement does not become noticeable except when there is increased demand for the hormone during periods of rapid growth, as in adolescence and during pregnancy. The neurologic syndrome is characterized by mental retardation, deaf-mutism, disturbances in standing and gait, and pyramidal signs such as clonus of the foot, the Babinski sign, and patellar hyperreflexia. Affected individuals are goitrous but euthyroid, have normal pubertal development and adult stature, and have little or no impaired thyroid function. Individuals with the myxedematous syndrome also are mentally retarded and deaf and have neurologic symptoms, delayed sexual development and growth, myxedema, and absence of goiter; serum T_4 levels are low, and thyroid-stimulating hormone levels are markedly elevated.

TREATMENT. Administration of a single intramuscular injection of iodinated poppy seed oil to children younger than 4 yr of age with myxedematous cretinism results in a euthyroid state in 5 mo. Older children require treatment with T_4.

CHAPTER 273

Hyperthyroidism

(Nelson Textbook, Chapter 578)

Hyperthyroidism results from excessive secretion of thyroid hormone and, with few exceptions, is due to diffuse toxic goiter (Graves disease) during childhood.

ETIOLOGY. Enlargement of the thymus, splenomegaly, lymphadenopathy, infiltration of the thyroid gland and retro-orbital tissues with lymphocytes and plasma cells, and peripheral lymphocytosis are well-established findings in Graves disease. In the thyroid gland, T helper cells (CD4+) tend to predominate in dense lymphoid aggregates.

CLINICAL MANIFESTATIONS. The clinical course in children is highly variable but usually is not as fulminant as it is in many adults. Symptoms develop gradually. The earliest signs in children may be emotional disturbances accompanied by motor hyperactivity. The children become irritable and excitable and cry easily because of emotional lability. Their schoolwork suffers as a result of a short attention span. Tremor of the fingers can be noticed if the arm is extended. There may be a voracious appetite combined with loss of or no increase in weight. With careful examination, a goiter is found in almost all patients. Exophthalmos is noticeable in most patients but is usually mild. The skin is smooth and flushed, with excessive sweating. Tachycardia, palpitations, dyspnea, and cardiac enlargement and insufficiency cause discomfort but rarely endanger the patient's life. Thyroid "crisis," or "storm," is a form of hyperthyroidism manifested by an acute onset, hyperthermia, and severe tachycardia and restlessness. There may be rapid progression to delirium, coma, and death.

LABORATORY FINDINGS. Serum levels of thyroxine (T_4), triiodothyronine (T_3), free T_4, and free T_3 are elevated.

TREATMENT. Most pediatric endocrinologists recommend medical therapy rather than radioiodine or subtotal thyroidectomy. The two thionamide drugs in widest use are propylthiouracil (PTU) and methimazole (Tapazole).

SECTION 3

Disorders of the Parathyroid Glands

(Nelson Textbook, Chapters 580–583)

CHAPTER 274

Hypoparathyroidism

(Nelson Textbook, Chapter 581)

CLINICAL MANIFESTATIONS. There is a spectrum of parathyroid deficiencies with clinical manifestations varying from no symptoms to those of complete and long-standing deficiency (Table 274–1). Mild deficiency may be revealed only by appropriate laboratory

TABLE 274–1 Etiologic Classification of Hypocalcemia

Parathyroid Hormone (PTH) Deficiency

Aplasia or hypoplasia of parathyroids
  With 22q11 deletion
    DiGeorge syndrome
    Velocardiofacial syndrome
    Conotruncal-face syndrome
  With 10p13 deletion
    DiGeorge syndrome
  With maternal diabetes mellitus or retinoic acid treatment during pregnancy
  With CHARGE syndrome
  With X-linked isolated hypoparathyroidism
Preproparathyroid hormone gene mutation
  Autosomal dominant
Autoimmune parathyroiditis
  Isolated
  With type 1 autoimmune polyendocrinopathy
    Mutation of *AIRE* gene
    Calcium-sensing receptor antibodies
Infiltrative lesions
  Hemosiderosis (treatment of thalassemia)
  Copper deposition (Wilson disease)
Unknown causes of hypoparathyroidism
  With dysmorphic features in Middle Eastern children
    Autosomal recessive
  Kenny-Caffey syndrome
    Autosomal recessive

PTH Receptor Defects (Pseudohypoparathyroidism)

Type IA (inactivating mutation of $G_{s\alpha}$)
  With gonadotropin-independent precocious puberty
Type IB (normal $G_{s\alpha}$)
Type II (normal cyclic adenosine monophosphate response)

Ca²⁺-Sensing Receptor Activating Mutation

Sporadic
Autosomal dominant

Mitochondrial DNA Mutations

Kearns-Sayre syndrome and other mutations

Magnesium Deficiency

Absorption defect
Renal tubular defect
Aminoglycoside therapy

Exogenous Inorganic Phosphate Excess

Laxatives
Soft drinks with phosphoric acid

Vitamin D Deficiency

Nutritional
Vitamin D deficiency (rickets)
  Mutation of 1α(OH)ase (P450$^{vd1\alpha}$)

AIRE = autoimmune regulator.

studies. Muscular pain and cramps are early manifestations; they progress to numbness, stiffness, and tingling of the hands and feet. There may be only a positive Chvostek or Trousseau sign or laryngeal and carpopedal spasms. Convulsions with loss of consciousness may occur at intervals of days, weeks, or months. These episodes may begin with abdominal pain, followed by tonic rigidity, retraction of the head, and cyanosis. Headache, vomiting, increased intracranial pressure, and papilledema may be associated with convulsions and may suggest a brain tumor. Permanent physical and mental deterioration occur if initiation of treatment is long delayed.

LABORATORY FINDINGS. The serum calcium level is low (5–7 mg/dL), and the phosphorus level is elevated (7–12 mg/dL). Levels of parathyroid hormone are low when measured by immunometric assay.

TREATMENT. Emergency treatment for neonatal tetany consists of intravenous injections of 5–10 mL of a 10% solution of calcium gluconate at the rate of 0.5–1 mL/min while heart rate is monitored. Additionally, 1,25-dihydroxycholecalciferol (calcitriol) should be given.

CHAPTER 275

Hyperparathyroidism

(Nelson Textbook, Chapter 581)

Excessive production of parathyroid hormone (PTH) may result from a primary defect of the parathyroid glands such as an adenoma or hyperplasia *(primary hyperparathyroidism)*. More often, the increased production of PTH is compensatory, usually aimed at correcting hypocalcemic states of diverse origins *(secondary hyperparathyroidism)* (Table 275–1).

CLINICAL MANIFESTATIONS. At all ages, the clinical manifestations of hypercalcemia of any cause include muscular weakness, anorexia, nausea, vomiting, constipation, polydipsia, polyuria, loss of weight, and fever. When hypercalcemia is of long duration, calcium may be deposited in the renal parenchyma (nephrocalcinosis), with progressively diminished renal function.

LABORATORY FINDINGS. The serum calcium level is elevated. Serum levels of PTH are elevated.

TREATMENT. Surgical exploration is indicated in all instances. Most neonates with severe hypercalcemia require total parathyroidectomy; severe hypercalcemia may remit spontaneously in others.

TABLE 275–1 Etiologic Classification of Hypercalcemia

Parathyroid Hormone (PTH) Excess

Primary hyperparathyroidism
  Adenoma
    Sporadic
    Autosomal dominant
    Hyperparathyroidism–jaw tumor syndrome
  Hyperplasia or adenoma
    Multiple endocrine neoplasia type I
      Mutation in *MEN1* gene (11q13)
    Multiple endocrine neoplasia 2A and 2B
      Mutation in *RET* proto-oncogene
    Parathyroid hyperplasia of infancy
      Inactivating mutation of Ca^{2+}-sensing receptor
      Secondary to maternal hypoparathyroidism
  Ectopic PTH production
    Nonendocrine malignancies

Parathyroid Hormone–Related Peptide (PTHrP) Excess

Nonendocrine malignancies
Benign hypertrophy of breasts

Ca^{2+}-Sensing Receptor Inactivating Mutation

Heterozygous-familial hypocalciuric hypercalcemia
Neonatal hyperparathyroidism

Activating Mutation of PTH/PTHrP Receptor

Jansen-type metaphyseal chondrodysplasia

Inactivating Mutations of PTH/PTHrP Receptor

Blomstrand Chondrodysplasia

Vitamin D Excess

Iatrogenic
Ectopic production
  Sarcoidosis, tuberculosis, granulomatous lesions, subcutaneous fat necrosis
  Excessively fortified milk

Unknown Cause

Williams syndrome (7q11.23 deletion)

Other

Hypophosphatasia
  Mutation of tissue nonspecific alkaline phosphatase gene
Prolonged immobilization
Thyrotoxicosis
Hypervitaminosis A
Leukemia

Disorders of the Adrenal Glands

(Nelson Textbook, Chapters 584–591)

CHAPTER 276

Adrenocortical Insufficiency

(Nelson Textbook, Chapter 585)

Deficient production of cortisol or aldosterone may result from a wide variety of congenital or acquired lesions of the hypothalamus, pituitary gland, or adrenal cortex (Table 276–1). Depending on the pathologic lesions, symptoms may be severe or mild, appear abruptly or insidiously, begin in infancy or later, and be permanent or temporary.

CLINICAL MANIFESTATIONS. In patients with adrenal hypoplasia, defects in steroidogenesis, or pseudohypoaldosteronism, symptoms and signs begin shortly after birth and are characteristic of salt loss. Failure to thrive, vomiting, lethargy, anorexia, and dehydration occur; circulatory collapse may be fatal. In older children with Addison disease, the onset is usually more gradual and is characterized by muscular weakness, lassitude, anorexia, loss of weight, general wasting, and low blood pressure. Abdominal pain may simulate an acute abdominal process, and there may be an intense craving for salt. If the condition is not recognized and treated, adrenal crisis may supervene. The patient suddenly becomes cyanotic, the skin is cold, and the pulse is weak and rapid. The blood pressure falls, and respirations are rapid and labored. In the absence of immediate and intensive therapy, the course is rapidly fatal. The presenting manifestations may be those of hypoglycemia, particularly in the neonate with congenital adrenal hypoplasia.

LABORATORY FINDINGS. When salt-losing manifestations are present, the levels of sodium and chloride in the serum are usually low and those of potassium elevated, with increased plasma renin activity. Urinary excretion of sodium and chloride is increased, urinary potassium is decreased, and there is acidosis. The most definitive test is measurement of the plasma or serum levels of cortisol before and after administration of adrenocorticotropic hormone (ACTH); resting levels are low, and no increase occurs after administration of ACTH.

TREATMENT. Intravenous administration of 5% glucose in 0.9% saline solution should be given to correct the hypoglycemia and the sodium loss. Concomitantly, a water-soluble form of hydrocortisone, such as hydrocortisone hemisuccinate, should be given intravenously. After the acute manifestations are under control,

TABLE 276–1 Etiologic Classification of Adrenocortical Hypofunction

Corticotropin-Releasing Hormone Deficiency

Isolated deficiency
Multiple deficiencies
    Congenital defects (e.g., anencephaly, septo-optic dysplasia)
    Destructive lesions (e.g., tumor)
    Idiopathic (e.g., idiopathic hypopituitarism)

Corticotropin Deficiency

Isolated
Autosomal recessive
Multiple deficiencies
    Pituitary hypoplasia or aplasia
    Destructive lesions (e.g., craniopharyngioma)
    Autoimmune hypophysitis

Primary Adrenal Hypoplasia or Aplasia

X-linked
    With Duchenne muscular dystrophy and glycerol kinase deficiency (Xp21 deletion)
    With hypogonadotropic hypogonadism (DAX-1 mutation)

Familial Glucocorticoid Deficiency

Corticotropin-receptor mutations
    With alacrima, achalasia, and neurologic disorders (triple A syndrome)

Defects of Steroid Biosynthesis

Lipoid adrenal hyperplasia (StAR mutation)
3β-Hydroxysteroid dehydrogenase deficiency
    Classic
      Salt loser
      Non-salt loser
    Mild or nonclassic
21-Hydroxylase (P450C21) deficiency
    Classic
      Salt loser
      Non-salt loser
    Nonclassic or mild
Isolated aldosterone (P450C18) deficiency

Pseudohypoaldosteronism (Aldosterone Unresponsiveness)

Adrenoleukodystrophy (Peroxisomal Membrane Protein Defect)

Isolated adrenal involvement
With neurologic involvement

Acid Lipase Deficiency

Wolman disease, fatal neonatal form

Destructive Lesions of Adrenal Cortex

Granulomatous lesions (e.g., tuberculosis)

Table continued on following page

TABLE 276–1   Etiologic Classification of Adrenocortical Hypofunction *Continued*

Autoimmune Adrenalitis (Idiopathic Addison Disease)

Isolated
Associated with hypoparathyroidism or mucocutaneous candidiasis (type I autoimmune polyglandular syndrome), or both
Associated with autoimmune thyroid disease and insulin-dependent diabetes (type II autoimmune polyglandular syndrome)

Neonatal Hemorrhage

Acute Infection (Waterhouse-Friderichsen Syndrome)

Mitochondrial Disorders

Acquired Immunodeficiency Syndrome

Iatrogenic

Abrupt cessation of exogenous corticosteroids or corticotropin
Removal of functioning adrenal tumor
Adrenalectomy for Cushing disease
Drugs
    Aminoglutethimide
    Mitotane (o, p-DDD)
    Metyrapone
    Ketoconazole

Fetal Adrenal Suppression–Maternal Hypercortisolism

Endogenous
Therapeutic

most patients require chronic replacement therapy for their aldosterone and cortisol deficiencies.

CHAPTER 277

Adrenal Disorders and Genital Abnormalities

(Nelson Textbook, Chapter 586)

Disorders of adrenal hormone synthesis with signs of adrenal hyperfunction or hypofunction, or both, and associated genital abnormalities occur in patients with congenital adrenal hyperplasia and virilizing adrenal tumors (Table 277–1).

CONGENITAL ADRENAL HYPERPLASIA (CAH)

PATHOGENESIS. The deficiency of cortisol results in increased secretion of corticotropin, which, in turn, leads to adrenocortical hyperplasia and overproduction of intermediary metabolites. De-

TABLE 277–1   Etiologic Classification of Adrenocortical Hyperfunction

Excess Androgen

Congenital adrenal hyperplasia
   21-Hydroxylase (P450c21) deficiency
   11β-Hydroxylase (P450c11) deficiency
   3β-Hydroxysteroid dehydrogenase defect
Tumor
   Carcinoma
   Adenoma

Excess Cortisol (Cushing Syndrome)

Bilateral adrenal hyperplasia
   Hypersecretion of corticotropin (Cushing disease)
   Ectopic secretion of corticotropin
   Exogenous corticotropin
Adrenocortical nodular dysplasia
Pigmented nodular adrenocortical disease (Carney complex)
Tumor
   Carcinoma
   Adenoma

Excess Mineralocorticoid (Hypertensive Hypokalemic Syndrome)

Primary hyperaldosteronism
   Aldosterone-secreting adenoma
   Bilateral micronodular adrenocortical hyperplasia
   Glucocorticoid-suppressible aldosteronism
   Tumor
      Adenoma
      Carcinoma
Desoxycorticosterone excess
   Congenital adrenal hyperplasia
      11β-Hydroxylase (P450c11)
      17α-Hydroxylase (P450c17)
   Tumor (carcinoma)
Apparent mineralocorticoid excess
   11β-Hydroxysteroid dehydrogenase deficiency

Excess Estrogen (Adrenal Feminization Syndrome)

Carcinoma
Adenoma

Mixed Hypercorticism–Tumor

pending on the enzymatic step that is deficient, there may be signs, symptoms, and laboratory findings of mineralocorticoid deficiency or excess; incomplete virilization or premature androgenization of the affected male; and virilization or sexual infantilism in the affected female. *Deficiency of 21-hydroxylase* accounts for 90% of affected patients.

CLINICAL MANIFESTATIONS

Non–Salt-Losing Congenital Adrenal Hyperplasia. In the male with 21-hydroxylase deficiency, the main clinical manifestations are those of premature isosexual development. The infant usually appears normal at birth, but signs of sexual and somatic precocity may appear within the first 6 mo of life or develop more gradually, becoming evident at 4–5 yr of age or later. Enlargement of the penis, scrotum, and prostate; appearance of pubic hair; and development of acne and a deep voice are noted. Muscles are well developed, and bone age is advanced for chronological age.

Salt-Losing Congenital Adrenal Hyperplasia. In patients with the salt-losing variants, symptoms begin shortly after birth with failure to regain birth weight loss and with dehydration. Vomiting is prominent, with anorexia. Without treatment, collapse and death may occur within a few weeks.

TREATMENT. Administration of glucocorticoids inhibits excessive production of androgens and prevents progressive virilization. Patients with disturbances of electrolyte regulation (salt-losing disease) and elevated plasma renin activity require a mineralocorticoid and sodium supplementation in addition to the glucocorticoid.

SECTION 5

Disorders of the Gonads

(Nelson Textbook, Chapters 592–598)

CHAPTER 278

Hypofunction of the Testes

(Nelson Textbook, Chapter 593)

Testicular hypofunction may be primary in the testis (primary hypogonadism) or secondary to deficiency of pituitary gonadotropic hormones (secondary hypogonadism). Patients with primary hypogonadism have elevated levels of gonadotropin (hypergonadotropic); those with secondary hypogonadism have low or absent levels (hypogonadotropic).

KLINEFELTER SYNDROME

ETIOLOGY. One in 500 to 1000 male newborns has a 47,XXY chromosome complement, representing the most common sex chromosomal aneuploidy in males. The incidence approximates 1% among the mentally retarded.

CLINICAL MANIFESTATIONS. The diagnosis is rarely made before puberty because of the paucity or subtleness of clinical manifestations in childhood. Because behavioral or psychiatric disorders may often be apparent long before defects in sexual development, the condition should be considered in all boys with mental retardation and in children with psychosocial, learning, or school adjustment problems. Affected children may be anxious, immature, excessively shy, or aggressive, and they may engage in antisocial acts. The patients tend to be tall, slim, and underweight and to have relatively long legs, but body habitus can vary markedly. The testes tend to be small for age, but this sign may become apparent only after puberty, when normal testicular growth fails to occur. The phallus tends to be smaller than average.

TREATMENT. Replacement therapy with long-acting testosterone preparation depends on the age of the patient. It should begin at 11–12 yr of age.

Chapter 279

Hypofunction of the Ovaries
(Nelson Textbook, Chapter 596)

Hypofunction of the ovaries may be caused by congenital failure of development, postnatal destruction (primary or hypergonadotropic hypogonadism), or lack of stimulation by the pituitary (secondary or hypogonadotropic hypogonadism). Many chronic diseases may result in the latter type of hypofunction.

TURNER SYNDROME

CLINICAL MANIFESTATIONS. Many patients with Turner syndrome are recognizable at birth because of a characteristic edema of the dorsa of the hands and feet and loose skinfolds at the nape of the neck. Low birth weight and decreased length are common. Clinical manifestations in childhood include webbing of the neck, a low posterior hairline, small mandible, prominent ears, epicanthal folds, high arched palate, a broad chest presenting the illusion of widely spaced nipples, cubitus valgus, and hyperconvex fingernails. The diagnosis is often first suspected at puberty when sexual maturation fails to occur. Short stature is the cardinal finding in all girls with Turner syndrome. Sexual maturation fails to occur at the expected age.

TREATMENT. Treatment with recombinant human growth hormone increases height velocity and ultimate stature in most but not all children. Replacement therapy with estrogens is indicated, but there is little consensus about the optimal age at which to initiate treatment.

Diabetes Mellitus in Children

CHAPTER 280

Diabetes Mellitus

(Nelson Textbook, Chapter 599)

Diabetes mellitus is a syndrome of metabolic disease characterized by hyperglycemia. It is caused by deficiency of insulin secretion or insulin action, or both, and results in abnormal metabolism of carbohydrate, protein, and fat. It is the most common endocrine-metabolic disorder of childhood and adolescence, with important consequences for physical and emotional development.

TYPE I DIABETES. This condition is characterized by severe insulinopenia and dependence on exogenous insulin to prevent ketosis and to preserve life.

TYPE II DIABETES. Persons in this subclass (formerly known as adult-onset diabetes, maturity-onset diabetes [MOD], or non–insulin-dependent diabetes mellitus [NIDDM]) are not insulin dependent and only infrequently develop ketosis; however, some may need insulin for correction of symptomatic hyperglycemia and ketosis may develop in some during severe infections or other stress.

TYPE I DIABETES MELLITUS (IMMUNE MEDIATED)

CLINICAL MANIFESTATIONS. The classic presentation of diabetes in children is a history of polyuria, polydipsia, polyphagia, and weight loss. The duration of these symptoms varies but is often less than 1 mo. An insidious onset characterized by lethargy, weakness, and weight loss is also common. Ketoacidosis is responsible for the initial presentation of many (approximately 25%) diabetic children. The early manifestations may be relatively mild and consist of vomiting, polyuria, and dehydration. In more prolonged and severe cases, Kussmaul's respiration is present, and there is an odor of acetone on the breath. Abdominal pain or rigidity may be present and may mimic appendicitis or pancreatitis. Cerebral obtundation and ultimately coma ensue. Laboratory findings include glucosuria, ketonuria, hyperglycemia, ketonemia, and metabolic acidosis.

DIAGNOSIS. The diagnosis of diabetes mellitus is dependent on the demonstration of hyperglycemia in association with glucosuria with or without ketonuria. When classic symptoms of polyuria and polydipsia are associated with hyperglycemia and glucosuria, the glucose tolerance test is not needed to support the diagnosis.

TREATMENT. The management of IDDM may be divided into three phases depending on the initial presentation: that of ketoacidosis, the postacidotic or transition period for establishment of metabolic control, and the continuing phase of guidance of the diabetic child and his or her family.

Ketoacidosis. The immediate aims of therapy are expansion of intravascular volume; correction of deficits in fluid, electrolyte, and acid-base status; and initiation of insulin therapy to correct intermediary metabolism.

Fluid and Electrolyte Therapy. The expansion of reduced intravascular volume and correction of depleted fluid and electrolyte stores are most important in the treatment of diabetic ketoacidosis. The amount of dehydration is commonly about 10%; initial fluid therapy can be based on this estimate, with subsequent adjustments related to clinical and laboratory data. The initial hydrating fluid should be isotonic saline (0.9%).

Insulin Therapy. The continuous low-dose intravenous infusion method involves a priming dose of 0.1 U/kg of regular insulin followed by a constant infusion of 0.1 U/kg/hr.

Postacidotic Phase or Transition Period for Establishment of Metabolic Control. Diabetic ketoacidosis is usually corrected within 36 to 48 hr by the foregoing therapeutic regimen. At this time, food and fluids are usually tolerated orally and insulin can be given by subcutaneous injection. The child who presents with classic symptoms and documented hyperglycemia, in the absence of clinical dehydration and ketoacidosis, can be considered as requiring treatment at this transition stage. For such children, subcutaneous injections of fast-acting insulin are begun at doses of 0.1–0.25 U/kg every 6–8 hr before meals with simultaneous monitoring of blood glucose concentration and adjustment of the insulin dose for 1–2 days. One to 2 days of fast-acting insulin therapy is needed to estimate the total daily insulin requirement as a guide to subsequent use of combined intermediate and short-acting forms.

TYPE II DIABETES

Type II diabetes mellitus is increasing dramatically among children, especially adolescents in the United States, accompanying the rise in obesity in the pediatric population. Treatment of type II diabetes should target weight loss and increasing physical activity as an initial approach. These approaches, however, are frequently unsuccessful. Sulfonylurea compounds that stimulate endogenous insulin secretion and biguanides that diminish hepatic glucose production may be used in these children and adolescents.

PART 25

The Nervous System

(Nelson Textbook, Chapters 600–613)

CHAPTER 281

Congenital Anomalies of the Central Nervous System

(Nelson Textbook, Chapter 601)

Neural tube defects account for most congenital anomalies of the central nervous system (CNS) and result from failure of the neural tube to close spontaneously between the 3rd and 4th wk of in utero development. The major neural tube defects include spina bifida occulta, meningocele, myelomeningocele, encephalocele, anencephaly, dermal sinus, tethered cord, syringomyelia, diastematomyelia, and lipoma involving the conus medullaris.

MYELOMENINGOCELE

Myelomeningocele represents the most severe form of dysraphism involving the vertebral column and occurs with an incidence of approximately 1 in 1000 live births.

ETIOLOGY. The cause of myelomeningocele is unknown, but studies have provided strong evidence that maternal periconceptional use of folic acid supplementation reduces the incidence of neural tube defects in pregnancies at risk by at least 50%.

CLINICAL MANIFESTATIONS. The condition produces dysfunction of many organs and structures, including the skeleton, skin, and genitourinary tract, in addition to the peripheral nervous system and the CNS. A myelomeningocele may be located anywhere along the neuraxis, but the lumbosacral region accounts for at least 75% of the cases. The extent and degree of the neurologic deficit depend on the location of the myelomeningocele. *Hydrocephalus* in association with a type II Chiari defect develops in at least 80% of patients with myelomeningocele.

TREATMENT. Management and supervision of a child and family with a myelomeningocele require a multidisciplinary team approach, including surgeons, physicians, and therapists, with one individual (often a pediatrician) acting as the advocate and coordinator of the treatment program.

PROGNOSIS. For a child who is born with a myelomeningocele and who is treated aggressively, the mortality rate is 10–15%, and most deaths occur before age 4 yr. At least 70% of survivors have normal intelligence, but learning problems and seizure disorders are more common than in the general population.

DISORDERS OF NEURONAL MIGRATION

Disorders of neuronal migration may result in minor abnormalities with little or no clinical consequence (e.g., small heterotopia of neurons) or devastating abnormalities of the CNS (e.g., mental retardation, lissencephaly, schizencephaly).

HYDROCEPHALUS

Hydrocephalus is not a specific disease; rather, it represents a diverse group of conditions that result from impaired circulation and absorption of cerebrospinal fluid or, in the rare circumstance, from increased production by a choroid plexus papilloma.

CLINICAL MANIFESTATIONS. In an infant, an accelerated rate of enlargement of the head is the most prominent sign. In addition, the anterior fontanel is wide open and bulging and the scalp veins are dilated. The forehead is broad, and the eyes may deviate downward because of impingement of the dilated suprapineal recess on the tectum, producing the setting-sun eye sign. Long-tract signs including brisk tendon reflexes, spasticity, clonus (particularly in the lower extremities), and Babinski sign are common. In an older child, the cranial sutures are partially closed so that the signs of hydrocephalus may be more subtle. Irritability, lethargy, poor appetite, and vomiting are common to both age groups, and headache is a prominent symptom in older patients. Serial measurements of the head circumference indicate an increased velocity of growth.

DIAGNOSIS. Computed tomography and/or magnetic resonance imaging along with ultrasonography in an infant are the most important studies to identify the specific cause of hydrocephalus.

TREATMENT. Most cases of hydrocephalus require extracranial shunts, particularly a ventriculoperitoneal shunt.

CRANIOSYNOSTOSIS

Craniosynostosis is defined as premature closure of the cranial sutures. *Primary craniosynostosis* refers to closure of one or more sutures due to abnormalities of skull development, whereas *secondary craniosynostosis* results from failure of brain growth and expansion. The cause is unknown in the majority of children; however, genetic syndromes account for 10–20% of cases.

CLINICAL MANIFESTATIONS AND TREATMENT. Most cases of craniosynostosis are evident at birth and are characterized by a skull deformity that is a direct result of premature suture fusion. Palpation of the suture reveals a prominent bony ridge, and fusion of the suture may be confirmed by plain skull radiographs or bone scan in ambiguous cases. Premature closure of the sagittal suture produces a long and narrow skull, or *scaphocephaly,* the most common form of craniosynostosis. Scaphocephaly is associated with a prominent occiput, a broad forehead, and a small or absent anterior fontanel. Scaphocephaly does not produce increased intracranial pressure or hydrocephalus, and results of neurologic examination of affected patients are normal. *Frontal plagiocephaly* is the next most common form of craniosynostosis and is characterized by unilateral flattening of the forehead, elevation of the ipsilateral orbit and eyebrow, and a prominent ear on the corresponding side. Surgical intervention produces a cosmetically pleasing result.

CHAPTER 282

Seizures in Childhood

(Nelson Textbook, Chapter 602)

Seizures do not constitute a diagnosis but are a symptom of an underlying central nervous system (CNS) disorder that requires a thorough investigation and management plan. A *seizure* (convulsion) is defined as a paroxysmal involuntary disturbance of brain function that may be manifested as an impairment or loss of consciousness, abnormal motor activity, behavioral abnormalities, sensory disturbance, or autonomic dysfunction. *Epilepsy* is defined as recurrent seizures unrelated to fever or to an acute cerebral insult.

CLASSIFICATION OF SEIZURES

Clinical classification of seizures may be difficult because the manifestations of different seizure types may be similar (Table 282–1). Epilepsy in children has also been classified by syndrome.

Partial Seizures

Partial seizures account for a large proportion of childhood seizures, up to 40% in some series.

SIMPLE PARTIAL SEIZURES (SPS). Motor activity is the most common symptom of SPS. The movements are characterized by asynchronous clonic or tonic movements, and they tend to involve the face, neck, and extremities. *The distinguishing characteristic of SPS is that the patients remain conscious and may verbalize during the seizure. Furthermore, no postictal phenomenon follows the event.* The electroencephalogram (EEG) may show spikes or sharp waves unilaterally or bilaterally or a multifocal spike pattern in patients with SPS.

COMPLEX PARTIAL SEIZURES (CPS). A CPS may begin with a simple partial seizure with or without an aura, followed by impaired consciousness; conversely, the onset of the CPS may coincide with an altered state of consciousness. *The presence of an aura*

TABLE 282–1 International Classification of Epileptic Seizures

Partial Seizures

Simple partial (consciousness retained)
   Motor
   Sensory
   Autonomic
   Psychic
Complex partial (consciousness impaired)
   Simple partial, followed by impaired consciousness
   Consciousness impaired at onset
Partial seizures with secondary generalization

Generalized Seizures

Absences
   Typical
   Atypical
Generalized tonic-clonic
Tonic
Clonic
Myoclonic
Atonic
Infantile spasms

Unclassified Seizures

---

always indicates a focal onset of the seizure. Automatisms are a common feature of a CPS in infants and children. A CPS is associated with interictal EEG anterior temporal lobe sharp waves or focal spikes, and multifocal spikes are a frequent finding.

BENIGN PARTIAL EPILEPSY WITH CENTROTEMPORAL SPIKES (BPEC). BPEC is a common type of partial epilepsy in childhood and has an excellent prognosis. The seizures are usually partial, and motor signs and somatosensory symptoms are often confined to the face. Oropharyngeal symptoms include tonic contractions and paresthesias of the tongue, unilateral numbness of the cheek (particularly along the gum), guttural noises, dysphagia, and excessive salivation. BPEC occurs during sleep in 75% of patients, whereas CPS tends to be observed during waking hours. The EEG pattern is diagnostic for BPEC and is characterized by a repetitive spike focus localized in the centrotemporal or rolandic area with normal background activity.

Generalized Seizures

ABSENCE SEIZURES. Simple (typical) absence (petit mal) seizures are characterized by a sudden cessation of motor activity or speech with a blank facial expression and flickering of the eyelids. They are never associated with an aura; they rarely persist longer than 30 sec; and they are not associated with a postictal state. Children with absence seizures may experience countless seizures daily, whereas complex partial seizures are usually less frequent.

Automatic behavior frequently accompanies simple absence seizures.

GENERALIZED TONIC-CLONIC SEIZURES. These seizures are extremely common and may follow a partial seizure with a focal onset (second generalization) or occur de novo. They may be associated with an aura, suggesting a focal origin of the epileptiform discharge. Patients suddenly lose consciousness and in some cases emit a shrill, piercing cry. Their eyes roll back, their entire body musculature undergoes tonic contractions, and they rapidly become cyanotic in association with apnea. The clonic phase of the seizure is heralded by rhythmic clonic contractions alternating with relaxation of all muscle groups.

Tight clothing and jewelry around the neck should be loosened, the patient should be placed on one side, and the neck and jaw should be gently hyperextended to enhance breathing. Postictally, children initially are semicomatose and typically remain in a deep sleep from 30 min to 2 hr.

INFANTILE SPASMS. Infantile spasms usually begin between the ages of 4 and 8 mo and are characterized by brief symmetric contractions of the neck, trunk, and extremities. There are at least three types of infantile spasms: flexor, extensor, and mixed. Clusters or volleys of seizures may persist for minutes, with brief intervals between each spasm. The EEG that is most commonly associated with infantile spasms is referred to as *hypsarrhythmia,* which consists of a chaotic pattern of high-voltage, bilaterally asynchronous, slow-wave activity, or a modified hypsarrhythmia pattern.

Febrile Seizures

Febrile convulsions rarely develop into epilepsy, and they spontaneously remit without specific therapy. They are the most common seizure disorder during childhood, with a uniformly excellent prognosis. Febrile seizures are age dependent and are rare before 9 mo and after 5 yr of age.

CLINICAL MANIFESTATIONS. The convulsion is associated with a rapidly rising temperature and usually develops when the core temperature reaches 39°C or greater. The seizure is typically generalized, tonic-clonic of a few seconds to 10-min duration and followed by a brief postictal period of drowsiness.

TREATMENT. Routine treatment of a normal infant who has simple febrile convulsions includes a careful search for the cause of the fever, active measures to control the fever including the use of antipyretics, and reassurance of the parents. Short-term anticonvulsant prophylaxis is not indicated.

Treatment of Epilepsy

The first step in the management of epilepsy is to ensure that the patient has a seizure disorder and not a condition that mimics epilepsy. Most would concur that antiepileptics should be withheld from a previously healthy child with the first afebrile convulsion if there is a negative family history, normal results of an examination and EEG, and a cooperative and compliant family. A recurrent seizure, particularly if it occurs in close proximity to the first seizure, is an indication to begin anticonvulsant therapy. The second step involves choosing an anticonvulsant. The drug of choice depends on the classification of the seizure, determined by the history and EEG findings. A loading dose is indicated for drugs that are useful for the treatment of status epilepticus.

Neonatal Seizures

Neonates are at particular risk for the development of seizures because metabolic, toxic, structural, and infectious diseases are more likely to be manifested during this time than at any other period of life. Generalized tonic-clonic convulsions tend not to occur during the 1st mo of life.

CLINICAL MANIFESTATIONS AND CLASSIFICATION. *Focal seizures* consist of rhythmic twitching of muscle groups, particularly those of the extremities and face. *Multifocal clonic* convulsions are similar to focal clonic seizures but differ in that many muscle groups are involved, frequently several simultaneously. Tonic seizures are characterized by rigid posturing of the extremities and trunk and are sometimes associated with fixed deviation of the eyes. Myoclonic seizures are brief focal or generalized jerks of the extremities or body that tend to involve distal muscle groups. Subtle seizures consist of chewing motions, excessive salivation, and alterations in the respiratory rate including apnea, blinking, nystagmus, bicycling or pedaling movements, and changes in color.

ETIOLOGIC DIAGNOSIS. Hypoxic-ischemic encephalopathy is the most common cause of neonatal seizures. Many additional disorders are likely to cause seizures, including metabolic, infectious, traumatic, structural, hemorrhagic, embolic, and maternal disturbances.

TREATMENT. Anticonvulsants should be used in the treatment of infants with seizures secondary to hypoxic-ischemic encephalopathy or an acute intracranial hemorrhage.

Status Epilepticus

Status epilepticus is defined as a continuous convulsion lasting longer than 30 min or the occurrence of serial convulsions between which there is no return of consciousness. Generalized tonic-clonic seizures predominate in cases of status epilepticus. Status epilepticus is a medical emergency that requires an organized and skillful approach to minimize the associated mortality and morbidity.

TREATMENT. Initial treatment of patients begins with an assessment of the respiratory and cardiovascular systems. Children should be transferred to an intensive care unit if possible. The oral airway is secured and inspected for patency, and the pulse, temperature, respirations, and blood pressure are recorded. Excessive oral secretions are removed by gentle suction, and a properly fitting face mask attached to oxygen is applied. If patients do not respond to oxygen by mask or are difficult to ventilate by an Ambu bag, consideration should be given to intubation and assisted ventilation. A nasogastric tube is placed in position, and an intravenous catheter is immediately inserted.

Drugs should always be delivered intravenously in the management of status epilepticus. Benzodiazepines (diazepam, lorazepam, or midazolam) may be used initially, because these are effective for immediate control of prolonged tonic-clonic seizures in most children. Diazepam should be given intravenously directly into the vein (not the tubing) in a dose of 0.1–0.3 mg/kg at a rate no greater than 2 mg/min for a maximum of three doses. After administration of diazepam or lorazepam, several options are available for further management.

Chapter 283

Headaches

(Nelson Textbook, Chapter 604)

Headache is a common problem in pediatrics. The effect that headaches have on a child's academic performance, memory, personality, and interpersonal relationships, as well as school attendance, depends on their etiology, frequency, and intensity. A headache may occasionally indicate a severe underlying disorder (e.g., a brain tumor), and thus careful evaluation of children with recurrent, severe, or unconventional headaches is mandatory. Infants and children respond to a headache in an unpredictable fashion. Most toddlers cannot communicate the characteristics of a headache, but rather they may become irritable and cranky, vomit, prefer a darkened room because of photophobia, or repeatedly rub their eyes and head. The most important causes of headache in children include migraine, increased intracranial pressure, and psychogenic factors or stress.

CHAPTER 284

Movement Disorders

(Nelson Textbook, Chapter 606)

Abnormalities of movement in children constitute a wide range of conditions with multiple causes. The type of movement disorder assists in localization of the pathologic process, whereas the onset, age, and degree of the abnormal motor activity and associated neurologic findings help to classify the disorder and organize the investigation. Movement disorders are rarely limited to one form such as ataxia; the examination usually demonstrates additional abnormal movements, such as tremor or chorea.

The major infectious causes of ataxia include cerebellar abscess, acute labyrinthitis, and acute cerebellar ataxia. *Acute cerebellar ataxia* occurs primarily in children 1–3 yr of age and is a diagnosis by exclusion. The condition often follows a viral illness, such as varicella or coxsackievirus or echovirus infection, by 2–3 wk and is thought to represent an autoimmune response to the viral agent affecting the cerebellum. The onset is sudden, and the truncal ataxia can be so severe that the child is unable to stand or sit. Vomiting may occur initially, but fever and nuchal rigidity are absent. Horizontal nystagmus is evident in approximately 50% of cases, and if the child is able to speak, dysarthria may be impressive. Later in the course, the cerebrospinal fluid protein level undergoes a moderate elevation. The ataxia begins to improve in a few weeks but may persist for as long as 2 mo. *Acute labyrinthitis* may be difficult to differentiate from acute cerebellar ataxia in a toddler. The condition is associated with middle ear infections and intense vertigo, vomiting, and abnormalities in labyrinthine function, particularly ice water caloric testing.

CHAPTER 285

Encephalopathies

(Nelson Textbook, Chapter 607)

Encephalopathy is a generalized disorder of cerebral function that may be acute or chronic, progressive or static. The etiology of the encephalopathies in children includes infectious, toxic (e.g., carbon monoxide, drugs, lead), metabolic, and ischemic (hypoxic-ischemic encephalopathy) causes.

CEREBRAL PALSY

Cerebral palsy (CP) is a static encephalopathy that may be defined as a nonprogressive disorder of posture and movement, often associated with epilepsy and abnormalities of speech, vision, and intellect resulting from a defect or lesion of the developing brain.

CLINICAL MANIFESTATIONS. CP may be classified by a description of the motor handicap in terms of physiologic, topographic, and etiologic categories and functional capacity. The physiologic classification identifies the major motor abnormality, whereas the topographic taxonomy indicates the involved extremities. CP is also commonly associated with a spectrum of developmental disabilities, including mental retardation, epilepsy, and visual, hearing, speech, cognitive, and behavioral abnormalities.

Infants with *spastic hemiplegia* have decreased spontaneous movements on the affected side and show hand preference at a very early age. The arm is often more involved than the leg, and difficulty in hand manipulation is obvious by 1 yr of age. Walking is usually delayed until 18–24 mo, and a circumductive gait is apparent. *Spastic diplegia* is bilateral spasticity of the legs. The first indication of spastic diplegia is often noted when an affected infant begins to crawl. The child uses the arms in a normal reciprocal fashion but tends to drag the legs behind more as a rudder (commando crawl) rather than using the normal four-limbed crawling movement. If the spasticity is severe, application of a diaper is difficult, owing to excessive adduction of the hips. *Spastic quadriplegia* is the most severe form of CP because of marked motor impairment of all extremities and the high association with mental retardation and seizures. Swallowing difficulties are common, owing to supranuclear bulbar palsies, and they often lead to aspiration pneumonia.

TREATMENT. A team of physicians from various specialties as well as the occupational and physical therapists, speech pathologist, social worker, educator, and developmental psychologist provide important contributions to the treatment of these children.

CHAPTER 286

Neurodegenerative Disorders of Childhood

(Nelson Textbook, Chapter 608)

Neurodegenerative disorders of childhood encompass a large number of heterogeneous diseases that result from specific genetic and biochemical defects, chronic viral infections, and toxic substances and a significant group of conditions of unknown cause. The hallmark of a neurodegenerative disease is progressive deterioration of neurologic function with loss of speech, vision, hearing, or locomotion, often associated with seizures, feeding difficulties, and impairment of intellect. A precise history confirms regression of developmental milestones, and the neurologic examination localizes the process within the nervous system. Although the outcome is invariably fatal and current therapeutic attempts have been unsuccessful, it is important to make the correct diagnosis so that genetic counseling may be offered and prevention strategies can be implemented. The inherited neurodegenerative disorders include the sphingolipidoses, neuronal ceroid lipofuscinosis, adrenoleukodystrophy, and sialidosis.

CHAPTER 287

Brain Tumors in Children
(Nelson Textbook, Chapter 611)

Brain tumors are second only to leukemia as the most prevalent malignancy in childhood, and they account for the most common solid tumors in this age group. Brain tumors can present at any age, but each tends to have a peak age incidence.

CLINICAL MANIFESTATIONS. Brain tumors present in many ways, depending on the location, type, and rate of growth of the tumor and the age of the child. Generally, there are two distinct patterns of presentation: symptoms and signs of increased intracranial pressure (ICP) and focal neurologic signs. Tumors located within the posterior fossa primarily produce symptoms and signs of increased ICP due to obstruction of cerebrospinal fluid pathways and the development of hydrocephalus. Supratentorial tumors are more likely to be associated with focal abnormalities, including long-tract signs and seizures.

Alterations in personality are often the first symptoms of a brain tumor, irrespective of its location. The child, beginning weeks or months before the discovery of the tumor, may have become lethargic, irritable, hyperactive, or forgetful or may perform poorly academically. After the tumor has been removed and there is amelioration of the increased ICP, significant reversal of the behavioral problems usually occurs.

Increased ICP is characterized by headache, vomiting, diplopia, and papilledema; and in infants a bulging fontanel and increasing head size (macrocrania) develop. The headache initially tends to occur in the morning and is relieved with standing. The headache is described as dull, generalized, and steady and may be intermittent and worsened by coughing or sneezing or during defecation. The headache is typically associated with vomiting, which often relieves the headache. Diplopia is a common symptom of posterior fossa tumors. Nystagmus is a prominent sign associated with posterior fossa tumors. Supratentorial tumors may also be associated with symptoms and signs of increased ICP. However, focal neurologic signs including hemiparesis and complex partial seizures predominate, particularly with a temporal lobe tumor.

INFRATENTORIAL TUMORS. The *cerebellar astrocytoma* is the most common posterior fossa tumor of childhood and has the best prognosis. The treatment is surgical resection, and the 5-yr survival is greater than 90%. The *medulloblastoma* is the next most common posterior fossa tumor in the pediatric age group and is the most prevalent brain tumor in children younger than 7 yr. All patients are treated with surgical extirpation, followed by irradiation. Many centers treat all patients with a combination of chemotherapy and radiation. *Brain stem gliomas* are the third most frequent posterior fossa tumor in children. The symptoms and signs result from invasion and destruction of cranial nerve nuclei and the pyramidal tracts. The most common cranial nerve symptoms include diplopia and facial weakness due to abducens and facial nerve involvement. The surgical treatment of brain stem gliomas is controversial.

SUPRATENTORIAL TUMORS. *Craniopharyngioma* is one of the most common supratentorial tumors in children. The tumor may be confined to the sella turcica, or it can extend through the diaphragma sella and compress the optic nerve system, pons, or third ventricle, producing hydrocephalus. Approximately 90% of craniopharyngiomas show calcification on the plain skull radiograph or CT scan. Pressure or injury to the optic chiasm typically produces bitemporal visual field defects, although most children are unaware of peripheral visual loss until the time of testing. Papilledema and symptoms of increased ICP are evident when hydrocephalus is prominent. The treatment is a craniotomy using a subfrontal approach.

PART 26

Neuromuscular Disorders

(Nelson Textbook, Chapters 614–624)

CHAPTER 288

Evaluation and Investigation

(Nelson Textbook, Chapter 614)

The term *neuromuscular disease* refers to disorders of the motor unit and excludes suprasegmental disorders, such as cerebral palsy, even though muscle tone, strength, function, and reflexes are influenced by cerebral disease.

CLINICAL MANIFESTATIONS. Examination of the neuromuscular system includes an assessment of muscle bulk, tone, and strength. Tone and strength should not be confused: passive tone is range of motion around a joint; active tone is physiologic resistance to movement. Hypotonia may be associated with normal strength or with weakness. A few specific clinical features are important in the diagnosis of some neuromuscular diseases. Fasciculations of muscle, which are often best seen in the tongue, are a sign of denervation. Sensory abnormalities indicate neuropathy. Fatigable weakness is characteristic of neuromuscular junctional disorders. Myotonia is specific for a few myopathies. Generalized hypotonia and motor developmental delay are the most common presenting manifestations of neuromuscular disease in infants and young children.

LABORATORY FINDINGS

Serum Enzymes. Several lysosomal enzymes are released by damaged or degenerating muscle fibers and may be measured in serum. The most useful of these enzymes is *creatine phosphokinase* (CK), which is found in only three organs and may be separated into corresponding isozymes: MM for skeletal muscle, MB for cardiac muscle, and BB for brain.

Nerve Conduction Velocity (NCV). Neuropathies of various types are detected by decreased conduction.

Muscle Biopsy. The muscle biopsy is the most important and specific diagnostic study of muscle.

CHAPTER 289

Developmental Disorders of Muscle

(Nelson Textbook, Chapter 615)

A heterogeneous group of congenital neuromuscular disorders is sometimes known as the *congenital myopathies* (Table 289–1). Most congenital myopathies are nonprogressive conditions, but some patients show slow clinical deterioration accompanied by additional changes in their muscle biopsy material. Although clinical features, including phenotype, may raise a strong suspicion of a congenital myopathy, the definitive diagnosis is determined by the histopathologic findings in the muscle biopsy sample. In general, only supportive treatment is available for these disorders.

TABLE 289–1 Inheritance Patterns and Chromosomal or Mitochondrial Loci of Neuromuscular Diseases Affecting the Pediatric Age Group

Disease	Transmission	Locus
Duchenne/Becker muscular dystrophy	XR	Xp21.2
Emery-Dreifuss muscular dystrophy	XR	Xq28
Myotonic muscular dystrophy (Steinert)	AD	19q13
Facioscapulohumeral muscular dystrophy	AD	4q35
Limb-girdle muscular dystrophy	AD	5q
Limb-girdle muscular dystrophy	AR	15q
Congenital muscular dystrophy with merosin deficiency	AR	6q2
Congenital muscular dystrophy (Fukuyama)	AR	8q31-33
Myotubular myopathy	XR	Xq28
Myotubular myopathy	AR	Unknown
Nemaline rod myopathy	AD	1q21-q23
Nemaline rod myopathy	AR	2q21.2-q22
Congenital muscle fiber-type disproportion	AR	Unknown
Central core disease	AD	19q13.1
Myotonia congenita (Thomsen)	AD	7q35
Myotonia congenita (Becker)	AR	7q35
Paramyotonia congenita	AD	17q13.1-13.3
Hyperkalemic periodic paralysis	AD	17q13.1-13.3
Hypokalemic periodic paralysis	AD	1q31-q32
Glycogenosis II (Pompe; acid maltase deficiency)	AR	17q23
Glycogenosis V (McArdle; myophosphorylase deficiency)	AR	11q13

TABLE 289–1 Inheritance Patterns and Chromosomal or Mitochondrial Loci of Neuromuscular Diseases Affecting the Pediatric Age Group *Continued*

Disease	Transmission	Locus
Glycogenosis VII (Tarui; phosphofructokinase deficiency)	AR	1cenq32
Glycogenosis IX (phosphoglycerate kinase deficiency)	XR	Xq13
Glycogenosis X (phosphoglyceromutase deficiency)	AR	7p12-p13
Glycogenosis XI (lactate dehydrogenase deficiency)	AR	11p15.4
Muscle carnitine deficiency	AR	Unknown
Muscle carnitine palmitoyltransferase deficiency 2	AR	1p32
Spinal muscular atrophy (Werdnig-Hoffmann; Kugelberg-Welander)	AR	5q11-q13
Familial dysautonomia (Riley-Day)	AR	9q31-33
Hereditary motor-sensory neuropathy (Charcot-Marie-Tooth; Déjerine-Sottas)	AD	17p11.2
Hereditary motor-sensory neuropathy (axonal type)	AD	1p35-p36
Hereditary motor-sensory neuropathy (Charcot-Marie-Tooth-X)	XR	Xq13.1
Mitochondrial myopathy (Kearns-Sayre)	Maternal; sporadic	Single large mtDNA deletion
Mitochondrial myopathy (MERRF)	Maternal	tRNA point mutation at position 8344
Mitochondrial myopathy (MELAS)	Maternal	tRNA point mutation at positions 3243 and 3271

AD = autosomal dominant; AR = autosomal recessive; XR = X-linked recessive; MERRF = mitochondrial encephalomyopathy with ragged-red fibers; MELAS = mitochondrial encephalomyopathy with lactic acidosis and strokelike episodes; mtDNA = mitochondrial deoxyribonucleic acid; tRNA = transfer ribonucleic acid.

CHAPTER 290

Muscular Dystrophies

(Nelson Textbook, Chapter 616)

A muscular dystrophy is distinguished from all other neuromuscular disease by four obligatory criteria: (1) it is a primary myopathy; (2) it has a genetic basis; (3) the course is progressive; and (4) degeneration and death of muscle fibers occur at some stage in the disease. Some metabolic myopathies may fulfill the definition of a progressive muscular dystrophy but are not traditionally classified as dystrophies.

Muscular dystrophies are a group of unrelated diseases, each transmitted by a different genetic trait and each differing in its clinical course and expression. Some are severe diseases at birth or lead to early death; others follow very slow progressive courses over many decades, may be compatible with normal longevity, or may not even become symptomatic until late adult life. Some categories of dystrophies, such as limb-girdle muscular dystrophy, are not homogeneous diseases but rather syndromes encompassing several distinct myopathies.

DUCHENNE AND BECKER MUSCULAR DYSTROPHIES

Duchenne muscular dystrophy is the most common hereditary neuromuscular disease affecting all races and ethnic groups.

CLINICAL MANIFESTATIONS. Infant boys are only rarely symptomatic at birth or in early infancy, although some are already mildly hypotonic. Poor head control in infancy may be the first sign of weakness. Toddlers may assume a lordotic posture when standing to compensate for gluteal weakness. An early Gowers sign is often evident by age 3 yr and is fully expressed by age 5 or 6 yr. A Trendelenburg gait, or hip waddle, appears at this time. The length of time that a patient remains ambulatory varies greatly. The relentless progression of weakness continues into the 2nd decade. Respiratory muscle involvement is expressed as a weak and ineffective cough, frequent pulmonary infections, and decreasing respiratory reserve. Intellectual impairment occurs in all patients, although only 20–30% have an intelligence quotient (IQ) less than 70. The degenerative changes and fibrosis of muscle constitute a painless process. Death occurs usually at about 18 yr of age. The causes of death are respiratory failure in sleep, intractable heart failure, pneumonia, or occasionally aspiration and airway obstruction.

In *Becker muscular dystrophy*, boys remain ambulatory until late adolescence or early adult life. Death often occurs in the mid to late 20s; fewer than half of patients are still alive by age 40 yr; these survivors are severely disabled.

TREATMENT. There is now neither medical cure for this disease nor a method of slowing its progression. Much can be done to treat complications and to improve the quality of life of affected children.

CHAPTER 291

Guillain-Barré Syndrome

(Nelson Textbook, Chapter 623)

Guillain-Barré syndrome is a postinfectious polyneuropathy that causes demyelination in mainly motor but sometimes also sensory nerves.

CLINICAL MANIFESTATIONS. The paralysis usually follows a nonspecific viral infection by about 10 days. The original infection may have caused only gastrointestinal (especially *Campylobacter jejuni)* or respiratory tract (especially *Mycoplasma pneumoniae)* symptoms. Weakness begins usually in the lower extremities and progressively involves the trunk, the upper limbs, and finally the bulbar muscles. Proximal and distal muscles are involved relatively symmetrically, but asymmetry is found in 9% of patients. The onset is gradual and progresses over days or weeks. Particularly in cases with an abrupt onset, tenderness on palpation and pain in muscles is common in the initial stages. *Bulbar involvement* occurs in about half of cases. Respiratory insufficiency may result. Dysphagia and facial weakness are often impending signs of respiratory failure.

The clinical course is usually benign, and spontaneous recovery begins within 2–3 wk. Most patients regain full muscular strength, although some are left with residual weakness. Improvement usually follows a gradient inverse to the direction of involvement, with recovery of bulbar function first and lower extremity weakness resolving last. Bulbar and respiratory muscle involvement may lead to death if the syndrome is not recognized and treated.

LABORATORY FINDINGS AND DIAGNOSIS. The cerebrospinal fluid protein is elevated to more than twice the upper limit of normal, glucose level is normal, and there is no pleocytosis.

TREATMENT. Patients in early stages of this *acute* disease should be admitted to the hospital for observation because the ascending paralysis may rapidly involve respiratory muscles during the next 24 hr. Rapidly progressive ascending paralysis is treated with intravenous immunoglobulin (IVIG), administered for 2, 3, or 5 days. Plasmapheresis, corticosteroids, and/or immunosuppressive drugs are alternatives if IVIG is ineffective. Supportive care, such as respiratory support, prevention of decubiti in children with flaccid tetraplegia, and treatment of secondary bacterial infections, is important.

PART 27

Disorders of the Eye

(Nelson Textbook, Chapters 625–641)

CHAPTER 292

Disorders of the Eye Movement and Alignment

(Nelson Textbook, Chapter 630)

STRABISMUS

Strabismus, or misalignment of the eyes, is one of the most common eye problems encountered in children. This important ocular disorder can result in vision loss (amblyopia) in one eye and can have significant psychologic effects. Early detection and treatment of strabismus is essential to prevent permanent visual impairment.

DEFINITIONS. The word *strabismus* means "to squint or to look obliquely." Many terms are used in discussing strabismus. *Heterophoria* is a latent tendency for the eyes to deviate. Some degree of heterophoria is found in normal individuals; it is usually asymptomatic. *Heterotropia* is a misalignment of the eyes that is apparent. The undeviated eye becomes the preferred eye, resulting in loss of vision or amblyopia of the deviated eye.

Esophorias and *esotropias* are inward or convergent deviations of the eyes, commonly known as *crossed eyes*. *Exophorias* and *exotropias* are divergent or outward-facing eye deviations, with *"walleyed"* being the lay term. Hyperdeviations and hypodeviations designate upward or downward deviation of an eye.

CLINICAL MANIFESTATIONS AND TREATMENT

Nonparalytic Strabismus. This is the most common type. The individual extraocular muscles usually have no defect. The amount of deviation is constant, or relatively constant, in the various directions of gaze. *Esodeviations* are the most common type of ocular misalignment in children and represent well over 50% of all ocular deviations.

Congenital esotropia is a confusing term. Few children who are diagnosed with this disorder are actually born with an esotropia. Most reports in the literature have therefore considered infants with confirmed onset earlier than 6 mo as having the same condition, which some observers have redesignated infantile esotropia. The primary goal of treatment in congenital esotropia is to eliminate or reduce the deviation as much as possible. Once any associated amblyopia is treated, surgery is performed to align the eyes. It is important that parents realize that early successful surgical alignment is only the beginning of the treatment processes. Because many children may redevelop strabismus or amblyopia, they need to be monitored closely during the visually immature period of life.

Exodeviations are the second most common type of misalignment. The divergent deviation may be intermittent or constant. *Intermittent exotropia* is the most common exodeviation in childhood. It is characterized by outward drifting of one eye, which usually occurs when a child is fixating at distance. The decision to perform eye muscle surgery is based on the amount and frequency of the deviation. *Constant exotropia* may rarely be congenital. Surgery can restore binocular vision even in long-lasting cases.

Paralytic Strabismus. When an eye muscle is paretic or palsied, a characteristic muscle imbalance occurs in which the deviation of the eye varies according to the direction of gaze. It is important to differentiate an extraocular muscle paresis or palsy from a concomitant deviation because nonconcomitant forms of strabismus are oftean associated with trauma, systemic disorders, or neurologic abnormalities.

CHAPTER 293

Disorders of the Lacrimal System

(Nelson Textbook, Chapter 632)

DACRYOSTENOSIS AND DACRYOCYSTITIS. *Congenital nasolacrimal duct obstruction* (CNLDO), or dacryostenosis, is the most common disorder of the lacrimal system, occurring in up to 6% of newborns. Signs of CNLDO include an excessive tear lake, overflow of tears onto the lid and cheek, and reflux of mucoid material that is produced in the lacrimal sac. Erythema or maceration of the skin may result from irritation and rubbing produced by dripping of tears and discharge. If the blockage is complete, these signs may be severe and continuous.

The primary treatment of uncomplicated nasolacrimal obstruction is a regimen of nasolacrimal massage, usually two to three times a day, accompanied by cleansing of the lids with warm water. Topical antibiotics are used for significant mucopurulent drainage. Most cases of CNLDO resolve spontaneously, 96% before 1 yr of age. For cases that do not resolve by 1 yr, the nasolacrimal duct may be probed, with a cure rate of approximately 90%.

CHAPTER 294

Disorders of the Conjunctiva

(Nelson Textbook, Chapter 633)

CONJUNCTIVITIS

The conjunctiva reacts to a wide range of bacterial and viral agents, allergens, irritants, toxins, and systemic diseases. Conjunctivitis is common in childhood and may be infectious or noninfectious.

Ophthalmia Neonatorum

Ophthalmia neonatorum, a form of conjunctivitis occurring in infants younger than 4 wk, is the most common eye disease of newborns. Its many different etiologic agents vary greatly in their virulence and outcome.

CLINICAL MANIFESTATIONS. The clinical manifestations of the various forms of ophthalmia neonatorum are not specific enough to allow an accurate diagnosis. Regardless of its cause, ophthalmia neonatorum is characterized by redness and chemosis (swelling) of the conjunctiva, edema of the eyelids, and discharge, which may be purulent. Ophthalmia neonatorum is a potentially blinding condition.

DIAGNOSIS. Conjunctivitis appearing after 48 hr should be evaluated for a possibly infectious cause. Gram stain of the purulent discharge should be performed, and the material should be cultured.

TREATMENT. Treatment of infants in whom gonococcal ophthalmia is suspected and the Gram stain shows the characteristic intracellular gram-negative diplococci should be initiated immediately with ceftriaxone, 50 mg/kg/24 hr for one dose not to exceed 125 mg. In addition, the eye should be irrigated initially with saline every 10–30 min, gradually increasing to 2-hr intervals, until the purulent discharge has cleared. Inclusion blennorrhea is treated with oral erythromycin (50 mg/kg/24 hr in four divided doses) for 2 wk. *Pseudomonas* neonatal conjunctivitis is treated with systemic antibiotics, including an aminoglycoside, plus local saline irrigation and gentamicin ophthalmic ointment. Staphylococcal conjunctivitis is treated with parenteral methicillin and local saline irrigation.

PREVENTION. Drops of 0.5% erythromycin or 1% silver nitrate are instilled directly into the open eyes at birth using wax or plastic single-dose containers.

Acute Purulent Conjunctivitis

This is characterized by more or less generalized conjunctival hyperemia, edema, mucopurulent exudate, and various degrees of ocular discomfort. It is usually a result of bacterial infection. Common forms of acute purulent conjunctivitis usually respond well to warm compresses and frequent topical instillation of antibiotic drops. *Neisseria gonorrhoeae* and *Chlamydia* are relatively common causes of acute purulent conjunctivitis in children beyond the newborn period, especially when it occurs in adolescents. These infections require specific testing and treatment.

Viral Conjunctivitis

This is generally characterized by a watery discharge. These inflammations are self-limited.

CHAPTER 295

Disorders of the Retina and Vitreous

(Nelson Textbook, Chapter 637)

RETINOPATHY OF PREMATURITY

Retinopathy of prematurity (ROP) is a retinal vasculopathy that occurs almost exclusively in preterm infants. Clinical manifestations range from mild, usually transient changes of the peripheral retina to severe progressive vasoproliferation, scarring, and potentially blinding retinal detachment.

PATHOGENESIS. The risk factors associated with ROP are not fully known, but prematurity and the associated retinal immaturity at birth represent the major factors. Hyperoxia is also a major factor, but other problems, such as respiratory distress, apnea, bradycardia, heart disease, infection, hypoxia, hypercarbia, acidosis, anemia, and the need for transfusion are thought by some to be contributory factors.

CLINICAL MANIFESTATIONS AND PROGNOSIS. In more than 90% of at-risk infants, the course is one of spontaneous arrest and regression of the usually asymmetric disease process, with little or no residual effects or visual disability. Fewer than 10% of infants have progression toward severe disease, with significant extraretinal vasoproliferation, cicatrization, detachment of the retina, and impairment of vision.

TREATMENT. In selected cases, cryotherapy or laser photocoagulation of the avascular retina reduces the more severe complications of progressive ROP. Advances in vitreoretinal surgical techniques have led to limited success in reattaching the retina in infants with total retinal detachment (stage 5 ROP), but the visual results are often disappointing.

PART 28

The Ear

(Nelson Textbook, Chapters 642–649)

CHAPTER 296

Hearing Loss

(Nelson Textbook, Chapter 643)

TYPES OF HEARING LOSS. Hearing loss can be peripheral or central in origin. Peripheral hearing loss is commonly caused by dysfunction in the transmission of sound through the external or middle ear or by the dysfunction in the transduction of sound energy into neural activity at the inner ear and the 8th nerve. Peripheral hearing loss can be conductive (CHL), sensorineural (SNHL), or mixed. CHL, the most common type of hearing loss in children, occurs when sound transmission through the external or middle ear or both is physically impeded. Damage to or maldevelopment of structures in the inner ear and lesions of the acoustic division of the 8th nerve cause SNHL. A combined CHL and SNHL is considered a *mixed* hearing loss. Auditory deficits originating along the central auditory nervous system pathways from the proximal 8th nerve to the cerebral cortex are generally considered *central* (also called retrocochlear) hearing losses. These causes of hearing loss are rare in children.

EFFECTS OF HEARING IMPAIRMENT. These depend on the nature and degree of the hearing loss and on the individual characteristics in the child. Most hearing-impaired children have some usable hearing. Only 6% of those in the hearing-impaired population have bilateral profound hearing loss. Hearing loss very early in life can affect the development of speech and language, social

TABLE 296–1   Criteria for Referral for Audiologic Assessment

Age (mo)	Referral Guidelines for Children with "Speech" Delay
12	No differentiated babbling or vocal imitation
18	No use of single words
24	Single-word vocabulary of ≤10 words
30	Fewer than 100 words; no evidence of two-word combinations; unintelligible
36	Fewer than 200 words; no use of telegraphic sentences, clarity <50%
48	Fewer than 600 words; no use of simple sentences; clarity ≤80%

From Matkin ND: Early recognition and referral of hearing-impaired children. Pediatr Rev 6:151, 1984. Reproduced by permission of Pediatrics.

TABLE 296–2 Guidelines for Referral of Children Suspected of Having Hearing Loss

Age (mo)	Normal Development
0–4	Should startle to loud sounds, quiet to mother's voice, momentarily cease activity when sound is presented at a conversational level
5–6	Should correctly localize to sound presented in a horizontal plane, begin to imitate sounds in own speech repertoire or at least reciprocally vocalize with an adult
7–12	Should correctly localize to sound presented in any plane Should respond to name, even when spoken quietly
13–15	Should point toward an unexpected sound or to familiar objects or persons when asked
16–18	Should follow simple directions without gestural or other visual cues; can be trained to reach toward an interesting toy at midline when a sound is presented
19–24	Should point to body parts when asked; by 21–24 mo, can be trained to perform play audiometry

From Matkin ND: Early recognition and referral of hearing-impaired children. Pediatr Rev 6:151, 1984. Reproduced by permission of Pediatrics.

and emotional development, behavior, attention, and academic achievement.

HEARING SCREENING. Because hearing impairment can have a major impact on the development of a child and because the earlier the impairment is identified the better is the prognosis, early identification through screening programs is widely and strongly advocated.

Identification of Hearing Impairment. Table 296–1 presents guidelines for screening language development in young children, and Table 296–2 provides guidelines for identifying children with abnormal auditory behavior.

TREATMENT. Once a hearing loss is identified, a full developmental and speech and language evaluation is needed. A conductive hearing loss can often be corrected through treatment of a middle ear effusion or surgical correction of the abnormal sound-conducting mechanism. Children with SNHL should be evaluated for possible hearing aid use. Identification and amplification before age 6 mo makes a very significant difference in the speech and language abilities of affected children.

CHAPTER 297

Disease of the External Ear

(Nelson Textbook, Chapter 645)

EXTERNAL OTITIS (OTITIS EXTERNA)

ETIOLOGY. External otitis (also called "swimmer's ear," although it occurs without swimming) is most commonly caused by *Pseudomonas aeruginosa*. External otitis results from the loss of protective cerumen and chronic irritation and maceration from excessive moisture in the canal.

CLINICAL MANIFESTATIONS. The predominant symptom is ear pain, which is often severe and accentuated by manipulation of the pinna and especially by pressure on the tragus. The severity of the pain and tenderness may be disproportionate to the degree of inflammation. Itching is a frequent precursor of pain and is usually characteristic of chronic inflammation of the canal or resolving acute otitis externa. Edema of the ear canal, erythema, and thick, clumpy otorrhea are prominent signs of the acute disease. The cerumen is usually white and soft, as opposed to its usual yellow, gold, or brown color and firmer consistency. The canal frequently is so tender and swollen that the entire ear canal and tympanic membrane cannot be adequately visualized. Other physical findings may include palpable and tender lymph nodes in the periauricular and, especially, preauricular areas.

TREATMENT. Topical otic preparations containing neomycin (active against gram-positive organisms and some gram-negative organisms, notably *Proteus* species) with either colistin or polymyxin (active against gram-negative bacilli, notably *Pseudomonas* species) and corticosteroids are effective in treating most forms of acute diffuse external otitis. If canal edema is marked, a wick should be inserted into the outer third of the ear canal and the topical drops applied to the wick several times a day for 24–48 hr.

CHAPTER 298

Otitis Media and Its Complications

(Nelson Textbook, Chapter 646)

After respiratory tract infections, inflammation of the middle ear, otitis media (OM), is the most prevalent disease of childhood. OM is inflammation of the middle ear, without reference to pathogenesis or etiology.

ACUTE OTITIS MEDIA (AOM)

CLINICAL MANIFESTATIONS. Children with an upper respiratory tract infection often develop the symptoms of AOM, which include otalgia, fever, hearing loss, and generalized malaise. Other symptoms may include otorrhea, irritability, and lethargy, followed less often by anorexia, nausea, vomiting, diarrhea, and headache. Fever occurs in 30–50% of patients; temperatures exceeding 40°C (104°F) are uncommon and suggest bacteremia or another complication. In infants, the symptoms may be less localizing, and fever, irritability, diarrhea, vomiting, or malaise may be quite prominent.

DIAGNOSIS. The diagnosis of AOM is based on clinical symptoms combined with visualization of the tympanic membrane. Examination with a pneumatic otoscope reveals a hyperemic, opaque, bulging tympanic membrane with poor mobility; purulent otorrhea with tympanic membrane perforation may be present. The usual middle ear landmarks frequently are obscured.

TREATMENT. Amoxicillin is the initial antibiotic of choice. Patients with AOM may be treated with high-dose amoxicillin (80–90 mg/kg/24 hr in three divided doses), which is well tolerated. Treatment is continued for 10 days. Patients assessed to be at low risk for resistant *Streptococcus pneumoniae* may be treated with the traditional dose of amoxicillin (40–45 mg/kg/24 hr in three divided doses). Treatment failure can be defined by lack of clinical improvement, such as persistent ear pain or fever, and by objective findings, such as tympanic membrane bulging or otorrhea, after 3 days of therapy. Few comparative studies are available to guide therapy for treatment failures. There are compelling data for effectiveness of treatment of AOM with cefuroxime axetil (30 mg/kg/24 hr in 2 divided doses) orally; or ceftriaxone (50 mg/kg) as a single intramuscular injection daily for 3 days.

Supportive therapy, including analgesics, antipyretics, and local heat, is usually helpful. An oral decongestant (pseudoephedrine hydrochloride) may relieve some nasal congestion, and antihistamines may help patients with known or suspected nasal allergy.

If a patient's clinical manifestations of acute infection increase during the first 24 hr despite antimicrobial therapy, a suppurative complication of OM should be suspected. Because it is well established that middle ear fluid often persists after an episode of AOM, follow-up for a single episode of AOM can occur several weeks after the initial diagnosis if the child is otherwise clinically well.

PERSISTENT MIDDLE EAR EFFUSION

It is reasonable to observe children who have asymptomatic (except for hearing loss) middle ear effusion still present after an acute episode of OM, examining the patient 2 mo after the initial visit, at which time most patients are effusion free. Treatment with another antimicrobial, which is effective against resistant bacteria, may be indicated if a child has any signs or symptoms of persistent infection, such as otalgia, or if such organisms have been isolated from subacute effusions in the community. If at 3 mo the middle ear fluid is still present, either as a result of AOM or middle ear effusion that occurred secondary to an upper respiratory tract infection, further therapy should be considered.

RECURRENT ACUTE OTITIS MEDIA

Some children suffer recurrent episodes of AOM with almost every upper respiratory tract infection, have moderate symptoms, respond well to therapy, and have fewer episodes with advancing age. Others have end-to-end otitis, severe symptoms, or persistent middle ear effusion with superimposed episodes of AOM. If the episodes are frequent and close together (three to four episodes in 6 mo or six episodes in a year), especially if they are very symptomatic, further evaluation and management are warranted. Myringotomy and ventilating tubes are also effective and should be considered for children failing to respond to medical management.

OTITIS MEDIA WITH EFFUSION

Otitis media with effusion (OME) is a middle ear effusion lacking the clinical manifestations of acute infection, such as otalgia and fever. It is often a result of AOM and in this situation generally clears by 3 mo in 90% of children.

CLINICAL MANIFESTATIONS. These children often seem inattentive, complain of hearing loss, or have hearing loss documented by audiometric evaluation. They may appear to be off balance or dizzy and sometimes complain of otalgia or tinnitus. Children who are otherwise asymptomatic in the daytime may be restless sleepers at night.

PHYSICAL EXAMINATION. The tympanic membrane is often retracted and moves poorly or not at all with pneumatic otoscopy. If a significant amount of middle ear fluid is found, the middle ear landmarks may be obscured; if the tympanic membrane is very retracted, the malleus may be very prominent, and the incudostapedial joint may be seen as the eardrum drapes tightly over it. The tympanic membrane is usually opaque but may also be translucent, with an air-fluid level or air bubbles seen behind it. The middle ear fluid may be whitish, yellow, or almost bluish.

AUDIOMETRIC FINDINGS. Conductive hearing loss of various degree is usually present.

TREATMENT. If the fluid has persisted for 3 mo or less and the child is not significantly symptomatic, treatment other than watchful waiting may not be indicated, because the fluid often resolves. However, if the fluid has persisted longer than 3 mo, is bilateral, and is associated with hearing loss, treatment should be considered. If a child has an underlying sensorineural hearing loss or is significantly symptomatic, treatment should be considered sooner than 3 mo. Either observation or a trial of antibiotics and control of environmental risk factors are indicated treatment options for children with acute or subacute effusions. Antibiotics should especially be considered for symptomatic effusions. In clinical trials, both amoxicillin and amoxicillin-clavulanate have been shown to be somewhat more effective than placebo.

If a child has significant hearing loss, myringotomy with insertion of tympanostomy tubes is an additional option after a trial of antibiotics. Myringotomy and insertion of ventilation tubes may also be helpful in patients with atelectasis of the tympanic membrane or when pain, hearing loss, vertigo, or tinnitus is present in association with OME. Adenoidectomy for chronic OME may benefit some children.

PART 29

The Skin

CHAPTER 299

Eczema

(Nelson Textbook, Chapter 661)

Eczema is a generic designation for a particular type of reaction pattern in the skin, which includes exudation, lichenification, and pruritus. Acute eczematous lesions are characterized by erythema, weeping, oozing, and the formation of microvesicles within the epidermis. Chronic lesions are generally thickened, dry, and scaly, with coarse skin markings (lichenification) and altered pigmentation. Many types of eczema occur in children; the most common is atopic dermatitis, although seborrheic dermatitis, allergic and irritant contact dermatitis, nummular eczema, and dyshidrosis also are relatively common in childhood. Various dermatoses that have pruritus as a common feature may become eczematized as a result of scratching. Atopic skin is sensitive to many factors that increase pruritus, such as soap, wool, cool air, and food allergens. Once the diagnosis of eczema has been established, it is important to classify the eruption more specifically for proper management.

CONTACT DERMATITIS. This form of eczema can be subdivided into irritant dermatitis, resulting from nonspecific injury to the skin, and allergic contact dermatitis, in which the mechanism is a delayed hypersensitivity reaction. Irritant dermatitis is more frequent in children, particularly during the early years of life. Clinically, irritant contact dermatitis may be indistinguishable from atopic dermatitis or allergic contact dermatitis. In general, irritant contact dermatitis clears after removal of the stimulus and after temporary treatment with a topical corticosteroid preparation.

Acute allergic contact dermatitis is an erythematous, intensely pruritic, eczematous dermatitis, which, if severe, may be edematous and vesiculobullous. The essential principle in treatment is elimination of contact with the allergen. Acute dermatitis responds to cool compresses and topical application of a corticosteroid ointment. An antihistamine may be useful when taken orally.

NUMMULAR ECZEMA. This disorder is unrelated to other types of eczema and is characterized by more or less coin-shaped eczematous plaques. Control of pruritus is usually achieved with a fluorinated corticosteroid preparation. Sedation with an antihistamine may be helpful, particularly at night. Antibiotics are indicated for secondary infection.

SEBORRHEIC DERMATITIS. This chronic inflammatory disease is most common in the pediatric age group, during infancy and adolescence, paralleling the distribution, size, and activity of the sebaceous glands.

Clinical Manifestations. The disorder may begin within the 1st mo of life and may be most troublesome during the 1st yr. Diffuse or focal scaling and crusting of the scalp, sometimes called cradle cap, may be the initial and at times the only manifestation. A greasy, scaly, erythematous papular dermatitis, which is usually nonpruritic, may involve the face, neck, retroauricular areas, axillae, and diaper area. During adolescence, seborrheic dermatitis is more localized and may be confined to the scalp and intertriginous areas.

Treatment. Scalp lesions should be controlled with an antiseborrheic shampoo (selenium sulfide, sulfur, salicylic acid, zinc pyrithione, tar), used daily if necessary. Inflamed lesions usually respond promptly to topical corticosteroid therapy given two to four times daily. Wet compresses should be applied to the moist or fissured lesions before application of the corticosteroid ointment. Response to therapy is usually rapid.

CHAPTER 300

Cutaneous Bacterial Infections

(Nelson Textbook, Chapter 671)

Bacterial skin infection is the single most common diagnosis among children with skin problems. The most common bacterial skin infection of children is impetigo, which makes up approximately 10% of all skin problems.

IMPETIGO

CLINICAL MANIFESTATIONS

Nonbullous Impetigo. There are two classic forms of impetigo: nonbullous and bullous. Lesions typically begin on skin of the face or extremities that has been traumatized. The most common lesions that precede nonbullous impetigo include insect bites, abrasions, lacerations, chickenpox, scabies pediculosis, and burns. A tiny vesicle or pustule forms initially and rapidly develops into a honey-colored crusted plaque that is generally less than 2 cm in diameter. Lesions are associated with little to no pain or surrounding erythema, and constitutional symptoms are generally absent. *Staphylococcus aureus* is the predominant organism of non-bullous impetigo in the United States.

Bullous Impetigo. This is mainly an infection of infants and young children. Bullous impetigo is always caused by coagulase-positive *S. aureus.* Flaccid, transparent bullae develop most commonly on skin of the face, buttocks, trunk, perineum, and extremities; neonatal bullous impetigo can begin in the diaper area. Rupture of bullae occurs easily, leaving a narrow rim of scale at the edge of a shallow, moist erosion.

DIAGNOSIS. Cultures of fluid from an intact blister or moist plaque should yield the causative agent; when the patient appears ill, blood cultures should also be obtained.

TREATMENT. Topical or systemic antibiotic treatment is superior to placebo or cleansing with 3% hexachlorophene soap. Mupirocin is an ointment that is bactericidal. Applied topically three times daily for 7–10 days, it is equal or greater in effectiveness, with fewer side effects, than oral erythromycin ethylsuccinate. Systemic therapy with a β-lactamase–resistant oral antibiotic should be prescribed for patients with widespread involvement.

CHAPTER 301

Acne

(Nelson Textbook, Chapter 675)

ACNE VULGARIS

Acne, particularly the comedonal form, occurs in approximately 80% of adolescents.

CLINICAL MANIFESTATIONS. Acne vulgaris is characterized by four basic types of lesions: open and closed comedones, papules, pustules, and nodulocystic lesions. One or more types of lesions may predominate; in its mildest form, which is often seen early in adolescence, lesions are limited to comedones on the central area of the face. Lesions may also involve the chest, upper back, and deltoid areas. Lesions often heal with temporary postinflammatory erythema and hyperpigmentation; pitted, atrophic, or hypertrophic scars may be interspersed, depending on the severity, depth, and chronicity of the process.

TREATMENT. No evidence shows that early treatment, with the exception of isotretinoin, alters the course of acne. Acne can be controlled and severe scarring prevented, however, by judicious maintenance therapy that is continued until the disease process has abated spontaneously.

Cleansing. Only superficial drying and peeling are achieved by cleansing, and almost any mild soap or astringent is adequate.

Topical Therapy. *Tretinoin (Retin-A)*, a derivative of retinoic acid, is the single most effective agent for treatment of comedonal acne. Erythema and peeling may be expected, particularly on initiation of therapy, and pustular flares from rupture of microcomedones are common. It may be applied once daily, 30 min after washing, in the form best tolerated. Typically, 0.025% cream is prescribed initially; the strength of the formulation is increased sequentially until adequate control, without undue irritation, is achieved. Optimal results are not seen for 3–6 mo.

Systemic Therapy. *Antibiotics*, especially tetracycline and its derivatives, are indicated for treatment of patients who cannot tolerate or have not responded to topical medications, who have moderate to severe inflammatory papulopustular and nodulocystic acne, and who have a propensity for scarring. For most adolescent patients, therapy may be initiated with tetracycline, 1 g/24 hr, divided twice daily, for at least 6 wk, followed by a gradual decrease to the minimal effective dose. The drugs are best administered in combination with topical benzoyl peroxide or tretinoin but not topical antibiotics.

Isotretinoin (13-*cis*-retinoic acid, Accutane) is indicated for moderate to severe nodulocystic acne that has not responded to conventional therapy or has recurred quickly after several successful courses of conventional therapy; for severe, scarring acne such as acne conglobata and acne fulminans; and for acne that is associated with severe psychologic disturbance. The recommended dosage is 0.5–1.0 mg/kg/24 hr. Four months of therapy is required for most patients. Isotretinoin use has many side effects. It is teratogenic and is contraindicated in pregnancy.

PART 30

Bone and Joint Disorders

SECTION 1

Orthopedic Problems
(Nelson Textbook, Chapters 678–689)

CHAPTER 302

Evaluation of the Child
(Nelson Textbook, Chapter 679)

The key to an accurate diagnosis is a careful history, a thorough physical examination, appropriate radiographic imaging, and occasionally laboratory testing. A glossary of common orthopedic terminology is provided in Table 302–1.

TABLE 302–1 Glossary of Orthopedic Terminology

Term	Definition
Abduction	Movement away from the midline
Adduction	Movement toward and possibly across the midline
Anteversion	Increased angulation of the femoral head and neck with respect to the knee in the frontal plane
Apophysis	Bone growth center that is not a growth plate or physis and that has a strong muscle insertion (e.g., greater trochanter of femur)
Arthroplasty	Surgical reconstruction of a joint
Arthrotomy	Surgical incision into a joint
Calcaneovalgus	Dorsiflexion of hindfoot
Cavovarus	High longitudinal or medial arch of foot with plantarflexed supinated forefoot and hindfoot varus
Cavus	High longitudinal arch of the foot (usually plantarflexed forefoot)
Dislocation	Complete loss of contact between two joint surfaces
Equinus	Plantarflexion of the forefoot, hindfoot, or entire foot
Extension	To straighten; is the reverse of flexion
External or lateral rotation	Outward rotation away from the midline
Flexion	To bend

TABLE 302–1 Glossary of Orthopedic Terminology *Continued*

Term	Definition
Internal or medial rotation	Inward rotation toward the midline
Subluxation	Incomplete loss of contact between two joint surfaces
Valgum	Angulation of a bone or joint in which the apex is toward the midline; genu valgum results in knock-knee because the angulation of the knee is toward the midline
Varum	Angulation of a bone or joint away from the midline; genu varum results in bowleg because the angulation is away from the midline

CHAPTER 303

The Knee

(Nelson Textbook, Chapter 683)

Pain around the knee is one of the most common presenting complaints in older children and adolescents. This may be insidious in onset or the result of trauma. *Accumulation of fluid* (effusion) in the knee is indicative of an abnormal intra-articular process. Fluid accumulating after injury is usually blood (hemarthrosis) and is indicative of a potentially serious injury to one or more of the ligaments or menisci or an occult fracture. Recurrent effusions may indicate a chronic internal derangement such as a meniscal tear. Unexplained accumulation of fluid may occur with arthritis (septic, viral, postinfectious, juvenile rheumatoid arthritis, systemic lupus erythematosus), hemorrhage secondary to hemophilia, and overactivity. Occasionally, this fluid requires aspiration to relieve discomfort and to help establish the diagnosis. The presence of purulent material indicates septic arthritis or osteomyelitis.

OSTEOCHONDRITIS DISSECANS

Osteochondritis dissecans commonly involves the knee and occurs when an area of bone adjacent to the articular cartilage becomes avascular and ultimately separates from the underlying bone.

CLINICAL MANIFESTATIONS AND DIAGNOSIS. The child or adolescent typically presents with a vague knee pain. With the knee fully flexed, it is possible to palpate the involved area directly on the articular cartilage of the medial femoral condyle. This is usually tender. Anteroposterior, lateral, and tunnel radiographs of the knee are necessary to establish the diagnosis and to follow the disease process. As revascularization occurs, the bone heals spontaneously.

TREATMENT. In children 11 yr of age and younger, the treatment is primarily by observation. In adolescents 13 yr of age and older, especially those with a suspected loose body, arthroscopic surgical intervention may be necessary.

OSGOOD-SCHLATTER DISEASE

The patellar tendon inserts into the tibia tubercle, which is an extension of the proximal tibial epiphysis. This area is vulnerable to microfracture during late childhood or adolescence, especially in athletes, producing Osgood-Schlatter disease. Physical examination demonstrates swelling, tenderness, and increased prominence of the tibia tubercle. Radiographs are usually necessary to rule out other lesions. Rest, restriction of activities and, occasionally, a knee immobilizer may be necessary, combined with an isometric exercise program. Complete resolution of symptoms usually requires 12–24 mo.

CHAPTER 304

The Hip
(Nelson Textbook, Chapter 684)

DEVELOPMENTAL DYSPLASIA OF THE HIP

Developmental dysplasia of the hip usually occurs in the neonatal period. The hips at birth are rarely dislocated but rather "dislocatable."

CLINICAL MANIFESTATIONS. The Barlow test is the most important maneuver in examining the newborn hip. This provocative test to dislocate an unstable hip is performed by stabilizing the pelvis with one hand and then flexing and adducting the opposite hip and applying a posterior force. If the hip is dislocatable, it is usually readily felt. After release of the posterior force, the hip usually relocates spontaneously. The Ortolani test is a maneuver to reduce a recently dislocated hip. It is most likely to be positive in infants who are 1–2 mo of age because adequate time must have passed for the true dislocation to have occurred. In performing this test, the thigh is flexed and abducted and the femoral head is lifted anteriorly into the acetabulum. If reduction is possible, the relocation will be felt as a "clunk," not an audible "click."

Limitation of hip abduction is indicative of soft tissue contractures and may indicate developmental dysplasia. Conversely, hip abduction contractures may indicate dysplasia of the contralateral hip. An asymmetric number of thigh skinfolds and apparent shortening of an extremity and uneven knee levels when the supine infant's feet are placed together on the examining table with the hips and knees flexed indicate developmental dysplasia with proximal displacement of the femoral head.

RADIOGRAPHIC EVALUATION. Hip stability as well as acetabular development may be assessed accurately in neonates and young infants by dynamic ultrasonography. Radiographic evaluation in older infants and children includes anteroposterior and frog-leg lateral radiographs of the pelvis.

TREATMENT

Birth. When an unstable hip is recognized at birth, maintenance of the hip in the position of flexion and abduction ("human" position) for 1–2 mo is usually sufficient.

Age 1–6 Months. During this age, a true dislocation may develop. As a consequence, treatment is directed toward reduction of the femoral head into the acetabulum. The Pavlik harness is the treatment of choice in this age group.

Age 6–18 Months. In the older infant, surgical closed reduction is the major method of treatment.

Age 18 Months–8 Years. After 18 mo of age, the progressive deformities are so severe that open reduction followed by pelvic (innominate) osteotomy or femoral osteotomy, or both, are necessary to realign the hip.

SLIPPED CAPITAL FEMORAL EPIPHYSIS

Slipped capital femoral epiphysis (SCFE) is the most common adolescent hip disorder. Its cause is unknown.

CLINICAL MANIFESTATIONS. In the acute or acute-on-chronic unstable SCFE, the physical examination is limited as a result of severe pain with any attempted hip motion. In a chronic, stable SCFE, the patient has an antalgic gait and the affected extremity is externally rotated. Hip range of motion demonstrates a lack of internal rotation and increased external rotation. Also, as the hip is flexed, it becomes progressively externally rotated.

TREATMENT. The goals of treatment for SCFE are to prevent further slippage and minimize complications. This is accomplished by performing an epiphysiodesis (closure) of the capital femoral epiphysis.

CHAPTER 305

The Spine

(Nelson Textbook, Chapter 685)

Abnormalities in the vertebral column are a common nontraumatic pediatric musculoskeletal problem. A simple classification of the common spinal abnormalities is presented in Table 305–1.

TABLE 305–1 Classification of Spinal Deformities

Scoliosis

Idiopathic

Infantile
Juvenile
Adolescent

Congenital

Failure of formation
  Wedge vertebrae
  Hemivertebrae
Failure of segmentation
  Unilateral bar
  Bilateral bar
Mixed

Neuromuscular

Neuropathic diseases
  Upper motor neuron
    Cerebral palsy
    Spinocerebellar degeneration (Friedreich ataxia, Charcot-Marie-Tooth disease)
    Syringomyelia
    Spinal cord tumor
    Spinal cord trauma
  Lower motor neuron
    Poliomyelitis
    Spinal muscular atrophy
Myopathic diseases
  Duchenne muscular dystrophy
  Arthrogryposis
  Other muscular dystrophies

Syndromes

Neurofibromatosis
Marfan syndrome

Compensatory

Leg-length discrepancy

Kyphosis

Postural round-back
Scheuermann disease
Congenital kyphosis

Adapted from the Terminology Committee, Scoliosis Research Society: A glossary of scoliosis terms. Spine 1:57, 1976.

IDIOPATHIC SCOLIOSIS

ETIOLOGY AND EPIDEMIOLOGY. Idiopathic scoliosis is the most common form of scoliosis. It occurs in healthy, neurologically normal children, but its exact cause is unknown.

CLINICAL MANIFESTATIONS. Asymmetry of the posterior chest wall on forward bending (the Adams test) is the most striking and consistent abnormality in patients with scoliosis. Associated findings include asymmetry in shoulder height, apparent leg-length discrepancy, flank asymmetry, and asymmetry of the anterior chest wall. A careful neurologic evaluation is essential, especially in patients with apparent juvenile-onset scoliosis, atypical curve patterns, or back pain.

RADIOGRAPHIC EVALUATION. If there is clinical evidence of spinal deformity, standing posteroanterior and lateral standing radiographs of the entire spine should be obtained. The degree of curvature is determined by measuring the angular relationships between the most tilted vertebra at either end of the apparent curve (the Cobb method).

TREATMENT. The risk for curve progression varies according to sex, age, menarchal status, and curve magnitude at initial discovery. Premenarchal girls with curves between 20 and 30 degrees have a significantly higher risk for progression than do girls 2 yr after menarche with similar curves. Boys with curvature of the same magnitude appear to have similar risks of progression when judged by other maturation standards. Curves less than 30 degrees rarely progress after skeletal maturation is complete; curves greater than 45 or 50 degrees often continue to progress during adult life.

The generally accepted methods of treatment of progressive idiopathic adolescent scoliosis are bracing and surgical correction. Most orthopedic surgeons recommend a trial of brace treatment for immature patients with curves less than 40 degrees. Surgical treatment is usually considered for patients with idiopathic curves greater than 45 degrees. Surgical treatment usually combines correction of deformity with permanently implanted internal fixation rods and posterior fusion of the involved vertebrae.

CHAPTER 306

The Neck
(Nelson Textbook, Chapter 686)

TORTICOLLIS

Torticollis is the term applied to the clinical finding of a twisted neck. In most instances, the head is tipped toward one side and the chin rotated toward the other. Torticollis is a sign, not a disease, and may be the result of a wide range of underlying pathophysiologic processes.

Muscular torticollis is the most common variety and is presumed to result from injury to the sternocleidomastoid muscle during delivery. Large infants who have had difficult vertex deliveries are at special risk. Swelling within the sternocleidomastoid muscle may be palpable in neonates with muscular torticollis; swelling diminishes shortly after birth, and the lesion may not be present in older infants. Contracture of the muscle results in the typical head tilt and rotation. In patients with a suggestive history and appropriate physical findings, a program of gentle passive stretching exercises started within the first month of life often results in resolution. When deformity persists, the patient should be referred for orthopedic evaluation. Surgical release of the sternomastoid muscle is occasionally required in such patients and should be performed before the development of secondary facial asymmetry (plagiocephaly).

SECTION 2

Sports Medicine
(Nelson Textbook, Chapters 690–696)

CHAPTER 307

Management of Musculoskeletal Injury
(Nelson Textbook, Chapter 691)

Sports injuries in young children are predominantly due to sprains, strains, fractures, contusions, and overuse syndromes.

INITIAL EVALUATION OF THE INJURED EXTREMITY. Initially, the examiner should determine the quality of the peripheral pulses and capillary refill rate as well as the gross motor and sensory function to assess neurovascular injury.

Criteria for immediate attention and rapid orthopedic consultation include vascular compromise (blood flow may be obstructed by a dislocated structure, so a skilled physician should reduce any obstructing dislocated joint); nerve compromise (peripheral nerve damage can be repaired after vascular and skeletal stability have been achieved); and open fracture (an open fracture should not be reduced immediately because of the risk of further contamination). The exposed wound should be covered with sterile saline-soaked gauze, and the injured limb should be padded and splinted. Pressure should be applied to any site of bleeding.

THE TRANSITION FROM IMMEDIATE MANAGEMENT TO RETURN TO PLAY

Phase 1: Limit further injury, control swelling and pain, and minimize strength and flexibility losses. This requires the use of an appropriate device such as crutches or a sling, ice, compression, elevation, and analgesia. Ice in a plastic bag is placed directly on the skin for 20 min continuously, three to four times per day until the swelling resolves. Compression limits further bleeding and swelling but should not be so tight that it limits perfusion. Elevation of the extremity promotes venous return and limits swelling. Nonsteroidal anti-inflammatory medication or acetaminophen is indicated for analgesia. Pain-free isometric strengthening and range of motion should be initiated as soon as possible.

Phase 2: Improve strength and range of motion (i.e., flexibility) while allowing the injured structures to heal. Protective devices are removed when the patient's strength and flexibility improve and activities of daily living are pain free.

Phase 3: Achieve near normal strength and flexibility of the injured structures and further improve or maintain cardiovascular fitness.

Phase 4: Return to exercise or competition without restriction.

Chapter 308

Head and Neck Injuries

(Nelson Textbook, Chapter 692)

Head and neck injuries account for 90% of traumatic deaths and are the primary cause of permanent disability resulting from sports.

HEAD INJURY. The most common head injury is the concussion, which is characterized by immediate and transient alteration of consciousness, disturbance of vision and equilibrium, and other similar symptoms. The cumulative effect of chronic concussions can cause permanent injury.

An *epidural hematoma* is a rapidly accumulating hematoma between the dura and the cranium. Eighty-five percent are associated with a skull fracture, and the most serious lacerate the middle meningeal artery. Most victims suffer loss of consciousness followed by a lucid, awake interval often associated with a severe headache. If untreated, this abruptly evolves to deterioration and death within 15–30 min. A *subdural hematoma* occurs when an artery or bridging vein is torn between the dura and the brain parenchyma. It is the most frequent, identifiable focal brain injury in sports and the most common cause of death in sports-related head injuries because it is also associated with cerebral contusion and edema. Patients may lose consciousness at the time of injury but recover in the acute setting.

NECK INJURIES. *Fracture with or without dislocation* is considered when a player has any head or neck injury or loss of consciousness but more specifically when the athlete has midline cervical pain, painful range of motion, tenderness over the cervical spine, or bilateral neurologic signs or symptoms after neck trauma. Patients should be immobilized and should have a full radiographic evaluation with anteroposterior, lateral, oblique, and open-mouth views.

Transient quadriplegia (<36 hr) is manifested as sensory changes that may be associated with motor paresis involving both arms, both legs, or all four extremities. Patients with a neck injury can return to contact sports when they have full, pain-free range of motion, strength and sensation, and normal lordosis of their cervical spine.

TREATMENT. In the acute management of head and neck injuries, the principles of advanced life support are followed. Airway, breathing, circulation, and disability (ABCD) are the primary concerns. Other management principles are as follows: Assume a neck injury is present in an unconscious athlete. Cervical spine immobilization is mandatory. Do not use ammonia smelling salts. The noxious stimulant causes involuntary withdrawal, which may cause secondary injury to an unstable cervical spine. Perform serial neurologic examinations. If the athlete is lucid, look for the signs indicative of a neck injury before the athlete is permitted to move.

Athletes with a head injury require transfer for evaluation and observation if they have a suggested skull fracture, deteriorating mental status or worsening headache, focal neurologic deficits or seizure, loss of consciousness for more than 5 min, confusion lasting longer than 30 min, persistent emesis, more than one concussion in a practice/game, or inadequate postinjury supervision.

Skeletal Dysplasia

(Nelson Textbook, Chapters 697 and 713)

CHAPTER 309

General Considerations in Disorders of Skeletal Development

(Nelson Textbook, Chapter 697)

The terms skeletal dysplasias, bone dysplasias, and osteochondrodysplasias refer to a genetically and clinically heterogeneous group of disorders of skeletal development and growth. They can be divided into the osteodysplasias typified by osteogenesis imperfecta and the chondrodysplasias. The clinical picture is dominated by skeletal abnormalities. The manifestations may be restricted to the skeleton, but in most cases nonskeletal tissues are also involved.

The chondrodysplasias are distinguished from other forms of short stature by a disproportionality of skeletal manifestations. They have been separated into individuals with predominantly short limbs and those with predominantly short trunks. The better-defined chondrodysplasia groups, such as the achondroplasia and type II collagenopathy groups, contain graded series of disorders that range from very severe to very mild. This may be true for other groups as more mutations are found and the full spectrum of clinical phenotypes associated with mutations of a given gene are defined. The emerging view is that they are clinical phenotypes distributed along spectra of phenotypic abnormality associated with mutations of particular genes. Although a few chondrodysplasias can be easily diagnosed, most require the analysis of information from the history, physical examination, skeletal radiographs, family history, and laboratory testing. The process involves recognizing complex patterns that are characteristic of the different disorders (Table 309–1).

Bone is a dynamic organ capable of rapid turnover, weight bearing, and withstanding the stresses of various physical activities. It is constantly being formed (modeling) and re-formed (remodeling). It is the major body reservoir for calcium, phosphorus, and magnesium. Disorders that affect this organ and the process of mineralization are designated metabolic bone disease. Advances in our knowledge of bone metabolism, the process of mineralization, interactions of the vitamin D/parathyroid hormone (PTH)/endocrine axis, and metabolism of vitamin D to active compounds have led to improved treatment of metabolic bone diseases.

DIAGNOSIS AND TREATMENT. Establishing a diagnosis helps to distinguish between lethal and nonlethal disorders in premature or

TABLE 309–1 Major Problems Associated with Skeletal Dysplasias

Problem	Example
Lethality*	Thanatophoric dysplasia
Associated anomalies	Ellis-van Creveld syndrome
Short stature	Spondyloepiphyseal dysplasia congenita
Cervical spine dislocations	Larsen syndrome
Severe limb bowing	Metaphyseal dysplasia type Schmid
Spine curvatures	Metatrophic dysplasia
Clubfeet	Diastrophic dysplasia
Fractures	Osteogenesis imperfecta
Pneumonias, aspirations	Camptomelic dysplasia
Hydrocephalus	Achondroplasia
Joint problems (hips, knees)	Most skeletal dysplasias
Hearing loss	Common (greatest with cleft palate)
Myopia/cataracts	Stickler syndrome
Immune deficiency†	Cartilage-hair hypoplasia
Sudden infant death syndrome	Achondroplasia (rare)
Poor body image	Variable, but common to all
Sex reversal	Camptomelic dysplasia

*Mostly due to severely reduced size of thorax.

†At least four additional disorders, all involving the metaphyses, can have immunodeficiency.

TABLE 309–2 Lethal Neonatal Dwarfism

Usually Fatal*

Achondrogenesis (different types)
Thanatophoric dysplasia
Short rib polydactyly, Majewski type
Short rib polydactyly, Saldino-Noonan type
Homozygous achondroplasia
Osteopetrosis (congenital form)
Camptomelic dysplasia
Dyssegmental dysplasia, Silverman-Handmaker type
Osteogenesis imperfecta, type II
Hypophosphatasia (congenital form)
Chondrodysplasia punctata (rhizomelic form)

Often Fatal

Asphyxiating thoracic dystrophy (Jeune syndrome)

Occasionally Fatal

Ellis-van Creveld syndrome
Diastrophic dysplasia
Metatropic dwarfism
Kniest dysplasia

*A few prolonged survivors have been reported in most of these disorders.

TABLE 309–3 Usually Nonlethal Dwarfing Conditions Recognizable at Birth or Within First Few Months of Life

Most Common

Achondroplasia
Osteogenesis imperfecta (types I, III, IV)
Spondyloepiphyseal dysplasia congenita
Diastrophic dysplasia
Ellis-van Creveld syndrome

Less Common

Chondrodysplasia punctata (some forms)
Kniest dysplasia (not severe congenital forms)
Metatrophic dysplasia
Langer mesomelic dysplasia

newborn infants (Tables 309–2 and 309–3). Because there is no definitive therapy to normalize bone growth in any of the disorders, management is directed at preventing and correcting skeletal deformities, treating nonskeletal complications, genetic counseling, and helping patients and families learn to cope.

PART 31

Unclassified Diseases

(Nelson Textbook, Chapters 714–717)

CHAPTER 310

Sudden Infant Death Syndrome

(Nelson Textbook, Chapter 714)

Sudden infant death syndrome (SIDS) is defined as the sudden death of an infant that is unexpected by history and unexplained by a thorough postmortem examination that includes a complete autopsy, investigation of the scene of death, and review of the medical history.

PATHOPHYSIOLOGY. The most compelling hypothesis to explain SIDS is a brain stem abnormality in cardiorespiratory control, including arousal responsiveness, and perhaps other autonomic controls such as blood pressure and sleep-wake regulation. The clinical data to support this hypothesis were initially inferred from assessments of patients with idiopathic apparent life-threatening events or other infants at increased epidemiologic risk for SIDS (preterm infants, subsequent siblings of a previous SIDS victim), a few of whom later died of SIDS.

Clinical Risk Groups. Infants with idiopathic apparent life-threatening events are at increased risk for SIDS (Table 310–1). There are no data about the extent, if any, to which home monitoring or any other intervention might decrease the risk of SIDS in infants with these events.

Sleeping Position. A significant decrease in prone prevalence is

TABLE 310–1 General Incidence of SIDS in Infant Groups at Increased Epidemiologic Risk for SIDS*

Risk Group	Incidence of SIDS
Idiopathic apparent life-threatening event	Risk increased 3–5 times
Siblings	Risk increased at least 4–5 times
Preterm infants:	
1500–2499 g birth weight	Relative risk (RR) 2.64†
1000–1499 g birth weight	RR 3.68†
Racial:	
African-Americans	RR 1.7–2.0‡
Native Americans	RR 2.1‡
Intrauterine drug exposure	Risk increased 3–5 times

*The incidence of SIDS in the United States in 1996 was 0.74 deaths/1000 live births.
†RR 1.0 for full-term infants.
‡RR 1.0 for whites.

associated with a decrease in SIDS rates. The current back-to-sleep recommendations call for the supine position for sleeping in all infants without medical contraindications (e.g., micrognathia or obstructive sleep apnea). Supine is also the recommended sleeping position for all preterm infants, and supine sleeping should begin in the hospital before discharge from the neonatal intensive care unit. The mechanism for the epidemiologic association between decreased prone/side prevalence and decreased risk for SIDS has not been established.

INTERVENTION. The apnea hypothesis led to the hope that home electronic surveillance would reduce the risk for SIDS. A major problem related to determining the efficacy of home monitoring has been uncertainty about the extent of monitor use or compliance.

PART 32

Environmental Health Hazards

(Nelson Textbook, Chapters 718–724)

CHAPTER 311

Lead Poisoning

(Nelson Textbook, Chapter 721)

PATHOPHYSIOLOGY. The high toxicity of lead results from its avidity for the sulfhydryl (SH) group of proteins. Lead irreversibly binds to the SH group of a protein and thus impairs its function.

CLINICAL MANIFESTATIONS. In practice, the probability of severe symptoms increases as the exposure to lead and blood lead levels rise. The most serious manifestation of lead poisoning is acute encephalopathy. This may appear without a prodrome or may be preceded by behavioral changes or lead colic, characterized by occasional vomiting, intermittent abdominal pain, and constipation. Encephalopathy includes persistent vomiting, ataxia, seizures, papilledema, impaired consciousness, and coma. The symptoms of childhood lead poisoning in the absence of clear signs of encephalopathy are usually nonspecific and vague. Abdominal colic, behavioral abnormalities, attention disorders, hyperactivity, or severe unexplained retardation should lead one to suspect clinical lead poisoning. Neurobehavioral abnormalities, demonstrated at low levels of lead exposure by epidemiologic studies, include lower intelligence and poor school performance.

DIAGNOSIS. Of critical importance in the diagnosis is an accurate environmental history, particularly of exposure to lead-containing paint. History of pica, when present, is strongly suggestive. Unless the symptoms of lead poisoning are obviously severe and evident, in most cases, the diagnosis needs to be established by blood lead testing.

DEFINITION AND CLASSIFICATION OF LEAD POISONING. The proposed CDC classification based on blood lead level (Table 311–1) is useful for providing approximate management guidelines and for helping large programs establish priorities.

TREATMENT

Removing the Source of Lead Exposure. The most important aspect of therapy is to remove the child from the source of exposure to lead.

Symptomatic Children and Children with Blood Lead Levels of More Than 70 µg/dL. In symptomatic children, regardless of blood lead level, the treatment is always given in a hospital. Children with blood lead

TABLE 311–1 Centers for Disease Control and Prevention 1991 Classification and Recommendations

Blood Lead Level (μ/dL)	Action Recommended	
0–9		No immediate concern
≥10		"Lead poisoning"
10–14	Environmental survey	If found in too many children, survey the community
15–19	Environmental survey	Education about lead exposure
20–24	Remove from lead source	Bring to medical attention
25–54	Remove from lead source	EDTA test: if positive, 25–44 EDTA; 45–54 EDTA or DMSA
55–69	Remove from lead source	Treat with EDTA or DMSA
≥70 or symptomatic	Emergency hospitalization	Treat with BAL and EDTA
	Always return the child to a clean house.	

EDTA = edetate calcium-disodium; DMSA = succimer; BAL = dimercaprol.

levels of 70 μg/dL or more, even if asymptomatic, should always be considered as posing a medical emergency and should immediately be hospitalized for treatment. Treatment should consist of dimercaprol (BAL, 75 mg/m² every 4 hr; total daily dose of 450 mg/m²), followed by edetate calcium-disodium (EDTA) (1500 mg/m²/24 hr by continuous infusion.

Asymptomatic Children with Blood Lead Levels of 10–19 μg/dL. At these levels, no treatment or medical intervention is necessary; only general education is recommended.

CHAPTER 312

Poisonings: Drugs, Chemicals, and Plants

(Nelson Textbook, Chapter 722)

More than 90% of toxic exposures in children occur in the home, and most involve only a single substance. Ingestion is the most common route of poisoning exposure (75% of cases).

MANAGEMENT PLAN FOR POISONING AND OVERDOSE

Progression of Symptoms. Knowing the nature and progression of symptoms is helpful for assessing the need for immediate life support, the prognosis, and the type of intervention that may need to be performed. Several characteristic toxic syndromes (Ta-

TABLE 312–1 Toxic Syndromes

Syndrome	Symptoms	Causes
Anticholinergic	Exocrine gland hyposecretion, thirst, flushed skin, mydriasis, hyperthermia, urinary retention, delirium, hallucinations, tachycardia, respiratory insufficiency	Belladonna alkaloids, jimsonweed, some mushrooms, antihistamines, tricyclic antidepressants, scopolamine
Cholinergic (muscarinic and nicotinic)	Exocrine gland hypersecretion, urination, nausea, vomiting, diarrhea, muscle fasciculations, miosis, weakness or paralysis, bronchospasm, tachycardia or bradycardia, convulsions, coma	Organophosphate and carbamate insecticides, some mushrooms, tobacco, black widow spider bites (severe)
Extrapyramidal	Tremor, rigidity, opisthotonos, torticollis, dysphonia, oculogyric crisis	Phenothiazines, haloperidol, metoclopramide
Hypermetabolic	Fever, tachycardia, hyperpnea, restlessness, convulsions, metabolic acidosis	Salicylates, some phenols, triethyltin, chlorophenoxy herbicides
Narcotic	Central nervous system depression, hypothermia, hypotension, hypoventilation, miosis	All narcotics, propoxyphene, heroin
Sympathomimetic	Excitation, psychosis, seizures, hypertension, tachypnea, hyperthermia, mydriasis	Amphetamines, phencyclidine, cocaine, crack cocaine, phenylpropanolamine, methylphenidate, theophylline, caffeine
Withdrawal	Abdominal cramps, diarrhea, lacrimation, sweating, "goose flesh," yawning, tachycardia, restlessness, hallucinations	Cessation of alcohol, barbiturates, benzodiazepines, narcotics

ble 312–1) are described, and evaluation of signs and symptoms may assist in identifying the offending agent.

Initial Medical Care. If the patient is treated at home, follow-up assessment calls must be made approximately 0.5, 1, and 4 hr after exposure. If a patient requires hospital treatment, the probability of the development of life-threatening symptoms dictates the mode of transportation used. Once a patient has arrived in the appropriate medical care setting, initial attention should focus on life support, with primary emphasis on cardiorespiratory care. Shock, dysrhythmias, and seizures should be treated as for any other critically ill patient. There are few poisons for which there is an antidote.

Preventing Absorption. Most toxins are rapidly absorbed from the gastrointestinal tract or the lungs. Many may also be well absorbed on dermal contact. Prompt action to remove the toxin from contact with the absorptive surface is crucial and may make the difference between no toxicity and major toxicity. Dermal and ocular decontamination can be accomplished by flushing the affected area with tepid water. A minimum of 10 min is recommended for ocular exposure. For inhaled toxins, decontamination is generally accomplished by removing the patient to fresh air or, if necessary, administering oxygen. In addition to supportive care, a few specific antidotes are used for some specific inhaled toxins. Several procedures are used to prevent absorption of toxin from the stomach and gastrointestinal tract, and each has limitations and risks.

Emesis. The only emetic routinely used is *syrup of ipecac,* which contains two emetic alkaloids that work both in the central nervous system and locally in the gastrointestinal tract to produce vomiting.

Gastric Lavage. This technique involves placing a tube into the stomach to aspirate contents, followed by flushing with aliquots of fluid, usually normal saline. Although gastric lavage has been widely used for many years, objective data do not document its efficacy, particularly in children.

Activated Charcoal. The use of activated charcoal to prevent absorption of toxins has increased dramatically in the past 2 decades as data demonstrating its efficacy have accumulated.

Cathartics. Cathartics are commonly used in conjunction with activated charcoal-toxin complex, although no evidence shows that this is of value.

Enhancing Elimination. In practice, enhancing excretion is useful for only a minority of toxins.

Index

Note: Page numbers followed by the letter f refer to figures; page numbers followed by the letter t refer to tables.